W9-CEX-482

The American Health Foundation

is a non-profit biomedical research and health education institution dedicated to reducing disease and medical care costs through prevention.

The Mahoney Institute for Health Maintenance, the clinical arm of the American Health Foundation, conducts research and clinical programs aimed at the prevention of disease through population studies, health economics, health promotion services and public education.

The Naylor Dana Institute for Disease Prevention is the American Health Foundation's center for basic biomedical and biochemical research. Laboratory studies are conducted to uncover the causes and mechanisms of chronic diseases and to develop strategies for their prevention and control.

Through research and the application of its knowledge through public education, the American Health Foundation is filling a major role in the development and practice of preventive health care.

THE BOOK OF
HEALTH

THE BOOK OF
HEALTH

The American Health Foundation

EDITOR IN CHIEF
Ernst L. Wynder, M.D.

SPECIAL EDITOR
Sidney Hertzberg

ASSOCIATE EDITOR
Ellen Parker

A GROLIER COMPANY

Franklin Watts

NEW YORK LONDON TORONTO SYDNEY 1981

*Book design and illustrations
by Anne Canevari Green*

Library of Congress Cataloging in Publication Data

Main entry under title:

The Book of health.

Bibliography: p.
Includes index.
1. Health.   I. Wynder, Ernst L.
II. American Health Foundation.
RA776.B666   613   81–10325
ISBN 0–531–09929–6   AACR2

This book is dedicated to Eleanor Naylor Dana and David Mahoney for their help in founding and building the American Health Foundation and to our staff for their dedication to disease prevention

Contents

PART II
Environment

PART III
Knowing Your Body

Tables

Figures

Contributors

THE USES OF EPIDEMIOLOGY

*ERNST L. WYNDER, M.D.
American Health Foundation, New York, New York

MARGARET MUSHINSKI, M.A.
American Health Foundation, New York, New York

NUTRITION

*BARRY LEWIS, M.D.
St. Thomas's Hospital Medical School, London

*ANGELICA CANTLON, R.D., M.S.
American Health Foundation, New York, New York

MYRON BRIN, PH.D.
Hoffmann-LaRoche, Inc., Nutley, New Jersey
(vitamins)

RUTH M. KAY, PH.D.
University of Toronto, Toronto, Canada
(fiber, pregnancy, the young)

ELIZABETH RICHTER, R.D., M.A.
New York, New York
(obesity)

MORTON SCHWARTZ, PH.D.
Memorial Sloan-Kettering Cancer Center, New York, New York
(trace elements)

JOHN H. WEISBURGER, PH.D., M.D. h.c.
American Health Foundation, Valhalla, New York
(additives and contaminants)

GERALD N. WOGAN, PH.D.
Massachusetts Institute of Technology, Cambridge, Massachusetts
(additives and contaminants)

ALCOHOL

*FRANK A. SEIXAS, M.D.
Norwood Hospital, Norwood, Massachusetts

*LIRIO COVEY, M.S.
American Health Foundation, New York, New York

DRUGS

*MITCHELL S. ROSENTHAL, M.D., and IRA MOTHNER
Phoenix House Foundation, New York, New York

*DONALD B. LOURIA, M.D.
College of Medicine and Dentistry, New Jersey Medical School, Newark, New Jersey

H. WINTER GRIFFITH, M.D.
Tucson, Arizona
(drug interactions)

TOBACCO

*ERNST L. WYNDER, M.D.
American Health Foundation, New York, New York

*MARGARET MUSHINSKI, M.A.
American Health Foundation, New York, New York
(cancer epidemiology)

GILBERT BOTVIN, M.D.
American Health Foundation, New York, New York
(smoking cessation)

SHELDON G. COHEN, M.D.
National Institute of Allergy and Infectious Disease, Bethesda, Maryland
(allergy and immunity)

SADJA GOLDSMITH GREENWOOD, M.D.
University of California, San Francisco
(pregnancy and infant development)

MORTON I. GROSSMAN, PH.D.
UCLA School of Medicine, Los Angeles, California
(peptic ulcer)

IAN T.T. HIGGINS, M.D.
   University of Michigan, Ann Arbor
   (chronic obstructive pulmonary disease)

DIETRICH HOFFMANN, PH.D.
   American Health Foundation, Valhalla, New York
   (low yield cigarettes)

GARDNER C. MACMILLAN, M.D.
   National Heart, Lung, and Blood Institute, Bethesda, Maryland
   (cardiovascular disease)

DON POWELL, PH.D.
   American Health Foundation, New York, New York
   (smoking cessation)

JEROME L. SCHWARTZ, PH.D.
   University of California, Davis, California
   (smoking cessation)

PHYSICAL FITNESS

*ARTHUR S. LEON, M.D.
   University of Minnesota, Minneapolis, Minnesota

*SAMUEL M. FOX III, M.D.
   Georgetown University School of Medicine, Washington, D.C.

FAMILY PLANNING AND CHILDBEARING

*SALLY KILBY, R.N.
   American Journal of Nursing, New York, New York

NANCY CUDDIHY, R.N.
   Roosevelt Hospital, New York, New York
   (birth methods)

ROBERT HOOVER, M.D.
   National Cancer Institute, Bethesda, Maryland
   (hormones)

ROXANNE LITTNER, M.S.
   American Health Foundation, New York, New York

VINCENT RICCARDI, M.D.
   Kleberg Genetics Center, Baylor College of Medicine, Houston, Texas
   (genetic counseling)

STRESS

*KENNETH GREENSPAN, M.D., ELAINE POMERANZ, and MARTIN WEINSTOCK
   College of Physicians and Surgeons of Columbia University, New York, New York

*JAMES S.J. MANUSO, PH.D.
   Equitable Life Assurance Society of the United States, New York, New York

WILLIAM P. CASTELLI, M.D.
National Heart, Lung, and Blood Institute, Framingham, Massachusetts
(heart attacks)

SHELDON G. COHEN, M.D.
National Institute of Allergy and Infectious Diseases, Bethesda, Maryland
(asthma)

ARI KIEV, M.D.
Social Psychiatry Research Institute, New York, New York
(suicide)

HERBERT SPIEGEL, M.D.
College of Physicians and Surgeons of Columbia University, New York, New York
(perspective on stress)

DENTAL HYGIENE

*JAMES P. CARLOS, D.D.S.
National Institute of Dental Research, Bethesda, Maryland

HOME ACCIDENTS

*NORVIN C. KIEFER, M.D., M.P.H.
New York, New York

TRAFFIC ACCIDENTS

*JAMES O'DAY
Highway Safety Research Institute, Ann Arbor, Michigan

GEOFFREY KABAT, PH.D.
American Health Foundation, New York, New York

AIR POLLUTION

*CARL M. SHY, M.D.
University of North Carolina, Chapel Hill, North Carolina

MERRIL EISENBUD
New York University, New York, New York

WATER POLLUTION

*ROBERT G. TARDIFF, PH.D.
National Academy of Sciences, Washington, D.C.

*HERMAN F. KRAYBILL, PH.D.
National Cancer Institute, Bethesda, Maryland

RADIATION

*JEAN ST. GERMAIN, M.S.
   Memorial Sloan-Kettering Cancer Center, New York, New York

VILMA HUNT, PH.D.
   Environmental Protection Agency, Washington, D.C.

FREDERICK URBACH, M.D.
   Temple University School of Medicine, Philadelphia, Pennsylvania (ultra-violet radiation)

NOISE

*THOMAS FAY, PH.D.
   Columbia-Presbyterian Hospital, New York, New York

INFECTIOUS DISEASES

*STEPHEN B. THACKER, M.D.
   Center for Disease Control, Atlanta, Georgia

MARIA C. CORSARO, M.S.
   New York City Department of Health, New York, New York

ROXANNE LITTNER, M.S.
   American Health Foundation, New York, New York

OCCUPATIONAL HEALTH

*B. DWIGHT CULVER, M.D.
   University of California, Irvine

WILLIAM DALTON
   New York University, New York, New York (accidents)

DEBORAH ENSIGN, M.ED.
   American Health Foundation, New York, New York

JOAN SPIVAK, M.S.
   American Health Foundation, New York, New York

JAMES H. STERNER, M.D.
   University of California, Irvine (noise)

LEGISLATIVE MEDICINE

RICHARD B. KLARBERG, J.D.S.
   American Health Foundation, New York, New York

KNOWING YOUR BODY

ERNEST L. WYNDER, M.D.
   American Health Foundation, New York, New York

* Chief contributors/editors.

Consultants

HENRY BLACKBURN, M.D.
University of Minnesota, Minneapolis, Minnesota (Nutrition)

DUANE BLOCK, M.D.
Ford Motor Company, Dearborn, Michigan (Highway Accidents)

VICTOR B. BOND
Brookhaven National Laboratory, Upton, New York (Radiation)

GILBERT BOTVIN, PH.D.
American Health Foundation, New York, New York (Stress)

JUDITH E. BROWN, R.D., M.P.H., PH.D.
University of Minnesota, Minneapolis, Minnesota (Nutrition)

JOHN D. CAPLAN
General Motors Research Laboratory, Warren, Michigan (Air Pollution, Highway Accidents)

KATHERINE L. CLANCY, R.D., PH.D.
Arlington, Virginia (Nutrition)

JOAN CLAYBROOK
National Highway Traffic Safety Administration, Washington, D.C. (Highway Accidents)

JEFFREY P. COHN, M.A., M.S.
Washington, D.C. (Water Pollution)

DORLAND J. DAVIS, M.D.
Bethesda, Maryland (Infections)

VICTOR A. DRILL, M.D.
University of Illinois, Chicago, Illinois (Family Planning and Childbearing)

NANCY EYLER, M.D.
American Health Foundation, New York, New York (Knowing Your Body)

ALVIN H. FREIMAN, M.D.
Memorial Sloan-Kettering Cancer Center, New York, New York (Tobacco)

STANLEY E. GITLOW, M.D.
Mt. Sinai Hospital, New York, New York (Alcohol)

JEROME GOODMAN, PH.D.
American Health Foundation, New York, New York (Radiation)

GIO B. GORI, PH.D.
National Cancer Institute, Bethesda, Maryland (Tobacco, Radiation)

PETER GREENWALD, M.D.
State of New York Department of Health, Albany, New York (Family Planning and Childbearing)

SAMI HASHIM, M.D.
St. Luke's Hospital Center, New York, New York (Nutrition)

IAN T.T. HIGGINS, M.D.
University of Michigan, Ann Arbor, Michigan (Air Pollution)

JOSEPH HIXSON
Red Hook, New York (Radiation)

DIETRICH HOFFMANN, PH.D.
American Health Foundation, Valhalla, New York (Air Pollution)

ILSE HOFFMANN
American Health Foundation, Valhalla, New York (Tobacco)

ARTHUR HOLLEB, M.D.
American Cancer Society, New York, New York (Radiation)

SEYMOUR JABLON
National Research Council, Washington, D.C. (Radiation)

ANN JACOBS, M.S.
American Health Foundation, New York, New York (Nutrition)

WILLIAM B. KANNEL, M.D.
National Heart, Lung, and Blood Institute, Framingham, Mass. (Tobacco)

SUSAN KAPASSO, M.S.
St. Christopher's Hospital for Children, Philadelphia, Pennsylvania (Family Planning and Childbearing)

JOHN F. KING, M.D.
Equitable Life Assurance Society of the United States, New York, New York (Family Planning and Childbearing)

BARRY LEWIS, M.D.
St. Thomas's Hospital Medical School, London (Tobacco, Stress, Physical Activity)

JOYCE LOWINSON, M.D.
Albert Einstein College, New York, New York (Alcohol, Drugs, Stress)

ALAN A. McLEAN, M.D.
International Business Machines, Inc., New York, New York (Stress)

JOHN McLEAN MORRIS, M.D.
Yale University School of Medicine, New Haven, Conn. (Family Planning and Childbearing)

MARGARET MUSHINSKI, M.A.
American Health Foundation, New York, New York (Air Pollution, Water Pollution)

NEW YORK STATE DEPARTMENT OF MOTOR VEHICLES
Albany, New York (Highway Accidents)

NEW YORK STATE DEPARTMENT OF TRANSPORTATION
Albany, New York (Highway Accidents)

OCCUPATIONAL SAFETY AND HEALTH ADMINISTRATION
Washington, D.C. (Occupational Health)

JANE OGLE
Vogue magazine, New York, New York (Nutrition, Tobacco, Home Accidents)

PATRICIA O'GORMAN, PH.D.
National Institute on Alcohol Abuse and Alcoholism, Rockville, Maryland (Alcohol)

NORBERT J. ROBERTS, M.D.
Exxon, New York, New York (Occupational Health)

HERBERT D. SARETT, PH.D.
Mead Johnson, Evansville, Indiana (Nutrition)

M.J. SLOAN, PH.D.
Shell Oil Company, Washington, D.C. (Air Pollution, Highway Accidents)

JOEL SOLOMON, M.D.
Downstate Medical Center, New York, New York (Alcohol)

A. LOUIS SOUTHREN, M.D.
New York Medical College, New York, New York (Family Planning and Childbearing)

STEVEN STELLMAN, PH.D.
American Health Foundation, New York, New York (Water Pollution)

JAMES H. STERNER, M.D.
University of California, Irvine, California (Noise)

BARRY STIMMEL, M.D.
Mt. Sinai Hospital, New York, New York (Alcohol)

RICHARD L. TIPPIE
National Safety Council, Chicago, Illinois (Highway Accidents)

ARTHUR UPTON, M.D.
New York University, New York, New York (Radiation)

ANTHONY R. VOLPE, D.D.S.
Colgate Palmolive Company, Piscataway, New Jersey (Dental Hygiene)

HEATHER WALTER, M.D., M.P.H.
American Health Foundation, New York, New York (Knowing Your Body)

JOHN H. WEISBURGER, PH.D.
American Health Foundation, Valhalla, New York (Occupational Health)

JOYCE YAEGER
Planned Parenthood of New York City, New York (Family Planning and Childbearing)

THE BOOK OF

HEALTH

Introduction

"To die young as late in life as possible" is how the ancient Greeks expressed a common goal. Most of us, unfortunately, conduct ourselves in ways that make us old before our time and dead before our possible full life span has been attained. We eat, drink, smoke, and neglect exercise to the point where we rob ourselves, our families, and our country of a large part of our potential creativity and productivity.

Traditional medicine—including physicians, surgeons, nurses, public health departments, and all the up-to-date sophisticated drugs and devices—has gone about as far as it can go in extending our life span. Over the past 150 years, in the developed nations at least, we have cleaned up our sewage systems, purified our water, discovered vaccination, and achieved a standard of living that frees most of us from the threat of starvation. Modern medicine has given us the means of eradicating the terrible diseases of our ancestors—cholera, typhoid, smallpox, tuberculosis, and the deficiency diseases such as scurvy, beriberi, and rickets.

Paradoxically, however, the higher standard of living we have achieved in our industrial civilization, although permitting more people to live longer than in previous generations, has led to sharp increases in the incidence of a new generation of major killers: heart disease, cancer, emphysema, diabetes, high blood pressure, and cirrhosis of the liver.

All of us are at least vaguely aware that rich foods, smoking, drinking alcohol, lack of exercise, and pollution of our work places and our general environment are contributing factors in bringing on these killer diseases, that significantly shorten our lives. Yet few of us are aware of the specific relationships between these risk factors and poor health, or early mortality.

All of us, too, are aware that we are mortal beings. From earliest childhood, we hear about death, about the fact that "no one lives forever." Yet, deep down inside each of us we do not actually believe in our *own* deaths, at least not *now*. It is very hard, therefore, for us to change our lifelong habits to meet a threat that seemingly has no reality. It is an incontrovertible fact, however, that changing our individual behavior, our particular lifestyles, is today the **best way we can prolong our lives** so as to maintain health throughout a lifetime.

How can we overcome the frustration of wanting to do something we know we must do but just can't do? The basic element is knowledge. We must know what risk to life and health we take by putting fudge sauce on our ice cream or by eating the ice cream itself. We must understand the risk factors involved in the next cigarette we smoke. We must realize just how much life we lose because of the extra weight we carry around. If we can obtain accurate information about how our own behavior affects our health, then we can be responsible for how we maintain our health.

This book is designed to provide such information in a clear, concise, and accurate manner, so that we may act on this knowledge, maintain our own good health, and increase our own life span. The book is not intended to provide bedtime reading or to be read in one sitting; it is a lifetime reference guide. The information in this volume is the best currently available, as interpreted by our contributors and editors and the staff of the American Health Foundation.

One word of caution: Medicine cannot be an exact science. Many of the most important medical advances in the treatment of yellow fever and typhoid, for example, were made before the mechanisms of these diseases were fully understood.

Medicine can and must act on reasonable, common sense assumptions that a particular course of action might work even if all the facts have not been isolated. Thus, while we do not know *all* the answers, each one of us is able to evaluate the particular risk factors in our lives and understand the preventive measures that may eliminate, or at the least reduce them. An increasingly informed public, particularly among the younger generations, will go a long way toward developing a nation of healthier lifestyles than we enjoy today.

The underlying premise of the book is that each of us is the master of our own body. In the final analysis, when it comes to maintaining our health, we must be responsible for ourselves, although medicine, society, industry, and government clearly must and can help. We must accept responsibility for our well-being by acknowledging and acting upon the fact that there is a cause-and-effect relationship between how we act and how we feel. If we are to remain healthy as late in life as possible, our informed minds must channel our health action into the proper directions. This volume attempts to inform and point us toward that goal but, ultimately, we will be required to achieve it on our own. This book is basically concerned with what happens *before* disease takes hold, before symptoms are observed. We describe the risk factors that *lead* to disease and disability and suggest the steps to be taken to prevent their onset.

Three years have elapsed from inception to the final printing of this volume. The task of distilling much knowledge, and appropriately translating scientific and medical information into a language readily understood by lay readers has been a challenging enterprise and a constructive experience for the editors and for the various contributors.

If this volume prolongs the full, productive, and useful life of one reader, we will be pleased. We will not be satisfied, however, until all humans can live out the lives they were designed to live. Health, after all, is the foundation upon which all other desires and all other capacities are built. We know that health, if properly maintained, can last a lifetime.

The Uses of Ep'i-de'mi-ol'o-gy

Because of its resemblance to the word *epidermis*, meaning skin, epidemiology is probably one of the most misunderstood concepts in the medical dictionary. The word comes from the Greek: *epi* ("upon"), and *demos* ("the people"). Epidemiology is the study of disease and its relationship to various environmental conditions. Determining the occurrence rates of diseases in population groups and isolating the factors associated with them is what epidemiology is all about.

You yourself may be an epidemiologist of sorts without knowing it. For example, have you and your family ever experienced an upset stomach, headache or fever, and then realized that each symptom directly followed consumption of certain foods or drinks? Did you observe that the symptoms disappeared once you stopped eating or drinking the suspected product? Discovering such factors associated with disease development is the activity epidemiologists routinely engage in. The factors studied are not only those associated with diet, but also include such diverse factors as water impurities, smoking, drinking, and exposure to chemicals and dusts at home or at work. One of the earliest applications of epi-

demiology occurred during an outbreak of cholera in London in 1854. A physician named John Snow traced the disease to a pump on Broad Street that was supplying Londoners with what he assumed was contaminated water. He could only assume, rather than "prove" the association between contaminated water and cholera because the germ theory of disease causation had not yet been discovered. But his epidemiological evidence was sound: people who drank water from other sources did not come down with cholera nor did Londoners who drank beer instead of water. Snow suggested a simple but historic measure to control the disease: take the handle off the Broad Street pump and thus cut off the supply of contaminated water. With this action, the cholera epidemic was effectively controlled.

From such simple beginnings, the discipline of epidemiology has advanced to the point where it now uses advanced scientific tools and refined study methods. Epidemiologists bring together the work of many other disciplines—biology, pathology, geology, nutrition, chemistry, statistics, and sociology—in their efforts to trace the development of disease. Masses of statistical data

43

are collected and analyzed. Studies are no longer restricted to epidemics of acute infectious diseases, which, like cholera, have been largely conquered. Epidemiologists are now also studying the increasing incidence of modern-day killers—the chronic, noninfectious diseases such as cancer, cardiovascular disorders, and birth defects.

Epidemiologic findings can only be as good as the accuracy and comprehensiveness of the data collected. This data reaches epidemiologists from a variety of official and nonoffical sources. Epidemiologists need to have the overall figures on births and causes of deaths, disease and injuries on a current, ongoing basis. They also need figures from old records for comparison. They need such figures for both the specific disease group under investigation and the "control" group in order to make the comparisons that reveal disease patterns. Comparisons are central to the epidemiological approach. In order to determine if the association of a disease with a place, with a habit, with a particular population, or with particular factors in those populations is more or less than expected, one must know what is "usually" expected.

In general there are two ways of tracking a disease. Take the example of lung cancer. You can use a group of people with lung cancer and another group without it and investigate their lifestyles. If you find, for example, that cigarette smoking is much more common among the lung cancer victims than among the others, you have reason to investigate this clue in more depth. This was the initial step taken in establishing the causative relationship between cigarette smoking and lung cancer.

Or, you can track the disease another way. Take a random group of people typical of the population as a whole and follow them for a few years, checking on their habits and noting the number of persons who develop lung cancer. If a larger number of cigarette smokers than nonsmokers develop lung cancer, the likelihood that a causal association exists is strengthened.

If both study methods point to a similar culprit, one can be fairly certain that an important discovery is about to be made. The time will now be ripe for laboratory scientists to pursue this lead to find the biological reason for the association between cigarette smoking and lung cancer.

Obviously, the sophistication and validity of epidemiologic findings will vary with the richness of the available data. If the original tobacco/lung cancer studies had included data about working environments or exposure to insulating material, an additional connection might have been pursued—that those who smoked cigarettes and were also exposed to asbestos fibers were even more likely to get lung cancer than smokers of nonfiltered cigarettes. This is exactly what epidemiologists later discovered.

Of course, the fact that there is a statistical association between a risk factor (cigarette smoking) and a disease (lung cancer) does not necessarily mean that the risk factor causes the disease. But if the epidemiological data are sound, if the degree of association is consistent and strong, and if the data make biological and common sense, it is safe to assume that the statistical connection is not accidental. In the London cholera case, although four decades were needed before germ theory confirmed John Snow's epidemiological suspicion that contaminated water caused cholera, many lives were saved by not waiting for the final proof.

It is now more than three decades since the statistical connection between tobacco and cancer was firmly established. Modern-day epidemiologists are now monitoring the decline of the rate of lung cancer in ex-smokers and following the rates among smokers of high-filtration (low tar and nicotine) cigarettes. The ultimate goal of epidemiology is to suggest preventive measures and provide clues to causes of disease.

Epidemiologists, then, may be considered medical detectives in search of the causes of disease and hence of ways to prevent diseases from occurring. This book will enable readers to make full use of epidemiologic advances in medical understanding and to apply the appropriate lessons and remedial actions to themselves.

PART

I

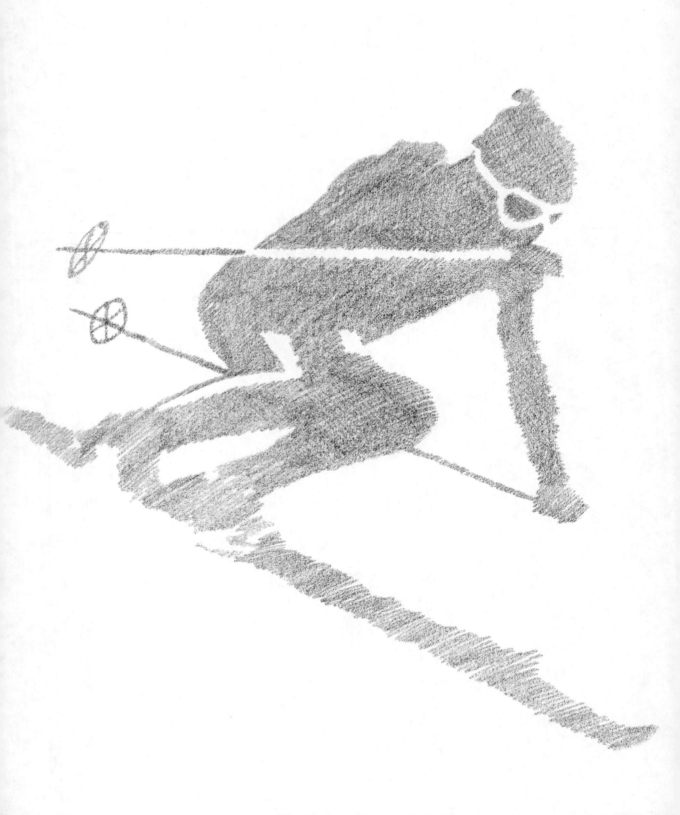

LIFESTYLE

CHAPTER

1

Nutrition

"You are what you eat." Virtually every modern language contains a version of this piece of folk wisdom. Today, at least in the developed countries, the cliché misses a major issue in nutrition. How much food is enough?

Primitive people, not aware that they were what they ate, possessed an advantage. Because they had to forage for their food, they were forced to be physically active. There was no escaping it. In order to eat, they had to work hard.

In today's world there are two types of malnutrition. There is the traditional form in which people suffer from a lack of calories, protein, minerals, and vitamins. Another form of malnutrition, however, exists in the developed countries in which people are largely overfed.

Most of us in the industrialized nations eat too much. Anthropologists and biochemists have speculated that nature did not design our bodies to consume so much fat, so many refined car-

bohydrates, so much sugar, so much salt—so much, period. We all know that hard work requires hearty meals, but somehow we seem to have forgotten the obverse: our normally sedentary lives demand fewer calories. If our metabolic capabilities are overloaded with excess fats, sugars, and calories, we must expect to pay a price—and we do, in diabetes, heart disease, strokes, and perhaps even in premature senility.

If we are what (and how much) we eat, then how we eat affects how we live and how long we live. Our bodies can no longer be trusted to tell us when to eat and when to stop. We have to determine what, as the scientists say, an optimal diet should be for our way of life. Only with such knowledge can we hope to overcome some of the chronic diseases that afflict us.

Glossary

BASAL METABOLIC RATE (BMR)   The minimum metabolic activity required to maintain life processes such as heartbeat and respiration, or the "cost of living."

CALORIE   The measure of the potential energy or fuel value of a food.

CARBOHYDRATE LOADING   A technique to increase the storage of energy in the muscle tissue. This is done prior to a long endurance type of activity.

CELLULOSE   A nondigestible carbohydrate found in the skins of fruits and vegetables.

CHOLESTEROL   A fatlike substance that is required by all the cells in the body. It is a normal component of the blood but is of concern when present in excessive amounts. Cholesterol is derived from two sources: (1) the liver manufactures cholesterol and (2) foods of animal origin contain cholesterol.

DIETARY FIBER   That portion of food that is resistant to digestive enzymes and passes through the bowel undigested. The cellulose, hemicellulose, gum, pectin, and lignin of vegetables, cereals, and fruits are the major sources of dietary fiber.

EMULSIFIER   A chemical used to prevent separation of oil and water. It is often found in salad dressings.

ESSENTIAL FATTY ACIDS   The polyunsaturated fatty acids, linolenic, linoleic, and arachidonic, which must be obtained from the diet for good health.

HYDROGENATED FATS   Liquid vegetable oils that have been combined with additional hydrogen to become solid, saturated fats. Examples are stick margarine and some vegetable shortening.

INGREDIENT LIST   List of components of a food in order of predominance by weight. This must be on a food package that does not have a specific standard for ingredient content.

LACTATION   The period following childbirth during which the breasts secrete milk.

LEGUMES   Plants having seed-containing pods used as food.

MONOUNSATURATED FATS   Fats that contain a predominance of monounsaturated fatty acids that chemically are capable of absorbing additional hydrogen but not as much hydrogen as polyunsaturated fatty acids. These fats have little effect on blood cholesterol. Examples include olive oil and peanut oil.

NATURAL FOODS   Foods that have been minimally processed or not processed at all. These foods may have a shorter shelf life than processed since they contain no artificial ingredients.

NUTRIENT   The chemical constituents of foods that are utilized in the body: proteins, carbohydrates, fats, vitamins, minerals, water.

NUTRIENT DENSITY   The ratio of nutrient composition of a food to its caloric content.

ORGANIC FOODS   All foods are organic from a chemical standpoint since they are composed of carbon, hydrogen, oxygen, and sometimes nitrogen.

POLYUNSATURATED FATS   Fats that contain a predominance of polyunsaturated fatty acids that chemically are capable of absorbing additional hydrogen. These fats are usually of vegetable origin, are liquid at room temperature, and tend to lower the cholesterol in the blood. Examples include safflower oil and corn oil. Also, the fat in fish is predominantly polyunsaturated.

P:S RATIO   The relationship between polyunsaturated and saturated fats. This ratio can be used to describe the fats in a particular food since most foods contain more than one type of fat. Also, the ratio can be used to describe the type of fats in an entire diet. The present P:S ratio for the American diet is approximately .4 or 1:2.5. Generally, the ratio should approach 1:1.

PRESERVATIVE   The generic term for substances added to food to prevent spoilage.

PROCESSED FOODS   These are foods that have been treated in some way to inhibit deterioration and increase the shelf life of the food. Food processing is an ancient method dating back to the drying of foods 5,000–6,000 years ago. Freezing, canning, and other methods are a result of relatively new technologies.

RDA (RECOMMENDED DIETARY ALLOWANCES)   A list devised by the National Academy of Sciences of the recommended levels of seventeen essential nutrients that should be consumed daily to meet the nutritional needs of practically all healthy persons. This guide incorporates a safety margin to compensate for any individual differences and normal stresses of daily living.

ROUGHAGE   A coarse, bulky food, high in fiber, which is nondigestible and stimulates the gastrointestinal tract. An example is cellulose.

SATURATED FATS   Fats that contain a predominance of saturated fatty acids that chemically are not capable of absorbing any more hydrogen. These fats usually are of animal origin, are solid at room temperature, and tend to increase the amount of cholesterol in the blood. Examples include butter and the fat of meat and poultry.

VEGETARIANS   Those who (1) eat only plant foods ("strict vegetarians" or "vegans"), (2) eat only dairy products, eggs, and plant foods ("lacto-ovo-vegetarians"), or (3) avoid red meat but eat fish and/or poultry. Vegetarianism stems from religious beliefs, health motives, and ethical, ecological, and economic reasons.

VITAMINS   Organic compounds present in minute amounts in food and needed for good health, normal growth, and reproduction.

From Scarcity to Plenty

Our remote ancestors ate from a limited supply of available food simply to satisfy hunger. By contrast, today's menus result from many factors other than the basic nutritional needs left us by millions of years of human evolution. We have so much food in the developed world that undernutrition is quite rare as compared with overnutrition. We eat not only to allay our hunger but also for pleasure as well as to satisfy our social and emotional needs. Our choice of food is subject to convenience as well as to the commercial, promotional, and marketing interests of the food industry. These forces are all potent influences in food choice today.

In primitive societies, hunting and gathering were the only skills available to people for acquiring their nourishment. It was not necessarily such a mean existence, for the few hunter-gatherers still in the world today are remarkably healthy. Like their ancestors, they eat nuts and other fruits and vegetables and the lean meat of wild animals. Salt is unavailable, sugar nearly so. As a result, they get few of the diseases common in affluent societies today, including high blood pressure, heart disease, and tooth decay. A typical hunter-gatherer has a blood cholesterol level just over half that of Western man. In one classic study of the African Bushman essentially no vitamin deficiencies were found.

When humans harnessed fire and learned to cook, the range of food that could be rendered edible by cooking was greatly increased. Farming, a late chapter in human history dating back only some 400–500 generations, added still more variety to the human diet. At first, farming meant growing food for direct consumption only—subsistence farming—but eventually societies developed in which farm families raised surpluses for sale on the open market.

The large-scale, mechanized industrial farm that dominates agriculture today has developed only very recently. Together with modern ways of food storage, industrial farming has brought us security of food supply as well as important changes in our dietary patterns. Modern food technology has greatly simplified the homemaker's role in food preparation and has made available many convenience foods. As a side effect, an increasing portion of our meals are now eaten out, as proven by the rising popularity of fast food restaurants.

Over the years nutrition has gradually improved in many ways in the industrial countries of the world. Food hygiene, refrigeration, and other techniques for preventing bacterial growth have reduced food-borne infections and have permitted prolonged storage of formerly perishable goods. On the other hand, the evidence is mounting that some serious and even fatal diseases common in the modernized societies are due in part to our new food habits. These new disease trends have accompanied our increasing consumption of foods rich in fat, salt, and sugar, while our intake of roughage has gone down. Our nutritional patterns today differ sharply from the habits man evolved through hundreds of thousands of generations, and may go along way toward explaining many of our medical woes.

Obesity, a widespread problem in many parts of the world, clearly pinpoints dietary and lifestyle patterns as the culprit. Many factors in our lives make it far too easy to put on weight. These include the increasing mechanization of life and labor that has led to more and more sedentary habits. Also, the sheer quantity of food now available to many of us encourages eating and drinking to excess.

Food habits differ widely among different countries and social groups, but except where undernutrition is a problem, the world's various eating patterns each provide sufficient nutrients for growth. There is more to eating than growth however, and some dietary habits may be among the causes of common serious illnesses. For example, people growing up in Western countries usually consume a diet high in fat. Such people are prone to coronary heart disease, and to cancer of the colon, breast, prostate, ovary, uterus, and pancreas. The Japanese, until recently ate food containing much less fat than we do, only about 10–20 percent of the calories consumed (figure 1.1), which may be why they are less prone to these diseases. (This is also true for the central and western Latin Americans.) As of the early 1980s, however, fat intake in Japan has doubled (from 10 percent of calories to 20 percent of calories).

Our Western diet includes more highly milled and refined starches—white flour, white bread, breakfast cereals made from such flour—and fewer sources of roughage or fiber, than it did a century ago. Comparisons of countries with differing food patterns show that diseases such as diverticulitis, appendicitis, and colon cancer occur more often where people consume such low-fiber diets. We may need to resume a diet containing more fiber as found in whole grain breads, cereals containing bran, and fresh fruits, vegetables, and salads.

Eating is not only necessary for life, it is also one of life's greatest pleasures. Little is known about the reasons why people choose the kinds and amounts of food they do, but we do know that eating and drinking retain powerful emotional overtones throughout life. In our society today,

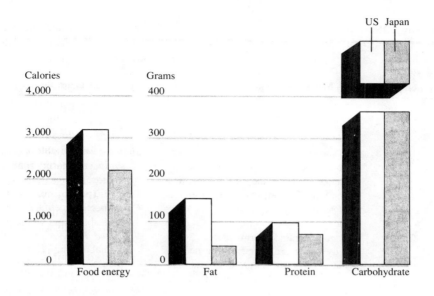

FIGURE 1.1

Intake of food energy and nutrients per person—
the contrast between the USA and Japan
SOURCE: *National Nutritional Survey, Ministry of Health and Welfare, Japan, 1969;*
National Food Situation, Department of Agriculture, USA, 1968

hunger in fact often becomes a minor factor in determining our eating habits. Good health and good nutrition go hand in hand however, and optimal weight is a matter for science, not for subjective judgment made according to the dictates of fashion. This chapter provides guidelines for prudent, pleasurable, and affordable eating, aimed at demonstrating optimal weight for each individual. The optimal weight for each of us is that which provides a *minimum* chance of developing serious illness while encouraging a *maximum* life span.

The Food We Eat

Before we can understand the relationship of food to health, we must understand something about the energy yield of food and its nutrients.

ENERGY How much food energy is required for health? Quantities of potential food energy are measured in calories. Naturally, persons who do the hardest physical work need the most calories. A lumberjack may need, on the average, 3,700 calories a day, a household worker 2,100. During half an hour, while walking you may spend 120–140 calories; while lying down, 40 calories; and while running, 600 calories. Thus, your physical activity substantially affects the amount of food energy—calories—you need.

Food energy is also needed for processes of which we are seldom conscious: the heart's action in pumping blood, breathing, keeping an erect posture, the replacement of body cells. The energy requirement for these functions is known as the basal metabolic rate. Women have slightly lower basal metabolic rates than men, and older people have lower rates than younger people.

Table 1.1
MACRO- AND MICRONUTRIENTS

Nutrients	Calorie yield per gram	Main functions	Types and examples
Macronutrients			
Carbohydrate	4	Main source of energy for the body. Carbohydrate foods are often accompanied by fiber and certain vitamins and minerals, but fiber is not a source of food energy for man.	*Simple Sugars* (table sugar, sucrose, corn syrup, dextrose, honey, brown sugar, fructose) *Starches* (potato, rice, grain) *Fiber* (pectins, celluloses as found in fruits, vegetables, and whole grains)
Fat	9	Most concentrated energy source. Some fatty acids are essential for health. Fatty foods carry a group of vitamins known as fat-soluble vitamins (A, D, E, and K).	*Saturated Fatty Acids* (found in foods of animal origin, i.e., meats, cream, butter, cheese, egg yolk, and in hard margarine and shortenings) *Monounsaturated Fatty Acids* (found in foods like olive oil, peanut oil, olives) *Polyunsaturated Fatty Acids* (found in foods of vegetable origin, i.e., corn, safflower, sesame seed oils)
Protein	4	Needed for growth, maintenance, and repair of cells and tissues. Necessary for the formation of hormones, antibodies, and enzymes. Can also yield energy.	*Animal Proteins* (chicken, meats, fish, dairy) *Vegetable Proteins* (legumes: split peas, nuts, kidney beans, etc.)
Micronutrients			
Vitamins	–	Involved in the chemical reactions of life processes, often as catalysts or activators.	*Fat Soluble*—vitamins A, D, E, K (dairy products, yellow and dark green vegetables, polyunsaturated oils) *Water Soluble*—B complex, ascorbic acid (C), folacin, pantothenic acid (found in small quantities in many foods)
Minerals	–	Needed for proper composition of body fluids, bone and blood formation, nerve function.	*Needed in Quantity* - calcium, phosphorus, sodium, chloride, potassium, magnesium sulfur *Trace Elements* - iron, iodine, magnesium, copper, zinc, cobalt, molybdenum, flouride, selenium, chromium
Water	–	Most abundant component of living tissues. Needed for internal temperature regulation and for maintaining fluid balance.	All foods

During certain phases of life, our calorie needs go up. Infants and children need relatively high amounts of calories per kilogram of body weight to grow and develop. Pregnancy and lactation require extra energy for the growth of the fetus and of the mother's reproductive tissues. See section on Infancy.

The way we regulate food intake to balance our energy needs is not completely understood. We do know that excess body fat can only come from excess food energy. On the average, a pound of fatty tissue is gained by eating approximately 3,500 calories beyond the body's requirements; conversely, if you spend or "burn" approximately 3,500 calories more than you eat, you will, on average, shed one pound.

We are only moderately efficient at using food energy. Like generators in power stations, we convert some of this energy to heat, which is partly wasted but which allows humans and other animals to maintain optimal body temperature.

The foods from which we obtain energy are discussed in the following sections on proteins, carbohydrates, sugars, and fats. Fat is the most concentrated source of energy, providing 9 calories per gram. Carbohydrate provides 4 calories per gram, and protein 4 calories per gram. Alcohol also yields energy—7 calories per gram—but, unlike fat, carbohydrate or protein, it often stimulates the appetite, thereby encouraging the consumption of still more food energy. Thus alcohol is often an indirect source of surplus food energy.

The energy value of a meal is only partly determined by the size of a helping; it is also affected by the mix of nutrients. Hence the energy value of a meal should be thought of in terms of "caloric density." For detailed comparisons of caloric contents of some common foods, see the food composition tables (table 1.2).

NUTRIENTS

There are two broad nutrient groups: macronutrients and micronutrients. Macronutrients include protein, carbohydrates, and fat, all of which provide energy. Micronutrients are the vitamins and minerals, each essential to the body in relatively small amounts. Foods contain these nutrients in widely varying proportions. For specific details refer to table 1.2.

Proteins

Living cells contain many different proteins. An adequate supply of protein in the diet is essential for good health. Proteins are long chains of building blocks called amino acids, which contain nitrogen, carbon, hydrogen, oxygen, and often sulfur. The dietary proteins provide the amino acids necessary for cell growth in the infant and child, for tissue maintenance and repair at all ages, and for reproduction and lactation. These body proteins are in an active state of change, continuously being broken down and rebuilt.

The body has more than 2,000 enzymes, which are themselves proteins, each with a specific role in promoting the chemical reactions necessary for the life processes. Other proteins circulate in the blood plasma. Albumin, for instance, maintains the volume of fluid in the blood vessels. Twelve or more proteins take part in the blood-clotting process that stops bleeding. The circulating antibodies are plasma proteins that specifically protect us from infections and from poisoning by bacterial toxins. Many of the hormones that are transported in the bloodstream are proteins or protein-like.

For all these functions we need the right kinds of protein in the diet as well as an adequate total amount. The right kind is determined by the particular mix of amino acids contained in the protein and by the digestibility of the foods providing the protein.

Table 1.2
FOOD COMPOSITION: THE NUTRITIVE VALUE OF FOODS

Food, Approximate Measure, and Weight (in grams)		gm.	Food Energy calories	Pro-tein (gm.)	Fat (gm.)	Carbo-hydrate (gm.)
Dairy Products						
Milk:						
Fluid:						
Whole, 3.5% fat	1 cup	244	160	9	9	12.0
Lowfat, 2%	1 cup	246	145	10	5	14.8
Nonfat (skim)	1 cup	245	90	9	trace	12.5
Dry, nonfat instant	1 cup	68	245	24	trace	35.1
Buttermilk:						
Cultured from skim milk	1 cup	245	90	9	trace	12.5
Evaporated, unsweetened	1 cup	252	345	18	20	24.4
Condensed, sweetened	1 cup	306	980	25	27	166.2
Cream:						
Half & Half	1 tbsp.	15	20	1	2	.7
Light	1 tbsp.	15	30	1	3	.6
Whipping, heavy	1 tbsp.	15	45	trace	6	.5
Sour Cream	2 tbsp.	30	57	trace	6	1.0
Cheese:						
Blue or Roquefort	1 oz.	28	105	6	9	.6
Camembert	1⅓ oz.	38	115	7	9	.5
Cheddar	1 oz.	28	115	7	9	.6
Cottage:						
creamed	1 cup	245	260	33	10	7.1
uncreamed	1 cup	200	170	34	1	5.4
Cream Cheese	1 oz.	28	100	2	10	.6
Parmesan, grated	1 tbsp.	5	25	2	2	.2
Swiss	1 oz.	28	105	8	8	.5
Imitation cream products (made with vegetable fat)						
Creamers:						
Powdered	1 tsp.	2	10	trace	1	trace
Liquid (frozen)	1 tbsp.	15	20	trace	2	trace
Milk Beverages:						
Cocoa, homemade	1 cup	250	245	10	12	27.3
Chocolate-flavored drink (made with skim milk)	1 cup	250	190	8	6	27.3
Malted milk powder	1 oz.	28	115	4	2	20.1

Calcium (mg.)	Iron (mg.)	Vitamin A Value (I.U.)	Thiamine (mg.)	Riboflavin (mg.)	Niacin (mg.)	Ascorbic Acid (mg.)	Sodium (mg.)	Potassium (mg.)
288	0.1	350	0.07	0.41	0.2	2	122	351
352	0.1	200	0.10	0.52	0.2	2	150	431
296	0.1	10	0.09	0.44	0.2	2	127	355
879	0.4	20	0.24	1.21	0.6	5	358	1,173
296	0.1	10	0.10	0.44	0.2	2	319	343
635	0.3	810	0.10	0.86	0.5	3	297	764
802	0.3	1100	0.24	1.16	0.6	3	343	961
16	trace	70	trace	0.02	trace	trace	7	19
15	trace	130	trace	0.02	trace	trace	6	18
11	trace	230	trace	0.02	trace	trace	5	13
31	— *	230	trace	0.04	trace	—	12	17
89	0.1	350	0.01	0.17	0.3	0	—	—
40	0.2	380	0.02	0.29	0.3	0	—	42
213	0.3	370	0.01	0.13	trace	0	198	23
230	0.7	420	0.07	0.61	0.2	0	560	210
180	0.8	20	0.06	0.56	0.2	0	580	140
23	0.3	400	trace	0.06	trace	0	71	21
68	trace	60	trace	0.04	trace	0	44	9
251	0.3	310	trace	0.11	trace	0	200	29
1	trace	trace	—	—	trace	—	31	—
2	—	10	0	0	—	—	1	—
295	1.0	400	0.10	0.45	0.5	3	128	363
270	0.5	210	0.10	0.40	0.3	3	115	355
82	0.6	290	0.09	0.15	0.1	0	125	104

*Reliable information unavailable.

Table 1.2

FOOD COMPOSITION: THE NUTRITIVE VALUE OF FOODS

Food, Approximate Measure, and Weight (in grams)		gm.	Food Energy calories	Pro-tein (gm.)	Fat (gm.)	Carbo-hydrate (gm.)
Milk Desserts:						
Custard	1 cup	265	305	14	15	29.4
Ice Cream						
Regular 10% fat	1 cup	133	255	6	14	27.7
Rich 16% fat	1 cup	148	330	4	24	26.6
Ice Milk						
Hardened	1 cup	131	200	6	7	29.3
Soft-serve	1 cup	175	265	8	9	39.2
Yogurt						
Partially skim	1 cup	245	125	8	4	12.7
Whole milk	1 cup	245	150	7	8	12.0
Eggs						
Large, 24 oz./dozen						
Raw:						
Whole, without shell	1 egg	50	80	6	6	.5
White of egg	1 egg	33	15	4	trace	.3
Yolk of egg	1 egg	17	60	3	5	.1
Cooked:						
Scrambled w/fat	1 egg	64	110	7	8	1.5
Meat, poultry, fish, shellfish; related products						
Roast, oven-cooked, no liquid added:						
Lean and fat	3 oz.	85	375	17	34	0
Lean only	1.8 oz.	51	125	14	7	0
Steak, broiled:						
Relatively fat, i.e. sirloin						
Lean and fat	3 oz.	85	330	20	27	0
Lean only	2 oz.	56	115	18	4	0
Relatively lean, i.e. round						
Lean and fat	3 oz.	85	220	24	13	0
Lean only	2.4 oz.	68	130	21	4	0
Beef, canned:						
Corned beef	3 oz.	85	185	22	10	0
Corned beef hash	3 oz.	85	155	7	10	9

Calcium (mg.)	Iron (mg.)	Vitamin A Value (I.U.)	Thiamine (mg.)	Riboflavin (mg.)	Niacin (mg.)	Ascorbic Acid (mg.)	Sodium (mg.)	Potassium (mg.)
297	1.1	930	0.11	0.50	0.3	1	209	387
194	0.1	590	0.05	0.28	0.1	1	84	241
115	trace	980	0.03	0.16	0.1	1	49	141
204	0.1	280	0.07	0.29	0.1	1	89	255
273	0.2	370	0.09	0.39	0.2	2	119	341
294	0.1	170	0.10	0.44	0.2	2	125	350
272	0.1	340	0.07	0.39	0.2	2	115	323
27	1.1	590	0.05	0.15	trace	0	61	65
3	trace	0	trace	0.09	trace	0	48	46
24	0.9	580	0.04	0.07	trace	0	9	17
51	1.1	690	0.05	0.18	trace	0	164	93
8	2.2	70	0.05	0.13	3.1	—	41	189
6	1.8	10	0.04	0.11	2.6	—	35	161
9	2.5	50	0.05	0.16	4.0	—	48	220
7	2.2	10	0.05	0.14	3.6	—	42	192
10	3.0	20	0.07	0.19	4.8	—	60	272
9	2.5	10	0.06	0.16	4.1	—	52	238
17	3.7	20	0.01	0.20	2.9	—	—	—
11	1.7	—	0.01	0.08	1.8	—	474	176

Table 1.2

FOOD COMPOSITION: THE NUTRITIVE VALUE OF FOODS

Food, Approximate Measure, and Weight (in grams)		gm.	Food Energy calories	Pro-tein (gm.)	Fat (gm.)	Carbo-hydrate (gm.)
Beef and Vegetable Stew	1 cup	235	210	15	10	16.5
Beef Pot Pie (= 8 oz.)	1 pie	227	560	23	33	43.0
Chicken, cooked:						
Flesh only, broiled	3 oz.	85	115	20	3	2.0
Breast, fried, ½ w/bone	3.3 oz.	94	155	25	5	1.2
Flesh & skin only	1.3 oz.	76	155	25	5	2.5
Drumstick, fried: w/bone	2.1 oz.	59	90	12	4	1.5
Flesh & skin only	1.3 oz.	38	90	12	4	.5
Chicken, canned, boneless	3 oz.	85	170	18	10	2.0
Chicken Pot Pie (= 8 oz.)	1 pie	227	535	23	31	41.0
Chili con carne, canned:						
W/Beans	1 cup	250	335	19	15	31.1
W/O Beans	1 cup	255	510	26	38	16.0
Heart, beef, lean, braised	3 oz.	85	160	27	5	.6
Lamb, cooked:						
Chop, thick, w/bone, broiled	4.8 oz.	137	400	25	33	.8
Lean & fat	4 oz.	112	400	25	33	.8
Lean only	2.6 oz.	74	140	21	6	.5
Leg, roasted:						
Lean & fat	3 oz.	85	235	22	16	.8
Lean only	2.5 oz.	71	130	20	5	1.3
Shoulder, roasted:						
Lean & fat	3 oz.	85	285	18	23	1.5
Lean only	2.3 oz.	64	130	17	6	2.0
Liver, beef, fried	2 oz.	57	130	15	6	4.0
Pork, cured, cooked:						
Ham, lean & fat, roasted	3 oz.	85	245	18	19	.8
Luncheon meat:						
Boiled ham, sliced	2 oz.	57	135	11	10	.3
Canned, spiced, or unspiced	2 oz.	57	165	8	14	1.8
Pork, fresh, cooked:						
Chop, thick, w/bone	3.5 oz.	98	260	16	21	1.8
Lean & fat	2.3 oz.	66	260	16	21	1.8
Lean only	1.7 oz.	48	130	15	7	1.8

Calcium (mg.)	Iron (mg.)	Vitamin A Value (I.U.)	Thiamine (mg.)	Riboflavin (mg.)	Niacin (mg.)	Ascorbic Acid (mg.)	Sodium (mg.)	Potassium (mg.)
28	2.8	2310	0.13	0.17	4.4	15	91	613
32	4.1	1860	0.25	0.27	4.5	7	644	361
8	1.4	80	0.05	0.16	7.4	—	56	233
9	1.3	70	0.04	0.17	11.2	—	—	—
9	1.3	70	0.04	0.17	11.2	—	—	—
6	0.9	50	0.03	0.15	2.7	—	—	—
6	0.9	50	0.03	0.15	2.7	—	—	—
18	1.3	200	0.03	0.11	3.7	3	—	117
68	3.0	3020	0.25	0.26	4.1	5	581	336
80	4.2	150	0.08	0.18	3.2	—	1,354	594
97	3.6	380	0.05	0.31	5.6	—	37.7	—
5	5.0	20	0.21	1.04	6.5	1	87	198
10	1.5	—	0.14	0.25	5.6	—	66	302
10	1.5	—	0.14	0.25	5.6	—	61	280
9	1.5	—	0.11	0.20	4.5	—	51	232
9	1.4	—	0.13	0.23	4.7	—	53	241
3	1.4	—	0.12	0.21	4.4	—	60	273
9	1.0	—	0.11	0.20	4.0	—	45	207
8	1.0	—	0.10	0.18	3.7	—	43	196
6	6.0	30,280	0.15	2.37	9.4	15	104	216
8	2.2	0	0.40	0.16	3.1	—	636	199
6	1.6	0	0.25	0.09	1.5	—	—	—
5	1.2	0	0.18	0.12	1.6	—	700	126
8	2.2	0	0.63	0.18	3.8	—	41	188
8	2.2	0	0.63	0.18	3.8	—	39	180
7	1.9	0	0.54	0.16	3.3	—	37	167

Table 1.2
FOOD COMPOSITION: THE NUTRITIVE VALUE OF FOODS

Food, Approximate Measure, and Weight (in grams)		gm.	Food Energy calories	Pro- tein (gm.)	Fat (gm.)	Carbo- hydrate (gm.)
Roast, oven-cooked, no liquid added:						
Lean & fat	3 oz.	85	310	21	24	11.5
Lean only	2.4 oz.	68	175	20	10	1.3
Cuts, simmered:						
Lean & fat	3 oz.	85	320	20	26	1.5
Lean only	2.2 oz.	63	135	18	6	2.3
Sausage:						
Bologna, 3″ diam. by ⅛″ thick slice	2 slices	26	80	3	7	1.3
Braunschweiger, 2″ × ¼″ slice	2 slices	20	65	3	5	2.0
Deviled ham, canned	1 tbsp.	13	45	2	4	.3
Frankfurter	1 frank	56	170	7	15	.8
Pork links, cooked, 16 per pound, raw	2 links	26	125	5	11	1.5
Salami, dry type	1 oz.	28	130	7	11	.8
Salami, cooked	1 oz.	28	90	5	7	1.8
Vienna, canned (7 sausages per 5 oz. can)	1 sausage	16	40	2	3	1.3
Veal, medium fat, cooked, bone removed:						
Cutlet	3 oz.	85	185	23	9	3.0
Roast	3 oz.	85	230	23	14	3.0
Fish & Shellfish:						
Bluefish, baked with table fat	3 oz.	85	135	22	4	2.8
Clams:						
Raw, meat only	3 oz.	85	65	11	1	3/0
Canned, solids and liquid	3 oz.	85	45	7	1	1.0
Crabmeat, canned	3 oz.	85	85	15	2	1.8
Fish sticks, breaded, cooked, frozen	8 oz.	227	400	38	20	17.0
Haddock, breaded, fried	3 oz.	85	140	17	5	1.8
Ocean Perch, breaded, fried	3 oz.	85	195	16	11	8.0
Oysters, raw, meat only	1 cup	240	160	20	4	11.0
Salmon, pink, canned	3 oz.	85	120	17	5	1.8
Sardines, Atlantic, canned in oil, drained	3 oz.	85	175	20	9	3.5

Cal-cium (mg.)	Iron (mg.)	Vita-min A Value (I.U.)	Thia-mine (mg.)	Ribo-flavin (mg.)	Niacin (mg.)	Ascor-bic Acid (mg.)	Sodium (mg.)	Potas-sium (mg.)
9	2.7	0	0.78	0.22	4.7	—	51	233
9	2.6	0	0.73	0.21	4.4	—	49	224
8	2.5	0	0.46	0.21	4.1	—	34	158
8	2.3	0	0.42	0.19	3.7	—	31	145
2	0.5	—	0.04	0.06	0.7	—	338	60
2	1.1	1310	0.03	0.29	1.6	—	—	—
1	0.3	—	0.02	0.01	0.2	—	—	—
3	0.8	—	0.08	0.11	1.4	—	—	—
2	0.6	0	0.21	0.09	1.0	—	250	70
4	1.0	—	0.10	0.07	1.5	—	—	—
3	0.7	—	0.07	0.07	1.2	—	—	—
1	0.3	—	0.01	0.02	0.4	—	—	—
9	2.7	—	0.06	0.21	4.6	—	55	251
10	2.9	—	0.11	0.26	6.6	—	57	259
25	0.6	40	0.09	0.08	1.6	—	87	—
59	5.2	90	0.08	0.15	1.1	8	173	263
47	3.5	—	0.01	0.09	0.9	—	—	119
38	0.7	—	0.07	0.07	1.6	—	851	94
25	0.9	—	0.09	0.16	3.6	—	—	—
34	1.0	—	0.03	0.06	2.7	2	150	297
28	1.1	—	0.08	0.09	1.5	—	129	243
226	13.2	740	0.33	0.43	6.0	—	175	290
167	0.7	60	0.03	0.16	6.8	—	329	307
372	2.5	190	0.02	0.17	4.6	—	699	501

Table 1.2

FOOD COMPOSITION: THE NUTRITIVE VALUE OF FOODS

Food, Approximate Measure, and Weight (in grams)		gm.	Food Energy calories	Pro-tein (gm.)	Fat (gm.)	Carbo-hydrate (gm.)
Shad, baked, w/table fat and bacon	3 oz.	85	170	20	10	0
Shrimp, canned, meat	3 oz.	85	100	21	1	1.8
Swordfish, broiled with butter	3 oz.	85	150	24	5	2.3
Tuna, canned in oil, drained solids	3 oz.	85	170	24	7	2.8

Dry legumes

Beans, dry:						
Common varieties as Great Northern, navy & others:						
Cooked, drained:						
Navy (pea)	1 cup	190	225	15	1	40.0
Canned, solids & liquid:						
White with—						
Frankfurters	1 cup	255	365	19	18	32.0
Pork and Tomato Sauce	1 cup	255	310	16	7	46.0
Red kidney	1 cup	255	230	15	1	48.0
Black beans, cooked	1 cup	100	337	22	1.4	25.0
Black-eyed peas (cowpeas), cooked	1 cup	250	190	13	0.8	33.0
Fava beans (broad beans), raw	1 lb	454	1533	110	7.7	256.0
Garbanzo beans (chickpeas), cooked	1 cup	100	338	20	4.6	54.0
Great northern beans, cooked	1 cup	180	212	14	1.1	37.0
Lentils, cooked	1 cup	200	212	16	trace	37.0
Lima beans, cooked, large or small	1 cup	190	262	16	1.1	47.0
Mung beans, cooked	1 cup	105	355	25	1.3	61.0
Mung bean sprouts,						
Raw	1 cup	105	37	4	0.2	5.0
Cooked	1 cup	125	35	4	0.3	7.0
Navy beans (small white), cooked	1 cup	190	224	15	1.1	39.0
Peanuts (see Nuts and Seeds)						
Peas:						
Whole, cooked	1 cup	100	338	24	1.2	58.0
Split, cooked	1 cup	200	230	16	0.6	40.0
Pinto or Calico Beans, cooked	1 cup	95	330	22	1.1	58.0

Calcium (mg.)	Iron (mg.)	Vitamin A Value (I.U.)	Thiamine (mg.)	Riboflavin (mg.)	Niacin (mg.)	Ascorbic Acid (mg.)	Sodium (mg.)	Potassium (mg.)
20	0.5	20	0.11	0.22	7.3	—	66	321
98	2.6	50	0.01	0.03	1.5	—	—	103
23	1.1	1750	0.03	0.04	9.3	—	—	—
7	1.6	70	0.04	0.10	10.1	—	—	—
95	5.1	0	0.27	0.13	1.3	0	13	790
94	4.8	330	0.18	0.15	3.3	trace	1374	668
138	4.6	330	0.20	0.08	1.5	5	1181	536
74	4.6	10	0.13	0.10	1.5	—	8	673
140	7.9	30	0.35	.18	1.9	—	25	1000
43	3.3	30	0.40	.10	1.0	—	20	570
460	32.0	320	2.3	1.4	11.0	—	—	—
150	6.9	50	0.20	.13	1.8	—	26	800
90	4.9	0	0.25	.13	1.3	0	13	750
50	4.2	40	0.14	.12	1.2	0	—	500
55	5.9	—	0.25	.11	1.3	—	4	1200
120	8.1	80	0.25	.20	2.4	—	6	1100
20	1.4	20	0.14	.14	0.8	20	5	230
21	1.1	30	0.11	.13	0.9	8	5	200
95	5.1	0	0.27	.13	1.3	0	13	790
64	5.1	120	0.47	.26	2.7	—	35	1000
22	3.4	80	0.30	.18	1.8	—	26	590
130	6.1	—	0.51	.18	1.9	—	10	940

Table 1.2

FOOD COMPOSITION: THE NUTRITIVE VALUE OF FOODS

Food, Approximate Measure, and Weight (in grams)		gm.	Food Energy calories	Pro-tein (gm.)	Fat (gm.)	Carbo-hydrate (gm.)
Peanut Butter, small amount of fat and salt added	1 tbsp.	16	93	4	7.9	1.5
Moderate amount of sugar, fat, and salt added	1 tbsp.	16	94	4	8.1	1.3
Pecans, halves	1 cup	108	742	10	77	2.3
Pine nuts:						
Pignolias	1 oz.	28	156	9	13	.8
Pinon Nuts	1 oz.	28	180	4	17	2.8
Pistachio nuts	30	15	88	3	8	1.0
Pumpkin or Squash seed kernels, dried	2 tbsp.	18	97	5	8.2	.8
Sesame seeds:						
Whole	2 tbsp.	18	101	3	8.8	2.5
Hulled	2 tbsp.	16	94	3	8.6	1.2
Sesame meal, home-ground	½ cup	46	259	9	23.0	4.0
Sunflower seed kernels	2 tbsp.	18	102	4	8.6	2.2
Sunflower meal, home-ground	½ cup	45	252	11	21	4.8
Walnuts, black, chopped	1 tbsp.	8	50	2	4.8	0
English or Persian, chopped	1 tbsp.	8	52	1	5.1	.5
Vegetables & vegetable products						
Asparagus, green:						
Cooked, drained:						
Spears	4	60	10	1	trace	1.5
Pieces	1 cup	145	30	3	trace	4.5
Canned, solids and liquid	1 cup	244	45	5	1	4.0
Beans:						
Lima, cooked, drained, immature seeds	1 cup	170	190	13	1	32.3
Snap:						
Green:						
Canned, solids and liquid	1 cup	239	45	2	trace	9.3
Beets:						
Diced or sliced	1 cup	170	55	2	trace	11.8

Calcium (mg.)	Iron (mg.)	Vitamin A Value (I.U.)	Thiamine (mg.)	Riboflavin (mg.)	Niacin (mg.)	Ascorbic Acid (mg.)	Sodium (mg.)	Potassium (mg.)
10	.3	—	.02	.02	2.5	0	97	110
9	.3	—	.02	.02	2.4	0	97	100
79	2.6	140	.93	.14	1.0	2	trace	650
—	—	—	.18	—	—	—	—	—
3	1.5	10	.36	.07	1.3	trace	—	—
20	1.1	30	.10	—	0.2	0	—	150
9	2.0	10	.04	.03	0.4	—	—	—
210	1.9	trace	.18	.04	1.0	0	11	130
18	.4	—	.02	.02	0.8	0	—	—
530	4.8	10	.45	.11	2.5	0	28	330
22	1.2	10	.36	.04	1.0	—	6	160
54	3.2	20	.88	.10	2.4	—	14	410
trace	.5	20	.02	.01	0.1	—	trace	37
8	.2	trace	.03	.01	0.1	trace	trace	36
13	0.4	540	0.10	0.11	0.8	16	1	110
30	0.9	1310	0.23	0.26	2.0	38	1	260
44	4.1	1240	0.15	0.22	2.0	37	576	405
80	4.3	480	0.31	0.17	2.2	29	2	720
81	2.9	690	0.07	0.10	0.7	10	564	227
24	0.9	30	0.05	0.07	0.5	10	73	350

Table 1.2
FOOD COMPOSITION: THE NUTRITIVE VALUE OF FOODS

Food, Approximate Measure, and Weight (in grams)		gm.	Food Energy calories	Protein (gm.)	Fat (gm.)	Carbohydrate (gm.)
Beet greens, leaves and stem, cooked & drained	1 cup	145	25	3	trace	3.3
Broccoli, cooked, drained:						
Whole stalks, medium sized	1 stalk	80	45	6	1	3.0
Brussel sprouts	1 cup	155	55	7	1	4.5
Cabbage:						
Raw, chopped	1 cup	90	20	1	trace	4.0
Red, raw, shredded	1 cup	70	20	1	trace	4.0
Savoy, raw, coarsely shredded	1 cup	70	15	2	trace	1.8
Cabbage, celery	1 cup	75	10	1	trace	1.5
Carrots:						
Raw, whole	1 carrot	50	20	1	trace	4.0
Cauliflower, cooked	1 cup	120	25	3	trace	3.3
Celery, raw:						
Stalk, large outer	1 stalk	40	5	trace	trace	1.0
Collards, cooked	1 cup	190	55	5	1	6.5
Corn, sweet:						
Cooked, ear	1 ear	140	70	3	1	12.3
Canned, solids and liquid	1 cup	256	170	5	2	33.0
Cucumber, 10 oz., raw, pared	1 cuke	207	30	1	trace	6.5
Dandelion greens, cooked	1 cup	180	60	4	1	8.8
Endive, curly (including escarole)	2 oz.	57	10	1	trace	1.5
Kale, cooked	1 cup	110	30	4	1	1.3
Lettuce, raw:						
Butterhead, as Boston types, 4-in. diam.	1 head	220	30	3	trace	4.5
Crisphead, as Iceberg, 4¾-in. diam.	1 head	454	60	4	trace	11.0
Mushrooms, canned, solids and liquids	1 cup	244	40	5	trace	5.0
Mustard greens, cooked	1 cup	140	35	3	1	3.5
Okra, cooked	8 pods	85	25	2	trace	4.3
Onions:						
Mature, raw, 2½″ diam.	1 onion	110	40	2	trace	8.0
Parsley, raw, chopped	1 tbsp.	4	trace	trace	trace	trace
Parsnips, cooked	1 cup	155	100	2	1	21.0

Calcium (mg.)	Iron (mg.)	Vitamin A Value (I.U.)	Thiamine (mg.)	Riboflavin (mg.)	Niacin (mg.)	Ascorbic Acid (mg.)	Sodium (mg.)	Potassium (mg.)
144	2.8	7400	0.10	0.22	0.4	22	110	480
158	1.4	4500	0.16	0.36	1.4	162	18	480
50	1.7	810	0.12	0.22	1.2	135	16	420
34	0.3	90	0.04	0.04	0.2	33	16	185
44	0.4	120	0.05	0.05	0.3	42	18	190
47	0.6	140	0.04	0.06	0.2	39	15	190
32	0.5	110	0.04	0.03	0.5	19	17	190
18	0.4	5500	0.03	0.03	0.3	4	20	148
25	0.8	70	0.11	0.10	0.7	66	11	260
16	0.1	100	0.01	0.01	0.1	4	50	140
289	1.1	10,260	0.27	0.37	2.4	87	—	460
2	0.5	310	0.09	0.08	1.0	7	trace	150
10	1.0	690	0.07	0.12	2.3	13	500	200
35	0.6	trace	0.07	0.09	0.4	23	17	450
252	3.2	21,060	0.24	0.29	—	32	74	384
46	1.0	1870	0.04	0.08	0.3	6	7	150
147	1.3	8140	—	—	—	68	47	240
77	4.4	2130	0.14	0.13	0.6	18	15	430
91	2.3	1500	0.29	0.27	1.3	29	41	794
15	1.2	trace	0.04	0.60	4.8	4	1066	—
193	2.5	8120	0.11	0.19	0.9	68	25	310
78	0.4	420	0.11	0.15	0.8	17	2	228
30	0.6	40	0.04	0.04	0.2	11	11	174
8	0.2	340	trace	0.01	trace	7	2	25
70	0.9	50	0.11	0.12	0.2	16	12	590

Table 1.2
FOOD COMPOSITION: THE NUTRITIVE VALUE OF FOODS

Food, Approximate Measure, and Weight (in grams)		gm.	Food Energy calories	Pro- tein (gm.)	Fat (gm.)	Carbo- hydrate (gm.)
Peas, green:						
Cooked	1 cup	160	115	9	1	17.5
Canned, solids and liquid	1 cup	249	165	9	1	30.0
Peppers, hot, red, w/o seeds, dried	1 tbsp.	15	50	2	2	6.0
Peppers, sweet:						
Raw, about 5 per lb:						
Green pod w/o stem and seeds	1 pod	74	15	1	trace	2.7
Cooked, boiled	1 pod	73	15	1	trace	2.7
Potatoes, medium (about 3 per lb.):						
Baked, peeled	1	99	90	3	trace	19.5
Boiled:						
Peeled after boiling	1	136	105	3	trace	23.3
Peeled before boiling	1	133	80	2	trace	18.0
French-fried, $2 \times \frac{1}{2} \times \frac{1}{2}''$:						
Cooked in deep fat	10 pce.	57	155	2	7	21.0
Frozen, heated	10 pce.	57	125	2	5	18.0
Mashed:						
Milk added	1 cup	195	125	4	1	25.0
Milk & butter added	1 cup	195	185	4	8	24.3
Potato chips, medium	10 chips	20	115	1	8	9.8
Pumpkin, canned	1 cup	228	75	2	1	14.5
Radishes, raw, small	4	40	5	trace	trace	1.3
Sauerkraut, canned	1 cup	235	45	2	trace	9.3
Spinach, cooked	1 cup	180	40	5	1	2.8
Squash, cooked:						
Summer, diced	1 cup	210	30	2	trace	5.5
Winter, baked, mashed	1 cup	205	130	4	1	26.3
Sweetpotatoes:						
Cooked, medium, 6 oz:						
Baked, peeled after baking	1 pot.	110	155	2	1	34.5
Boiled, peeled after boiling	1 pot.	147	170	2	1	38.3
Candied	1 pot.	175	195	2	6	33.3
Tomatoes:						
Raw, 7 oz.	1 tom.	200	40	2	trace	8.0
Canned	1 cup	241	50	2	1	8.3

Calcium (mg.)	Iron (mg.)	Vitamin A Value (I.U.)	Thiamine (mg.)	Riboflavin (mg.)	Niacin (mg.)	Ascorbic Acid (mg.)	Sodium (mg.)	Potassium (mg.)
37	2.9	860	0.44	0.17	3.7	33	2	310
50	4.2	1120	0.23	0.13	2.2	22	588	239
40	2.3	9750	0.03	0.17	1.3	2	236	140
7	0.5	310	0.06	0.06	0.4	94	10	157
7	0.4	310	0.05	0.05	0.4	70	7	109
9	0.7	trace	0.10	0.04	1.7	20	4	400
10	0.8	trace	0.13	0.05	2.0	22	4	556
7	0.6	trace	0.11	0.04	1.4	20	3	385
9	0.7	trace	0.07	0.04	1.8	12	4	450
5	1.0	trace	0.08	0.01	1.5	12	2	369
47	0.8	50	0.16	0.10	2.0	19	632	548
47	0.8	330	0.16	0.10	1.9	18	695	525
8	0.4	trace	0.04	0.01	1.0	3	—	226
57	0.9	14,590	0.07	0.12	1.3	12	5	588
12	0.4	trace	0.01	0.01	0.1	10	6	116
85	1.2	120	0.07	0.09	0.4	33	1755	329
167	4.0	14,580	0.13	0.25	1.0	50	90	580
52	0.8	820	0.10	0.16	1.6	21	2	250
57	1.6	8610	0.10	0.27	1.4	27	2	1248
44	1.0	8910	0.10	0.07	0.7	24	11	267
47	1.0	11,610	0.13	0.09	0.9	25	15	367
65	1.6	11,030	0.10	0.08	0.8	17	64	287
24	0.9	1640	0.11	0.07	1.3	42	5	444
14	1.2	2170	0.12	0.07	1.7	41	313	523

Table 1.2
FOOD COMPOSITION: THE NUTRITIVE VALUE OF FOODS

Food, Approximate Measure, and Weight (in grams)		gm.	Food Energy calories	Pro-tein (gm.)	Fat (gm.)	Carbo-hydrate (gm.)
Tomato catsup	1 tbsp.	15	15	trace	trace	3.8
Tomato juice, canned	1 cup	243	45	2	trace	9.3
Turnips, cooked, diced	1 cup	155	35	1	trace	7.8
Turnip greens, cooked	1 cup	145	30	3	trace	4.5
Fruit and fruit products						
Apples, raw (3 per lb.)	1 ap.	150	70	trace	trace	17.5
Apple juice	1 cup	248	120	trace	trace	30.0
Applesauce, canned:						
Sweetened	1 cup	255	230	1	trace	56.5
Unsweetened or artificially sweetened	1 cup	244	100	1	trace	24.0
Apricots:						
Raw (12 per lb.)	3 apr	114	55	1	trace	12.8
Canned in heavy syrup	1 cup	259	220	1	trace	54.0
Dried, uncooked	1 cup	150	390	8	1	87.3
Cooked, unsweetened, fruit & liquid	1 cup	285	240	5	1	52.8
Apricot nectar, canned	1 cup	251	140	1	trace	34.0
Avocados, whole fruit, raw:						
California	1 avo.	284	370	5	37	4.3
Bananas, raw, medium	1 ban.	175	100	1	trace	24.0
Blackberries, raw	1 cup	144	85	2	1	17.0
Blueberries, raw	1 cup	140	85	1	1	18.0
Cantaloupes, raw; medium, about $1\frac{2}{3}$ lb.	$\frac{1}{2}$	385	60	1	trace	14.0
Cherries, canned, red, sour, pitted	1 cup	244	105	2	trace	24.3

Cal-cium (mg.)	Iron (mg.)	Vita-min A Value (I.U.)	Thia-mine (mg.)	Ribo-flavin (mg.)	Niacin (mg.)	Ascor-bic Acid (mg.)	Sodium (mg.)	Potas-sium (mg.)
3	0.1	210	0.01	0.01	0.2	2	156	54
17	2.2	1940	0.12	0.07	1.9	39	486	552
54	0.6	trace	0.06	0.08	0.5	34	53	290
252	1.5	8270	0.15	0.33	0.7	68	—	—
8	0.4	50	0.04	0.02	0.1	3	1	152
15	1.5	—	0.02	0.05	0.2	2	2	250
10	1.3	100	0.05	0.03	0.1	3	5	166
10	1.2	100	0.05	0.02	0.1	2	5	190
18	0.5	2890	0.03	0.04	0.7	10	1	300
28	0.8	4510	0.05	0.06	0.9	10	3	600
100	8.2	16,350	0.02	0.23	4.9	19	34	1300
63	5.1	8550	0.01	0.13	2.8	8	20	800
23	0.5	2380	0.03	0.03	0.5	8	trace	380
22	1.3	630	0.24	0.43	3.5	30	9	1303
10	0.8	230	0.06	0.07	0.8	12	1	440
46	1.3	290	0.05	0.06	0.5	30	1	240
21	1.4	140	0.04	0.08	0.6	20	1	120
27	0.8	6540	0.08	0.06	1.2	63	24	498
37	0.7	1660	0.07	0.05	0.5	12	5	317

Table 1.2
FOOD COMPOSITION: THE NUTRITIVE VALUE OF FOODS

Food, Approximate Measure, and Weight (in grams)		gm.	Food Energy calories	Pro-tein (gm.)	Fat (gm.)	Carbo-hydrate (gm.)
Cranberry juice cocktail, canned	1 cup	250	165	trace	trace	41.0
Cranberry sauce, sweetened, canned,						
strained	1 cup	277	405	trace	1	99.0
Dates, pitted, cut	1 cup	178	490	4	1	116.3
Figs, dried, $1 \times 2''$	1 fig	21	60	1	trace	14.0
Fruit cocktail, canned in heavy syrup	1 cup	256	195	1	trace	47.8
Grapefruit:						
Raw, medium:						
White	½	241	45	1	trace	10.3
Pink or red	½	241	50	1	trace	11.5
Canned, syrup pack	1 cup	254	180	2	trace	43.0
Grapefruit juice:						
Fresh	1 cup	246	95	1	trace	22.8
Canned, white:						
Unsweetened	1 cup	247	100	1	trace	24.0
Sweetened	1 cup	250	130	1	trace	31.5
Frozen, concentrate,						
unsweetened:						
Undiluted, can, 6 fluid oz.	1 can	207	300	4	1	68.8
Diluted, with 3 parts water	1 cup	247	100	1	trace	24.0
Grapes, raw:						
American, i.e. Concord,						
Delaware, Niagara	1 cup	153	65	1	1	13.0
European, i.e. Muscat, Malaga,						
Sultana	1 cup	160	95	1	trace	22.8
Grapejuice, canned or bottled	1 cup	253	165	1	trace	40.3
Grapejuice drink, canned	1 cup	250	135	trace	trace	33.7
Lemons, raw	1 lem.	110	20	1	trace	4.0
Lemon juice, raw	1 cup	244	60	1	trace	14.0
Lemonade concentrate:						
Diluted w/water	1 cup	248	110	trace	trace	27.5
Lime juice:						
Fresh	1 cup	246	65	1	trace	15.3
Canned, unsweetened	1 cup	246	65	1	trace	15.3

Cal-cium (mg.)	Iron (mg.)	Vita-min A Value (I.U.)	Thia-mine (mg.)	Ribo-flavin (mg.)	Niacin (mg.)	Ascor-bic Acid (mg.)	Sodium (mg.)	Potas-sium (mg.)
13	0.8	trace	0.03	0.03	0.1	40	3	25
17	0.6	60	0.03	0.03	0.1	6	3	83
105	5.3	90	0.16	0.17	3.9	0	2	1200
26	0.6	20	0.02	0.02	0.1	0	7	125
23	1.0	360	0.05	0.03	1.3	5	13	411
19	0.5	10	0.05	0.02	0.2	44	1	180
20	0.5	540	0.05	0.02	0.2	44	1	190
33	0.8	30	0.08	0.05	0.5	76	3	343
22	0.5	20	0.09	0.04	0.4	92	2	400
20	1.0	20	0.07	0.04	0.4	84	2	400
20	1.0	20	0.07	0.04	0.4	78	3	405
70	0.8	60	0.29	0.12	1.4	286	8	1250
25	0.2	20	0.10	0.04	0.5	96	2	420
15	0.4	100	0.05	0.03	0.2	3	3	160
17	0.6	140	0.07	0.04	0.4	6	5	263
28	0.8	—	0.10	0.05	0.5	trace	5	293
8	0.3	—	0.03	0.03	0.3	—	3	88
19	0.4	10	0.03	0.01	0.1	39	1	102
17	0.5	50	0.07	0.02	0.2	112	2	344
2	trace	trace	trace	0.02	0.2	17	1	40
22	0.5	20	0.05	0.02	0.2	79	2	260
22	0.5	20	0.05	0.02	0.2	52	2	256

Table 1.2
FOOD COMPOSITION: THE NUTRITIVE VALUE OF FOODS

Food, Approximate Measure, and Weight (in grams)		gm.	Food Energy calories	Pro-tein (gm.)	Fat (gm.)	Carbo-hydrate (gm.)
Limeade concentrate, frozen, diluted						
w/water	1 cup	247	100	trace	trace	25.0
Oranges, raw	1 or.	180	65	1	trace	15.3
Orange juice, fresh	1 cup	248	110	2	1	23.3
Canned, unsweetened	1 cup	249	120	2	trace	28.0
Diluted w/water	1 cup	249	120	2	trace	28.0
Orange-apricot juice drink	1 cup	249	125	1	trace	30.3
Orange and grapefruit juice, diluted						
w/water	1 cup	248	110	1	trace	26.5
Papayas, raw, ½" cubes	1 cup	182	70	1	trace	16.5
Peaches:						
Raw, whole, medium	1 peach	114	35	1	trace	7.8
Canned, water-pack	1 cup	245	75	1	trace	17.8
Dried, uncooked	1 cup	160	420	5	1	97.8
Pears:						
Raw	1 pear	182	100	1	1	21.8
Canned, syrup-pack	1 cup	255	195	1	1	45.5
Pineapple:						
Raw, diced	1 cup	140	75	1	trace	17.8
Canned, heavy syrup-pack, crushed	1 cup	260	195	1	trace	47.8
Pineapple juice, canned	1 cup	249	135	1	trace	32.8
Plums:						
Raw, 2" diameter	1 plum	60	25	trace	trace	6.3
W/pits and juice	1 cup	256	205	1	trace	50.3
Prunes, dried, "softenized":						
Uncooked, medium	4 pr.	32	70	1	trace	16.5
Cooked, unsweetened	1 cup	270	295	2	1	69.5
Prune juice, canned or bottled	1 cup	256	200	1	trace	49.0
Raisins, seedless:						
½ oz. package	1 pkg.	14	40	trace	trace	10.0
Cup, pressed down	1 cup	165	480	4	trace	116.0
Raspberries, red, raw	1 cup	123	70	1	1	14.3
Rhubarb, cooked, sugar added	1 cup	272	385	1	trace	95.3
Strawberries, raw, capped	1 cup	149	55	1	1	10.5

Calcium (mg.)	Iron (mg.)	Vitamin A Value (I.U.)	Thiamine (mg.)	Riboflavin (mg.)	Niacin (mg.)	Ascorbic Acid (mg.)	Sodium (mg.)	Potassium (mg.)
2	trace	trace	trace	trace	trace	5	trace	32
54	0.5	260	0.13	0.05	0.5	66	1	263
27	0.5	500	0.22	0.07	1.0	124	2	500
25	1.0	500	0.17	0.05	0.7	100	2	500
25	0.2	550	0.22	0.02	1.0	120	2	500
12	0.2	1140	0.05	0.02	0.5	40	trace	234
20	0.2	270	0.16	0.02	0.8	102	2	454
36	0.5	3190	0.07	0.08	0.5	102	6	433
9	0.5	1320	0.02	0.05	1.0	7	1	202
10	0.7	1100	0.02	0.06	1.4	7	5	334
77	9.6	6240	0.02	0.31	8.5	28	26	1520
13	0.5	30	0.04	0.07	0.2	7	3	213
13	0.5	trace	0.03	0.05	0.3	4	3	214
24	0.7	100	0.12	0.04	0.3	24	1	226
29	0.8	120	0.20	0.06	0.5	17	3	245
37	0.7	120	0.12	0.04	0.5	22	3	373
7	0.3	140	0.02	0.02	0.3	3	1	96
22	2.2	2970	0.05	0.05	0.9	4	4	725
14	1.1	440	0.02	0.04	0.4	1	2	193
60	4.5	1860	0.08	0.18	1.7	2	10	800
36	10.5	—	0.03	0.03	1.0	5	5	602
9	0.5	trace	0.02	0.01	0.1	trace	4	107
102	5.8	30	0.18	0.13	0.8	2	45	1259
27	1.1	160	0.04	0.11	1.1	31	1	207
212	1.6	220	0.06	0.15	0.7	17	5	548
31	1.5	90	0.04	0.10	1.0	88	1	244

Table 1.2
FOOD COMPOSITION: THE NUTRITIVE VALUE OF FOODS

Food, Approximate Measure, and Weight (in grams)		gm.	Food Energy calories	Protein (gm.)	Fat (gm.)	Carbohydrate (gm.)
Tangerines, raw	1 med.	116	40	1	trace	9.0
Tangerine juice, canned, unsweetened	1 cup	249	125	1	1	28.0
Watermelon, raw, wedge, 4×8 inches	1 wdge.	925	115	2	1	24.5
Grains and flours						
Bagel, 3-in. diameter						
Egg	1 bgl.	55	165	6	2	30.8
Water	1 bgl.	55	165	6	2	30.8
Barley, whole-grained, hulled, raw	1 cup	204	936	27	5.7	194.0
Pot or Scotch, dry	1 cup	200	696	19	2.2	150.0
Pearl, light, dry	1 cup	200	698	16	2.0	154.0
Biscuits, baking powder, from mix, 2″ diam.	1 bisc.	28	90	2	3	13.8
Bran flakes, (40% bran) + thiamin & iron	1 cup	35	105	4	1	20.0
Bran flakes w/raisins, + thiamin & iron	1 cup	50	145	4	1	30.0
Breads:						
Boston brown	1 slice	48	100	3	1	19.8
Cracked wheat	1 slice	25	65	2	1	12.0
Raisin	1 slice	25	65	2	1	12.0
Rye, Amer. light	1 slice	25	60	2	trace	13.0
White, enriched						
Soft-crumb type	1 slice	25	70	2	1	13.3
Firm-crumb type	1 slice	20	65	2	1	12.0
Whole wheat, soft-crumb						
16 slices/loaf	1 slice	28	65	3	1	11.0
Slice, toasted	1 slice	24	65	3	1	11.0
Whole wheat, soft-crumb						
18 slices/loaf	1 slice	25	60	3	1	9.8
Slice, toasted	1 slice	21	60	3	1	9.8

Cal-cium (mg.)	Iron (mg.)	Vita-min A Value (I.U.)	Thia-mine (mg.)	Ribo-flavin (mg.)	Niacin (mg.)	Ascor-bic Acid (mg.)	Sodium (mg.)	Potas-sium (mg.)
34	0.3	360	0.05	0.02	0.1	27	2	100
45	0.5	1050	0.15	0.05	0.2	55	2	440
30	2.1	2510	0.13	0.13	0.7	30	4	426
9	1.2	30	0.14	0.10	1.2	0	—	—
8	1.2	0	0.15	0.11	1.4	0	—	—
180	1.2	—	1.2	0.45	13	0	41	1280
68	5.4	0	.42	0.14	7.4	0	—	590
32	4.0	0	.24	0.10	6.2	0	6	320
19	0.6	trace	0.08	0.07	0.6	trace	272	32
25	12.3	0	0.14	0.06	2.2	0	207	137
28	13.5	trace	0.16	0.07	2.7	0	212	154
43	0.9	0	0.05	0.03	0.6	0	113	131
22	0.3	trace	0.03	0.02	0.3	trace	132	34
18	0.3	trace	0.01	0.02	0.2	trace	91	58
19	0.4	0	0.05	0.02	0.4	0	139	36
21	0.6	trace	0.06	0.05	0.6	trace	127	26
22	0.6	trace	0.06	0.05	0.6	trace	114	28
24	0.8	trace	0.09	0.03	0.8	trace	148	72
24	0.8	trace	0.09	0.03	0.8	trace	148	72
25	0.8	trace	0.06	0.03	0.7	trace	148	72
25	0.8	trace	0.06	0.03	0.7	trace	148	72

Table 1.2
FOOD COMPOSITION: THE NUTRITIVE VALUE OF FOODS

Food, Approximate Measure, and Weight (in grams)		gm.	Food Energy calories	Pro- tein (gm.)	Fat (gm.)	Carbo- hydrate (gm.)
Breadcrumbs, dry grated	1 cup	100	390	13	5	73.3
Buckwheat, whole grain raw, ⅓ cup						
rounded (makes 1 cup cooked)		65	218	7	1.6	43.9
Buckwheat flour, dark,						
sifted	1 cup	98	326	12	2.4	64.1
light, sifted	1 cup	98	340	6	1.2	76.3
Cakes made from cake mixes:						
Angel Food, ¹⁄₁₂ of 10″ diam. cake	1 pce.	53	135	3	trace	30.8
Cupcakes, 2½″ diam. w/o icing	1 small	25	90	1	3	14.8
w/choco. icing	1 small	36	130	2	5	19.3
Devil's food, 2-layer w/choco. icing						
¹⁄₁₆ of 9-in. diam. cake	1 pce.	69	235	3	9	35.5
Gingerbread, ⅑ of 8″ square cake	1 pce.	63	175	2	4	32.8
Cakes made from home recipes						
Fruitcake, dark, made w/enriched						
flour, ¹⁄₃₀ of 8″ loaf	1 pce.	15	55	1	2	8.3
Plain sheet cake,						
w/o icing, ⅑ of 9″ square cake	1 pce.	86	315	4	12	47.8
Pound, ½″ thick	1 slice	30	140	2	9	12.8
Sponge, ¹⁄₁₂ of 10″ diam. cake	1 pce.	66	195	5	4	34.8
Yellow, 2-layer, ¹⁄₁₆ of 9″ diam.						
cake:						
w/o icing	1 pce.	54	200	2	7	32.3
w/chocolate icing	1 pce.	75	275	3	10	43.3
Cookies:						
Brownies w/nuts, made from						
a mix	1 pce.	20	85	1	4	11.3
Chocolate chip:						
Made from home recipe						
w/enriched flour	1 ckie.	10	50	1	3	4.8
Commercial	1 ckie.	10	50	1	2	7.0
Fig bars, commercial	1 ckie.	14	50	1	1	9.3
Sandwich, chocolate or vanilla,						
commercial	1 ckie.	10	50	1	2	7.0
Corn flakes, added nutrients:						
Plain	1 cup	25	100	2	trace	23.0
Sugar-covered	1 cup	40	155	2	trace	36.8

Calcium (mg.)	Iron (mg.)	Vitamin A Value (I.U.)	Thiamine (mg.)	Riboflavin (mg.)	Niacin (mg.)	Ascorbic Acid (mg.)	Sodium (mg.)	Potassium (mg.)
122	3.6	trace	0.22	0.30	3.5	trace	736	152
74	2.0	0	.39	0.10	6.2	0	—	290
32	2.7	0	.57	0.15	2.8	0	—	—
11	1.0	0	.08	0.04	0.4	0	—	310
50	0.2	0	trace	0.06	0.1	0	77	32
40	0.1	40	0.01	0.03	0.1	trace	113	21
47	0.3	60	0.01	0.04	0.1	trace	121	42
41	0.6	100	0.02	0.06	0.2	trace	181	90
57	1.0	trace	0.02	0.06	0.5	trace	192	173
11	0.4	20	0.02	0.02	0.1	trace	24	74
55	0.3	150	0.02	0.08	0.2	trace	258	68
6	0.2	80	0.01	0.03	0.1	0	33	18
20	0.8	300	0.03	0.09	0.1	trace	110	57
39	0.2	80	0.01	0.04	0.1	trace	140	42
51	0.5	120	0.02	0.06	0.2	trace	156	81
9	0.4	20	0.03	0.02	0.1	trace	48	36
4	0.2	10	0.01	0.01	0.1	trace	35	12
4	0.2	10	trace	trace	trace	trace	42	14
11	0.2	20	trace	0.01	0.1	trace	35	28
2	0.1	0	trace	trace	0.1	0	48	4
4	0.4	0	0.11	0.02	0.5	0	251	30
5	0.4	0	0.16	0.02	0.8	0	267	27

Table 1.2
FOOD COMPOSITION: THE NUTRITIVE VALUE OF FOODS

Food, Approximate Measure, and Weight (in grams)		gm.	Food Energy calories	Pro- tein (gm.)	Fat (gm.)	Carbo- hydrate (gm.)
Corn flour, sifted	1 cup	117	431	9	3.0	92.0
Corn grits (hominy grits) degermed, enriched,						
dry	1 cup	160	579	14	1.3	127.9
cooked	1 cup	245	125	3	0.1	28.0
Cornmeal, unbolted, dry	⅓ cup	41	144	4	1.6	28.4
bolted	1 cup	122	442	11	4.1	90.9
degermed, enriched	1 cup	138	502	11	1.7	108.2
Corn muffins, made w/enriched degermed cornmeal & enriched flour, 2⅜″ diam.	1 mufn.	40	125	3	4	19.3
Corn, puffed, presweetened, added nutrients	1 cup	30	115	1	trace	7.8
Corn, shredded, added nutrients	1 cup	25	100	2	trace	23.0
Crackers:						
Graham, 2½″ square	4 cr.	28	110	2	3	48.3
Saltines	4 cr.	11	50	1	1	9.3
Danish pastry, plain (w/o fruits or nuts):						
Packaged ring, 12 oz.	1 ring	340	1435	25	80	153.8
Doughnuts, cake type	1 donut	32	125	1	6	16.8
Farina, quick-cooking, enriched, cooked	1 cup	245	105	3	trace	23.3
Macaroni, cooked, enriched:						
Cooked:						
Firm stage (8–10 min)	1 cup	130	190	6	1	39.3
Until tender (11–15 min.)	1 cup	140	155	5	1	31.5
Macaroni (enriched) and cheese, baked	1 cup	200	430	17	22	41.0
Millet, whole grain, raw (makes 1 cup cooked)	¼ cup	58	190	6	1.7	37.7
Muffins, w/enriched white flour, 3″ diam.	1 mufn.	40	120	3	4	18.0
Noodles (egg), cooked, enriched	1 cup	160	200	7	2	38.5

Cal-cium (mg.)	Iron (mg.)	Vita-min A Value (I.U.)	Thia-mine (mg.)	Ribo-flavin (mg.)	Niacin (mg.)	Ascor-bic Acid (mg.)	Sodium (mg.)	Potas-sium (mg.)
7	2.1	400	.23	.07	1.6	0	1	—
6	4.6	700	.70	.42	5.6	0	2	130
2	.7	150	.10	.07	1.0	0	500	27
8	1.0	210	.15	.04	0.8	(0)	—	120
(21)	2.2	590	.37	.10	2.3	(0)	1	300
8	4.6	610	.61	.36	4.8	(0)	1	170
42	0.7	120	0.08	0.09	0.6	trace	192	54
3	0.5	0	0.13	0.05	0.6	0	90	27
1	0.6	0	0.11	0.05	0.5	0	269	—
11	0.4	0	0.01	0.06	0.4	0	190	110
2	0.1	0	trace	trace	0.1	0	123	13
170	3.1	1050	0.24	0.51	2.7	trace	1244	381
13	0.4	30	0.05	0.05	0.4	trace	168	31
147	0.7	0	0.12	0.07	1.0	0	466	25
14	1.4	0	0.23	0.14	1.8	0	1	103
8	1.3	0	0.20	0.11	1.5	0	1	85
362	1.8	860	0.20	0.40	1.8	trace	1086	240
20	1.6	30	0.19	0.06	1.0	0	—	250
42	0.6	40	0.07	0.09	0.6	trace	176	50
16	1.4	110	0.22	0.13	1.9	0	3	70

Table 1.2
FOOD COMPOSITION: THE NUTRITIVE VALUE OF FOODS

Food, Approximate Measure, and Weight (in grams)		gm.	Food Energy calories	Pro-tein (gm.)	Fat (gm.)	Carbo-hydrate (gm.)
Oats (w/ or w/o corn), puffed, added						
nutrients	1 cup	25	100	3	1	19.8
Oatmeal or rolled Oats, cooked	1 cup	240	130	5	2	23.0
Pancakes, 4″ diam:						
Wheat, enriched flour, (home						
recipe)	1 cake	27	60	2	2	8.5
Buckwheat (made from mix w/egg						
& milk)	1 cake	27	55	2	2	7.3
Plain or buttermilk, made from mix						
w/egg & milk	1 cake	27	60	2	2	8.5
Pie (piecrust made w/unenriched flour)						
⅐ of 9″ diam. pie:						
Apple (2-crust)	1 pce.	135	350	3	15	50.8
Cherry (2-crust)	1 pce.	135	350	4	15	49.8
Custard (1-crust)	1 pce.	130	285	8	14	31.8
Lemon meringue	1 pce.	120	305	4	12	45.3
Mince (2-crust)	1 pce.	135	365	3	16	52.3
Pecan (1-crust)	1 pce.	118	490	6	27	55.8
Pumpkin (1-crust)	1 pce.	130	275	5	15	30.0
Piecrust, baked shell for pie made						
w/enriched flour	1 shell	180	900	11	60	79.0
Pizza (cheese), ⅛ of 14″ diam. pie	1 pce.	75	185	7	6	25.8
Popcorn, popped, w/oil and salt	1 cup	9	40	1	2	4.5
Potato flour, whole	1 cup	184	646	15	1.5	143.13
Pretzels:						
Dutch, twisted	1 pr.	16	60	2	1	10.8
Thin, twisted	1 pr.	6	25	1	trace	5.3
Sticks, small, 2¼ inches	10 st.	3	10	trace	trace	2.5
Rice, brown, raw						
Long-grain	1 cup	185	666	14	4.3	143.8
Short-grain	1 cup	200	720	15	3.8	156.5
Rice, converted cooked	1 cup	175	186	4	0.2	42.1
Rice, white, enriched:						
Cooked	1 cup	205	225	4	trace	52.3
Instant, ready to serve	1 cup	165	180	4	trace	41.0

Cal-cium (mg.)	Iron (mg.)	Vita-min A Value (I.U.)	Thia-mine (mg.)	Ribo-flavin (mg.)	Niacin (mg.)	Ascor-bic Acid (mg.)	Sodium (mg.)	Potas-sium (mg.)
44	1.2	0	0.24	0.04	0.5	0	317	—
22	1.4	0	0.19	0.05	0.2	0	520	150
27	0.4	30	0.05	0.06	0.4	trace	115	32
59	0.4	60	0.03	0.04	0.2	trace	125	66
58	0.3	70	0.04	0.06	0.2	trace	152	42
11	0.4	40	0.03	0.03	0.5	1	416	110
19	0.4	590	0.03	0.03	0.7	trace	420	145
128	0.8	300	0.07	0.21	0.4	0	382	182
17	0.6	200	0.04	0.10	0.2	4	346	62
38	1.4	trace	0.09	0.09	0.5	1	619	246
55	3.3	190	0.19	0.08	0.4	trace	267	149
66	0.7	3210	0.04	0.13	0.7	trace	285	213
25	3.1	0	0.36	0.25	3.2	0	1100	89
107	0.7	290	0.04	0.12	0.7	4	525	98
1	0.2	—	—	0.01	0.2	0	175	—
61	32.0	trace	0.77	0.26	6.3	35	63	2900
4	0.2	0	trace	trace	0.1	0	269	21
1	0.1	0	trace	trace	trace	0	101	8
1	trace	0	trace	trace	trace	0	50	4
59	3.0	0	0.63	0.09	8.7	0	17	400
64	3.2	0	0.68	0.10	9.4	0	18	430
33	1.4	0	0.19	0.02	2.1	0	630	75
21	1.8	0	0.23	0.02	2.1	0	767	57
5	1.3	0	0.21	—	1.7	0	450	—

Table 1.2
FOOD COMPOSITION: THE NUTRITIVE VALUE OF FOODS

Food, Approximate Measure, and Weight (in grams)		gm.	Food Energy calories	Protein (gm.)	Fat (gm.)	Carbohydrate (gm.)
Rice flour, brown	1 cup	120	432	9	2.8	92.7
Rice bran	1 tbsp.	6	18	1	1.2	.8
Rice polishings	1 tbsp.	7	17	1	0.9	1.2
Rolls, enriched:						
Home recipe	1 roll	35	120	3	3	20.3
Frankfurter or hamburger	1 roll	40	120	3	2	20.3
Hard, round or rectangular	1 roll	50	155	5	2	29.3
Rye berries, raw	⅓ cup	71	237	9	1.6	46.7
Rye flour						
Dark	1 cup	128	419	21	3.3	76.3
Light	1 cup	88	319	8	0.9	69.7
Rye wafers, whole-grain						
1⅞″ × 3½″	2 waf.	13	45	2	trace	9.3
Soybean flour, stirred						
Full-fat	1 cup	70	295	26	14.0	16.2
Low-fat	1 cup	88	313	38	5.9	26.9
Defatted	1 cup	100	326	47	0.9	32.5
Spaghetti, cooked, tender stage, enriched	1 cup	140	155	5	1	31.5
Spaghetti w/meat balls, & tomato sauce, canned	1 cup	248	330	19	12	36.5
Spaghetti in tomato sauce w/cheese, canned	1 cup	250	190	6	2	37.0
Waffles, w/enriched flour, 7-in. diameter	1 wafl.	75	210	7	7	29.75
Wheat berries, raw:						
Hard red spring	1 cup	175	578	24	4.7	109.9
Hard red winter	1 cup	175	578	22	4.4	112.6
Soft red winter	1 cup	175	571	18	4.2	115.3
White	1 cup	175	586	16	3.5	122.6
Durum	1 cup	175	581	22	5.8	110.2
Wheat, cracked, dry	⅓ cup	66	217	7	1.4	44.1
Wheat, puffed, added nutrients	1 cup	15	55	2	trace	11.8
Wheat, rolled, dry	1 cup	85	289	8	1.7	64.8

Cal-cium (mg.)	Iron (mg.)	Vita-min A Value (I.U.)	Thia-mine (mg.)	Ribo-flavin (mg.)	Niacin (mg.)	Ascor-bic Acid (mg.)	Sodium (mg.)	Potas-sium (mg.)
38	1.9	0	0.41	0.06	5.6	0	11	260
5	1.2	0	0.14	0.02	1.9	0	trace	96
4	1.1	0	0.12	0.01	1.8	0	trace	47
16	0.7	30	0.09	0.09	0.8	trace	98	41
30	0.8	trace	0.11	0.07	0.9	trace	202	38
24	1.2	trace	0.13	0.12	1.4	trace	313	49
27	2.6	0	0.31	0.16	1.1	0	1	330
69	5.8	0	0.78	0.28	3.5	0	1	1100
19	1.0	0	0.13	0.06	0.5	0	1	140
7	0.5	0	0.04	0.03	0.2	0	110	—
140	5.9	80	0.60	0.22	1.5	0	1	1200
230	8.0	70	0.73	0.32	2.3	0	1	1600
270	11.0	40	1.1	0.43	2.6	0	1	1800
11	1.3	0	0.20	0.11	1.5	0	1	85
124	3.7	1590	0.25	0.30	4.0	22	1009	665
40	2.8	930	0.35	0.28	4.5	10	955	303
85	1.3	250	0.13	0.19	1.0	trace	356	109
63	5.4	0	1.0	.21	7.5	0	5	650
81	6.0	0	0.91	.21	7.5	0	5	650
74	6.1	0	0.75	.19	6.3	0	5	660
63	5.3	0	0.93	.21	9.3	0	5	680
65	7.5	0	1.2	.21	7.7	0	5	760
28	2.4	0	0.29	.07	2.4	0	1	—
4	0.6	0	0.08	0.03	1.2	0	1	51
31	2.7	0	0.31	.10	3.5	0	2	323

Table 1.2

FOOD COMPOSITION: THE NUTRITIVE VALUE OF FOODS

Food, Approximate Measure, and Weight (in grams)		gm.	Food Energy calories	Pro-tein (gm.)	Fat (gm.)	Carbo-hydrate (gm.)
Wheat, bulgur, dry	¾ cup	128	452	14	1.9	94.7
Wheat flour, whole wheat, stirred	1 cup	120	400	16	1.8	87.5
80% extraction	1 cup	110	402	13	1.4	84.5
Whole wheat pastry	1 cup	148	496	14	3.0	103.3
Gluten	1 cup	140	528	58	2.7	66.1
All-purpose, (white), enriched	1 cup	115	419	12	1.6	89.2
Wheat bran, crude	1 tbsp.	5	19	1	0.1	3.5
Wheat gluten	3½ oz.	100	—	89	5.4	—
Wild rice, raw	¼ cup	40	141	6	0.3	28.6

Fats & oils

Butter:						
Regular, 4 sticks/lb:						
Tablespoon (⅛ st.)	1 tbsp.	14	100	trace	12	.1
Whipped	1 tbsp.	9	65	trace	8	trace
Fats, cooking:						
Lard	1 tbsp.	13	115	0	13	0
Vegetable fats	1 tbsp.	13	110	0	13	0
Margarine:						
Regular, 4 sticks/lb:						
Tablespoon	1 tbsp.	14	100	trace	12	.1
Soft	1 tbsp.	14	100	trace	11	trace
Oils, salad or cooking:						
Corn	1 tbsp.	14	125	0	14	0
Cottonseed	1 tbsp.	14	125	0	14	0
Olive	1 tbsp.	14	125	0	14	0
Peanut	1 tbsp.	14	125	0	14	0
Safflower	1 tbsp.	14	125	0	14	0
Soybean	1 tbsp.	14	125	0	14	0
Salad Dressing:						
Blue Cheese	1 tbsp.	15	75	1	1	15.5

Calcium (mg.)	Iron (mg.)	Vitamin A Value (I.U.)	Thiamine (mg.)	Riboflavin (mg.)	Niacin (mg.)	Ascorbic Acid (mg.)	Sodium (mg.)	Potassium (mg.)
37	4.7	0	0.36	.18	5.8	0	—	290
49	4.0	0	0.66	.14	5.2	0	4	440
26	1.4	0	0.28	.08	2.2	0	2	100
53	4.4	0	0.78	.18	7.8	0	4	580
56	—	0	—	—	—	0	3	84
18	10.0	0	0.74	.45	6.0	0	2	110
4	0.5	0	0.02	.01	0.7	0	trace	36
—	0.6	0	—	—	2.4	0	trace	57
8	1.7	0	0.18	.25	2.5	0	3	88
3	0	470	—	—	—	0	140	3
2	0	310	—	—	—	0	94	2
0	0	0	0	0	0	0	0	0
0	0	—	0	0	0	0	0	0
3	0	470	—	—	—	0	140	3
3	0	470	—	—	—	0	94	2
0	0	—	0	0	0	0	0	0
0	0	—	0	0	0	0	0	0
0	0	—	0	0	0	0	0	0
0	0	—	0	0	0	0	0	0
0	0	—	0	0	0	0	0	0
0	0	—	0	0	0	0	0	0
12	trace	30	trace	0.02	trace	trace	164	6

Table 1.2

FOOD COMPOSITION: THE NUTRITIVE VALUE OF FOODS

Food, Approximate Measure, and Weight (in grams)		gm.	Food Energy calories	Protein (gm.)	Fat (gm.)	Carbohydrate (gm.)
Commercial, mayonnaise type:						
Regular	1 tbsp.	15	65	trace	6	10.2
Special dietary, Low calorie	1 tbsp.	16	20	trace	2	.5
French:						
Regular	1 tbsp.	16	65	trace	6	2.7
Home-cooked, boiled	1 tbsp.	16	25	1	2	.7
Mayonnaise	1 tbsp.	14	100	trace	11	.2
Thousand Island	1 tbsp.	16	80	trace	8	2.0
Sugars & sweets						
Candy:						
Caramels, plain or chocolate	1 oz.	28	115	1	3	21.0
Chocolate, milk, plain	1 oz.	28	145	2	9	14.0
Chocolate-coated peanuts	1 oz.	28	160	5	12	8.0
Fondant; mints, uncoated; candy corn	1 oz.	28	105	trace	1	24.0
Fudge, plain	1 oz.	28	115	1	4	18.8
Gum drops	1 oz.	28	100	trace	trace	25.0
Hard	1 oz.	28	110	0	trace	27.0
Marshmallows	1 oz.	28	90	1	trace	21.0
Chocolate-flavored syrups or topping:						
Thin type	1 oz.	38	90	1	1	19.2
Fudge type	1 oz.	38	125	2	5	18.0
Chocolate-flavored beverage powder (4 heaping tspn./oz.):						
W/non-fat dry milk	1 oz.	28	100	5	1	17.7
W/out nonfat dry milk	1 oz.	28	100	1	1	21.7
Honey, strained or extracted	1 tbsp.	21	65	trace	0	16.0
Jams and preserves	1 tbsp.	20	55	trace	trace	13.0
Jellies	1 tbsp.	18	50	trace	trace	12.5
Molasses, cane:						
Light (1st extraction)	1 tbsp.	20	50	—	—	12.5
Blackstrap (3rd extraction)	1 tbsp.	20	45	—	—	11.2

Cal-cium (mg.)	Iron (mg.)	Vita-min A Value (I.U.)	Thia-mine (mg.)	Ribo-flavin (mg.)	Niacin (mg.)	Ascor-bic Acid (mg.)	Sodium (mg.)	Potas-sium (mg.)
2	trace	30	trace	trace	trace	—	84	5
3	trace	40	trace	trace	trace	—	105	17
2	0.1	—	—	—	—	—	219	13
14	0.1	80	0.01	0.03	trace	trace	116	19
3	0.1	40	trace	0.01	trace	—	84	5
2	0.1	50	trace	trace	trace	trace	112	18
42	0.4	trace	0.01	0.05	0.1	trace	64	54
65	0.3	80	0.02	0.10	0.1	trace	27	109
33	0.4	trace	0.10	0.05	2.1	trace	17	143
4	0.3	0	trace	trace	trace	trace	60	1
22	0.3	trace	0.01	0.03	0.1	trace	54	42
2	0.1	0	0	trace	trace	0	10	1
6	0.5	0	0	0	0	0	9	1
5	0.5	0	0	trace	trace	0	11	2
6	0.6	trace	0.01	0.03	0.2	0	20	106
48	0.5	60	0.02	0.08	0.2	trace	33	107
167	0.5	10	0.04	0.21	0.2	1	150	230
9	0.6	—	0.01	0.03	0.1	0	76	140
1	0.1	0	trace	0.01	0.1	trace	1	11
4	0.2	trace	trace	0.01	trace	trace	2	18
4	0.3	trace	trace	0.01	trace	1	3	14
33	0.9	—	0.01	0.01	trace	—	7	213
137	3.2	—	0.02	0.04	0.4	—	19	585

Table 1.2

FOOD COMPOSITION: THE NUTRITIVE VALUE OF FOODS

Food, Approximate Measure, and Weight (in grams)		gm.	Food Energy calories	Protein (gm.)	Fat (gm.)	Carbohydrate (gm.)
Syrups:						
Table blends, chiefly corn, light & dark	1 tbsp.	21	60	0	0	15.0
Sugars:						
Brown, firm packed	1 cup	220	820	0	0	205.0
White:						
Granulated	1 tbsp.	11	40	0	0	10.0
Miscellaneous items						
Barbecue sauce	1 cup	250	230	4	17	15.2
Beverages, alcoholic:						
Beer	12 oz.	360	150	1	0	13.7
Gin, rum, vodka, whiskey:						
80 proof, 1½ fl. oz.	jigger	42	100	—	—	trace
86 proof, 1½ fl. oz.	jigger	42	105	—	—	trace
90 proof, 1½ fl. oz.	jigger	42	110	—	—	trace
94 proof, 1½ fl. oz.	jigger	42	115	—	—	trace
100 proof, 1½ fl. oz.	jigger	42	125	—	—	trace
Wines:						
Dessert, 3½ fl. oz.	glass	103	140	trace	0	8.0
Table, 3½ fl. oz.	glass	102	85	trace	0	4.3
Beverages, carbonated, sweetened, nonalcoholic, 12 fl. oz.:						
Carbonated water		366	115	0	0	29.3
Cola type		369	145	0	0	36.9
Fruit-flavored sodas and Tom Collins mixes		372	170	0	0	44.6
Ginger ale		366	115	0	0	28.8
Root beer		370	150	0	0	37.5
Bouillon cubes, ½-in.	1 cube	4	5	1	trace	trace
Chocolate:						
Bitter or baking	1 oz.	28	145	3	15	.5
Semisweet, small pieces	1 cup	170	860	7	61	70.7

Cal-cium (mg.)	Iron (mg.)	Vita-min A Value (I.U.)	Thia-mine (mg.)	Ribo-flavin (mg.)	Niacin (mg.)	Ascor-bic Acid (mg.)	Sodium (mg.)	Potas-sium (mg.)
9	0.8	0	0	0	0	0	14	1
187	7.5	0	0.02	0.07	0.4	0	66	757
0	trace	0	0	0	0	0	trace	trace
53	2.0	900	0.03	0.03	0.8	13	2038	435
18	trace	—	0.01	0.11	2.2	—	24	96
—	—	—	—	—	—	—	trace	1
—	—	—	—	—	—	—	trace	1
—	—	—	—	—	—	—	trace	1
—	—	—	—	—	—	—	trace	1
—	—	—	—	—	—	—	trace	1
8	—	—	0.01	0.02	0.2	—	4	77
9	0.4	—	trace	0.01	0.1	—	5	94
—	—	0	0	0	0	0	—	—
—	—	0	0	0	0	0	—	—
—	—	0	0	0	0	0	—	—
—	—	0	0	0	0	0	—	—
—	—	0	0	0	0	0	—	—
—	—	—	—	—	—	—	960	4
22	1.9	20	0.01	0.07	0.4	0	1	235
51	4.4	30	0.02	0.14	0.9	0	3	553

Table 1.2

FOOD COMPOSITION: THE NUTRITIVE VALUE OF FOODS

Food, Approximate Measure, and Weight (in grams)		gm.	Food Energy calories	Pro-tein (gm.)	Fat (gm.)	Carbo-hydrate (gm.)
Gelatin:						
Plain, dry powder in envelope	1 env.	7	25	6	trace	trace
Olives, pickled:						
Green, 4 med., 3 extra large		16	15	trace	2	trace
Ripe: Mission, 3 small		10	15	trace	2	trace
Pickles, cucumber:						
Dill, medium	1	65	10	1	trace	1.5
Fresh, sliced	2 slices	15	10	trace	trace	2.0
Sweet, gherkin	1 small	15	20	trace	trace	5.0
Popcorn. See Grain Products						
Popsicle, 3-fl. oz.	1 pop.	95	70	0	0	17.5
Sherbet	1 cup	193	260	2	2	58.5
Soups:						
Canned, ready-to-serve:						
Beef broth, bouillon consomme	1 cup	240	30	5	0	2.5
Beef noodle	1 cup	240	70	4	3	6.7
Clam chowder, Manhattan type (w/tomatoes, w/o milk)	1 cup	245	80	2	3	11.2
Cream of chicken	1 cup	240	95	3	6	7.2
Cream of mushroom	1 cup	240	135	2	10	9.2
Minestrone	1 cup	245	105	5	3	14.5
Split pea	1 cup	245	145	9	3	20.5
Tomato	1 cup	245	90	2	3	13.75
Vegetable beef	1 cup	245	80	5	2	10.5
Tapioca, dry, quick cooking	1 cup	152	535	1	trace	132.0
Vinegar	1 tbsp.	15	trace	trace	0	trace
White sauce, medium	1 cup	250	405	10	31	21.5
Yeast:						
Bakers' dry, active	1 pkg	7	20	3	trace	2.0
Brewers', dry	1 tbsp	8	25	3	trace	3.0

Calcium (mg.)	Iron (mg.)	Vitamin A Value (I.U.)	Thiamine (mg.)	Riboflavin (mg.)	Niacin (mg.)	Ascorbic Acid (mg.)	Sodium (mg.)	Potassium (mg.)
—	—	—	—	—	—	—	—	—
8	0.2	40	—	—	—	—	315	7
9	0.1	10	trace	trace	—	—	73	3
17	0.7	70	trace	0.01	trace	4	928	130
5	0.3	20	trace	trace	trace	1	101	—
2	0.2	10	trace	trace	trace	1	—	—
0	trace	0	0	0	0	0	7	2
31	trace	120	0.02	0.06	trace	4	19	42
trace	0.5	trace	trace	0.02	1.2	—	782	130
7	1.0	50	0.05	0.07	1.0	trace	917	77
34	1.0	880	0.02	0.02	1.0	—	938	184
24	0.5	410	0.02	0.05	0.5	trace	970	79
41	0.5	70	0.02	0.12	0.7	trace	955	98
37	1.0	2350	0.07	0.05	1.0	—	995	314
29	1.5	440	0.25	0.15	1.5	1	941	270
15	0.7	1000	0.05	0.05	1.2	12	970	230
12	0.7	2700	0.05	0.05	1.0	—	845	240
15	0.6	0	0	0	0	0	5	27
1	0.1	—	—	—	—	—	trace	15
228	0.5	1150	0.10	0.43	0.5	2	948	348
3	1.1	trace	0.16	0.38	2.6	trace	4	140
17	1.4	trace	1.25	0.34	3.0	trace	10	152

Source: Adapted from United States Department of Agriculture data in "Laurel's Kitchen" by Laurel Robertson, Carol Flinders and Bronwen Godfrey, Nilgiri Press, Berkeley, California, 1976, and "Recommended Dietary Allowances," The National Research Council, National Academy of Sciences, Washington, D.C., 1980.

Twenty-two known amino acids make up all proteins. Each kind of protein has a specific number and sequence of amino acids in its structural chain. Of the twenty-two acids, nine have to be obtained preformed in the diet. These amino acids are called the *essential amino acids*: lysine, histidine, isoleucine, leucine, phenylalanine, methionine, tryptophan, threonine, and valine. An essential amino acid is one that cannot be made at a sufficient rate or quantity by the human body to meet its needs for growth and tissue maintenance. The other amino acids, the *nonessential amino acids*, are produced by the body when given an overall adequate supply of dietary protein.

When we eat protein, it is broken down by the process of digestion into small groups of amino acids. These are absorbed, carried to the cells of the body, and there recombined to form the proteins that make up the body's tissues.

In industrialized Western countries where dietary protein deficiency is rare, protein provides approximately 12 percent of food energy. Recommended Dietary Allowances (RDA), established by the Food and Nutrition Board of the National Academy of Sciences (see table 1.3), lists the daily protein requirement at 44 grams for women and 56 grams for men. Most people eat much more protein than these amounts, but there is no convincing evidence that there is any great health advantage in doing so. The body can store less than a pound of protein in reserve. After the protein and energy needs of the body are met, excess dietary protein is simply broken down. Eating large quantities of protein-rich foods of animal origin increases the amount of saturated fat and cholesterol in the diet because these foods also contain large amounts of fat.

The proportions of the various amino acids in food protein greatly affect its nutritional value. This is especially true of the essential amino acids. As a single source, protein of animal origin often has all the essential amino acids in the correct proportion, whereas most vegetable proteins do not (see Vegetarian Diets, page 178).

However by combining foods with amino acid patterns that complement each other, the amino acid value of the protein can be equivalent to that of animal origin. For example, rice and beans have complementary amino acids. Rice is somewhat short of the amino acid lysine and beans are somewhat short of the amino acid methionine. When eaten together at the same meal, rice and beans make up for each other's deficiencies and supply the essential amino acids equivalent to a single complete protein.

During growth, pregnancy, lactation, and convalescence, the body needs proportionately more food protein than at other times. In proportion to its weight, a rapidly growing infant needs two-and-one-half times more protein than an adult.

There is little reason to believe that a physically active person needs more protein than a sedentary one; only more calories are needed, some of which may be obtained from proteins.

Many nutritionists now recognize that it is acceptable and even desirable to obtain a substantial part of protein needs from vegetable sources as well as from animal foods. This increases the intake of fiber and some minerals and decreases the amount of saturated fat and cholesterol in the diet. At present, some 70 percent of our protein comes from animal sources and 30 percent from vegetables. (See the American Health Foundation Food Plan on page 158 for optimal balance.) The blood cholesterol level is lower when vegetable protein is consumed than when the protein is of animal origin. In addition, vegetable-eating populations are less often obese (see Vegetarian Diets, page 178).

Carbohydrates

Carbohydrate is the major source of food energy for most people. In many developing countries or industrialized nations such as Japan, some 80 percent of energy comes from carbohydrates while as little as 10 percent is derived from dietary fat. In Japan today this percentage of fat is changing, rising in the 1980s to more than 20 percent of total calories.

Table 1.3

RECOMMENDED DAILY DIETARY ALLOWANCES,[a] REVISED 1980

(Designed for the maintenance of good nutrition of practically all healthy people in the U.S.A.)

	Age (years)	Weight (kg.)	Weight (lb.)	Height (cm.)	Height (in.)	Protein (g.)	Fat-Soluble Vitamins Vitamin A (μg. RE)[b]	Vitamin D (μg.)[c]	Vitamin E (mg. α-TE)[d]	Water-Soluble Vitamins Vitamin C (mg.)	Thiamin (mg.)
Infants	0.0–0.5	6	13	60	24	kg × 2.2	420	10	3	35	0.3
	0.5–1.0	9	20	71	28	kg × 2.0	400	10	4	35	0.5
Children	1–3	13	29	90	35	23	400	10	5	45	0.7
	4–6	20	44	112	44	30	500	10	6	45	0.9
	7–10	28	62	132	52	34	700	10	7	45	1.2
Males	11–14	45	99	157	62	45	1000	10	8	50	1.4
	15–18	66	145	176	69	56	1000	10	10	60	1.4
	19–22	70	154	177	70	56	1000	7.5	10	60	1.5
	23–50	70	154	178	70	56	1000	5	10	60	1.4
	51+	70	154	178	70	56	1000	5	10	60	1.2
Females	11–14	46	101	157	62	46	800	10	8	50	1.1
	15–18	55	120	163	64	46	800	10	8	60	1.1
	19–22	55	120	163	64	44	800	7.5	8	60	1.1
	23–50	55	120	163	64	44	800	5	8	60	1.0
	51+	55	120	163	64	44	800	5	8	60	1.0
Pregnant						+30	+200	+5	+2	+20	+0.4
Lactating						+20	+400	+5	+3	+40	+0.5

[a]The allowances are intended to provide for individual variations among most normal persons as they live in the United States under usual environmental stresses. Diets should be based on a variety of common foods in order to provide other nutrients for which human requirements have been less well defined.

[b]Retinol equivalents. 1 retinol equivalent = 1 μg retinol or 6 μg β carotene.

[c]As cholecalciferol. 10 μg cholecalciferol = 400 IU of vitamin D.

[d]α-tocopherol equivalents. 1 mg d-α tocopherol = 1 α-TE.

[e]INE (niacin equivalent) is equal to 1 mg of niacin or 60 mg of dietary tryptophan.

μg = microgram = 1 millionth of a gram

IU = international units   TE = tocopherol equivalent

Table 1.3 *(continued)*

RECOMMENDED DAILY DIETARY ALLOWANCES,[a] REVISED 1980

(Designed for the maintenance of good nutrition of practically all healthy people in the U.S.A.)

Age (years)	Vitamins						Minerals					
	Riboflavin (mg.)	Niacin (mg. NE)[e]	Vitamin B-6 (mg.)	Folacin (μg.)	Vitamin B-12 (μg.)	Calcium (mg.)	Phosphorus (mg.)	Magnesium (mg.)	Iron (mg.)	Zinc (mg.)	Iodine (μg.)
0.0–0.5	0.4	6	0.3	30	0.5[f]	360	240	50	10	3	40
0.5–1.0	0.6	8	0.6	45	1.5	540	360	70	15	5	50
1–3	0.8	9	0.9	100	2.0	800	800	150	15	10	70
4–6	1.0	11	1.3	200	2.5	800	800	200	10	10	90
7–10	1.4	16	1.6	300	3.0	800	800	250	10	10	120
11–14	1.6	18	1.8	400	3.0	1200	1200	350	18	15	150
15–18	1.7	18	2.0	400	3.0	1200	1200	400	18	15	150
19–22	1.7	19	2.2	400	3.0	800	800	350	10	15	150
23–50	1.6	18	2.2	400	3.0	800	800	350	10	15	150
51+	1.4	16	2.2	400	3.0	800	800	350	10	15	150
11–14	1.3	15	1.8	400	3.0	1200	1200	300	18	15	150
15–18	1.3	14	2.0	400	3.0	1200	1200	300	18	15	150
19–22	1.3	14	2.0	400	3.0	800	800	300	18	15	150
23–50	1.2	13	2.0	400	3.0	800	800	300	18	15	150
51+	1.2	13	2.0	400	3.0	800	800	300	10	15	150
Pregnant	+0.3	+2	+0.6	+400	+1.0	+400	+400	+150	g	+5	+25
Lactating	+0.5	+5	+0.5	+100	+1.0	+400	+400	+150	g	+10	+50

[f]The recommended dietary allowance for vitamin B-12 in infants is based on average concentration of the vitamin in human milk. The allowances after weaning are based on energy intake (as recommended by the American Academy of Pediatrics) and consideration of other factors, such as intestinal absorption;

[g]The increased requirement during pregnancy cannot be met by the iron content of habitual American diets nor by the existing iron stores of many women; therefore the use of 30–60 mg of supplemental iron is recommended. Iron needs during lactation are not substantially different from those of nonpregnant women, but continued supplementation of the mother for 2–3 months after parturition is advisable in order to replenish stores depleted by pregnancy.

SOURCE: Food and Nutrition Board, National Academy of Sciences—National Research Council

By contrast, in the U.S., Great Britain, and most westernized countries, eating patterns have come to include progressively less carbohydrate and more and more fat during the present century. In the 1960s and 70s, Americans obtained only about 46 percent of energy from carbohydrate, and as much as 42 percent from fat. The optimal food pattern for man probably lies between these extremes.

Sugars and Starch The simplest form of carbohydrate are the sugars, of which there are several. Table sugar, known as sucrose, is one. Others are fructose and dextrose derived from fruit and plant sources, and lactose, or milk sugar. Most of the sugar in our Western diet is sucrose, purified from sugar cane or sugar beet and added to processed foods or used at the table. Milk is the only significant animal source of carbohydrate.

Starch, a more complex form of carbohydrate, differs from sugars in that it does not dissolve in cold water and is not sweet to taste. Starch comes from cereal grains such as wheat, from root vegetables such as potatoes, and from other plants.

Starch, and sugars such as sucrose and lactose, are rapidly digested and are absorbed efficiently from the small intestine. The main product of carbohydrate digestion is glucose, which enters the blood stream. It is used by all body tissues, much of it being broken down (oxidized) for the production of energy. Each gram of carbohydrate yields four calories of energy. Glucose that is surplus to the energy requirements of the moment is converted to other substances and stored. Some is converted to glycogen and stored in muscle and liver, but most of the glucose is converted to fat and stored in adipose tissue under the skin and elsewhere.

As a source of energy, glucose is especially important to the brain. Other tissues have alternate sources of chemical energy, but the brain relies chiefly on glucose. As it has negligible stores of energy, the brain depends almost from minute to minute on glucose derived from the blood.

Fortunately, the body's chemistry is well able to maintain a normal level of glucose in the blood. Fluctuations are controlled by the secretion of two hormones: insulin and glucagon, which are, in turn, affected by other hormonal systems such as the thyroid and the pituitary and adrenal glands. These changes encourage the use and storage of glucose after a meal. Between meals, especially overnight, these processes slow down and glucose is instead secreted into the blood by the liver, which produces it from glycogen, proteins, and other substances. If blood glucose regulation fails, its level may become abnormally high; this is diabetes mellitus, due to absolute or relative deficiency of insulin. Too low a level of blood glucose, hypoglycemia, may occur in diabetics receiving too much insulin or too little food. It occurs in other people from a variety of causes.

An increased intake of carbohydrate coupled with a reduced intake of fat leads over time to a persistent fall in the level of blood cholesterol; there is strong reason to believe that this is a desirable effect.

Fiber Cellulose is also a carbohydrate and is one of the substances that makes up the fiber in our diet (see tables 1.4 and 1.5). Dietary fiber is not digested by man's intestinal secretions. Studies of rural Africans who eat high fiber diets have led to suggestions that extra dietary fiber may reduce the risk of many common diseases. For example, an increased fiber intake may be helpful in the treatment of constipation and probably in the prevention of diverticular disease and hemorrhoids. Certain fibers characteristically increase stool bulk that contributes to the easy passage of stool and dilutes possible toxic agents.

Table 1.4
DIETARY FIBER IN COMMON FOODS
(Recommended daily intake is 20–40 gms.)

Food	Portion size	Dietary fiber (gm.)
Cereals		
white bread	1 slice	0.7
boiled rice	½ cup	0.8
60% whole wheat bread	1 slice	1.4
Rice Krispies	1 cup	1.4
oatmeal (cooked)	1 cup	1.9
whole wheat bread	1 slice	2.4
bran flakes	1 cup	4.8
Shredded Wheat	2 biscuits	6.2
natural bran	½ cup	6.6
All-Bran	¾ cup	12.0
Fruits		
fruit juice*	6 ounces	0.2
cherries	1 cup	2.0
peach	1 medium	2.1
orange	1 medium	2.3
raisins	¼ cup	2.7
apple	1 medium	4.0
Vegetables		
lettuce (raw)	1 cup	1.1
tomato (raw)	1 small	1.5
potato (boiled)	1 medium	2.0
carrots (7½″, raw)	1	2.3
green beans (cooked)	¾ cup	3.2
cauliflower (cooked)	1 cup	3.2
brussel sprouts (cooked)	1 cup	4.5
peas (cooked)	½ cup	6.2
spinach (cooked)	½ cup	6.3
kidney beans (cooked)	½ cup	7.4
broccoli (cooked)	2 small stalks	11.5
pork and beans	1 cup	18.6

SOURCE: adapted from *McCance and Widdowson's Composition of Foods*, by A. A. Paul and D. A. T. Southgate Elsevier, North Holland, Biomedical Press, London, 1978.
*Fruit juices have considerably less fiber than whole fruit.

Table 1.5
LOW vs. HIGH-FIBER DIETS

Low dietary fiber		# Grams	High dietary fiber		# Grams
Breakfast					
½ c. orange juice from concentrate		0.1	1 fresh valencia or navel orange		2.3
1 c. Rice Krispies		1.4	⅓ c. All Bran,		5.3
½ toasted English Muffin		0.7	1 slice whole wheat toast		2.0
	Total	2.2		Total	9.6
Lunch					
¼ lb. hamburger		0.6	¼ lb. 3-bean salad		3.0
1 portion french fries (4 oz.)		0.8	1 slice pumpernickel		0.4
Ice cream (any quantity)		–	1.3 oz. dried fruit		1.1
			1 oz. mixed nuts.		0.3
	Total	1.4		Total	4.8
Dinner					
8 oz. commercial split pea soup		0.8	salad*		1.3
8 oz. steak		–	4 oz. steak		–
⅓ c. potato		0.3	⅔ c. potato		0.5
¼ c. green beans		1.0	¾ c. green beans		3.2
½ tomato		0.7	1 c. broccoli		11.5
½ c. baked custard		–	Fresh fruit cup**		0.5
	Total	2.8		Total	17.0
Snack					
1 oz. potato chips		0.5	1 apple		4.0

*Salad		# Grams	**Fruit cup		# Grams
2 large leaves of Romaine lettuce		0.4	1 oz. each:		
¼ c. tomato		0.4	apple		0.2
6 slices cucumber 2″ x ⅛″ x 1.8 oz.		0.2	orange		0.1
¼ c. carrot sticks		0.3	banana		0.1
oil and vinegar		–	grapes		0.1
	Total:	1.3		Total:	0.5

SOURCE: American Health Foundation

Fats

Fats, a major source of food energy in the Western world, are a compact nutrient, yielding more than twice as many calories (9) per gram as do proteins or carbohydrates. Adipose tissue, the body's main store of energy, is made up of cells containing fat. Unlike protein and carbohydrate, fat can be stored in almost unlimited amounts.

Fatty foods are also carriers of the "fat-soluble" group of vitamins: A, D, E, and K. Fat-containing foods are the main sources of these substances.

The presence of fat in a meal or snack heightens feelings of fullness, possibly because fats stimulate the secretion of a hormone (cholecystokinin) that slows the rate at which the stomach empties into the small intestine. Fats are digested and absorbed more slowly than are proteins and carbohydrates.

Pure fats, like corn oil, or those in food, are made up of a variety of fatty acids that determine their differing consistency and taste and that differ in their effects on the chemistry of the body. Chemically, fatty acids contain long chains of carbon atoms attached to hydrogen atoms. One group, the saturated fatty acids, contains the maximum possible number of hydrogen atoms (they are "saturated" with hydrogen). Most fats made chiefly of saturated fatty acids are solid at room temperature. Butter and lard are rich in saturated fatty acids. The other group, with fewer than the maximum number of hydrogen atoms, are the unsaturated fatty acids. These fats are liquid at room temperature and are called oils. Safflower and corn oils are polyunsaturated oils. The fatty acid that makes up the bulk of olive oil and peanut oil has one double bond and is called monounsaturated.

Table 1.6
CHARACTERISTICS OF FATTY ACIDS

Type	Source	Characteristics	Example
polyunsaturated fatty acids	vegetable origin	liquid at room temperature	safflower oil sunflower oil corn oil cottonseed oil sesame oil soybean oil
monounsaturated	vegetable	liquid at room temperature	peanut oil rice oil olive oil
saturated	animal*	hard at room temperature	lard butter bacon drippings
hydrogenated	liquid vegetable oil processed by hydrogenation to make hard	hard at room temperature	stick margarine† shortening (like Crisco)

*exception: coconut and palm oils are of vegetable origin and both are highly saturated.
†contains various levels of hydrogenated fats among other components.

Some of the polyunsaturated fatty acids are essential to human health and are therefore called *essential fatty acids*. These are linoleic and linolenic fatty acids and have to be obtained from the diet. They are necessary for health in two interrelated ways. They form part of the structure of the delicate membranes that line cells and the minute components within cells. Also, they are required for the formation of a group of hormonelike substances known as prostaglandins; these regulate many bodily functions including blood clotting.

Saturated fatty acids are major components of the fat of meat, dairy products, hydrogenated shortenings, lard, artificial dairy substitutes, and are found in most commerically baked products. Two highly saturated fats, coconut and palm oils, are of vegetable origin. These are used in many processed foods to control deterioration.

Fats rich in polyunsaturated acids are the oils made from corn, sunflower seeds, safflower seeds, and soybeans. The fat of fish is also a rich source of unsaturated fatty acids. Walnuts are another source high in polyunsaturated fatty acids. Although each type of fatty acid has specific characteristics of its own (see table 1.6), they all yield about the same amount of energy (calories); therefore, excess calories can result in overweight whether the fat is saturated or unsaturated. Foods that are less obvious sources of fat are shown in table 1.7.

Cholesterol Foods of animal origin contain cholesterol, a waxy, fatlike substance that is chemically quite different from fat. Foods of plant origin do not contain cholesterol. All tissues of the body require cholesterol that forms part of the membranes surrounding the cells and is used in the production of many hormones and other essential substances. It is derived from two sources: some cholesterol is manufactured in the body and some is obtained from foods of animal origin. When we absorb food cholesterol we compensate by producing less cholesterol in the liver. As this

self-regulating mechanism is less effective in some people than in others, it is sensible to be cautious about the amount of cholesterol-rich foods eaten, for cholesterol appears to be harmful in excess (see Cardiovascular Disease, page 131). Foods containing large amounts of cholesterol include egg yolks, beef, liver, organ meats, fish roe, whole milk, lard, butter, cheese and cream (see table 1.8).

A great research effort is in progress to determine the most desirable intake of fat for health, the desirable proportions of the various kinds of fatty acids, and an acceptable intake of cholesterol. It is established that most saturated fats increase the blood cholesterol level, while the polyunsaturated type tends to reduce it. Monounsaturated fatty acids are "neutral" in this respect, as are carbohydrates. When the dietary intake of saturated fats is reduced, and replaced by carbohydrate or monounsaturated fat, cholesterol levels decrease. If saturated fat is replaced by polyunsaturated fat, the blood cholesterol level falls even further.

The average adult in most Western countries has a serum cholesterol level of about 225 mg%. Although physicians may hold that this is a "normal" level, it is really *average*, being neither normal nor optimal (see figure 1.2). Levels higher than this carry greater risk for atherosclerosis and its associated disorders. To be at lowest risk for these disorders, the optimal level should be 160 mg%, plus or minus 20.

Diets for reducing the blood cholesterol level, intended to diminish the risk of heart attack and other diseases (see Nutrition in Disease, page 125) have about half the usual content of saturated fat and contain moderate amounts of polyunsaturated fat. They lead to an average fall of 15 percent in the blood cholesterol. This change persists as long as the diet is followed. Additional ways of reducing the blood cholesterol include

Table 1.7:
HIDDEN FAT IN FOODS

Foods	Calories per serving	% Calories from fat	Grams fat per serving	Proportion of saturated fat
Dairy				
Cheddar cheese, 2 oz.	228	73	19	High
Swiss cheese, 2 oz.	214	73	16	High
Eggs, 1 large	164	64	12	Moderate
Ice cream, ¾ cup	143	48	11	High
Cream cheese, 2 tbsp.	99	88	10	High
Whole milk, 8 oz. (1 glass)	159	47	8	High

The following cheeses also contain a minimum of 60% calories from fat and 8 to 9 grams fat per ounce: Bleu, Brick, Brie, Caraway, Edam, Gouda, Gruyere, Limburger, Monterey, Muenster, Port du Salut, Provolone, Romano, Roquefort; also, pasteurized processed American, Pimento or Swiss.

Foods	Calories per serving	% Calories from fat	Grams fat per serving	Proportion of saturated fat
Fish				
Herring (Pacific), 4 oz.	235	59	16	Low
Sardines (Atlantic), in oil, drained, 4 oz.	230	49	12	Low
Sockeye (red) salmon, 4 oz.	194	49	11	Low
Mackerel (Pacific), 4 oz.	204	50	11	Low
Red meat*				
Pork, loin roast (well-trimmed), 4 oz.	287	50	16	High
Pork, Boston butt (well-trimmed), 4 oz.	275	53	16	High
Hot dog, 1 (2 oz.)	176	80	16	High
Beef, rib roast (well-trimmed), 4 oz.	273	50	15	High
Beef, club steak (well-trimmed), 4 oz.	277	48	15	High
Liverwurst, 2 oz.	174	75	14	High
Lamb chop (well-trimmed), 4 oz.	239	45	12	High
Nuts and seeds				
Peanut butter, 2 tbsp.	188	73	16	Low
Almonds, ⅛ cup	123	77	11	Low
Sunflower seeds, ⅛ cup	100	71	9	Low
Walnuts, black, ⅛ cup	98	79	9	Low
Baked goods				
Apple pie, ⅛ of pie	302	38	13	Usually high
Danish pastry, ⅛ of ring	179	49	10	Usually high
Croissant, 1, about 1 oz.	109	50	6	Usually high
Other				
Avocado, ½ fruit	188	82	19	Low
Coconut, 1 piece, 2" x 2" x ½"	156	85	16	High
Cream of mushroom soup, 10 oz.	150	66	11	Variable
Milk chocolate, 1 oz.	147	53	9	High

*All values for fresh meat represent cooked portions of choice grade. The information is based on average of samples analyzed by the U.S. Department of Agriculture. These figures represent the "lean" of the meat only; every possible bit of outside fat has been removed. Almost all the above information in this chart is based on USDA food tables. However, in a few cases, information supplied by food companies was used.

SOURCE: Adapted from *Nutrition Action Newsletter*, Center for Science in the Public Interest, Washington, D.C., 1979.

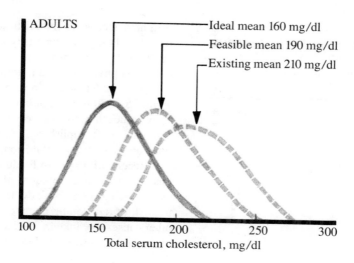

ADULTS
Ideal mean 160 mg/dl
Feasible mean 190 mg/dl
Existing mean 210 mg/dl

Total serum cholesterol, mg/dl

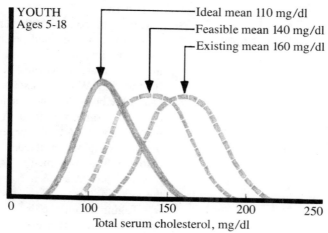

YOUTH
Ages 5-18
Ideal mean 110 mg/dl
Feasible mean 140 mg/dl
Existing mean 160 mg/dl

Total serum cholesterol, mg/dl

FIGURE 1.2

Ideal, feasible, and existing total serum cholesterol levels in adults and children.

This set of graphs compares the present distribution of cholesterol levels in the U.S. ("existing") with the range deemed optimal ("ideal") for adults (top) and youth ages 5–18 (bottom). Between these distribution curves is the range feasible for the U.S. public to achieve by a change in dietary habits over the next few years.

SOURCE: *American Health Foundation Conference on the Health Effects of Blood Lipids: Optimal Distributions for Populations. Workshop Report: Epidemiological Section (Henry Blackburn, ed.),* Preventive Medicine *8, 1979.*

Table 1.8
THE COMMON SOURCES OF CHOLESTEROL
IN THE AMERICAN DIET
(Recommended daily intake of cholesterol: 200 mg.)

Food and Description	Cholesterol (mg.)
Meat, poultry, fish	
Beef, lean, 8 oz.	206
Beef, lean, 4 oz.	103
Pork, lean, 6 oz.	150
Lamb, lean, 6 oz.	170
Veal, lean, 6 oz.	168
Chicken, white meat, 6 oz.	138
Chicken, dark meat, 6 oz.	156
Fish, flounder, 6 oz.	86
Fish, tuna, 3 oz.	56
Liver, beef, 3 oz.	372
Liver, chicken, 3 oz.	639
Dairy products	
Milk, whole, 1 cup	34
Milk, nonfat, 1 cup	5
Cheese, cheddar, 1 oz.	28
Cheese, lowfat cottage, 1 cup	23
Ice cream, rich, 1 cup	85
Yogurt, lowfat, 1 cup	17
Sour cream, 1 cup	152
Butter, 1 tbsp.	35
Eggs	
Egg, yolk	252
Egg, white	0
Baked goods	
Chocolate cake, with frosting, $\frac{1}{16}$ of 9 inch diameter cake	32
Sponge cake, $\frac{1}{12}$ of 10 inch diameter cake	162
Muffin, corn, average size	28
Brownie, 2 inch square	24
Bread pudding, 1 cup	170

SOURCE: Adapted from *Journal of the American Dietetic Association* vol. 61, no. 2 (August 1972).

weight reduction to diminish obesity and eating more foods high in certain types of fiber, especially pectins obtained from fruit.

Most physicians and nutritionists concur that reduction of fat intake from over 40 percent to about 25 to 30 percent of our food energy would help reduce the risk of coronary heart disease. This can be accomplished by following the guidelines under Everyday Nutrition, page 158.

Recently it has been found that high-fat diets tend to increase the amount of bile acids in the stool. There is persuasive evidence to suggest that the risk of developing colon cancer may (among other causes) be linked with the level of bile acids in the stool, as discussed on page 138.

Vitamins

Vitamins are complex substances needed in very small amounts for good health, normal growth, and reproduction. There are thirteen, possibly more, that are indispensable for normal body functioning. With the exception of vitamins D and K the body does not manufacture them; thus they must come from food. A well-balanced diet with plenty of fruits and vegetables, whole grain or enriched grain products, vitamin D-enriched whole milk or skimmed milk, and other animal products provides the necessary amounts of all the vitamins.

Taking vitamin pills is not a substitute for proper nutrition. However, a multivitamin preparation may be taken as extra insurance by infants and growing children, pregnant and nursing mothers, people on reducing diets, and the elderly. Any simple inexpensive multivitamin is adequate. Do not be misled by the word "natural" in a vitamin supplement. Natural and synthetic vitamins have identical compositions.

So-called megavitamin treatment—taking massive doses of a particular vitamin—should be avoided. Vitamins are essential nutrients, but high dosages become drugs and should only be taken to treat a specific condition. Large doses of the fat-soluble vitamins A and D have well-recognized ill effects, and this may be true of others, too. Large doses of vitamin C are mainly excreted in the urine. In the absence of certainty that "megavitamins" are safe, they are better avoided.

Following are discussions of some important vitamins. The rest are listed in table 1.9.

Vitamin A Vitamin A is a fat-soluble vitamin obtained in two ways. Some is manufactured in the body from foods containing carotene, the most abundant sources of which are yellow fruits and vegetables. Preformed vitamin A is obtained from fish, liver, dairy products, and egg yolk.

Vitamin A is essential for maintaining normal mucous membranes, for proper night vision, for growth and tissue repair, and, according to recent research, possibly for protecting the body from some cancer-producing agents. It is highly toxic in excessive amounts. Overdosage causes skin damage, jaundice, hair loss, blurred vision, headaches, and bone problems.

Vitamin C Vitamin C is water soluble and is plentiful in citrus and other fruits (guava, papaya, strawberries, melon, etc.), green leafy vegetables, and potatoes. Some is lost in cooking, especially by boiling in large amounts of water, cooking in copper pots, and when baking soda is present.

Vitamin C deficiency weakens the delicate walls of fine blood vessels and causes scurvy which involves bleeding in the skin and from the gums, painful bleeding in muscles, anemia, and poor healing of wounds. The vitamin is needed for formation of the fibrous protein collagen, which strengthens many tissues.

The only certain value of vitamin C is the prevention and treatment of scurvy. The evidence that taking a huge quantity—1,000 milligrams a day or more—will avert the common cold is ten-

Table 1.9
VITAMINS AND THEIR FOOD SOURCES*

Vitamins	Food sources
Fat soluble	
Vitamin A (retinol)	Green and yellow vegetables, (for carotene) lowfat cheese and milk, eggs
Vitamin D (cholecalciferol)	Fish oils, vitamin D-fortified foods including lowfat milk
Vitamin E (alpha-Tocopherol)	Wheat germ, whole grains, vegetables
Vitamin K	Leafy vegetables
Water soluble	
Vitamin C (ascorbic acid)	Citrus fruits, potatoes, peppers, tomatoes, cabbage
Vitamin B_1 (thiamin)	Pork, meat, poultry, yeast, enriched flour
Vitamin B_2 (riboflavin)	Milk, eggs, enriched flour, leafy vegetables
Niacin	Meat, poultry, eggs, enriched flour, whole grains
Vitamin B_6 (pyridoxine)	Meat, fish, whole grains, wheat germ, vegetables
Folic acid	Meat, leafy vegetables
Vitamin B_{12} (cyanocobalamin)	Eggs, milk, and meat

*See table 1.3, pages 101–102 for intake level in infancy, childhood, adolesence, and adulthood.

uous. Some researchers have found slight protection against virus infections; others, using 3,000 milligrams a day found none. It is known that vitamin C can prevent the interaction between nitrates and the amines in foods that is suspected of a role in causing cancer, especially cancer of the stomach (see Cancer, page 135). There is no evidence that vitamin C plays a role in the treatment of cancer.

Vitamin D Vitamin D is essential for the normal functioning of bone and tooth dentine. It is fat-soluble and is obtained in two ways. One source is foods like fatty fish (sardines and herrings); also foods that are supplemented with vitamin D including margarine and fortified milk. The other source is our own skin. A substance related to cholesterol is present in the skin and is converted to vitamin D when we are exposed to sunlight, or other ultraviolet light. Infants and children who get too little sunlight are prone to vitamin D deficiency. Vitamin D requirements are proportionately greater when bone growth is rapid, i.e., in infancy and early childhood.

Vitamin D is needed for proper absorption of calcium from the intestine and also for the absorbed calcium to be used in formation of bone and teeth. In children, the bone disease caused by vitamin D deficiency is called rickets. Not only are bones prone to deformity, but also muscle spasms and even convulsions can occur.

Vitamin D deficiency can also be due to diseases of the small intestine that impair absorption. This deficiency can cause the bone disease osteomalacia in adults, with pains in the back and limbs, and proneness to fractures. Another cause of osteomalacia is drugs that stimulate the liver to break down the vitamin; drugs used to treat epilepsy can have this side effect.

We need vitamin D throughout life. Where the climate is even moderately sunny, enough vitamin D can usually be made in the skin of adults and older children; but for safety a daily intake of 400 international units is recommended at all ages. Excess of vitamin D—leading to kidney stones, digestive troubles, and heart damage—is as harmful as its deficiency.

Vitamin E Vitamin E is widely available from food; polyunsaturated oils are a rich source. Human deficiency only occurs in premature babies and in people with diseases of the small intestine who fail to absorb the vitamin.

Deficiency results in anemia. There is no reason to believe that deficiency causes human infertility nor that large doses help sufferers from arterial or muscle diseases; wheat germ oil, high in vitamin E, is no panacea.

The B vitamins This group of vitamins is water-soluble. Thiamin (B_1) is needed for normal functioning of nerves, heart, and brain. Riboflavin (B_2) is needed for tissue repair. Niacin is needed for the healthy functioning of the skin, gastrointestinal tract, and the nervous system. Its deficiency leads to severe mental abnormalities, a peeling pigmented skin condition, a sore tongue, and diarrhea. Deficiency of these vitamins is common in alcoholism. Vitamin B_6 functions chiefly in the process of protein metabolism. B_6 in the diet is proportionate to protein intake.

Vitamin B_{12} and folic acid are needed for red blood cell formation; severe anemia arises from their deficiencies. Vitamin B_{12} deficiency also causes nerve damage and mental changes. Pure vegetarian diets may be deficient in B_{12} since it is found only in animal foods.

Vitamin B_{12} deficiency (pernicious anemia) can result from lack of a stomach secretion needed for its absorption, from stomach operations, and from disease of the small bowel. Folic acid deficiency, (megaloblastic anemia), can result from poor diets, intestinal disease, alcoholism, and from the use of drugs, such as those for treating epilepsy. This is also a cause of anemia during late pregnancy. Oral contraceptives have also caused deficiency in folic acid. (see chapter 6).

Deficiencies of B vitamins often occur together. A varied balanced diet ensures an adequate intake of these essential nutrients without the need for special vitamin supplements.

Minerals

Minerals present in relatively large amounts in the body are calcium, phosphorus, potassium, sodium, chloride, and magnesium. Other minerals, referred to as "trace elements," occur in tissues only in minute amounts. These include iron, zinc, copper, iodine, and others (see table 1.10), and are essential for many body processes. The average adult human body contains about 1,200,000 mg. of calcium and 21,000 mg. of magnesium, but only about 80 mg. of copper, a trace element.

Calcium Most of the body's one kilogram or more (2.2 pounds) of calcium (1.5 to 2 percent of body weight) is needed to give strength and rigidity to bones and teeth. Calcium-containing crystals together with protein fibers provide this strength. A very small amount of calcium is present in blood plasma and other fluids; this is essential for proper muscle contraction (including the heart muscle), for nerves to conduct their messages, and for blood to clot and stop bleeding.

Those on very high-fiber diets, such as vegetarians, should ensure sufficient calcium intake (see table 1.3) since a substance called phytic acid mostly found in unrefined grains decreases calcium absorption.

Important sources of calcium are milk, especially cow's milk (whole or skim), cheese, vegetables, fish that are normally eaten with their bones (canned fish and whitebait), enriched bread, and "hard" drinking water.

When bones are developing and growing, as in infancy and childhood and during pregnancy and nursing, when women are supplying calcium to the rapidly growing fetus and baby, especially large amounts of calcium are required in proportion to body weight.

The recommended intake for adults is 800 mg. per day. People vary widely in their needs

Table 1.10
COMMON MINERALS AND
THEIR FOOD SOURCES

Minerals	Major food sources
Calcium	dairy products, soybeans, seafood, leafy green vegetables
Chloride	all foods, table salt
Copper	meats, legumes, nuts, raisins, seafood
Fluoride	fluoridated water, dentifrices, milk
Iodine	iodized table salt, seafood
Iron	red meat, beans, nuts, raisins, poultry
Magnesium	green vegetables, milk, meat, nuts, seafood
Manganese	bananas, bran, leafy vegetables, whole grains, cereals, nuts, legumes
Molybdenum	cereals, leafy vegetables
Phosphorus	seafood, poultry, dairy products, meat, beans, grain
Potassium	all foods especially meat, vegetables, milk, dates, figs, seafood, bananas
Selenium	grains, seafood, seeds, nuts
Sodium	all foods, table salt, seafood
Sulfur	all protein-containing foods, nuts, wheat germ
Zinc	meat, seafood, legumes, milk, green vegetables, brewer's yeast

(the average is 500 mg.), and although most individuals keep healthy on this amount, some authorities believe 1,000 mg. per day is a safer allowance. Given time, some, but not all people are able to adapt to lower amounts.

The correct calcium intake in adults is that amount which balances losses (chiefly in the feces, also in urine). It is not yet clear whether thinning of bones (osteoporosis), a common disorder in elderly people, results partly from a lack of dietary calcium. Most people can tolerate a generous intake of calcium without harm, for the parathyroid gland regulates the amount of calcium in blood plasma and in bone. But some people (one to two percent in temperate climates) form calcium-containing kidney stones because they excrete too much calcium in the urine. A common cause of this is the overefficient absorption of calcium by the intestine. In this case, physicians may advise restriction of calcium-rich foods.

Calcium absorption is dependent on vitamin D; its deficiency is an important cause of bone disease.

Magnesium Adults need a substantial amount of magnesium, about 350 mg. per day. Magnesium is required for the action of many enzymes inside cells, especially those that release energy during the breakdown of foodstuffs.

Most magnesium is supplied in leafy green vegetables, nuts, soybeans, cereal products, and whole grains. Deficiency is usually due to abnormal losses from the body caused by alcoholism, prolonged diarrhea, or other intestinal diseases, rather than lack of intake in foods. It causes apathy, weakness, and twitching, with abnormal function of nerves, muscle, and brain.

Phosphorus Phosphorus in the form of phosphate is the second most abundant mineral in the body. It functions together with calcium to form the compound that makes bones and teeth strong and rigid. Approximately 85 percent of the body's phosphorus is in the bones and teeth.

Phosphorus also enables many chemical reactions to take place, allowing proteins, fats, and carbohydrates to be used to produce energy. It is important for fueling the contractions of heart and muscle.

Phosphorus is widely distributed in foods, but the high protein food sources, such as poultry, fish, meat, and eggs, are the most abundant sources. Cereal grains, especially whole grains, are also an excellent source. Phosphorus deficiency hardly ever arises from lack of intake in the diet.

Sodium and Chloride Most of the sodium in our diet is taken in the form of common salt (sodium chloride). Together, sodium and chloride help maintain proper fluid balance. Excessive sodium causes retention of fluid in the body and is believed to contribute to high blood pressure among those susceptible to it. Sodium deficiency decreases the volume of blood and tissue fluid and is one of the causes of low blood pressure and shock.

In the U.S., we eat 6–18 (average 15) grams of salt a day and get more sodium from baking powder, flavor enhancers, and other natural sources like vegetables. Since salt is 40 percent sodium, sodium intake averages 5 grams a day, considerably more than what our bodies require. Part of the reason for our heavy intake of salt is due to its traditional use as a preservative (in pickles, canned meats, smoked foods), and as an acquired taste in snacks (pretzels, salted nuts), spiced recipes, breakfast cereals, breads, crackers and other grains, fast foods (french fries, hamburgers), and, less obviously, in butter, margarine, and cheese. The habit of liking salt is prob-

Table 1.11

HIGH SODIUM FOODS IN OUR DIET, AND ALTERNATIVES

(A serving contains more than 400 mg.)

Foods	Daily sodium allowance:		Lower sodium food alternatives
	mg.	% of 3,000 mg.	
Hamburgers			
Burger King Whopper	909 mg.	30%	Fast food restaurants at present offer little substitu-
McDonald's Big Mac	962 mg.	32%	tion. Cook at home when the "fast food urge" hits. Use lean ground round and broil rather than fry.
Fish			
Arthur Treacher's fish sandwich	836 mg.	29%	Any fresh fish choices, i.e., halibut, trout, sea bass,
Burger King Whaler	735 mg.	25%	red snapper, filet of sole and salmon (fresh), etc.
McDonald's Filet-O-Fish	709 mg.	24%	
Chicken			
Kentucky Fried Original Dinner	2285 mg.	76%	Use margarine and bread crumbs to cover chicken
Kentucky Fried Crispy Dinner	1915 mg.	64%	and broil or bake.
Chicken TV Dinner	1164 mg.	39%	
Other fast food items			
Dairy Queen Brazier Dog	868 mg.	29%	chicken dog
Bologna, 1/8″ slice	585 mg.	20%	sliced chicken
Salami, 1 oz.	425 mg.	14%	lean roast beef
All ham except hamhock- 1 serv.	400–700 mg.	13–23%	sliced turkey
Hot dogs/frankfurters-1 serv.	1000–1250 mg.	33–42%	chicken dog
Pizza with sausage and extra cheese, 4 oz.	796 mg.	27%	pizza, plain with cheese
Tuna, salmon salad (canned), 1/2 cup	799 mg.	27%	fresh salmon or tuna salad, not canned
Olives, 6 small	792 mg.	26%	pieces of fresh fruit, cherries
Tomato Juice, 1 cup	448 mg.	15%	apple juice, grapefruit juice
Ketchup, 1 tbsp.	156 mg.	5%	
Other foods that contribute to our high sodium intake			
Salted nuts, 1 oz.	150–220 mg.	5–7%	walnuts, unsalted almonds
Dill pickle, 1 large (4″)	1200 mg.	40%	sliced cucumbers in vinegar
Potato chips, 1/2 cup	200 mg.	7%	unsalted popcorn
Pretzel, 1 large cracker	239 mg.	8%	unsalted pretzels
Cereal (with salt as a first ingredient), 2 oz.	660 mg.	22%	hot and cold cereals (with salt as one of the last ingredients)
Processed Swiss cheese, 1 oz.	361 mg.	12%	mozarrella, ricotta cheese
Salt, 1 tsp.	2300 mg.	77%	spices and herbs, avoid mixtures
Tomato soup, 1 cup	1980 mg.	66%	
Soy sauce, 1 tbsp.	1319 mg.	44%	

Read labels and avoid foods preserved with:
sodium benzoate, sodium citrate, sodium bicarbonate, sodium stearate, sodium nitrate, MSG

SOURCE: adapted from Barbara Kraus, *The Dictionary of Sodium, Fats and Cholesterol.* (New York: Grosset & Dunlap, Inc., 1974)

ably learned at an early age, though modern infant foods have been improved and are not as salty as they were in the past. Table 1.11 will give you some idea of the levels of sodium in common dietary sources.

It has been recommended that salt intake be limited to 5 grams a day, about one teaspoon, which includes about two grams of sodium. With sodium from other sources, the total intake of sodium should then be around 3 grams a day.

Potassium Potassium is an important component of the fluid inside cells where it produces the needed environment for muscles to contract, for nerves to carry their impulses, and for many enzymes to act in promoting chemical reactions.

Deficiency of potassium causes general weakness, even paralysis, and irregular or abnormal heartbeats. Potassium depletion may result from prolonged vomiting or diarrhea, especially in infants, from treatment with diuretic drugs used to control high blood pressure, and from cortisonelike drugs. Potassium is found in almost all plant and animal foods. More specific sources are bran, brewer's yeast, cocoa, coffee, dried legumes (peas, soybeans, and white beans), and potatoes and squash.

Trace elements Although the precise role of some trace elements is still unknown, it is well established that very small amounts of iron, iodine, fluoride, and copper, and probably manganese, zinc, chromium, selenium, cobalt, molybdenum, tin, vanadium, nickel, and silicon are essential for growth and continued good health. Problems arise both from deficiencies and excess, and the healthy range seems to be narrower than for other nutrients.

Iron In the United States, iron deficiency anemia tends to be found among infants, young children, and women, with a higher incidence among pregnant women, and less often among men. In infancy after six months of age (full-term infants usually have a sufficient store for the first six months), dietary iron is essential to replenish and meet iron requirements.

Anemia in women is often caused by large iron losses during menstruation and increased demands during pregnancy.

Iron is required to form hemoglobin, which enables the blood to transport oxygen to cells to meet energy needs. The iron stores in our body are relatively small, men having greater stores than women.

The amount of iron in our food supply has increased by 20 percent because of the enrichment laws passed in the 1950s.

Natural food sources of iron are liver (one of the richest), meats, egg yolk, legumes, and leafy green vegetables. Raisins and enriched breads and cereals contain a fair amount of iron.

Iron deficiency can arise not only from insufficient intake but also from poor availability for absorption. Substances in food can form an insoluble complex with food iron. For example, both phytates (alkaline compounds) and iron are present in leafy green vegetables but the phytates, by interacting to reduce acidity, prevent the body from absorbing iron.

Iron in foods of animal origin is better absorbed than that of plant origin. For example, 11 percent of iron from chicken is absorbed, while only one percent from spinach is absorbed. Generally, the body only absorbs 2–10 percent of iron from food.

The recommended allowances for iron at different ages are included in table 1.3. These figures assume that approximately 10 percent of the iron in food is absorbed.

Zinc is a component of certain enzymes; it is also involved in the storage and transmission of genetic information.

An adult contains about 1,800 mg. of zinc. High concentrations are present in the pigmented membrane of the eye and in the prostate gland. What zinc does in these tissues has not been clearly established. However, a cancerous prostate gland contains only one-third as much zinc as a normal one. Decreased amounts of zinc in the blood have been found in individuals taking certain drugs, including prednisone, oral contraceptives, and diuretics.

The richest sources of zinc are meat, seafood, nuts, wheat germ, dairy products, peanut butter, chocolate, and oatmeal. Vegetables and fruit are poor sources, and diets rich in fiber, by impairing zinc absorption, could lead to deficiency in people already on a marginally low zinc intake.

The established requirement for zinc is 15 mg. at eleven years of age and older. Diets containing the recommended amounts of animal protein will satisfy zinc needs, but those limited to vegetable protein may need additional wheat germ and nuts.

Copper is needed for several chemical reactions in the body, notably for the development of red blood cells. It is found especially in the liver and brain. Copper deficiency has been found in diseases of the small bowel and kidney, and in severe undernutrition (particularly in kwashiorkor). An ordinary balanced diet should satisfy the body's need for this nutrient (about 2 mgs.) since it is widely available in our food supply.

Much of the body's *iodine* is contained in the thyroid gland. This gland extracts iodide (a compound of iodine) from the blood plasma for it is an essential component of hormones secreted by the thyroid. Lack of thyroid hormone slows the body's chemical reactions. In infants, it slows growth and mental development, leading to cretinism. The need for iodine is somewhat greater in childhood, during the growth spurt of adolescence, and during pregnancy and nursing. Goiter is another consequence of iodine deficiency (see Cancer, page 135).

The iodine content of foods is relatively small and varies widely, but the requirements are minute. Fish is the best source of iodine, especially salt water fish. Iodized salt is now a major source of iodine.

Small amounts of *selenium* are essential to health, but the appropriate amount is critical. A well-balanced diet provides all the selenium needed—about 0.15 mg. a day. Amounts of 2.4 mg. or more a day are ultimately toxic. Grains, organ meats, and seafood are the best dietary sources.

Fluoride has been regarded as an essential nutrient since its importance is established in improving resistance to dental caries. There is also some evidence that fluoride may help prevent or retard the thinning of bones (osteoporosis) that occurs with aging. Dietary intake of fluoride ranges from 0.3 mg. in low-fluoride areas to 3.1 mg. in high-fluoride areas. The fluoride content of food varies widely according to where it is grown. Foods also absorb the mineral when cooked in fluoridated water.

Although very high intakes are toxic, there are no established ill-effects, including higher rates of cancer, when the intake is 1 mg. per day, an amount which has been shown to reduce dental disease to a low level. In certain areas, naturally occurring excess fluoride in the water causes mottled enamel in the permanent teeth of children where intake is several milligrams a day (see chapter 8).

Water

Water is an essential nutrient and by far the most abundant substance in the human body. An adult man has about 40–45 liters (10–12 gallons) representing about 60 percent of his body weight. He loses about 2 1/2 liters of water a day, chiefly in the urine, and as evaporation through the skin, and some through the lungs and in the feces. The

2 1/2 liters is replaced by drinking fluids, from the water present in foods, and by water derived from oxidation (burning) of foods.

Water intake is controlled by the hypothalmus in the brain, which adjusts thirst so as to keep constant the level of dissolved substances, mainly sodium. If we lose large amounts of salt and water, as by working or playing hard in an extremely hot climate, the sodium level in body fluids can fall, leading to weakness, apathy, muscle cramps, and collapse. On rare occasions this must be prevented by taking salt tablets, but only under severe circumstances and under medical direction. Usually hormonal adjustments maintain the body's sodium levels by controlling the rate at which the kidney excretes it.

The water in domestic water supplies is not a single substance, but contains dissolved salts and trace elements, some in nutritionally important amounts. The salts are derived from the soil and rocks through which the water has percolated. These minerals impart different degrees of "hardness" to water. The harder the water, the more lime will deposit in pots and pipes, and the less easily will soap lather. There may also be health implications in water hardness. People living in hard water regions tend to suffer less heart attack and stroke than people in regions where the water is naturally "soft" or is chemically treated to make it soft.

CAFFEINE

Coffee, tea, cola beverages, chocolate, and cocoa all contain caffeine, which stimulates the nervous system, acts on the heart, sometimes causing an increased tendency to abnormal rhythm, and stimulates the production of urine by the kidney. About 60 percent of American adults drink an average of more than two cups of coffee daily. Many people develop a caffeine dependence and feel unwell when abruptly deprived of it.

A small chocolate bar contains about 25 mg. of caffeine and many soft drinks contain from 32–65 mg. of caffeine per 12-ounce can. Thus a 70-pound, 10-year-old child who drinks 4 bottles of cola and eats 3 chocolate bars a day would be taking in proportionately more caffeine than a 170-pound man who drinks 7 cups of instant coffee (each containing 60 mg.) a day. The U.S. Food and Drug Administration limits caffeine in soft drinks to 50 mg. per 10-ounce can. A smaller but often highly significant amount of caffeine is present in over-the-counter drugs.

Caffeine has no nutritional value. Used in moderation, it is not harmful to most people. But excessive consumption of caffeine can lead to insomnia, lack of appetite, restlessness, and increased frequency of urination; in susceptible people it increases heart rate and can cause irregular heartbeats. Some studies have suggested an association between coffee and bladder cancer. This association would appear, however, to be a consequence of the fact that in general coffee drinkers tend to smoke more cigarettes than non-coffee-drinkers do. A causal relationship between cigarette smoking and bladder cancer has been established (see chapter 4).

Recently, epidemiological studies suggested an association between coffee and cancer of the pancreas. More definitive studies are required, however, and the evidence so far should not offset one's decision as to coffee drinking.

Standard average caffeine contents per cup

1. Roasted and ground coffee   85 mg.
2. Instant coffee   60 mg.
3. Tea   59 mg.
4. Cola   35–50 mg.
5. Instant tea   30 mg.
6. Cocoa   6–42 mg.
7. Decaffeinated coffee   3 mg.

There is no known relationship between coffee and other major diseases. But enough is known about its effects to limit its use to moderation.

ALCOHOL

Alcohol is a drug rather than a nutrient. However, it is thought to contribute from 5 to 12 percent of caloric intake in the U.S., and its prominence among beverages justifies its inclusion in the nutrition section. Its effects are dealt with comprehensively in the chapter 2.

The alcohol in beer, wine, and spirits is almost entirely ethyl alcohol (ethanol) formed by fermentation of sugar by yeast, and ranges from 3 percent (light beers) to more than 43 percent (liquors) of these beverages. It is used by the body for production of energy, yielding almost twice as many calories as the same weight of carbohydrate or protein. Alcohol contributes to obesity in some people, not only because of the calories directly obtained from it, but also because it appears to stimulate appetite.

FOOD ADDITIVES AND FOOD CONTAMINANTS

Additives are nonnutrient chemicals intentionally added to food to enhance its taste or appearance, to preserve it, and, in general, to make it more acceptable to the consumer.

The use of additives in food processing has a long history, beginning with the salting of meat for preservation, and has reached a high level of technological sophistication. Some 3,000 individual chemicals or mixtures are used in modern processing. In technologically developed countries, nearly all commonly eaten foods undergo some form of processing before they are consumed. Food processing technology is an integral, perhaps essential, feature of contemporary society. It would take more time and effort than most people are prepared to spend to construct a daily diet totally devoid of additives. In fact, such diets may not be more wholesome since they contain mold toxins and similar contaminants that additives are designed to counteract.

For the most part, additives are innocuous substances, but some have come under suspicion. Their use is carefully scrutinized by regulatory bodies. Serious issues are raised by the use of chemicals such as residues of pesticides, or contaminants that get into food indirectly and accidently. The kind of problem involved was dramatized by the widespread use of DDT, a chlorinated hydrocarbon and a powerful and very effective pesticide that has a long-term persistence in the environment. Eventually every item of food—plant or animal—was discovered to contain traces of DDT. The chemical is still found in the fatty tissues of people more than ten years after its use was sharply curtailed. Most pesticides currently used are less persistent but are often more acutely toxic and require more care in handling and spraying.

Other very effective specialized agricultural chemicals of the pesticide-insecticide class are similar chlorinated hydrocarbons. These include products such as Mirex, used to control fire ants in the southern United States; chlordane, effective termite control; or aldrin, used in treatment of plants normally eaten raw. Some of these products enter the environment, and, because of acutely sensitive chemical analytical technology, can be readily detected in trace amounts. Animal tests have shown that some of the chlorinated hydrocarbons can induce liver tumors in mice. Therefore, some of these products are used only for specific applications in order to avoid large-scale human contact as when used on vegetables.

Pesticides are considered essential in modern farming to produce large yields of wholesome produce, free of pests and worms. However, when improperly applied, excessive residual pesticide sometimes ends up in food products. In the United States, the federal Food and Drug Administration (FDA) regulates and controls food additives and contaminants, and in general, seeks to ensure a wholesome food supply. The FDA requires that intentional additives be used to achieve specific purposes and that the conditions under which their use is permitted be restricted to those purposes.

Intentional additives have many uses:

- Preservatives and antimicrobial agents to increase the wholesomeness or shelf-life of foods; some inhibit the growth of microorganisms. Examples are: calcium propionate added to bread and rolls, sulfur dioxide in preserved fruits, and sodium nitrate, the principal preservative for processed meat.

- Antioxidants to prevent rancidity of fats and discoloration, e.g., butylated hydroxytoluene (BHT), butylated hydroxyanisole (BHA), propyl gallate, and EDTA. The natural substance alpha tocopherol (vitamin E) has antioxidant properties and is also extensively used.

- Emulsifiers and vehicles or solvents to prevent the separation of oil and water in such products as mayonnaise, peanut butter, ice cream. Examples are: mono- and diglycerides, lecithin, polysorbate 60, sorbitan monostearate, and propylene glycol.

- Thickeners and gums to impart a desired texture, e.g., carrageenan, modified starches, methyl cellulose, sodium alginate, guar gum, and pectins. Foods in which they are used include canned soups and gravies, ice cream, puddings, salad dressing, sour cream, soft drinks, and beer.

- Acids, alkalis, and buffering agents to adjust and maintain the acidity of foods, and to serve as flavorings, antioxidants, and leavening agents. They are added to baked goods, gelatin desserts, processed cheeses, cocoa, baking powder, and ketchup. Examples are vinegar, cream of tartar, fumaric acid, carbonic acid, calcium citrate, sodium bicarbonate, and sodium hydroxide.

- Natural and synthetic flavoring agents and flavor potentiators include natural products such as citric acid, mannitol, and sorbital, dextrins and vanillin. Primary examples of flavor enhancers are monosodium glutamate (MSG) and hydrolyzed vegetable protein (HVP). Saccharin and cyclamates are additives whose safety is under debate, as discussed below.

- Coloring agents are often synthetic chemicals, e.g., FD&C Red No. 40. Natural coloring agents are beta-carotene (analogous to vitamin A) used to color margarine, ferrous gluconate in black olives, or beet juice.

The safety of some additives is sometimes a highly controversial issue. For example, the food and cosmetic dye, FD&C Red No. 2, has been declared unsafe in the United States on the basis of still controversial animal tests but is allowed on the market in Canada and in several other countries. On the other hand, the closely related FD&C Red No. 40 is banned in Canada but allowed in the United States.

Saccharin and cyclamates are artificial sweeteners that have been investigated as possible risk factors for bladder cancer in humans. In 1969, one test of cyclamates in rats showed an increased number of bladder cancers compared with the control animals. Thus, cyclamate was banned in the United States, though not in Canada. Since that time, several tests of cyclamate have not confirmed the original finding.

On the basis of experiments in which both the mother and the offspring were fed high doses of saccharin, and where an increased incidence of bladder cancer in male offspring was found, saccharin was banned for use in diet soft drinks in Canada, although not in the United States. In more recent experiments, animal data and laboratory tests have suggested that saccharin acts principally as a tumor promoter, that is, it enhances the tumor growth of cells initiated by a carcinogen. A characteristic of promoters is that their action depends highly on their concentration and continued long-term use, in contrast to potent carcinogens, where short-term exposure may lead to cancer.

It is for that reason, perhaps not surprising, that epidemiologic research on bladder cancer does not show a consistent increase of risk for human users of saccharin either in terms of pill and droplet form, or when taken in diet drinks. This is so when measured alone or when studied in cigarette smokers who do have an increased risk for bladder cancer. As yet, we do not have data on what happens to young children who drink a great number of diet drinks and who continue to do so most of their lives, nor what happens to pregnant women who consume diet drinks.

Since cyclamate does not have a slightly bitter aftertaste as does saccharin, a mixture of cyclamate and saccharin would provide a better sweetening compound while using a considerably smaller amount of saccharin and might be the best way to replace sugar in food and drinks. The fact that both diabetics, who use an unusually high amount of sweetener, and obese people, who use more artificial sweeteners than people of normal weight, do not have an increased risk of bladder cancer lends support to the present finding that sweeteners, as used so far, do not measurably increase the risk for bladder cancer.

The food preservative *nitrite* has also aroused conflicting views. Before the advent of effective refrigeration, pickling and salting (including the use of large amounts, up to 5,000 parts per million of nitrites and nitrates such as saltpeter) were traditional ways of preserving fish, meats, and certain vegetables. But nitrite reacts with chemicals often present in food to form cancer-inducing nitrosamines and nitrosamides. Current use limits nitrite to some meats or fish at levels of 80 to 160 parts per million. Small amounts of vitamins C or E inhibit the formation of nitrosamines and regulations now require that vitamin C be used together with nitrite in the treatment of pork and in the production of bacon.

Stomach cancer, which has been linked with nitrosamides, is becoming rarer in most Western countries. Perhaps the amount of refrigeration, increased use of fresh fruits and vegetables that provide vitamin C, and decreased use of pickling have contributed to this.

The potential for nitrite to form cancer-causing nitrosamines must be balanced against its benefits, particularly the prevention of the grave disease botulism.

Table 1.12
GUIDELINES FOR BODY WEIGHT

	Metric					WEIGHT	
	Men Weight (kg)[a]			**Women** Weight (kg)[a]			
Height[a] (m)	**Average**	**Acceptable weight range**		**Average**	**Acceptable weight range**		**KG LB**
1.45				46.0	42	53	150 340
1.48				46.5	42	54	140 320
1.50				47.0	43	55	130 300
1.52				48.5	44	57	120 280
1.54				49.5	44	58	110 260
1.56				50.4	45	58	100 240
1.58	55.8	51	64	51.3	46	59	95 220
1.60	57.6	52	65	52.6	48	61	90 200
1.62	58.6	53	66	54.0	49	62	85 190
1.64	59.6	54	67	55.4	50	64	80 180
1.66	60.6	55	69	56.8	51	65	75 170
1.68	61.7	56	71	58.1	52	66	70 160
1.70	63.5	58	73	60.0	53	67	65 150
1.72	65.0	59	74	61.3	55	69	60 140
1.74	66.5	60	75	62.6	56	70	55 130
1.76	68.0	62	77	64.0	58	72	50 120
1.78	69.4	64	79	65.3	59	74	45 110
1.80	71.0	65	80				40 100
1.82	72.6	66	82				35 95
1.84	74.2	67	84				30 90
1.86	75.8	69	86				25 85
1.88	77.6	71	88				80
1.90	79.3	73	90				75
1.92	81.0	75	93				70 65 60 55 50

	Nonmetric					
	Men Weight (lb)[a]			Women Weight (lb)[a]		
Height[a] (ft, in)	Average	Acceptable weight range		Average	Acceptable weight range	
4 10				102	92	119
4 11				104	94	122
5 0				107	96	125
5 1				110	99	128
5 2	123	112	141	113	102	131
5 3	127	115	144	116	105	134
5 4	130	118	148	120	108	138
5 5	133	121	152	123	111	142
5 6	136	124	156	128	114	146
5 7	140	128	161	132	118	150
5 8	145	132	166	136	122	154
5 9	149	136	170	140	126	158
5 10	153	140	174	144	130	163
5 11	158	144	179	148	134	168
6 0	162	148	184	152	138	173
6 1	166	152	189			
6 2	171	156	194			
6 3	176	160	199			
6 4	181	164	204			

[a]Height without shoes, weight without clothes.

SOURCE: adapted from "Obesity in America", (George A. Bray, ed.) U.S. Dept. of Health, Education and Welfare (now Department of Health and Human Services), Public Health Service, National Institutes of Health. November, 1979.

The synthetic hormone *diethylstilbestrol (DES)* has been used as a growth promoter in cattle since it has been found that cattle will grow faster with less feed when injected or fed relatively small amounts. The safety of eating meat from DES-treated cattle has been questioned because the direct exposure of humans to large doses of DES as a drug has caused some specific cancers (see Chapter 3). It is now known that hormones taken in large amounts for a long period of time, or exposure of the fetus to high levels of hormones, constitutes a cancer risk. It is also true that small amounts that do not significantly alter the normal hormone balance of humans do not usually lead to cancer. Its large-scale continued use as a drug to prevent threatened abortions, in doses of 5,000 mg., or more, the drug, presents a risk. However, the content of DES in the liver of cattle treated with DES as a growth promoter amounts, at the most, to a few parts per billion, which is not likely to pose any risk. The muscle or meaty parts of treated animals contains even less DES than liver. Nonetheless, the old practice of adding DES to the cattle feed, which led to the potential exposure of farm workers to relatively large amounts, may be harmful to these people. The current practice of injecting cattle with DES is much safer.

In the last twenty years, a number of specific powerful toxins produced by molds growing on certain foods have been discovered and identified. Proper harvesting and fungicide treatment of grains, peanuts, and other crops greatly reduces the occurrence of excessive amounts of such contaminants. An example is *aflatoxin*. This toxin, a mixture of four chemicals, can cause severe liver damage in humans, and is an extremely powerful cause of liver cancer in rats. Primary liver cancer (cancer that originates in the liver rather than spreads to it) in the United States has decreased markedly over the last eighty years. During the same time, contamination of the U.S. food supply with such toxins has also decreased. Such a decrease could, of course, be due to changes in other nutritional components leading to a better nutritional balance in the American food supply that could avoid or inhibit primary liver cancer. The FDA rejects any crop or food contaminated by more than 15 parts per billion of aflatoxin B_1, the most toxic of the four known aflatoxins. In this case the FDA permits a "threshold level" since without it many food crops could not be consumed. We see no danger for humans in this measure.

Nutrition in Disease

OBESITY AND UNDERNUTRITION

Obesity (not always synonymous with overweight) is the most common nutritional disorder in developed countries. While the social and cosmetic benefits of controlling weight are obvious, the damaging effects of obesity on health are far more serious.

Obesity means an excess of fat (adipose) tissue. As the amount of adipose tissue varies widely in apparently healthy people, a general definition of ideal weight or obesity is not easy. As life span is affected by weight, the best concept of ideal weight is that weight, in proportion to a particular height, that best promotes longevity. The weights shown in table 1.12 are ideal or desirable by this definition. If body weight is 20 percent or more above these figures, expected life span is measurably reduced; hence an excess weight of 20 percent or more constitutes medically significant obesity. On average, the chance of dying is increased by one-third in men aged fifteen to sixty-nine years who are obese by this standard.

Here are a few facts about people who are prone to obesity:

- About one in eight school children are obese, and 58 percent of them will become obese adults.

- Natural and adopted children whose parents are both obese are also likely to be obese. Obesity even in one parent increases the chance of the child being obese. To some extent this tendency seems to be inherited, but the influence of home environment is very important.

- In people of higher socioeconomic status, obesity is less common in women and slightly more common in men, compared with people of lower socioeconomic status.

- Only about 1.6 percent of obese people are fat because of an underlying cause such as a thyroid or adrenal glands disorder.

The overweight are prone to many illnesses—fatal, incapacitating, or simply uncomfortable. High blood pressure, with its potential consequences such as stroke and heart attack is one; it is especially likely to develop in people who gain weight during adult life. Heart attack risk is also enhanced because obese people tend to have high levels of blood cholesterol and blood fat and low levels of the apparently protective high-density lipoprotein (HDL) cholesterol. The risk of diabetes, which in turn may affect the heart, circulation, nerves, eyes, and kidneys, is increased in obese adults. Certain forms of cancer are more common in overweight people. These include cancer of the endometrium (interior wall of the uterus) and gallbladder, as well as cancer of the kidneys in women. The risk of gallstones and arthritis, venous thrombosis, and chronic bronchitis are all increased. Overweight persons frequently are accident-prone and are at increased risk of complications following surgery. Obesity, if pronounced, carries a severe social stigma and can also cause psychological as well as physical problems.

Weight control at different ages

We are especially prone to become overweight at certain times of life: in infancy, early childhood, adolescence, pregnancy, and early middle age. At each of these stages a number of social, cultural, environmental, and hereditary factors interact. It is known that the number of fat cells in adipose tissue is established during childhood and adolescence. One theory suggests that an excessive number of fat cells attained during these periods predisposes the adult to obesity; however, this supposition has not yet been backed by sufficient evidence.

Infancy　The breast-fed infant largely regulates its own caloric intake, which may vary from day to day. But bottle-feeding is regulated to a great extent by the person feeding the infant. Frequently the infant is subtly encouraged to empty the bottle, for, unfortunately, it is wrongly believed that a chubby baby is a healthy baby.

Overweight in infants may also be fostered by introducing solid foods before the age of four to six months. Strained baby food meats, egg yolks, or desserts have a higher "caloric density" than the volume of milk the food replaces. This means, for example, that a half cup of baby food yields more calories than the equivalent amount of milk. Some solid foods fed to babies, especially formula-fed babies, may stimulate thirst that is then likely to be quenched with another bottle of formula.

Overfeeding may also reflect the mother's inability to differentiate between signs of hunger in the infant and other sources of restlessness, crying, or discomfort, including thirst, for which water is required, not food.

Infants vary in their level of physical activity. One theory is that the quiet, inactive, and placid ones may gain weight rapidly with a moderate amount of food, while other infants who are very active from birth do not appear to gain as rapidly. Overweight infants do tend to set a weight pattern for their adult years, creating a lifetime problem of overweight. Obesity even in infancy should be avoided.

Early childhood　In early childhood (2–5 years) children usually become picky about food. They should be offered a wide variety of foods, frequently but in small portions, to ensure a balanced diet. They should not be given too many snacks, foods of high-caloric, low-nutrient density, or be encouraged to eat too rapidly. Children should never be forced to eat, nor should food ever be used as a reward or incentive.

Activity level is also an important factor in childhood weight. Overweight children do not necessarily eat more than others, but they may put on weight because they are less active than their ideal weight counterparts. Whether or not this is a major cause of obesity, there is no doubt that it helps it to persist.

Fat children tend to have a poor self-image and an expectation of rejection. Often they are rejected from social activities and tend to make fewer friends. Early overweight appears to create a vicious cycle.

Adolescence　Adolescence, like the first year of life, is a period of rapid growth when there is danger of overweight. Sex differences in the amount of fatty tissue and its placement emerge during adolescence. Boys who have been overweight often lose weight easily to become lean adolescents. During the adolescent years girls come to have about twice as much body fat as boys. Such changes are believed to be under hormonal control.

The psychological problems typical of this age can contribute to weight problems. Peer-group attitudes to food become increasingly influential. Adolescents must adjust to their new body and many who are overweight develop a poor self-image that they carry into their adult lives. Excessive weight can have profound effects on their emotional well-being. Some overweight adolescents develop a defeatist attitude, withdraw from social and physical activities, and develop unrestrained eating habits as a consolation. Or they may eat little during the day but devour calorie-rich, nutritionally poor food after school and on until late in the evening.

Conversely, some teenage girls strive for an excessive degree of slimness, which leads to an erratic and unbalanced diet with alternating periods of indulgence and denial. They are vulnerable to the latest diet fad, no matter how ill-advised.

Diet treatments for obesity in childhood and adolescence need careful judgment to permit growth and development while diminishing fat stores.

Adulthood As people enter their adult years and their lifestyles change, they become increasingly sedentary with a marked reduction in energy needs. Adult obesity most often commences between the ages of 20 to 30. Food intake increasingly revolves around social events and business activities; hence, eating becomes largely divorced from meeting biological needs and from satisfying appetite. For many Americans, alcohol becomes a substantial source of calories. In middle age eating all too often becomes a response to boredom. After childbirth, mothers often do not lose the weight gained in pregnancy. All in all, caloric intake ceases to be adjusted to energy expenditure, while energy output tends to diminish. In addition, the calorie needs of men and women for maintaining the basic life processes becomes gradually smaller as they age.

Dealing with overweight or the threat of it has become a major industry in this country. Each year a new, "instant" cure or fad diet appears—high-protein, high-fat, low-carbohydrate, single foods, liquid protein, or something else. Often the diet seems to work for a week or two. *But if any of these highly selective diets worked over the long term, the demands for new ones would cease.* Many fad diets obtain their reputations because they lead to an initial rapid weight loss;

in fact this loss is due chiefly to a mere loss of water, rather than from the needed reduction in fatty tissue. There is always the risk, too, that fad diets may be nutritionally unbalanced or that they may be misinterpreted by the uninformed dieter.

One group of popular reducing diets emphasizes foods high in protein, including animal protein, such as steaks, hamburgers, and lamb. Since these foods are high in saturated fats, such diets tend to raise blood cholesterol levels in susceptible individuals if this pattern of eating becomes established; this, in turn, increases the risk of heart disease (see page 106).

High-fat diets can cause an abnormal state called ketosis in the body, in which ketones, the end products of fatty-acid metabolism, accumulate in the blood and urine.

Another group of diets restricts the intake of carbohydrates while also limiting calories. This diet involves counting calories and grams of carbohydrates. When the carbohydrates are restricted, the dieter may seek fatty foods to satisfy the appetite.

There are also single food diets restricting the dieter to one or a limited number of foods such as grapefruit or bananas. Any diet that excludes a major food group will almost automatically decrease caloric intake and cause weight loss. *But these short-term, popular reducing diets are nutritionally unbalanced. Their profoundly important disadvantage is that they do not teach changes in dietary patterns and eating habits that last a lifetime. The lost weight is therefore likely to be regained when the diet is stopped. Avoid regimes that involve short-term radical changes in diet patterns.*

Suggestions for preventing overweight

People become overweight because they eat more food energy (calories) than their bodies require. The only sensible way to lose weight and keep it off permanently is to change the body's energy balance—to take in fewer calories by eating less and to expend more calories in physical activity.

Within a period of three to four weeks a person can be rewarded by a better appearance, better exercise capacity, and a sense of achievement.

The recommended plan for weight reduction and healthy eating habits is called the American Health Foundation Food Plan. (see page 158). It provides a nutritionally balanced regimen containing adequate proteins, fats (an equivalent combination of all three fatty acids), and carbohydrates (mostly complex), restricting food energy to match an individual's energy needs. For the obese person, food energy is further restricted until desirable body weight is reached. As outlined below, these eating patterns can be followed for a lifetime.

Treating obesity

The best diets are designed to let you lose 1–2 pounds per week. It may seem slow, but this is a rate you can maintain without becoming weak, fatigued, or irritable, and the weight loss will be permanent. The biochemical changes, including ketosis, rapid water loss, and loss of body protein that often accompany crash dieting will not occur. The steady loss of weight is due to the using up of fats stored in adipose tissue rather than to the loss of water, and the body's protein (chiefly in muscle tissue) is conserved because the diet is a balanced one. First, see the height/weight chart for your ideal body weight (table 1.12, pages 122–123). Then, follow the formula on page 160 for determining the caloric requirement for maintaining your ideal or desired weight.

Remember, a surplus of 250 calories per day, only 10 percent or so above needs, leads to an average gain of a pound of fat tissue in two weeks. At this rate, although people vary widely, in less than a year the normal amount of body fat will double, with an average weight gain of about 26 pounds. The principle of all successful reducing diets therefore, is to reverse this process. If you are very sedentary, you should choose a lower calorie diet than if you are active (see pages 161–170 for specific dietary plans at various calorie levels). It will take three to four days to get used to the diet, but you must persist. Make small gradual changes that you can stay with rather than overwhelming ones.

If you are more than twenty-five pounds overweight or have diabetes, heart trouble, or digestive problems, get your physician's approval before starting.

Foods such as vegetables, fruit, cereals, fish, and lean meat are satisfying and pleasurable; they provide far fewer calories than the same bulk of processed foods such as candies, cake, and pies. Do not keep the latter foods on hand where they will be accessible and tempting.

Couple your diet with a planned change in your eating patterns:

Eat only at mealtimes.

Never eat seconds.

Avoid bread, rolls, or crackers.

Slow down your pace of eating.

Stop eating before you feel full.

Put utensils down after each bite; chew and swallow each bite before cutting more food.

Never eat during an absorbing activity such as reading, watching television, or attending sports events.

Take small mouthfuls.

Leave the table as soon as you have finished.

Make smaller portions visually satisfying by using smaller plates and glasses. To help avoid cues for overeating:

> Store food in opaque containers or otherwise out of sight.
>
> Clear serving dishes from the table as soon as everyone has been served.
>
> Clear scraps immediately.
>
> Shop from a list and on a full stomach.

Put obstacles between the impulse to eat and actual eating so that there is time for you to reflect on whether you really need to eat. Always eat your food from a plate and drink all beverages from a glass. Never eat or drink from a serving box or container (unless, of course, you're eating out). Prepare only the number of portions needed for the meal.

Pack a suitable lunch instead of eating in restaurants. Minimize social occasions when the pressures to eat and drink are strong. Decide ahead of time what and how much you are going to eat and drink on such occasions.

Incorporate small, frequent increases in physical activity into your daily life: always walk a flight or two of stairs; park your car at a distance from your destination and walk (see chapter 5).

See figure 1.3 to determine how much exercise is necessary to burn up food calories of selected foods. For example, *an average person would have to walk vigorously for almost 1 1/2 hours to offset the calories consumed in one 12 oz. chocolate milk shake; a glass of skim milk is equivalent in calories to only 6 minutes of walking.*

Some people have unusually low energy needs because of inactivity or more subtle, little-understood biochemical reasons. To keep their weight constant such people have to eat less than average; and if they are overweight they will need a particularly low-calorie diet to lose weight. Such a diet should be supervised by a physician and/or nutritionist. But people whose metabolism works this way will still shed weight on an appropriate diet.

Problems of underweight

Anorexia nervosa A serious psychological disturbance, anorexia nervosa is mainly seen in adolescent girls who become emaciated from self-starvation. Severe anorexia can be fatal. It is thought that many anorexic girls, fearing puberty and the consequences of growing up, attempt to avert these changes by remaining a child. They avoid food and vomit if forced to eat. Often they cease menstruating. Anorexic behavior is also a way in which an adolescent can exert control over her environment. Treatment usually incorporates both nutritional and psychological therapy. It is prolonged and difficult, but can be effective. A less severe form of anorexia is an overresponse to social pressures favoring slenderness; this is easier to treat.

Protein/calorie malnutrition

Protein/calorie malnutrition is an infant disease caused by diets low in protein and calories. One example, kwashiorkor, is a major cause of often fatal illnesses in underdeveloped societies; it is primarily due to poverty and ignorance. There is evidence, not universally accepted, that some of those who recover from it may be left with irreversible mental damage. Protein/calorie malnutrition when seen in more privileged societies is secondary to other diseases or in children from families practicing extreme dietary eccentricities.

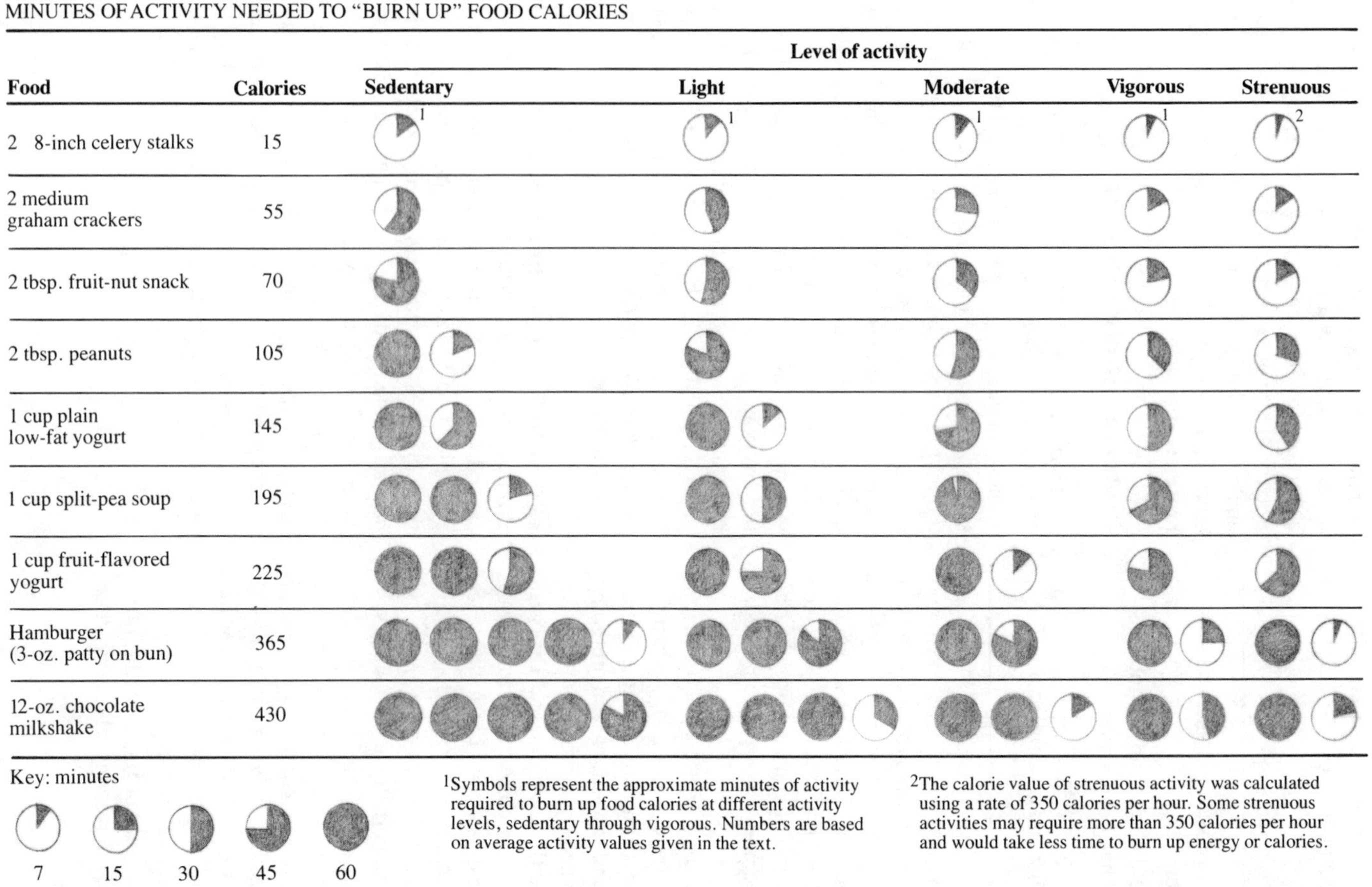

MINUTES OF ACTIVITY NEEDED TO "BURN UP" FOOD CALORIES

Food	Calories	Level of activity				
		Sedentary[1]	Light[1]	Moderate[1]	Vigorous[1]	Strenuous[2]
2 8-inch celery stalks	15					
2 medium graham crackers	55					
2 tbsp. fruit-nut snack	70					
2 tbsp. peanuts	105					
1 cup plain low-fat yogurt	145					
1 cup split-pea soup	195					
1 cup fruit-flavored yogurt	225					
Hamburger (3-oz. patty on bun)	365					
12-oz. chocolate milkshake	430					

Key: minutes   7   15   30   45   60

[1]Symbols represent the approximate minutes of activity required to burn up food calories at different activity levels, sedentary through vigorous. Numbers are based on average activity values given in the text.

[2]The calorie value of strenuous activity was calculated using a rate of 350 calories per hour. Some strenuous activities may require more than 350 calories per hour and would take less time to burn up energy or calories.

FIGURE 1.3

Calories and activity level

SOURCE: *adapted from "Food," Home and Garden Bulletin Number 228, U.S. Department of Agriculture*

CARDIOVASCULAR DISEASE

Heart attack and atherosclerosis

In Western countries, heart attack is the most common cause of death in men, especially in middle age; it also affects many women, especially after menopause. Most often, heart attack results from atherosclerosis of the coronary arteries, a patchy thickening of the artery walls from deposits of cholesterol and overgrowth of cells that narrows it and limits blood flow. The amount of cholesterol in the blood and the form in which it is carried in the blood are determining factors in atherosclerosis.

Cholesterol, which is required by the body (see page 107), has to be carried in the bloodstream to the many organs that use it. Since it does not dissolve in water, it is transported in minute soluble particles called lipoproteins, of which there are several forms. One is low-density lipoprotein (LDL), which supplies most parts of the body with cholesterol. Moderate levels of LDL in blood are necessary for health. Unfortunately, many of us have levels well in excess of those required. It appears that the greater the level of LDL in the blood, the greater the rate at which cholesterol is deposited on the walls of the arteries, thus favoring the development of atherosclerosis.

When amounts of these lipoproteins in the blood are excessive, levels of cholesterol or another kind of blood fat called triglyceride—or both—become abnormally high. This is common in many developed Westernized countries such as the U.S.

Another form of lipoprotein, high-density lipoprotein (HDL), has a different and apparently beneficial role. It seems to carry surplus cholesterol away from cells and may promote its excretion from the body. The more HDL there is in the blood, the less the risk of heart attack, perhaps because HDL reduces the tendency for cholesterol to accumulute on the walls of the arteries. This may explain why high LDL levels and low HDL levels both increase the risk of heart attack.

Women have higher levels of HDL than do men. In both sexes, HDL cholesterol levels can be increased by regular physical exercise. HDL levels tend to be low in obese people. During weight reduction they do not change much; but there is evidence that after the weight restabilizes at a lower level, high-density lipoprotein levels rise.

The importance of blood cholesterol and lipoprotein levels is dramatized by comparing populations with differing death rates from heart attack. With few exceptions, the higher the average cholesterol and LDL level, the higher the death rate; both rates are high in the U.S., Scotland, and Finland, for example, and low in Japan, Italy, and Greece.

There are many causes of high levels of cholesterol or triglycerides in the blood plasma. Genes play a part and account partially for the differences between individuals; high or low levels tend to run in families. There are also inherited disorders leading to very high cholesterol or triglyceride levels. These are relatively rare, but because of their severity it is important that they be recognized and treated.

Diet has major effects on blood cholesterol and triglyceride. One important factor is the amount and type of fat in the diet (see page 106). The more saturated fat (hard fats, often derived from animal products, e.g., lard, butter, hard margarine) in the diet, the higher the blood cholesterol level. Conversely, a low-fat diet in which most of the food energy comes from starches and other carbohydrates (in cereals, vegetables, fruit) leads to a low blood cholesterol. Unsaturated fats, which tend to be liquid vegetable oils or soft solids (like soft margarine) also tend to reduce blood cholesterol and blood triglyceride levels; this is especially true of polyunsaturated fats (e.g., corn oil, safflower oil, sunflower oil).

The amount of cholesterol in the diet has an effect on the blood cholesterol. People vary in their sensitivity to food cholesterol but, on average, a low-cholesterol diet will reduce the cholesterol level in the blood. Some types of food fiber also reduce the blood cholesterol—in particular the pectins present in apples, bananas, and most forms of fruit and vegetables. Other protein foods such as skim milk and soybeans have a small cholesterol-lowering effect.

Overweight people have a tendency to higher triglyceride and cholesterol levels, and weight reduction often decreases these levels. Apart from diet, the blood triglyceride and cholesterol levels is increased by diseases such as lack of thyroid hormone, alcoholism, and diabetes. Oral contraceptives tend to increase these levels too.

High cholesterol levels increase the risk of coronary heart disease and of atherosclerosis affecting the legs. In American men, those with blood cholesterol levels at the upper end of the range have a threefold greater risk of heart attack than those at the lower end. Another potential consequence in people with very high blood cholesterol is cholesterol deposits in the tendons (causing lumps on the back of the hands and behind the ankles). Recognizing these lumps helps to recognize the condition, which is readily treated by a physician. The effects of very high triglyceride levels also can include attacks of abdominal pain.

For all these reasons it is well worth knowing your blood cholesterol and triglyceride levels and having them checked regularly. If the results are borderline, the checkup should be repeated every year or two. People who are especially advised to have a cholesterol check are those who have a relative who has had a heart attack, angina, or poor circulation to the legs commencing before the age of sixty years, and those who have a relative with a high cholesterol level. The tendency is partly inherited. A checkup could lead to early diagnosis and treatment, or to a reassuring normal test result. People with diabetes, gout, or high blood pressure should also be checked.

The American Health Foundation sets an optimal blood cholesterol level at 160–180 mg./100 ml (160–180 milligrans per every 100 milliliters of blood); the upper limit is 220 mg./100 ml. Some 40–50 percent of American adults may have levels above this limit. At ages 5–18, the optimal level is 110–140 mg./100 ml. Many children have higher levels than this.

Most people who have heart attacks have two or more risk factors, each relatively mild in degree. The risk to a man with a mildly increased cholesterol of 260 mg./100 ml who smokes moderately (fifteen cigarettes a day) is far higher than the risk for a nonsmoker with a cholesterol of 225 mg./100 ml. Each risk factor strongly enhances the effect of the other risk factors (see figure 1.4).

Other risk factors for heart disease include high blood pressure, untreated diabetes, an aggressive, hurrying, impatient personality, and heredity (the relatives of people who have had a heart attack before age fifty-five years are at somewhat increased risk). Inheritance of this sort increases the chances of having high blood pressure, diabetes, high LDL levels and, perhaps, low HDL levels, all of which put one at a greater risk for heart attack. Obesity is important in that it predisposes one to all these risk factors; they are lessened by shedding surplus weight.

Angina pectoris

Angina, episodes of pain in the chest, arms, and lower jaw, is most often due to atherosclerosis. The narrowing of the coronary arteries is less severe than that which leads to heart attack and so the heart muscle is not irreversibly damaged. The lack of coronary blood flow usually becomes evident when the work of the heart is increased by exercise or cold, but the underlying factors are the same—high blood cholesterol levels, high blood pressure, diabetes, cigarette smoking, and others. In addition, obesity, smoking, and anemia make angina worse by increasing the work required of the heart.

Rates shown are for a group of 7,328 white men over a 10-year period, aged 30-59 at entry in Pooling Project

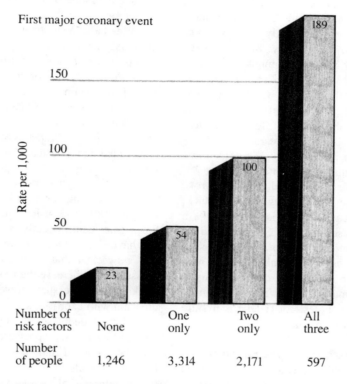

First major coronary event

Rate per 1,000

Number of risk factors	None	One only	Two only	All three
Number of people	1,246	3,314	2,171	597

Risk factors: Blood cholesterol more than 250 mg/dl.
Diastolic blood pressure more than 90 mmHg.
Any use of cigarettes (at entry)

FIGURE 1.4

Heart attack rate increases in relation to number of risk factors
SOURCE: *adapted from Inter-Society Commission for Heart Disease Resources. Atherosclerosis Study Group and Epidemiology Study Group. "Primary Prevention of Atherosclerotic Diseases." Circulation 42, A55, 1970, and Letter to the A.H.A. Journal 94, 539–540 (1977)*

Stroke

Stroke, a common cause of death and disability in many countries, can be due to a rupture of a fine blood vessel in the brain leading to hemorrhage in the brain or, particularly in the Western world, to blockage of an artery. Such blockage may be caused by a clot (thrombus) consisting of a plug of minute blood cells called platelets; it deprives part of the brain of its blood supply. Often the clot forms on an artery affected by atherosclerosis. A thrombus can form elsewhere and be carried in the bloodstream to the brain where it lodges in a tiny artery. Thrombi often form in the heart during a heart attack.

The factors that increase the risk of stroke are similar to those predisposing to heart attack, though not identical. High blood pressure is a very important cause of stroke. Smoking and diabetes increase the risk. Although the level of blood cholesterol is only weakly linked with stroke, the form in which it is carried seems to be important; in many stroke victims the high-density lipoprotein cholesterol (HDL) is usually low, as in patients with heart attack.

High blood pressure (hypertension)

An estimated 23 million adults in the United States have high blood pressure and until recently no more than 50 percent knew they were affected. Hypertension seldom produces symptoms until complications develop.

Hypertension occurs twice as frequently in blacks as in whites, particularly among children. More white women than white men are hypertensive. The frequency increases with age in the United States and similar countries, with the largest number being between 55–64 years. In other countries this rise with age is not seen; high blood pressure is not a normal consequence of aging. Nor is it seen in areas where dietary intake of salt is low.

High blood pressure increases the risk of heart attack and stroke. When very high, it can damage the kidneys and impair vision by injuring the retina.

When the heart beats, blood pressure rises to a maximum (the systolic pressure), the pressure then decreases to a minimum (the diastolic pressure). Although the normal range of blood pressure differs with age, a typical pressure in a healthy adult would be 120 mm. of mercury systolic and 75 mm. diastolic, usually written 120/75. When the fine branches of the arteries become constricted the resistance to blood flow is increased; as a result, blood pressure rises. If this is persistent, high blood pressure is diagnosed; a typical reading for high blood pressure would then be 180/110. A level of 145/95 would be borderline. Until recently, such a pressure would not have been thought to require treatment; but it is now clear that even a minimal increase in pressure may increase the risk of heart disease or stroke. Blood pressure, however, is variable, increasing with exertion, anger, or fear, and during digestion; it decreases during rest and sleep. A single elevated blood pressure reading is no cause for alarm, but it should be checked further at regular intervals.

A minority of people have high blood pressure as a consequence of other diseases, such as chronic kidney disease, hormone-producing tumors of the adrenal gland, or congenital narrowing (coarctation) of the aorta, the large artery leaving the heart. Drugs such as cortisone and prednisone, and in some women the oral contraceptive pill, can cause high blood pressure. One group of drugs used to treat depression, the amine oxidase inhibitors, can interact with foods such as cheese and yeast extract to cause severely raised blood pressure.

In most people with high blood pressure, however, three or four major factors are believed to operate:

First, high blood pressure tends to run in families; thus relatives of people with the condition should have blood pressure checks as often as the physician advises.

Second, obesity is often associated with high blood pressure; weight reduction often ameliorates it. There is also impressive evidence that people who become obese during early adult life have an increased chance of developing high blood pressure in middle age.

Third, the sodium in salt is linked with blood pressure. Most people eat much more salt than is good for them, and in susceptible persons (and in laboratory animals) it increases blood pressure.

Fourth, it is widely believed that stress leads to high blood pressure. There is no doubt that blood pressure rises temporarily during stress situations, but it is less clear that persisting high blood pressure is the result of stress (see chapter 7, Stress).

DIABETES

A lack of insulin, the substance that keeps blood sugar levels within normal ranges, is a major cause of diabetes. In this condition, affecting one adult in fifty, an excess of sugar (glucose) is found in the bloodstream, constantly or after eating. Sugar may also be present in the urine.

Glucose is used by the brain and other parts of the body to produce energy. It is derived from starch and sugar in the diet and from protein. Between meals it is secreted by the liver.

The most common form of diabetes occurs in middle age and in the elderly. This form is often inherited, with obesity as a very common predisposing factor. For obese diabetics, losing weight tends to restore the body's responsiveness to insulin. Diabetics are also especially prone to cardiovascular illness—heart attack, stroke, and high blood pressure. The eyes, kidneys, and nerves are prone to damage if diabetes is not carefully controlled.

Control of diabetes requires correction of obesity, and an evenly spaced, moderate intake of carbohydrate, such as starch, plus an avoidance of sugar. Insulin injections or blood-sugar lowering drugs may be needed. Pectin-type fiber (in vegetables and fruit) is recommended by some diabetes experts to stabilize the blood glucose level. Exercise may also aid in diabetes control but needs to be regular; insulin dosage is influenced by exercise habits.

CANCER

That diet plays a part in causing human cancer is suggested by the following statistical observations:

1. the differing rates of cancer incidence in different countries with different eating habits;
2. the altered rates of cancer occurrence in migrants from a country with a low rate of a particular cancer to one with a high rate of such cancer, and vice versa;
3. the cancer rates in populations with particular dietary habits;
4. the time trends of cancer incidence.

Most persuasive are the sharp differences in cancer rates between Japan and the U.S. (figure 1.5). These differences appear to be largely due to lifestyle (environment) since the rate changes among Japanese migrants to the United States. In fact, cancer rates are currently changing in Japan as the Japanese have moved in the last 20–30 years toward the Western style of diet.

Cancer of the oral cavity, larynx, and esophagus

Cancers of these three sites are closely linked in Western countries with both smoking and chewing tobacco and with high alcohol intake (see chapters 2 and 4). They may also be related to certain nutritional deficiencies. Alcohol could increase the risk of these cancers by leading to

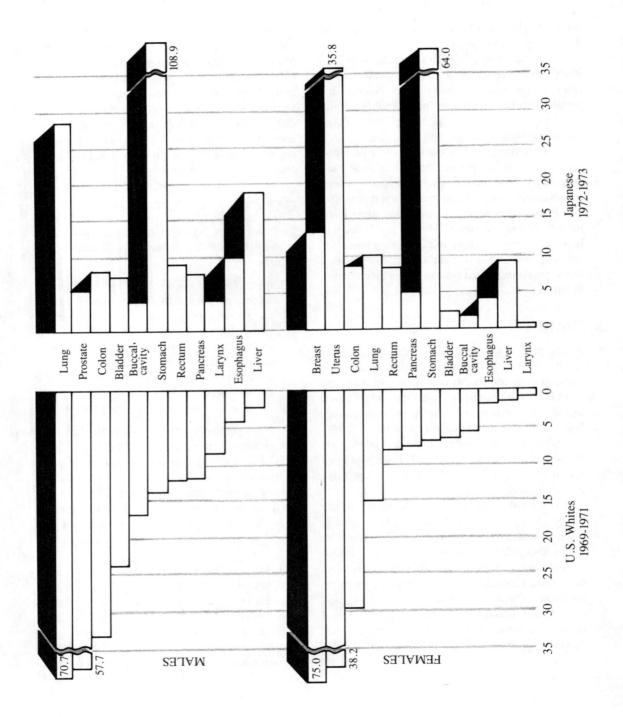

Japanese 1972-1973

Lung, Prostate, Colon, Bladder, Buccal cavity, Stomach, Rectum, Pancreas, Larynx, Esophagus, Liver

108.9

Breast, Uterus, Colon, Lung, Rectum, Pancreas, Stomach, Bladder, Buccal cavity, Esophagus, Liver, Larynx

35.8

64.0

U.S. Whites 1969-1971

MALES

70.7

57.7

FEMALES

75.0

38.2

FIGURE 1.5

Age-adjusted incidence rates for selected cancers for United States whites (1969–1971) and Japanese (1972–1973) by sex
SOURCE: *adapted from E.L. Wynder and T. Hirayama, "Special Report, Comparative Epidemiology of Cancers of the United States and Japan,"* Preventive Medicine 6, 1977

nutritional deficiencies, particularly of the vitamin B group.

Animal studies show that long-term lack of iron and riboflavin (B_2) leads to alterations in the cells lining the upper digestive and respiratory tracts, and it is thought that this applies to humans as well. In northern Sweden, cancers in these areas used to be relatively common, particularly in the mouth, perhaps because of low intake of iron and of fresh fruits and vegetables. With iron and vitamins now added to the flour in Sweden, such cancers are less common.

In some parts of China and around the Caspian Sea in Iran, as well as in the Transkei in southeastern Africa, a very high incidence of cancer of the esophagus is found. No specific cause has yet been discovered, although the very low intake of fruits and vegetables in these areas is thought to play a role.

Breast cancer

Breast cancer is the leading cause of cancer deaths among women in the United States and other developed nations. Although it occurs in men too, it is a hundred times more common in women, affecting one out of fifteen.

A disease so common is likely to result from factors that are widespread in the population. Research has as yet not revealed anything, with the possible exception of diet, that could explain the variation in occurrence of breast cancer among different people in the world. Total calories do not seem to play a role since most studies do not show an association of breast cancer with obesity.

Current research suggests that the total amount of fat in the diet, which in the United States accounts for 40–50 percent of daily calorie intake, relates to breast cancer development. Animal studies demonstrate that with chemically induced cancer in rats and mice, those animals on a high-fat diet (also 40 percent of calories) have enhanced breast tumor growth compared to animals on a lower fat diet (10 percent of calories). A high-fat intake increases the levels of the pituitary gland hormone prolactin, which is known to promote breast cancer development in rats. Although estrogen levels are not directly altered by fat, there is a relationship between nutrition and the endocrine system, and it is thought that, since prolactin and estrogen influence each other, changing the relative amounts of each hormone appears to have an effect on the growth of breast cancer cells. How the malignant process is initiated is not yet known. However, a promising line of research is the analysis of breast fluid of nonnursing women.

Whether a low-fat diet will slow down the growth or spread of breast cancer remains to be shown. The better survival of breast cancer patients in Japan, compared with the United States, would suggest that a low-fat diet may be of some benefit. If you have fibrocystic disease of the breast (multiple painful nodules), if breast cancer appears to run in your family (if your mother, sister, or an aunt have had breast cancer), or if you have had no pregnancies, or your first pregnancy after age 30, you have a higher risk for breast cancer. If you are in this category you should place particular emphasis on practicing self-examination of the breasts monthly. Your physician or your community cancer information center can demonstrate this simple technique.

Stomach cancer

Stomach cancer (gastric cancer) affects men more often than women; in U.S. men it is most common between the ages of 50–59. Fifty years ago, stomach cancer was the most common cancer in the U.S.; within the last twenty-five years the incidence has halved.

However, it still ranks high in Japan, some parts of central and western Latin America, and northern and eastern Europe. Migrants from a high-risk region, such as Japan or Scandinavia, to a low-risk region like the United States maintain their risk, even if they have lived in the high-risk area for only ten to fifteen years, indicating that the cancer process starts early in life. The second generation in migrant families acquires the low risk typical of the area of residence, indicating that environment is more important than inheritance.

Populations with a high rate of gastric cancer often have a high intake of nitrate and salt through the pickling of foods, in drinking and cooking water, and in vegetables grown in high nitrate soil. It is possible that nitrate is converted in foods or by metabolism in the mouth to nitrite, which reacts with food constituents in the stomach to produce substances such as nitrosamines that can start stomach cancer.

Since the residual content of nitrites in the liver is already relatively high, it is important that the possible conversion of nitrates to nitrites may be retarded by vitamins C and E, both antagonists of nitrite, particularly when taken in the form of salads, fresh vegetables, and fruits, and especially when taken as part of a meal (see page 110).

Populations prone to stomach cancer have a diet high in carbohydrates (such as rice and potatoes), pickled, salted foods, and low in fresh fruits and vegetables. In general, salt intake seems to be high. The high salt intake yields a parallel higher risk for stomach cancer and hypertension (high blood pressure).

Colon cancer

Cancer of the colon occurs with about equal frequency in men and in women and is one of the most common forms of cancer in the Western world, affecting one out of every fifteen persons.

The fact that this type of cancer is quite uncommon in Japan, other Asian countries, and in most developing societies suggests that environmental factors play a role in its incidence. Because colon cancer mortality rises in the Japanese and in others from low-risk areas when they immigrate to the United States, it would appear that factors in the United States environment are important among its causes. Total calories do not seem to be a factor since obesity does not affect risk for colon cancer.

The main difference between a low-incidence country such as Japan and a Western country is in the average total amount of fat consumed. In Western countries the total fat comes from standard dairy products—whole milk, cheese, butter, ice cream—and from meats such as beef, which provide mostly saturated fats, or from vegetable oils providing unsaturated fats. In this country, the total daily intake of fat accounts for 40–50 percent of calories consumed. In Japan, until recent years, the average diet included few products with saturated fat and the total intake was only 10–20 percent of calories. In the last few years, the Japanese have included more dairy products and some meats in their diet, so that now 20 percent of the calories consumed are from fat.

The colon cancer incidence in the West seems associated with the higher amounts of fat eaten. Laboratory tests on stool samples from people on a Western diet, or from rats on a Western-like diet, reveal more bile acids than in stools from Japanese, or rats on low-fat diets. When given a carcinogen, rats on a high-fat regimen also develop more colon cancer than those on a low-fat regimen, which can be explained by the higher level of cancer-promoting bile acids that are produced by fats.

A low-fiber intake in the diet is also important with regard to cancer of the colon. In Finland, despite a very high intake of fats (mainly from dairy products), there is a fairly low rate of colon cancer. There, the high intake of dietary fiber, three times the level consumed in the United States, leads to an increase in stool bulk. High-fiber bread, particularly whole wheat, is eaten at virtually every meal. It is thought that large stool bulk dilutes the cancer-inducing or cancer-promoting substances. Therefore, it is possible that the risk of this common disease could be lessened by consuming less fat and more fiber as suggested by the American Health Foundation Food Plan (see page 158).

When a cancer-producing substance is given to laboratory animals, its activity can be increased by a high-fat diet, either saturated or unsaturated fat (see page 106). Substances present in fried and broiled meat can induce mutations, although they have not yet been shown to cause cancer in experimental animals.

Prostate cancer

This type of cancer, while common in the U.S., is rare in developing countries, as well as in Japan. Prostate cancer, however, is increasing in Japan along with the increase in dietary fat; hence, diet may prove to play a role in this disease.

In the United States, prostate cancer is particularly common among blacks, in contrast to blacks in Africa, among whom it is quite uncommon. The reasons for this are not clear, although it appears to relate to the effect of dietary fat in the production and retention by the body and/or prostate of certain hormones. Some studies suggest that zinc is especially low in prostate cancer tissue as compared with normal prostate tissue. However, it is not known whether zinc deficiency is a factor causing prostate cancer.

Prostatic enlargement, a particularly common condition in middle-aged and elderly men, has not been shown to be related to prostate cancer, nor is obesity.

Liver cancer

In Western countries liver cancer is associated with prolonged alcoholism, largely as a consequence of cirrhosis (see chapter 2). In certain developing parts of the world where the incidence of liver cancer is quite high, it has been linked to a diet very low in protein and one that is contaminated with aflatoxins (see page 124).

Cancer of the uterus (endometrium)

This cancer, relatively uncommon among the Japanese, increases after they immigrate to the United States. It is also increasing in Japan concurrent with an increase in fat in the diet; hence, there is a possible link between endometrial cancer and nutrition.

Endometrial cancer chiefly affects older women and is strongly associated with overweight. It is thought that this may be caused by the accumulation of the hormone estrogen in fatty tissue and that the cancerous change is promoted by prolonged stimulation of endometrial tissue by estrogens. This is supported by the finding that prolonged and excessive use of estrogen replacement—for menopausal symptoms—increases the risk of cancer of the endometrium.

Miscellaneous

Dietary fat also may increase the risk for the highly fatal cancer of the pancreas. In animal experiments, the amino acid tryptophan has been proven to enhance the growth of bladder cancer produced with a cancer-inducing substance. This suggests that the proteins in high-meat intake, which produce a high level of tryptophan, may contribute to bladder cancer in humans. Areas where iodine deficiency is endemic have a high incidence of thyroid cancer and goiter.

DIVERTICULITIS AND DIVERTICULAR DISEASE

Diverticulitis is a common cause of recurrent abdominal pain and other complaints such as occasional fever, especially in the elderly and in those of middle age. It affects men and women equally and is more frequently encountered in overweight, sedentary persons who report a history of episodes of abdominal pain.

Research in tropical countries has shown how widely the frequency of diverticular disease varies in different communities. The low incidence of diverticular disease is often associated with the high intake of food fiber. Diverticula can develop in the colon of animals given a diet atypically low in fiber.

Diverticula are small saclike pouches that may develop in the large bowel or colon. These multiple pouches protude from the inner lining outward. Their presence does not always produce symptoms or ill-effects in the majority of people who have diverticula. Difficulties, however, can arise in two ways:

It is believed that the diverticula are caused by high pressure occurring within the colon cavity, in areas where strong contractions of the muscular walls take place. This spasm and the high pressure that it causes are believed to explain the symptomatic attacks of pain in the lower abdomen, which are often accompanied by temporary constipation or a narrowing of the stool.

The other, more serious source of illness arises when some of the diverticula become infected and inflamed, leading to more severe pain and slight fever. The pain is made worse by pressure over the affected part of the colon, most often in the lower abdomen or on the left side. Often the attacks recur and serious complications can ensue such as bleeding or perforation of the colon wall.

Diagnosis must be made by a physician, who will obtain X rays and/or perform other tests. The doctor may treat attacks of diverticulitis and their complications in a variety of ways and may also advise an appropriate diet to reduce symptoms and decrease the likelihood of further attacks.

The diet, designed to reduce the pressure within the colon, contains a high intake of fiber (roughage). When one eats a high-fiber diet the stools become softer, passing through the large bowel more easily without high pressures developing. Hence it is plausible to think that the proneness of people in affluent Western societies to diverticular disease is largely due to a deficiency of fiber in their diet. This possibility has not been proven at present, but sufferers from this disease can obtain a large measure of relief from attacks of pain and constipation when they adopt such a diet. In the U.S., average fiber intake is as little as 6 grams per day. It would not be difficult to increase this to 20–40 grams per day by dietary changes.

A relatively high-fiber diet in its various forms may have many advantages. An intake of wheat or bran (half to one ounce per day) improves bowel function in many people with chronic constipation. It is important to note that a high-fiber diet must include adequate liquids.

Such a high-fiber diet may increase the amount of intestinal gas present and the need to pass flatus, which is often only temporary. The need for fiber varies from person to person. If one is undertaking a high-fiber diet it is wise to be sure that any colonic symptoms have first been fully investigated by the physician. It is also wise to eat a diet containing adequate amounts of minerals such as iron, zinc, and calcium (see page 113). A higher fiber diet can lead to lower absorption by the body of essential minerals since they are transported by the fiber to the stool. A well-balanced diet with adequate vegetables, fruits, and nuts is not likely to yield mineral deficiencies even with a higher fiber diet.

GOUT

Gout is a common form of arthritis, especially in men. In 1976, more than 1.5 million Americans suffered from gout.

Gout first appears in acute attacks lasting two to three days with no symptoms in the intervals. These attacks are often extremely painful, typically affecting one joint at a time; the joint becomes red, swollen, and very tender to even a light touch. As the condition is easily treated, it is unfortunate that it is not always recognized promptly. Any joint can be affected: common sites are the base of the big toe, the ankle, knee, and wrist.

More men than women are affected (less than 5 percent of gout patients are women), and inheritance appears to play an important part in its causation. Blacks have a low incidence of gout. In gout, the level of uric acid in the blood rises too high, causing crystals of this rather insoluble substance to form in the joint fluid, bringing on the painful attack. Prevention of gout may require drug treatment to reduce uric acid levels, and includes dietary management.

High uric acid levels are common in heavy drinkers, but in more susceptible people, even moderate amounts of alcohol may have a similar effect. An upper limit is difficult to define but probably should be no more than two drinks per day. Another factor tending to raise the uric acid level is obesity; shedding excess weight often reduces uric acid. In addition, a measure of uric acid reduction can be achieved by avoiding foods such as liver, kidneys, sweetbreads, sardines, and tomatoes. These foods contain purines (protein substances) that are converted to uric acid.

Normal serum uric acid values vary between 3–7 mg./100 ml.

GALLSTONES

Gallstones are exceedingly common—as many as 25–30 percent of women in the U.S. are affected, and approximately 20 percent of the U.S. population over forty. It is more frequently encountered in the developed nations than in the less advanced countries.

Gallstone attacks may cause severe abdominal pain. Biliary colic or a "gallbladder attack," is the result of the painful spasms that occur when a gallstone lodges in the narrow bile duct or gallbladder duct. The pain is felt in the upper abdomen on the right side, and sometimes also in the back; there is usually vomiting and restlessness. A typical attack can last twelve hours or so unless treated. The stone ultimately dislodges or passes on into the bowel and is excreted.

There are many different kinds of gallstones, reflecting different causes. Some stones consist of bile pigments derived from excessive red blood cell breakdown (hemolytic anemia). The other, more common form of gallstones that tend to occur in later life, are composed chiefly of cholesterol (see page 107).

Certain nationalities and ethnic groups are more prone to gallstones of the common, cholesterol variety. American and British people tend to be quite susceptible, while gallstones are rare in Japan and almost unknown in some African countries. Environment appears to play a role.

Another important factor is obesity—obese people are roughly twice as prone to gallstones as lean ones. Use of oral contraceptives, especially after many years, increases the risk, while people with high blood fat levels (high triglycerides) are also prone to cholesterol stones.

We do not know with certainty which environmental factors influence the risk of gallstones. It is widely believed that diet is important, and various theories have involved the lack of fiber or roughage, excess food cholesterol, or fat in the diet.

Probably the most important step in reducing the risk of cholesterol gallstone disease is to avoid obesity, although this is not yet proven; it is known that fat people excrete more cholesterol into their bile than lean people, a condition largely corrected when they shed their excess weight. It is important to try to get rid of excess weight "once and for all" since repeated phases of crash-dieting may actually increase the level of cholesterol in the bile.

As oral contraceptives increase gallstone risk, it is especially necessary to avoid obesity when using the pill. It is probably unwise to continue using the pill beyond the age of thirty-five or forty years. Another drug that increases risk of gallstones, clofibrate, is used to treat high blood fat levels. Because of this side effect of clofibrate, an effort should be made to correct high blood fat levels by dietary means before trying drug treatment.

ANEMIA

Anemia is a below-normal count of the hemoglobin, the iron-containing pigment of the red blood cells. Hemoglobin transports oxygen from the lungs, via the bloodstream, to the tissues of the body. It also helps carry carbon dioxide waste from the tissues in the reverse direction for disposal.

Anemia has many causes; the treatment for one form will not work with another, and can have ill effects. Therefore, it must be diagnosed and classified by a physician.

The most common cause of anemia in developed countries is iron deficiency. Iron deficiency anemia affects persons of all ages, especially pregnant women, infants, adolescents, and older people.

Anemia can result from an inadequate intake of certain vitamins (B_{12}, folic acid, and vitamin C), protein, copper, and other minerals, all of which are necessary for the formation of red blood cells. Inadequate digestion, defects in absorption, and imperfect utilization of such nutrients may cause such deficiencies. To help avoid anemia, include iron-rich foods in the diet, such as iron-fortified foods, fish and poultry, dried fruits (apricots, prunes, raisins), dried peas and beans, nuts, green leafy vegetables, and whole grain breads and cereals. Include other nutrients necessary for red blood cell formation: folic acid, B_{12}, B_6, copper, and protein. Eat sufficient foods containing vitamin C, copper, and protein that help the body absorb more iron, since the body absorbs only 10 percent of the iron eaten. This is particularly important for people on a high-fiber diet.

Menstruating women may be advised by their physicians to take an iron supplement. Supplemental iron (ferrous sulfate) is used if anemia develops.

HYPOGLYCEMIA

Hypoglycemia means low blood sugar. The kind of hypoglycemia in which diet seems to play a role is usually called *reactive hypoglycemia*. One theory about its cause involves the excessive consumption of sugars, which stimulates an overproduction of insulin and produces symptoms of weakness, anxiety, sweating, and hunger. These conditions may occur three to four hours after eating large carbohydrate-rich meals. The reaction often seems connected with anxiety and stress, which in turn may intensify unless it is realized that the symptoms are benign and essentially harmless. If the symptoms are unequivocally relieved by a glucose drink within twenty to thirty minutes, they are likely to have been due to hypoglycemia. Low-sugar, high-fiber diets help to reduce the risk of attacks.

DISORDERS OF BONES AND JOINTS

Osteoarthritis

A major source of disability during and after middle age, osteoarthritis mostly affects the hips, knees, and the lower back, neck, and finger joints.

One of the long-held theories explaining osteoarthritis is that of excessive wear-and-tear on the joint surfaces. It is probably partially true. Grossly abnormal posture due to a paralysis, or loss of normal joint sensation can lead to troublesome osteoarthritis of the overstressed joints. Poor standing posture probably contributes to the development of arthritis of the spine. Obesity and osteoarthritis often coexist and are probably a common basis for pain in the weight-bearing joints in the lower spine, hips, and knees. Avoiding obesity and taking regular appropriate exercise are important in avoiding osteoarthritis.

Osteomalacia

Osteomalacia produces a softening of the bones leading to pains in the limbs, occasionally backache, and sometimes even deformities. It can arise from disorders of the small intestine, after stomach operations (partial gastrectomy), in severe kidney disease, and in epileptics as a side effect of some drug treatments. One of the common causes of osteomalacia is vitamin D deficiency. Since a major source of vitamin D is the action of sunlight on the skin, the elderly infirm who lead an indoor life and eat a limited diet are thus especially prone to osteomalacia. Risk can be reduced by including vitamin D in the diet, supplemented as necessary, but avoiding excessive dosages.

Osteoporosis

With advancing age, this form of bone disease becomes exceedingly common, almost universal, affecting women at an earlier age than men. The bony substance is reduced in amount, though remaining qualitatively normal; this leads to weakness and brittleness so that bone fractures result from relatively minor injuries that would not affect normal bone.

Controversy surrounds the effect of diet on human osteoporosis. The condition develops in rats deprived of calcium, but there is uncertainty as to the relevance of this. One study has indicated that human osteoporosis improves on a diet providing extra calcium, vitamin D, and fluoride.

It therefore seems a good idea to maintain a generous calcium intake, especially in the later years, by drinking a half-pint of milk or skimmed milk each day and by eating other calcium-rich foods such as cheese (including skimmed-milk cheese) and legumes. Regular exercise throughout life maintains bone strength. One of the main reasons for estrogen treatment of women who have an early menopause because of operations on, or disease of, the ovaries is to avoid subsequent osteoporosis.

Nutrition at Every Age

DIET IN PREGNANCY

The diet of a pregnant woman is closely linked to the health and development of her child both before and after birth. During pregnancy, all the nutrients required by the growing fetus should be derived from what the mother eats. Any nutrients lacking in the diet will be drawn in part from her body stores of nutrients; if her reserves are depleted the infant may not be adequately nourished.

A healthy woman who has practiced good eating habits can obtain most of her additional requirements during pregnancy by increasing the amounts of certain foods she has already been eating by 300 more calories per day, including 30 extra grams of protein. She will need supplemental iron, 30–60 mg. a day, and usually will need added folic acid.

Women who have had poor food habits or are underweight will require not only an improved general diet, but also appropriate multivitamin and multimineral supplements, which should be discussed with their physicians.

The pregnant adolescent is of particular concern since her own special needs continue along with her child's. Poor nutrition in an adolescent mother is a serious threat to the infant and to herself. This is a special problem because often the teenage mother is unmarried, or if married, comes from an unsupportive environment. These women need special supervision from appropriate health care sources.

Mothers who eat poorly and are underweight experience more complications during pregnancy and at time of delivery. Their infants sometimes weigh less than 5 1/2 pounds and survival rate is poor.

During pregnancy, nutrients and oxygen pass to the fetus across the thin walls of the placental blood vessels. How effectively oxygen, nutrients, and other substances reach the child depends largely on their concentration in the mother's blood and on the adequacy of blood flow through the placenta. Anything that decreases blood flow or its oxygen-carrying capacity, such as cigarette smoking, may affect fetal growth. Fetal circulation is less efficient than that which develops after birth. Infants born to mothers who smoke are significantly smaller, and their long-term physical and mental development may be affected. Drugs such as sleeping pills and alcohol may also be harmful to the fetus. High alcohol intake can cause permanent malformation and mental retardation. Thus, during pregnancy it is important to avoid smoking, alcohol, and drugs (see chapter 6).

Early pregnancy (the first three months) is a critical period for the development and differentiation of the fetal organs. At this time the mother's nutrient needs are not greatly increased and weight gain is slight (up to six pounds).

The brain begins to develop during the third month of gestation, with growth of the brain ending around the second to third year of life. After this time there is little change in the structure of the brain. Thus if the brain is significantly deprived of the nutrients it needs for growth during this time, permanent damage may result.

In the period from four to six months, a pregnant woman should gain 0.8 pounds (13 oz.) per week. Most of this gain will be due to the growth of breasts, uterus, and fat stores, plus an increased blood volume. In the last three months of pregnancy, the same weight gain can be accounted for by rapid growth of the fetus. An adequate weight gain for the entire pregnancy (24–28 pounds), is particularly critical (see table 1.13). A target weight gain during pregnancy is 24 pounds, which means an average of an extra 240 calories per day for nine months.

Table 1.13
OVERALL WEIGHT GAIN DURING PREGNANCY

Development	Weight gain (lb)
Infant	
infant at birth (approx.)	7½
placenta	1
surrounding fluid	2
Mother	
increased blood volume	4
fat reserves (energy store for lactation)	4
increased breast size	3
increased uterus size	2½
Total	24

If a woman is already overweight, pregnancy is not the time to attempt weight loss. Low-calorie diets, especially low-carbohydrate diets, are dangerous, possibly leading to a condition called *ketoacidosis*, which can cause permanent damage to the fetus.

The special dietary requirements of pregnancy are:

- Fifty percent more *protein*, obtainable from lean meat, poultry, fish, legumes, skim milk, and other dairy products.
- A significant increase in *calcium, folic acid*, and *iron. Calcium* is necessary for the skeletal structure, for teeth, for the function of the nervous system, for coagulation of blood, and for contraction of muscles. Milk, cheese, and other dairy products are good sources. For those who do not drink milk, dark green vegetables (kale, mustard greens, etc.), salmon, and sardines are other good sources of calcium. A pregnant woman must be sure she compensates from other sources of calcium if she does not drink milk (see table 1.2, page 60).

- *Folic acid*, like vitamin B_{12}, is necessary for the synthesis of deoxyribonucleic acid (DNA), and it is plentiful in almost all unprocessed foods. However, since it is easily destroyed through cooking, the actual amount consumed is considerably less. Therefore, most physicians give it as a supplement to ensure an adequate amount during pregnancy.
- *Iron* in significantly greater amounts in view of the need for more blood and red blood cells. Since iron is essential and many of the best sources of iron (like liver) are not frequently eaten, it is advisable for pregnant women to take an iron supplement.
- *Iodized salt* should be used since iodine is necessary for fetal development. Do not curtail salt excessively, and diuretics (water pills) should only be taken on a physician's advice.

Table 1.14 gives a daily food pattern to meet these requirements, and table 1.15 illustrates the reasons why extra nutrients are required and their sources.

For other complications of pregnancy in which diet may be involved, such as anemia, toxemia, nausea, constipation, and swelling (edema), see chapter 6.

THE NURSING MOTHER

The kinds of food the pregnant woman and the nursing mother need are similar, but the nursing mother should increase the amount to meet the new demands of milk production (see table 1.14).

The nursing mother needs 600–800 calories above normal each day; 400–500 of those calories should come from dietary sources and the remainder from fat stores she has built up during pregnancy to meet nursing needs. The calories needed from food sources may increase if the

Table 1.14
FOODS REQUIRED TO MEET
NUTRIENT NEEDS DURING PREGNANCY

Food	Number of servings per day	Amount per serving
Milk	3–4	1 cup skim milk (vitamins A and D fortified) or 1½ oz. cheese or 1 cup yogurt
Meat or Vegetable protein	2	3 oz. lean meat, chicken, or fish or 1 cup legumes (dried beans or peas)
Fruits	3	1 piece or 1 cup juice (at least 1 rich in vitamin C)
Vegetables	3	large servings at least 1 orange or yellow at least 1 dark green, leafy
Bread, Cereals	4	1 slice wholewheat bread ½ cup whole grain cereal
Fat	2	1 tbsp. soft margarine or 1 tbsp. mayonnaise or oil or 2 tbsp. salad dressing

mother nurses beyond three months, when her fat stores become depleted, or if her activity level demands more calories for her to maintain weight.

Dietary protein must meet maternal needs plus supply the essential amino acids through her breast milk to the baby. In order to prevent calcium depletion, the mother needs approximately 400 mg. above the normal 800 mg. per day; iron also frequently needs to be supplemented.

To meet these increased nutritional requirements, an additional cup of milk and another slice of bread or helping of cereal added to the diet during pregnancy is adequate. A daily intake of two quarts of fluid will maintain an adequate volume of the mother's milk.

EARLY INFANCY

Nutrition in infancy should do two things: satisfy the child's daily energy requirements and support growth and development of new tissues.

At no time in life are nutritional demands as great as in early infancy. Babies grow very rapidly. Birth weight is doubled within six months and tripled by twelve months. Development of the brain continues through this period. Both intellectual and physical achievement depend on an adequate diet. However, too rapid weight gain should be avoided since it can lead to obesity. In addition, overweight babies are more prone to respiratory illness.

The average American baby weighs 7 1/2 pounds at birth. Average weights by age for the first three years are shown in figures 1.6 and 1.7. Premature infants or very small babies, less than 5 1/2 pounds, tend to grow more rapidly than normal birth weight infants. Premature babies also require special attention because their nutrient needs differ, and digestive function and kidneys are often less well-developed.

> Breast milk from a well-nourished mother contains nearly all the nutrients that a baby needs in the right proportions for a normal growth pattern.

Commercial infant formulas modified from cow's milk or soybean milk can provide the best alternative when breast feeding is unsuccessful, inappropriate, or stopped early.

Comparison of the nutrients of human and cow's milk (see table 1.16) reveals that cow's milk contains more protein and less carbohydrate and polyunsaturated fat than human milk. The sodium level in cow's milk is three times that of human milk. Too much sodium and protein may be harmful to a baby, especially when diarrhea, vomiting, or excess water loss occurs. Cow's milk is also lower in vitamin C, which helps iron absorption, than is human milk. The protein and fat of cow's milk are both poorly absorbed by the infant. Cow's milk that has not been modified for infants is inappropriate for them at less than six months of age.

Commercial formula is made of cow's milk modified to contain essential nutrients in proportions similar to human milk and is now processed so it is better digested and absorbed. These formulas are available in powder, concentrated, and ready-to-feed form, and instructions should be followed precisely to avoid bacterial infection.

The milk-based formulas use nonfat dry milk as their protein source (casein) and vegetable oils as fat; the form of carbohydrate is lactose (milk sugar) and added sucrose. They are fortified to meet vitamin and mineral requirements and some are additionally supplemented with iron.

The soy-based formulas use soybeans as their protein source, but since the quality of soy protein is somewhat lower than that of milk the actual protein content must be higher to compensate.

Table 1.15
NUTRIENT NEEDS OF PREGNANCY

Nutrient	Amount	Reason for nutrient requirement	Good food source

Calories
Protein
	2,400
	74 gm.
		Increased rate of metabolism
		Rapid fetal tissue growth
		Amniotic fluid
		Placenta growth and development
		Maternal tissue growth: uterus, breasts
		Increased maternal circulating blood volume:
		    a. Hemoglobin increase
		    b. Plasma protein increase
		Maternal storage reserves for labor, delivery, and lactation
			All foods
			Low-fat milk
			Cheese
			Meat, poultry, fish
			Grains
			Legumes
			Nuts

Vitamin A	1,000 μg.RE	Essential for cell development and tissue growth Tooth bud formation (development of enamel-forming cells in gum tissue) Bone growth *CAUTION:* Too much vitamin A may injure the eyes of fetus and cause cleft palate.	Fortified margarine Green and yellow vegetables
Vitamin D	10 μg.	Needed for bones and teeth *CAUTION:* Too much vitamin D may cause dangerously high levels of calcium.	Fortified low-fat milk
Vitamin E	10 mg.α-TE	Needed for tissue growth and cell structure	Polyunsaturated vegetable oils Leafy vegetables Meat
Vitamin C	80 mg.	Needed in the formation and connection of tissue in the fetus. Increases iron absorption *CAUTION:* Too much vitamin C may cause scurvy in the newborn	Citrus fruits Berries Melons Tomatoes Green peppers Green leafy vegetables Broccoli Potatoes

Nutrient	Amount	Reason for nutrient requirement	Good food source
Folic Acid	800 μg.	Prevention of megaloblastic anemia in high-risk patients; increased heme production for hemoglobin; production of cell nucleus material	Green leafy vegetables
Niacin	15–16 mg.NE	All the B vitamins act as assistants to enzymes (catalysts). They are necessary for the enzymes for energy and protein metabolism.	Meat Peanuts
Riboflavin	1.6 mg.		Beans and peas Enriched grains
Thiamine	1.5 mg.		Low-fat milk Legumes
B_6 (pyridoxine)	2.6 mg.		Wheat, corn
B_{12}	4.0 μg.		
Minerals: Calcium	1,200 mg.	Fetal skeleton formation Fetal tooth bud formation Increased need for maternal calcium	Low-fat milk Cheese Whole grains Leafy green vegetables
Phosphorus	1,200 mg.	Fetal skeleton formation Fetal tooth bud formation Increased need for maternal phosphorus	Low-fat milk Cheese Lean meats
Iron	18+ mg. (+30–60 mg. supplement)	Increased maternal circulating blood volume and blood cells Fetal iron storage	Liver, meats Whole or enriched grain Leafy vegetables Nuts, legumes Dried fruits
Iodine	175 μg.	Increased basal metabolic rate–increased thyroid output	Iodized salt
Magnesium	450 mg.	Catalyst for energy and protein metabolism Tissue growth Muscle action	Nuts Soybeans Cocoa Seafood Whole grains Dried beans and peas

SOURCE: adapted from S. Williams, "Handbook of Maternal and Infant Nutrition," SRW Productions, Inc., Berkeley, California, 1976.

Table 1.16
NUTRIENT COMPARISONS OF HUMAN MILK, COW'S MILK, AND INFANT FORMULA (16 oz.)

Type of milk or formula		Protein		Carbohydrate		Total fat		Minerals			
	Calories	gm.	%	gm.	%	gm.	%	Calcium mg.	Phosphorus mg.	Sodium mg.	Iron mg.
Human	357	5	6	33	37	21	53	162	67	78	.09
Cow	319	17	21	23	29	17	48	580	457	237	trace
Infant formula* (milk based)	319	7	9	33	41	18	50	262	219	133	0.6
Infant formula* (soybean based)	323	10	12	32	40	17	47	333	238	143	5.7

*Choose formula in which the nutrients match these in quantity.

Infant formula makers are beginning to develop more formulas based on vegetable protein, which might be an important step since animal protein sources are becoming less plentiful. At present, this type of formula is most frequently used for infants who are allergic to milk.

Human milk is considered the optimal food for an infant not only because of its well-proportioned nutrient content but also for its natural protective qualities against bacterial infections of the intestine. The colostrum secretion, a substance excreted in the first two weeks in the breast milk, contains antibodies and proteins that destroy bacteria and viruses.

Human milk proteins are easier to digest and better absorbed by the infant than other foods. The lower protein and mineral content in human milk means less work for the kidneys. There is also evidence that iron in human milk is more efficiently absorbed because of the higher concentration of lactose and ascorbic acid and the lower concentration of phosphorus, each known to improve the potential for iron absorption.

The infant also controls its own food intake when breast fed, and thus is less likely to gain excessive weight. An advantage to the mother in breast feeding is that while supplying the infant's calories, she can lose some of the weight gained during pregnancy.

Many experts advise that breast feeding be continued for about six months. During the first year, a commercial formula or milk containing 2 percent fat or whole (not skim) milk may be used. After that, skim milk is an acceptable alternative.

Full-term babies are born with iron stores adequate for about four months. After that, iron supplements, iron-fortified cereals, or an iron-fortified formula should be used, as ordinary milk is low in iron. Physicians sometimes prescribe drops providing vitamins D and C, iron, and fluoride; but fluoride-containing drops should not be used if the baby is already getting a formula that contains fluoride, or a concentrated formula diluted with fluoridated tap water. Too much fluoride can be toxic.

Food allergies

A small but significant number of infants are sensitive to cow's milk protein, in which case a soy protein-based formula may be substituted. In some cases, a protein hydrolysate-based formula may be needed.

Other foods that may cause allergic reactions are wheat, eggs, chocolate, and citrus fruits. Symptoms of food allergy include diarrhea, vomiting, respiratory difficulties, skin rash, headache, general irritability, or poor growth. Since these symptoms may have many causes, it is important for the child to be examined by a physician.

If a food allergy appears likely, a process of elimination and reintroduction of suspected foods should be used to learn the cause. Strict avoidance of the allergenic food is then required. Substitute foods are usually available. For example, soy protein-based formula can replace milk-based formula, and rice cereal can replace wheat. Since the very young infant has a tendency to absorb

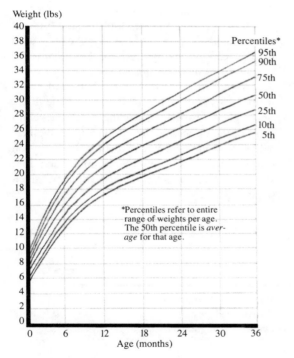

FIGURE 1.6

Weight of girls from birth to 36 months

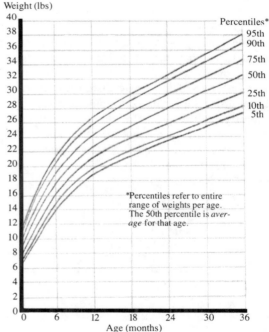

FIGURE 1.7

Weight of boys from birth to 36 months

SOURCE: adapted from National Center for Health Statistics, "NCHS Growth Charts, 1976." Monthly Vital Statistics Report, Vol. 25, No. 3 Supp. (HRA) 7S-1120 (Rockville, Md.: Health Resources Administration, June 1976). Data from the Fels Research Institute, Yellow Springs, Ohio

foreign proteins intact, breast feeding and the avoidance of solid foods during the first four to six months of life may be especially important for an infant with a family history of allergies.

Foods should be introduced into the diet individually rather than in combinations in order to determine whether or not the infant tolerates them well. As manufactured foods are introduced into the child's diet, it is important to read the list of ingredients and make sure that the product does not contain any potentially allergenic food. Once a child becomes allergic to a food, a minute quantity of the food is sufficient to cause symptoms.

Solid foods

Within a few weeks after birth infants can tolerate solid foods, but they should not be introduced earlier than four to six months. Too early introduction of solid food may disturb the nutrient balance of breast milk or formula diet and contribute excess calories. In addition, the infant's gastrointestinal tract is not ready to process the food properly nor is the oral musculature developed to handle solids in the mouth and push them back for efficient swallowing.

However, by four to six months both gastrointestinal tract and mouth muscles are more ready to accept and handle solids. At first, foods supplementing the formula should consist primarily of iron-fortified cereals, fruits, and juices. Foods containing added sugar should be avoided. Salt is also an ingredient of concern. An infant's kidneys are not mature enough to concentrate and excrete excessive salt, and the infant cannot distinguish between foods with and without salt. Use of salty foods should be avoided in infancy and, indeed, throughout life. Most commercial baby foods are low in salt; mothers who prepare baby foods at home should avoid it.

It is possible to make strained baby foods at home. Foods prepared for the family can be used for the baby by taking a portion before any salt is added and then grinding it.

A general scheme for the addition of solids in the first year of life is shown in table 1.17. This may be varied, depending on the development of the infant and the attitude of the mother. When new mothers begin feeding the baby on semisolids, it is strongly recommended that strained meats, vegetables, and fruits be given separately.

Table 1.17
RECOMMENDED FEEDING
DURING THE FIRST YEAR

At this age in months:	Following foods may be introduced (milk is needed throughout)
0 – 4	Breast milk or formula alone
4 – 6	Iron-enriched rice cereal and cooked cereals
7	Strained fruit
8	Strained vegetables
9	Minced meat and fish
10 – 12	Toast, biscuits, cottage cheese

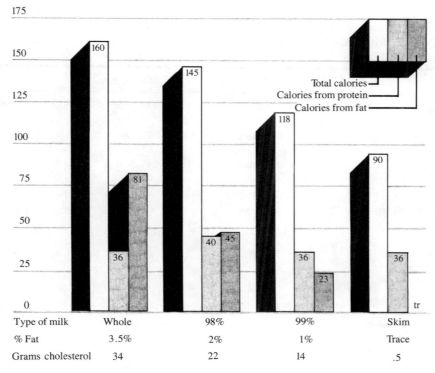

Total calories
Calories from protein
Calories from fat

Type of milk	Whole	98%	99%	Skim
% Fat	3.5%	2%	1%	Trace
Grams cholesterol	34	22	14	.5

FIGURE 1.8

Total calories, calories from protein, calories from fat, percentage of fat, and total cholesterol in different types of milk (8 oz.)
SOURCE: *adapted from USDA* Home and Garden Bulletin, *No. 72, 1971*

CHILDHOOD

As the child approaches one to two years, growth rate slows dramatically, accompanied by a decrease in appetite. In addition, the child who once accepted a large variety of foods now usually becomes more selective and independent. Fickle food habits during the preschool years can be trying for parents. Knowing that this is a normal phase can help avoid problems of force feeding or overeating. During this period, it is important to offer foods of high nutrient value and not resort to nutrient-poor substitutes. Suggested daily food requirements for the two- to twelve-year-old are listed in table 1.18.

The four- and five-year-old begins to acquire the food preferences and aversions of family members. From an early age the child makes emotional associations with foods that continue to affect choices through adult years. *Eating habits do not emerge spontaneously—they are learned.*

Table 1.18
RECOMMENDED DAILY FOODS,
2–12 YEARS

Food	2–5 years	6–9 years	10–12 years
Milk, low fat*	2 cups	2–3 cups	3 or more cups
Lean meat, poultry or fish	2 ounces	2–3 oz.	3–4 oz.
Dried beans, peas	3–4 tbsp.	4–5 tbsp.	5–6 tbsp.
Potatoes (macaroni, spaghetti, or rice)	3–4 tbsp.	4–5 tbsp	½ cup
Cooked vegetables (often including green, leafy, or deep yellow)	½ cup	⅓ cup	½ cup
Raw vegetables (lettuce, carrots, celery, etc.)	¼ cup	¼ cup	⅓ cup
Fruits	⅓ cup or more	1 cup or more	1 cup or more
Citrus fruits (orange, grapefruit, etc.)	1	1	1
Bread, whole grain, or enriched	2–3 slices	2–3 slices	2–3 slices
Cereal, whole grain, or enriched	½ cup	¾ cup	1 cup
Polyunsaturated margarine	1–2 tbsp.	1 or more tablespoons	1 or more tablespoons

*See figure 1.9 for a comparison of calories and cholesterol in whole, low-fat and skim milk.

This is an important lesson for parents who, as exemplars for their children, help to set their eating habits. If children routinely eat nutritious foods and have available nutrient-dense snacks, those will become their food choices.

By school age, eating habits generally change again as the parents' direct supervision is loosened. Breakfast all too often is eaten on the run, lunch may be traded for a high-calorie snack, or simply thrown away in favor of snacking after school. Calorie excesses or deficiencies may result from these haphazard patterns and will eventually be reflected in the weight and health of the child. Nutrients commonly falling short of requirements at this age are vitamins C and A, as well as calcium and protein.

The basics for school-aged children

The noon meal should include:
- 1/2 pint skim milk or yogurt
- 2 ounces, not including bones, of lean meat, poultry, or fish OR 1/2 cup cooked dried beans or peas OR 4 tablespoons of peanut butter, OR a combination of any of the above
- 2 or more vegetables, one dark leafy green
- 1–2 slices whole grain enriched bread

Sample school lunches

Nutritious lunches can be simple and delicious. Soups, leftovers, fresh fruits, and salads cost no more than potato chips, cokes, pastries, and doughnuts and are lower in calories and fat, higher in nutrients. Use a wide-mouthed thermos for hot items; use empty margarine tubs for cold items. Whole grain breads such as whole wheat, rye, cracked wheat, and pumpernickel are the best kinds of sandwich breads. If white bread is used be sure it is enriched. Also try pita pocket bread. Raw vegetables are fun to eat with the fingers.

Suggested all-time favorites

Peanut butter and banana sandwich
Carrots/celery sticks
1/2 apple
Skim milk

Try

Chicken wings or drumstick
Roll, muffin, or slice of bread with margarine
Fruit salad
Peanuts (in the shell or dry roasted)
Skim milk
OR
Cottage cheese and raisin sandwich
    on brown bread
Pepper rings
Orange
Skim milk

Variations

Cottage cheese and tomato on whole wheat
Cottage cheese and pineapple

Try

Skim milk semi-soft cheese and
    bean sprout sandwich
Cherry tomatoes and cucumbers
Plum or pear
Skim milk

Make salad sandwiches

Turkey, tuna,   on a roll or in a pita
chicken, ham,   pocket *OR* with crackers,
egg or salmon   and lots of vegetables
Skim milk
(add sunflower or pumpkin seeds, or an oatmeal cookie)

ADOLESCENCE AND TEENAGE

The years from twelve to eighteen are the second stage of rapid growth. The need for calories and protein increases. More calcium, phosphorus, and vitamin D for proper bone formation is required. Girls need more iron when menstruation starts (see table 1.3). An adequate amount of foods high in iron, such as lean meats or fish, green leafy vegetables, enriched breads, cereals and potatoes should also be included in the daily food intake of both boys and girls.

Dietary habits of teenagers are notoriously irregular. Nutrition often consists of skipped or sketchy meals, fast food orgies, and unwholesome snacking at any hour of the day or night. Teenagers suffer unnecessarily from their fashionable neglect of breakfast. A University of Iowa study of adolescent performance, energy, and alertness found that those who ate breakfast were less fatigued, more attentive, and achieved more than those who did not.

Adolescents yearn for peer approval of their appearance. Therefore, parents, doctors, nurses, teachers, and nutritionists should be able to exploit this yearning by emphasizing the importance of proper nutrition for beautiful skin, bright eyes, shiny hair, and strong bodies.

Adults should try to persuade adolescents that raw vegetables, fresh fruits, mini-sandwiches, and skim milk can be more fun as a lifestyle than food containing high fat and high sugar.

As mentioned earlier, this period of growth is one of the most active during one's life. Teenagers participating in sports require calories and nutrients from a well-balanced diet to meet their energy needs.

Snack list

- raisins or dates
- apple or banana slices
- chopped celery or shredded carrots
- graham crackers (unsalted)
- skim milk
- open-faced sandwiches made on whole grain breads, with leftover chicken, vegetables, etc.
- whipped cottage cheese dip with onion soup mix; dip in green pepper strips, radishes, cauliflower, broccoli
- tuna salad stuffed in celery sticks
- small piece of nut bread, carrot cake, pumpkin bread, banana bread, zucchini bread, etc.
- nuts and raisins
- sunflower seeds or pumpkin seeds (unsalted)
- 1 cup of soup using nonfat dry milk and water for more flavor and nutrition
- 2 bread sticks
- ice skim milk
- pizza
- cut tomato wedges sprinkled with dill
- fruit kabobs: banana wheels, pineapple chunks, strawberries, orange wedges on toothpicks
- low-fat yogurt with fresh fruit
- homemade popsicles or frozen cubes of fruit juices
- hot spiced cider with cloves and/or cinnamon
- if cookies are desired, try oatmeal
- if cake is desired, try angel food
- chilled fruit juices
- home-popped popcorn without added salt, butter or margarine

ADVANCING AGE

All the guidelines for healthy nutrition outlined above apply to the elderly; some nutritional problems are particularly common in this age group. Elderly people living on their own—men especially—tend to be careless about getting a balanced diet. This can often be due to difficulty in getting to food stores and restaurants. Weakness, arthritis, or depression may constrain these activities. There may be financial restraints, too—hence, the need to buy wisely. In others, weak teeth or pain from badly fitting dentures makes eating unpleasant. People who have had stomach operations often suffer from malnutrition. These problems need to be borne in mind not only by the elderly, but also by their relatives and any others with responsibilities for the care of the aged.

What can be done? In many communities there are public service groups that can offer aid. The problem of getting about may be eased by volunteers from various organizations to do the shopping or take the elderly out and help them do it themselves. Also, in many areas, organizations such as "Meals on Wheels" will deliver hot meals to the elderly.

With prudent buying, financial restraints can be eased and balanced nutrition still achieved. A banana costs less than any packaged junk food and is full of nutrients that benefit the elderly. Comparatively inexpensive high-fiber foods such as whole grains, dried beans, fruits, and vegetables can help counter problems among the elderly and possibly reduce the risk of colon cancer, diabetes, and constipation. Prudent diet principles apply throughout life, although they may be most important in early and middle age. Our tendency to overfeed the very young may be a factor in limiting life span, though this has been proven only in laboratory animals.

In populations with a high proportion of very old people, the lifestyle is often characteristically one of vigorous manual labor. In any case, keeping active throughout life may improve longevity, as well as help avoid obesity and heart disease.

To maintain ordinary nutritional requirements, older people should make sure they eat lean meat, fish, and poultry (high in protein, vitamins, and minerals), high protein derived from plants (such as dried beans, dried peas, nuts, and seeds), fruits, vegetables, whole grain breads and cereals, as well as dairy products.

Iron deficiency is common in the older population. When severe it leads to anemia. Not eating enough iron-rich foods is one cause. Another is bleeding due to stomach ulcer, piles, or more serious diseases of the bowel or uterus. The frequent use of aspirin is a common cause of unrecognized blood loss leading to anemia. The normal iron intake in the elderly continues to be 10 mg. per day. Some of the following foods should be a regular part of the diet: fortified cereals and bread, liver, lean meat, and fish.

Anemia in elderly people can also be due to other deficiencies, especially the lack of the B vitamin folic acid. We get this substance from green vegetables, whole wheat bread, and liver. Vitamin B_{12} deficiency is another cause of anemia; older vegetarians are very much at risk as this vitamin is obtained from meat, fish, liver, and eggs. Strict vegetarians should therefore take the vitamin in tablet form to avoid serious anemia. Moderate amounts of fish and meat give an adequate intake of the vitamin.

Vitamin C (ascorbic acid) frequently seems to be inadequate in the elderly, judging by blood tests measuring the level of this vitamin in the white cells. A healthy amount of ascorbic acid is supplied by fresh fruit and vegetables in the daily diet; in particular, an orange or a half grapefruit should be eaten every day.

Thinning and weakness of bones is common in elderly people. One form of bone disease, osteomalacia, is due to lack of vitamin D. We have a double source of this vitamin—from our skin, which can manufacture it if we get adequate sunlight, and from milk in various forms.

Deficiency of calories is seldom a problem. Beyond age sixty, physical activity tends to diminish though this is not necessarily desirable. Also, the amount of muscle mass in the body diminishes. Hence, energy needs also diminish.

However, elderly people who keep active may continue to need the same calorie intake as in middle age. Average needs in men aged seventy and older are 2,100 calories and in women 1,900 calories, compared with 2,600 and 2,200 calories in sedentary middle age. Many people tend to gain weight in middle age. However, body weight often diminishes in the elderly although fat tends to increase. This can be due to loss of muscle and bone.

Everyday Nutrition

THE AMERICAN HEALTH FOUNDATION FOOD PLAN

What is the optimal diet for the average sedentary person of today?

In industrialized Western countries, the average diet is generally adequate or more than adequate in its energy content (calories) and protein. The protein, however, is mostly derived from meat; meat and fish provide 70 percent, vegetable sources 30 percent, while calories are derived to a considerable extent from fat (40–45 percent). Much of this fat is of the hard, saturated type (16 percent of all calories), and the ratio of polyunsaturated to saturated fat is quite low (around 0.4). The average diet tends to be low in fiber due to the use of highly refined flour and cereal foods, and high in salt (6–18 gm./day) both as a spice and as a preservative. The diet contains about 500 mg. cholesterol per day and, often, a

considerable amount of alcohol. Many of these features in our diet have come about quite recently in our history.

The American Health Foundation Food Plan suggested below (see table 1.19) involves only moderate changes in our usual pattern of eating. For the most part, these changes amount to a return to earlier nutritional patterns and correspond with diets consumed in several Mediterranean countries whose inhabitants have less coronary disease and certain types of cancers and live longer than residents of the U.S.

1. A lower caloric intake—to maintain ideal body weight.
2. Fat intake should be no more than 25–30 percent of calorie consumption, and the ratio of polyunsaturated to saturated fats (P:S ratio) should be moderately increased (P:S ratio 1:1).
3. A reduced cholesterol intake. Recommended intake up to 200 mg.
4. The total protein intake is unchanged (12 percent), but the proportion taken from vegetable sources should be increased at least to 40 percent from the present 30 percent, following recommendations for suitable combinations (see Proteins, p.59); also, greater emphasis on fish is recommended.
5. A greater intake of whole-grain bread and cereals, and of fresh vegetables and fruit is suggested (58–63 percent, now 45 percent). This leads to the consumption of complex carbohydrates as a major source of calories (45 percent of the total) and to an increased intake of two major types of food fiber—the bran type and the pectins, which have different but potentially valuable health effects, and to a balanced intake of several vitamins and minerals.
6. A moderate usage of alcohol, limited to two average-size drinks per day.
7. Progressive reduction in intake of sodium as salt and from other sources. Three to five grams of salt per day is a suggested target.

Table 1.19

AMERICAN HEALTH FOUNDATION FOOD PLAN

Calories based on maintenance of ideal weight	1000 per day		1200 per day		1500 per day		1800 per day		2000 per day	
	% of total calories*	calories	% of total calories*	calories	% of total calories*	calories	% of total calories*	calories	% of total calories*	calories
Content:										
Protein (with an increase in vegetable protein)	12%	120	12%	144	12%	180	12%	216	12%	240
Fat	25–30%	250	25–30%	300–360	25–30%	375–450	25–30%	450–540	25–30%	500–600
saturated fat	8–10%	80	8–10%	100–120	8–10%	125–150	8–10%	149–180	8–10%	166–200
monounsaturated fat	8–10%	80	8–10%	100–120	8–10%	125–150	8–10%	149–180	8–10%	166–200
polyunsaturated fat	8–10%	80	8–10%	100–120	8–10%	125–150	8–10%	149–180	8–10%	166–200
Carbohydrate (with an increase in complex carbohydrate)	63%	630	58–63%	690–756	58–63%	870–945	58–63%	1044–1134	58–63%	1160–1260
Other dietary components:										
Dietary fiber (Table 1.4)	35 grams/day		35 grams/day		35 grams/day		35 grams/day		35 grams/day	
Salt (Table 1.11)	3–5 grams/day		3–5 grams/day		3–5 grams/day		3–5 grams/day		3–5 grams/day	
Cholesterol (Table 1.8)	200 mgs/day		200 mgs/day		200 mgs/day		200 mgs/day		200 mgs/day	

*Due to rounding off, figures may not add up to 100%.

A thumbnail sketch of The American Health Foundation Food Plan

1. Limit all sources of calories (including alcohol) to reach and maintain your ideal weight.
2. Use fish, chicken, very lean meat in place of fatty meats. Have occasional meatless meals (get protein from skim milk, low-fat cheese, lentils, beans, chick-peas, soy products).
3. Use skim milk or 2 percent fat milk instead of whole milk. Minimize cream, butter.
4. Use soft margarine, polyunsaturated oils; limit butter and solid shortening.
5. Egg whites may be used freely, but limit yolks to three per week.
6. Use low-fat cooking methods (steaming, broiling, etc).
7. Eat more vegetables, fruit, whole-grain bread; fewer baked goods, candies, sugar.
8. Spread calories evenly through the day.

Menus

The following menus offer samples for a variety of calorie plans, from 1,000 to 2,000 per day, figured at different fat percentages. Vegetarian menus are also included.

Choose the calorie count based on the intake that best correlates with your age and activity load. The fat content should be selected based on family history, cholesterol level, and other risk factors.

Here is a formula for estimating your daily caloric requirements:

Take your ideal (average) weight for height as shown in Table 1.12 in kilograms. Multiply by 24 (hours) to get your Basal Metabolic Rate (BMR). Multiply the kilogram weight by 8 to get calories spent during sleep and subtract from the BMR. If normally active (not strenuously active), take 50 percent of the result, which equals calories required for activity. Then add 10 percent of the same result to get "specific dynamic action," or energy required to digest food. Add these three figures to get total calories per day.

An example: A 5'6" woman ideally should weigh 128 lbs, or 58.1 kg. as determined from Table 1.12. Her BMR $= 24$ hrs. $\times$ 58.1 $=$ 1,394.4 calories/day. She expends 8 hrs $\times$ 58.1 $=$ 464.8 calories for sleeping. Therefore, $1{,}394.4 - 464.8 = 929.6$ calories are the basal (nonactive) calories she expends during waking hours. As she is normally active, she requires an additional 50 percent of this amount—$0.5 \times 929.6 = 464.8$ calories—for activity. She requires an additional 10 percent of "waking" basal calories—$0.1 \times 929.6 = 93.0$ calories—to digest her food. Therefore, her requirements for ideal weight $(929.6 + 464.8 + 93.0)$ indicate that she should follow a 1,487.4 calorie diet to achieve this weight. A 1,500 calorie menu is closest to this, and therefore she should choose one of these.

1,000 Calorie Plan

Carbohydrates[a] (61% of calories): 148 gm.
Protein[b] (20% of calories): 49 gm.
Fat (19% of calories): 20 gm.
Cholesterol: less than 200 mg.

Basic food groups (servings)	Sample menu A	Sample menu B
Breakfast		
1 protein	1 egg (2 per week)	½ cup oatmeal
1 fruit	½ small grapefruit	½ cup orange juice
1 carbohydrate	1 slice toast	1 slice toast
½ fat	½ tsp. margarine	½ tsp. margarine
½ non-fat milk	½ cup skim milk[c]	½ cup non-fat milk
Midmorning		
non-caloric beverage[d]	hot tea with lemon	hot coffee (black)
Lunch		
1 oz. protein	1 oz. baked chicken	1 oz. low-fat cheese melted over
1 carbohydrate	1 slice bread—or ½ pita	½ cup rice
½ fat	½ tsp. margarine	½ tsp. margarine
vegetables as desired[e]	mixed green salad w/ tomato wedge vinegar dressing	1 cup cole slaw w/ green pepper rings
1 vegetable	½ cup sprouts	¼ cup baked beans
1 fruit	½ cup fresh pineapple	½ cup cinnamon applesauce
½ cup non-fat milk	½ cup skim milk	½ cup skim milk
Midafternoon		
1 fruit	small orange	2 fresh plums
Dinner		
2 oz. protein	2 oz. broiled halibut	2 oz. veal roast
1 carbohydrate	3 tbsp. bread crumbs	½ cup barley soup
1 vegetable	1 cup yellow squash	1 cup carrots
vegetables as desired	1 cup fresh broccoli	1 cup asparagus spears
½ non-fat milk	½ cup skim milk	½ cup skim milk
Bedtime		
1 fruit	1 large tangerine	½ cup sliced peaches

[a]Carbohydrate group = bread, cereal, potato, rice, nuts, crackers, angel food cake, corn muffins, pasta grains, pastry.
[b]Protein group = meat, poultry, fish, eggs, (sometimes grain and dairy products). Note: serving size expressed in ounces because protein content varies with source.

[c]Reconstituted non-fat dried milk may substitute for skim milk.
[d]Non-caloric beverages = water, tea, coffee, etc. and should be consumed with every meal.
[e]As desired = unlimited.

1,200 Calorie Plan

Carbohydrates (56% of calories): 175 gm.
Protein (22% of calories): 66 gm.
Fat (22% of calories): 30 gm.
Cholesterol: less than 250 mg.

Basic food groups (servings)	Sample menu A	Sample menu B
Breakfast		
1 protein	1 egg (2 per week)	½ cup oatmeal
1 fruit	½ cup orange juice	½ cup applesauce
1 carbohydrate	1 corn muffin	1 slice toast
½ fat	½ tsp. margarine	½ tsp. margarine
1 non-fat milk	1 cup skim milk	1 cup skim milk
Midmorning		
non-caloric beverage	6 oz. diet lemonade	iced tea with lemon
Lunch		
2 oz. protein	low-fat chef's salad	½ cup vegetable bean lentil soup
vegetables as desired	with ½ oz. each of:	
	turkey, tuna, chicken,	
	low-fat cheese	
1 carbohydrate	1 slice bread	1 slice bread
1 fruit	½ cup fresh pineapple	1 large mandarin orange
1 cup non-fat milk	1 cup skim milk	1 cup skim milk
Midafternoon		
½ carbohydrate	¼ cup mixed walnuts and	2 soda crackers
1 fruit	raisins	½ cup sliced peaches
Dinner		
2 oz. protein	2 oz. broiled fish	2 oz. roast turkey
1 carbohydrate	1 small baked potato	½ cup steamed rice
vegetables as desired	fresh tomato salad with dill	1 cup brussels sprouts
		large mixed green salad with
		tomato juice dressing
1 vegetable	1 cup carrots, raw	1 cup turnips
½ cup non-fat milk	½ cup skim milk	½ cup skim milk
Bedtime		
1 fruit	12 fresh grapes	1 small pear
non-caloric beverage	coffee substitute	coffee substitute

1,500 Calorie Plan

Carbohydrates (70% of calories): 273 gm.
Protein (20% of calories): 65 gm.
Fat (10% of calories): 15 gm.
Cholesterol: 80 mg.

**Basic food groups
(servings)**   **Sample menu**

Breakfast

1 fruit   ½ broiled grapefruit
2 carbohydrate   2 slices whole wheat toast
1 non-fat milk   1 cup skim milk

Midmorning

1 carbohydrate   3 honey graham crackers

Lunch

3 oz. dairy protein   ½ cup low-fat, pot-style cottage cheese with paprika
1 carbohydrate   ½ a bagel or small hard roll
1 fruit   tangelo

Midafternoon

2 carbohydrate   1 piece angel food cake
3 fruit   1 cup pineapple juice

Dinner

3 oz. protein   3 oz. broiled halibut
2 carbohydrate   large baked potato
½ fat   ½ tsp. margarine
1 vegetable   tossed salad with lemon juice
1 vegetable   with ½ cup beets
2 fruit   2 peach halves, canned

Evening

2 carbohydrate   3 cups plain popcorn
1 fruit   ½ cup orange juice

1,500 Calorie Plan

Carbohydrates (65% of calories): 243 gm.
Protein (15% of calories): 53 gm.
Fat (20% of calories): 35 gm.
Cholesterol: 100 mg.

Basic food groups (servings)	Sample menu
Breakfast	
2 fruit	½ cup orange juice/2 tbsp. raisins
2 carbohydrate	½ cup oatmeal, 1 bran muffin
1 fat	1 tsp. margarine
1 non-fat milk	1 cup skim milk
Midmorning	
1 carbohydrate	3 honey grahams
½ fat	1 tsp. peanut butter
Lunch	
1½ carbohydrate	¾ cup cooked rice
1 vegetable	½ cup steamed Chinese vegetable
1 fat	1 tbsp. Italian dressing
2 fruit	1 cup cantaloupe balls
Midafternoon	
2 fruit	1 banana
2½ carbohydrate	
non-caloric beverage	herb tea
Dinner	
3 oz. protein	3 oz. broiled halibut
2 carbohydrate	1 cup potato
½ fat	½ tsp. margarine
vegetables as desired	lettuce and tomato salad with lemon
Evening	
2 fruit	⅔ cup pineapple juice

1,500 Calorie Plan

Carbohydrates (48% of calories): 182 gm.
Protein (22% of calories): 84 gm.
Fat (30% of calories): 50 gm.
Cholesterol: 200 mg.

Basic food groups (servings)	Sample menu
Breakfast	
1 fruit	½ cup orange juice
1 carbohydrate	1 slice toast
1 fat	1 tsp. margarine
1 non-fat milk	1 cup skim milk
Midmorning	
1 carbohydrate	3 graham crackers
2 fruit	⅔ cup apricot nectar
Lunch	
2 oz. protein	2 oz. sliced chicken
2 carbohydrate	½ cup rice, 1 sm. hard roll
2 fat	2 tsp. margarine
1 vegetable	½ cup green beans
1 fruit	½ cup mandarin oranges
Midafternoon	
1 carbohydrate	½ slice angel food cake
1 non-fat milk	1 cup skim milk
Dinner	
3 oz. protein	3 oz. fish with lemon
1 vegetable	½ cup cooked carrots
vegetables as desired	salad
1 fat	1 tsp. salad oil
Evening	
1 non-fat milk	1 cup skim milk
1 fat	2 tsp. peanut butter
1 carbohydrate	5 saltines

1,500 Calorie Plan

Carbohydrates (48% of calories): 183 gm.
Protein (17% of calories): 65 gm.
Fat (35% of calories): 60 gm.
Cholesterol: 200 mg.

**Basic food groups
(servings)**   **Sample menu**

Breakfast

1 fruit	½ cup orange juice
2 carbohydrate	2 slices of toast or English muffin
1 fat	1 tsp. margarine

Midmorning

1 fruit	1 small apple
1 carbohydrate	low cholesterol banana-bran muffin
2 fat	2 tsp. margarine

Lunch

2 oz. protein	2 oz. hamburger
1 fat	fried in vegetable oil (1 tsp.)
1 carbohydrate	hamburger bun
3 oz. dairy protein	½ cup low-fat cottage cheese
1 vegetable	with sliced tomatoes
1 vegetable	carrot/celery sticks

Midafternoon

1 carbohydrate	3 graham crackers
1 fat	2 tsp. peanut butter

Dinner

3 oz. protein	3 oz. salmon steak
2 fat	with margarine sauce
1 carbohydrate	½ baked potato
1 fat	1 tsp. margarine
1 vegetable	½ cup cooked peas
vegetables as desired	lettuce salad
1 fat	1 tsp. oil/vinegar dressing

Evening

2 fruit	⅓ cup strawberries
1 carbohydrate	½ slice angel food cake

1,800 Calorie Plan

Carbohydrates (63% of calories): 283 gm.
Protein (22% of calories): 97 gm.
Fat (15% of calories): 30 gm.
Cholesterol: less than 200 mg.

Basic food groups (servings)	Sample menu A	Sample menu B
Breakfast		
1 fruit	½ cup orange juice	½ cup grapefruit juice
2 eggs per week		
2 carbohydrate	½ cup cream of wheat	½ cup oatmeal
	1 slice toast	1 slice toast
½ fat unit	½ tsp. margarine	½ tsp. margarine
1 non-fat milk	1 cup skim milk	1 cup skim milk
Midmorning		
1 carbohydrate	4 slices melba toast	1 slice toast
Lunch		
4 oz. protein	½ cup split pea soup	½ cup navy bean soup
	2 oz. baked cod	2 oz. sliced chicken
3 carbohydrate	1 small baked potato	1½ cup steamed noodles
	2 slices bread	1 slice bread & ¼ cup stuffing
1 vegetable	lettuce & tomato salad	fresh cucumber & tomato salad
vegetables as desired		with vinegar dressing
1 fruit	½ cup pineapple	1 cup fresh watermelon cubes
1 non-fat milk	1 cup skim milk	1 cup skim milk
Midafternoon		
1 carbohydrate	4 soda crackers	1 slice toast
½ fat	½ tsp. margarine	½ tsp. margarine
1 cup non-fat milk	1 cup non-fat milk	1 cup non-fat milk
Dinner		
2 oz. protein	2 oz. roast turkey	2 oz. lean roast beef
3 carbohydrate	½ cup mashed yams	1 cup mashed potato
	1 slice bread	1 slice bread
1 vegetable	¼ cup black-eyed peas	½ cup pinto beans
vegetables as desired	fresh relish plate	celery hearts & radishes
1 non-fat milk	1 cup skim milk	1 cup skim milk
1 fruit	½ cup orange sections	⅔ cup blueberries
Bedtime		
1 fruit	1 small pear	½ cup orange juice
1 carbohydrate	4 whole wheat wafers	4 soda crackers

VEGETARIAN DIET

1,200 Calorie Plan

Carbohydrates (58% of calories): 174 gm.
Protein (22% of calories): 69 gm.
Fat (20% of calories): 26 gm.
Cholesterol: 200 mg.

**Basic food groups
(servings)**   **Sample menu**

Breakfast
1 fruit   ½ cup orange juice
1 carbohydrate   1 slice toast
½ fat   ½ tsp. margarine
1 non-fat milk   1 cup skim milk

Midmorning
½ non-fat milk   ½ cup skim milk

Lunch
2 oz. dairy protein   1 cup pea soup
1 carbohydrate   1 open-faced broiled cheese sandwich
½ fat   (2 oz. skim cheese: Mozzarella, or sapsago)
1 vegetable
vegetables as desired }   large cucumber, green pepper, carrot, onion and tomato salad
1 fruit   1 small fresh pear
1 non-fat milk   1 cup skim milk

Midafternoon
1 fruit   ½ small sliced banana
non-caloric beverage   iced or hot tea/lemon

Dinner
2 oz. dairy protein
1½ carbohydrate
½ fat   }   1 slice of broccoli or spinach quiche
1 vegetable
vegetables as desired   fresh relish plate
1 fruit   1 small apple
1 cup non-fat milk   1 cup non-fat milk

Bedtime
½ non-fat milk   ½ cup skim milk

VEGETARIAN DIET

1,500 Calorie Plan

Carbohydrates (60% of calories): 225 gm.
Protein (22% of calories): 84 gm.
Fat (18% of calories): 30 gm.
Cholesterol: 180 mg.

**Basic food groups
(servings)**   **Sample menu**

Breakfast

1 fruit   ½ cup applesauce
1 carbohydrate   1 slice toast
½ fat   ½ tsp. margarine
1 non-fat milk   1 cup skim milk

Midmorning

1 fruit   ½ cup dried apricots

Lunch

2 oz. dairy protein   ½ cup low-fat yogurt
2 carbohydrates   with herbs to make dressing for salad
1½ vegetables   steamed mixed vegetables with rice
½ fat   ½ tsp. margarine
vegetables as desired   large green salad with sprouts
1 fruit   1 cup fruit salad
1 non-fat milk   1 cup skim milk

Midafternoon

1 fruit   1 large tangerine

Dinner

2 oz. dairy protein and   1 egg omelette with ⅓ cup low-fat cottage cheese
    1 egg
2 carbohydrates   2 slices of bread
1 fat   1 tsp. margarine
2 vegetables   ⅔ cup black beans with large fresh spinach salad
                                         with chopped radishes and cucumbers
1 fruit   12 fresh grapes
1 non-fat milk   1 cup skim milk

Bedtime

1 non-fat milk   ½ cup yogurt sprinkled with wheat germ
1 carbohydrate   grapenuts

VEGETARIAN DIET—ADOLESCENT

2,000 Calorie Plan

Carbohydrates (64% of calories): 320 gm.
Protein (17% of calories): 87 gm.
Fat (19% of calories): 42 gm.
Cholesterol: less than 100 mg.

Basic food groups (servings)	Sample menu
Breakfast	
1 fruit	½ cup orange juice
3 carbohydrates	2 slices whole wheat toast ½ cup farina
1 fat	1 tsp. margarine
1 non-fat milk	1 cup skim milk
Midmorning	
1 fruit	1 small pear
1 carbohydrate	1 slice whole wheat toast
1 fat	1 tsp. margarine
Lunch	
2 oz. meatless protein 2 ½ fat	2 tbsp. peanut butter
2 carbohydrates	2 slices whole wheat bread
vegetables as desired	large tomato and cucumber salad
1 fat	1 tsp. salad dressing
1 dairy protein	1 cup low-fat yogurt with
1 fruit	½ cup fruit cocktail
1 non-fat milk	1 cup skim milk
Midafternoon	
1 fruit	½ cup sliced peaches
1 carbohydrate	4 saltines
1 oz. meatless protein 1 fat	1 tbsp. peanut butter
Dinner	
2 carbohydrates	1 cup spaghetti
1 vegetable	½ cup tomato sauce
1 dairy protein ½ fat	3 tbsp. grated parmesan cheese
1 meatless protein	½ cup 3-bean salad
vegetables as desired	½ cup cooked spinach
1 carbohydrate	1 slice whole wheat bread
1 fat	1 tsp. margarine
1 non-fat milk	1 cup skim milk
Bedtime	
1 carbohydrate	5 thin twisted pretzels
1 fruit	1 small apple
1 non-fat milk	1 cup skim milk

FOOD LABELING AND PREPARATION

You can't eat a healthy diet if you don't know what you're eating. Most packaged products provide some nutritional information for the conscientious consumer (see the explanation of a margarine label listing in table 1.20). Labels reveal the number of calories, the grams of protein, carbohydrates, and fat found in one serving of food. They also record the amount of cholesterol, sodium, vitamins, minerals, and sugar.

All products list ingredients in decreasing order. The higher the listing the more important the items in the product. When choosing products that contain fats, choose those where polyunsaturated fats are listed first and saturated fats are listed later.

Choose fats (margarines, salad oils, cooking oils) that list the first ingredient as *liquid* vegetable oil rather than as hydrogenated or partially hydrogenated vegetable shortening. Hydrogenated fats are more saturated (hard) than most liquid oils (excluding palm and coconut oils), which are highly unsaturated. Table 1.21 lists the variety of fats and oils available with their fatty acid content and cooking qualities.

Often sodium and cholesterol will be listed on food labels where appropriate. Keep in mind that the total daily cholesterol intake should not exceed 300 mg., and that the suggested total daily sodium intake is 3 grams, that is, 5 grams of salt.

The sugar content in foods is indicated by such words as: sucrose, glucose, fructose, maltose (malt), honey, corn syrup, maple syrup,

Table 1.20

LABEL EXAMPLE: 1 POUND MARGARINE

Nutrition information per serving		Interpretation
Serving size	14 gr. (1 tbsp.)	The weight may also be given in grams, ounces, slices, dependent on serving
Servings per container	32	This is the total quantity in container. It can also give you the cost per serving.
Calories	100	The energy content, given in calories per serving.
Protein	0	Given in gram measure per serving.
Carbohydrates	0	Given in grams per serving.
Fat	11 grams	Grams of fat per serving.
Percent of calories from fat over 99%		
Polyunsaturated fat	5 grams	There may be additional information given about fat and cholesterol. It may tell you amount of poly-
Saturated fat	2 grams	unsaturated and saturated fat content and milli-
Cholesterol 0	(0 per 100 gr.)	grams of cholesterol.
Percentage of U.S. Recommended Daily Allowances (U.S. RDA):		100% represents the highest amount of nutrient recommended for the normal person of any age and
Vitamin A	10%	sex. The percentage listed is the proportion of the
Vitamin D	10%	total 100% content that is necessary for daily nutrition.

Contains less than 2% of the U.S. RDA of protein, vitamin C, thiamine, riboflavin, niacin, calcium, and iron.

Table 1.21
COMPARISON OF FATS AND OILS AVAILABLE

Item	Calories	Cholesterol (milligrams)	Saturated Fat (grams)	Mono-unsaturated Fat (grams)	Poly-unsaturated Fat (grams)	Cooking qualities
Margarines*						
Tub margarine:**						Good as table spread
with liquid safflower oil	100	0	1.5	2.5	6.7	
with liquid corn oil	100	0	2.0	3.6	5.3	
Stick margarine with liquid corn oil	100	0	2.1	4.6	4.1	Can be used for table spread or for cooking
Stick or tub margarine with partially hardened or hydrogenated fat	100	0	2.4	6.2	2.0	
Imitation (diet) margarine	50	0	1.0	1.8	2.5	Good as table spread
Mayonnaise	100	8	2.0	2.0	6.0	Can be used for table spread and as salad dressing
Oils						
Polyunsaturated corn oil	125	0	2.0	4.0	8.0	All-purpose cooking oil

Cottonseed oil	125	0	4.0	3.5	6.5	Not readily available
Safflower oil	125	0	1.5	2.0	10.5	For salad dressings and baking
Sesame oil	125	0	2.0	6.0	6.0	Heavier concentrated oil (small amt.) goes a long way, good cooking oil, too heavy for baking
Soybean oil	125	0	2.0	3.5	8.5	Good for cooking
Sunflower oil	125	0	1.6	3.9	8.5	Cooking and salads
Monounsaturated Olive oil	125	0	2.8	7.0	3.9	Good for use in cooking or as salad dressing
Peanut oil	125	0	2.0	10.0	2.0	
Saturated products						
Vegetable shortening, hydrogenated	100	0	3.0	6.0	3.0	
Butter (1 tbsp.)	100	35	6.0	4.0	trace	
Lard	115	13	5.0	6.0	1.0	limited use suggested
Saturated Coconut oil	125	0	13.0	1.0	trace	

*Most margarines are made from polyunsaturated oil. However, many are partly hydrogenated (saturated) so they will be solid at room temperature. Margarines sold in tub containers are more unsaturated than those sold as sticks.

**Ingredients here are first ingredients listed for these products on package.

SOURCE: These figures are derived from the *American Heart Association Cookbook*.

brown sugar, and molasses. If any of these terms are listed at the beginning of the ingredients list, there is a large amount of sugar in the product.

See tables 1.22 and 1.23 for a guide to preparation and a list of substitutions.

Foods to have on hand

A low-fat kitchen contains:

Lean meats—fish, chicken, turkey, and veal more often than pork, ham, lamb, and beef, which contain larger amounts of saturated fats. Limit and/or restrict the use of luncheon meats, sausage, salami, frankfurters, and liverwurst.

Polyunsaturated oils made from vegetable sources—for cooking. Examples are safflower, soybean, corn, and cottonseed in descending order of amounts of polyunsaturates. Sesame and sunflower oils are fine as well. Use all of them sparingly.

Staples—whole-grain flours, corn meal, unflavored gelatin, vinegar. *Avoid*: bouillion cubes, as they are high in salt; and prepared bread crumbs.

Dried foods—beans (red, black, navy, pinto, kidney, lima); beans and seeds for sprouting (alfalfa, mung, lentil); peas (split peas, lentil, garbanzos); barley, millet, bulgar wheat, brown rice, kasha, oats; herbs and spices, which help make up for the loss of flavor that results from omitting high fat, salty, or sweet foods. *Avoid*: processed cereals where sugar is the main ingredient.

Breads—most commercial brands. *Avoid*: doughnuts, challah made with eggs, egg noodles, sweet rolls, cakes and mixes containing eggs and whole milk, as well as butter rolls, muffins, and biscuits.

Pastas—are low in fat and also in fiber, so be sure to include a crunchy vegetable or fruit in the meal. *Avoid*: egg noodle products.

Produce—all fresh fruits and most vegetables, excluding avocadoes, olives, and salted, roasted nuts. Also avoid canned vegetables packed in or with sugar, fat, or salt. Fresh foods, fruits, and vegetables offer a maximum source of nutrients.

Dairy—select low-fat or fat-free dairy products. This includes skim milk, low-fat milk, nonfat dry milk, and cheese made from skim milk. Cheeses worth noting are dry cottage cheese, part-skim ricotta, hoop cheese, pot cheese, and farmer's cheese.

Egg whites—restrict the use of egg yolks, which contain a large amount of cholesterol.

Equipment useful but not necessary in low-fat cooking

Steaming basket. This item is both inexpensive and easy to use for steaming vegetables and fish.

Pots, pans, casseroles, muffin tins, etc. with non-stick cooking surfaces. These are most helpful for low-fat cooking.

Wok. For low-fat cooking of vegetables.

DINING OUT

When eating out, order fresh fish, shellfish, chicken, turkey, lean meats, veal, vegetarian dishes, and low-fat dairy items, and limit the amount of fatty meats, cold cuts, and whole milk dairy products (if foods served have more fat than expected, trim off the excess). In other words, follow the same eating plan as you would at home.

More specifically, if you are trying to limit:

Cholesterol: Limit cream or cheese sauces, gravies, stews, soups made with cream or cheese, shrimp and shellfish dishes, butter, and sour cream.

Table 1.22
PREPARATION TABLE
A guide to methods and techniques of preparation for delicious, low-fat meals.
Check the substitutions list for alternatives to high-fat items.

Method	Technique	Foods
Steaming	Place food in a container that is put into a larger pot holding $1-2''$ of boiling water. The lid is placed on the pot and the food is cooked from 2 to 20 minutes; vegetables requiring less cooking time than chicken, for instance.	vegetables chicken fish
Roasting	A method using the oven in a pan without a lid. For meats and poultry, a rack may be useful to allow fat to drop into the pan during low temperature (350 degrees) cooking.	red meats turkey chicken
Broiling	Done under direct heat, also allowing fat to drip into a pan.	fish red meats poultry vegetables (tomatoes) fruits (grapefruit)
Baking	Another oven method that uses a lid to cover the container and usually requires some liquid. This method retains moisture and is good for less fatty meats and fish.	fruits (apples) red meats fish poultry casseroles with dairy products
Stewing	Similar to baking, stewing can be done on top of the stove or in the oven. Quite a bit of liquid is used here to tenderize tougher cuts of meat. A problem of fat accumulating in the liquid can be solved by cooking the dish ahead of time (hours or a day), refrigerating the pot so that the fat that hardens at the top can be removed easily.	fruit red meats chickens

Table 1.23
TABLE OF SUBSTITUTIONS

When recipe calls for:	Substitute:
Lard, hard (hydrogenated) vegetable shortening, chicken fat, butter, regular margarine, coconut and palm oil (found in processed foods) peanut oil, olive oil, rice oil	Polyunsaturated margarines (first ingredient *must* say "liquid vegetable oil"); corn oil, soybean oil, sunflower oil, safflower oil, sesame seed oil, cottonseed oil, or a commercial blend of these oils
Blue cheese and Roquefort salad dressing	Oil and vinegar, lemon juice, French, Russian, and Italian salad dressings
Butter (1 tbsp.)	1 tbsp. polyunsaturated margarine or ¾ tbsp. vegetable oil
Chocolate (1 oz.)	3 tbsp. cocoa + 1 tbsp. polyunsaturated oil or margarine
Sugar, honey, molasses	Fruit juice, natural strength or frozen concentrate; fresh fruit, frozen or canned fruit (unsweetened), grated, mashed, or liquidized in blender; raisins or other dried fruits (may be soaked in water or juice to plump fruit and obtain sweeter liquid)
Egg yolks	Egg whites (2 whites per yolk); 1 to 2 tbsp. liquid vegetable oil for each missing yolk
Cream, whole milk	Skim milk or low-fat milk; evaporated skim milk (comparable in heaviness to cream or whole milk, but contains much more protein than non-fat milk as well as questionable additives—restrict use); non-fat buttermilk (in some recipes)

Sour cream	100% uncreamed cottage cheese (e.g. hoop cheese or dry curd) blended with non-fat milk or buttermilk to sour cream consistency; blend of yogurt and cottage cheese
Whole milk yogurt	Non-fat yogurt (purchased or made at home)
Creamed cottage cheese, ricotta cheese	100% uncreamed cottage cheese, ricotta cheese, mozzarella (part skim milk); creamy non-fat cheese
Parmesan cheese, grated, romano cheese, grated	Sapsago cheese (also called green cheese), grated
Cream cheese	Hoop cheese (pressed brick form), sliced, as a spread 100% uncreamed cottage cheese (any kind)
Ice cream	Use home ice-cream maker to create your own or sherbets
Peanuts, almonds, Brazil nuts	Garbanzo "nuts"; roasted chestnuts; water chestnuts; Grape Nuts cereal; walnuts
Peanut butter	"Nut" butter (i.e. walnuts, sesame)
Egg noodles	Vegetable (eggless) noodles; yolk-free noodles; spaghetti, macaroni
Soy sauce	Low-salt soy sauce; regular soy sauce, diluted
Bouillon cubes	Fat-free stock, equivalent to volume each cube flavors
Salt	Spices of choice
Sugar-containing soft drinks	Mineral or carbonated or tap water; fruit juices

Calories: Limit sauces and gravies, salad dressings, sour cream, highly sugared items, breaded and fried dishes. Eat foods that are broiled, baked, roasted, steamed or cooked in wine (the wine's alcohol content, which contains the calories, evaporates and only the flavor is left). Eat moderate portions of all foods.

Salt: Avoid highly salted or smoked foods, gravies, and heavily salted soups.

Eat frequently at a favorite restaurant. Being a regular customer and knowing the staff may make you feel more comfortable when requesting a minor change in the food preparation. Don't hesitate to make a request.

Even slight modifications in the preparation of a dish make a nutritional difference. Fish and meats can be broiled plain or with polyunsaturated margarine rather than with butter if an added fat is essential. Salt can be omitted from many items if they are not precooked. Ask if foods can be served without the sauce or gravy. If it has already been cooked with gravy, push the gravy aside.

When ordering salads, ask for the salad dressing on the side so that you can decide how much to use.

Ask for margarine instead of butter. For your coffee, request skim milk or, if not available, whole milk, not cream.

Reduce the temptation to eat bread and butter before the meal. Take one slice and have the waiter remove the bread basket.

Order *a la carte* rather than a complete dinner so that you do not feel tempted to eat all foods included on the dinner just because you have paid for them.

Before you begin to eat, assess the size of the portion. If it is larger than what you should eat, divide the portion and put aside the remainder.

VEGETARIAN DIETS

The most popular type of vegetarian diets are plant foods supplemented with dairy foods and eggs. Other vegetarians limit their additions to dairy products. Total vegetarians or "vegans" eat only vegetable proteins (see vegetarian menus, pages 168–170).

The basis for a good vegetarian diet should include a variety of plant foods, particularly soybeans, which are rich in protein, B vitamins, iron, and fiber. Many vegetable oils are highly polyunsaturated. Grains provide complex carbohydrates, protein, thiamin, iron, and trace minerals. Fruits and vegetables contain many vitamins and trace minerals. A selection from these sources, plus dairy products, with or without eggs, provides a nutritious diet, in some respects better than one in which meat consumption is high.

Many nutritionists emphasize the importance of obtaining a substantial part of our protein needs from vegetable sources such as soybean products, lentils, peas, beans, and brown rice. Meat, fish, and dairy products are more expensive and are in limited world supply. They contain large amounts of predominantly saturated fat which gives extra calories, as well as cholesterol, which which tends to raise the blood cholesterol level. Research on humans and animals currently shows that the blood cholesterol level is lower when vegetable protein is consumed than when the protein is of animal origin. Vegetable protein foods contain some vitamins (C and A) and minerals in greater amounts than most animal foods and provide an important fiber content. Hence, the modern menu should include protein foods from both animal and vegetable sources.

Following are several means by which vegetarian diets may be nutritionally equivalent to the typical Western diets containing meat:

1. Substitute cheese, milk, and other dairy products (low-fat) for meat, poultry, and fish in the diet

2. A glass of low-fat or skim milk with an otherwise vegetarian meal will balance the plant proteins eaten
3. Combine vegetables so that the limited essential amino acid of one food complements the limited essential amino acid of the other food

For example:

Rice—combine with beans, nuts, low-fat dairy products, egg white, legumes, wheat germ, brewer's yeast.

Black beans—combine with corn, rice, dairy products, eggs, grains, nuts, seeds, wheat germ.

Common beans—combine with nuts, dairy products, egg white, grains, seeds, rice.

Noodles and spaghetti—combine with nuts, low-fat dairy products, egg white, wheat germ.

Peanuts and peanut butter—combine with low-fat dairy products, egg white, wheat germ.

Most vegetables—combine with nuts, low-fat dairy products, egg white, rice, sunflower seeds, wheat germ.

CHAPTER

2

Alcohol

In America today the arrival of guests usually means it's time to bring out the bottle. Celebrating? Have a drink. Hard day at the office? A couple of quick ones will fix you up. Depressed? Drown your sorrows. Lonely? Tense? Tired? Relax, have a drink. Even people violently opposed to the use of drugs seem to have few qualms about the use of alcohol, although it is also a drug.

Alcohol, in fact, is one of the oldest drugs known, and today it wreaks havoc in the lives of an estimated 10 percent of our citizens. The man or woman who "abuses" alcohol will, unless checked, destroy his or her liver. Even worse, at the wheel of an automobile the drinker is a danger to other people who may not drink at all or who use alcohol in moderation.

This powerful drug influences industrial productivity, destroys families and marriages, and contributes to many other diseases. A first step in learning how to control its use is education about what alcohol actually does in the body. Is it a stimulant or a depressant? How long do its effects last and how much is too much?

At long last some states are taking stern legislative measures to control the use of alcohol, through laws that regulate acceptable blood alcohol levels for drivers, and set legal drinking ages. Still, much more remains to be done both legislatively and educationally.

Perhaps most important of all, we must start treating the abuser of alcohol like the sick person he or she is, not as "that crazy, lovable drunk" or as someone who sometimes has "one too many." Until our children see this attitude toward alcohol abuse expressed openly in our society, until we stop seeing humor in drunkenness, we may expect many of them to adopt this destructive yet widely condoned drug habit.

Glossary

ALCOHOLIC (adapted from WHO definition)   An excessive drinker whose dependence on alcohol has attained such a degree that it shows a noticeable interference with bodily or mental health, personal relations and economic functioning, or who shows the prodromal (early) signs of such development.

ALCOHOLISM (National Council on Alcoholism)   A chronic relapsing disease ending in death, characterized by tolerance for alcohol, the presence of an alcohol withdrawal syndrome on the cessation or diminution of alcohol intake, and/or physical diseases consequent to alcohol ingestion.

BLOOD ALCOHOL CONCENTRATION (BAC)   The percentage of alcohol carried by the blood to the brain. The legal level of intoxication is a BAC of 0.10 percent in most states.

CONGENERS   Small amounts of aromatic and flavoring chemicals in distilled spirits that can exacerbate the intoxicating effects of alcohol and the resulting hangover.

CIRRHOSIS OF THE LIVER   The laying down of scar tissue causing decreased liver function; symptoms include jaundice, fluid retention, and bodily wasting.

FETAL ALCOHOL SYNDROME (FAS)   Birth defects including mental deficiency, facial abnormalities, birthmarks, defects of the heart, lungs, joints, and sexual organs that may occur in the children of women who drink heavily during pregnancy.

INTOXICATION   State of drunkenness. Rate and degree vary with amount and type of beverage, speed of drinking, body weight, tolerance level, rate of absorption, and mood.

PROOF   Measure of alcohol concentration in distilled spirits indicating twice the alcohol percentage.

TOLERANCE   Phenomenon in which more alcohol is required to produce an effect equal to that previously produced by a lesser amount of alcohol. (See Chapter 3, Drugs)

History and Definitions

The practice of drinking alcohol, the oldest form of drug use, is found in varying degrees in almost every culture. The sedative effect of alcohol, together with its taste, helps to account for its nearly universal appeal. Since alcohol is made under natural conditions by fermenting the sugar in plants, the custom of making alcoholic beverages arose independently throughout the world. Alcoholic drinks have been derived from such diverse crops as palm trees, bamboo, millet, and cactus by hundreds of preliterate cultures.

From earliest times, alcohol has played a role in religious and social rituals such as rites of passage, celebratory feasts, and treaty-signing occasions. In Judaism, wine is still consumed on all important occasions. In the sacrament of the Eucharist, Christians symbolically partake of the blood of Christ by drinking the consecrated wine.

The prescribed ceremonial uses of alcohol, along with its general availability, have always involved the danger of abuse. The first recorded efforts to regulate the use of alcohol appear in the Code of Hammurabi of Babylon (c. 1700 B.C.). In certain cultures, alcohol was effectively prohibited when the dominant religion prescribed abstinence, as in the case of Islam. In Europe, following the Reformation, some Christian sects made abstinence a fundamental tenet. Alcohol was viewed as an instrument of the devil and indulgence was looked upon as a sin. This attitude was the major impetus behind the temperance movement in the United States and in northern European countries.

In the United States, under the influence of fundamentalist religion, the temperance movement grew until it won the adoption of a constitutional amendment in 1919 prohibiting the manufacture and sale of alcoholic beverages. Although initially effective, Prohibition became increasingly unpopular and impossible to enforce as the decade wore on and was repealed in 1933. Other countries, notably India, have had similar experiences with efforts to enforce abstinence by legal means.

In most modern societies, there is little agreement about how much to regulate drinking and how to guard against the costly and destructive consequences of excessive alcohol use. This lack of consensus is evident in the wide variation in local regulations in the United States governing the sale of alcoholic beverages.

Recently, the concept of alcohol dependence or "alcoholism" as a disease, rather than as a crime or a sin, has been generally accepted. This acceptance raises the possibility of treating alcohol abuse dispassionately and scientifically rather than in an emotional, punitive, or moralistic manner.

WHAT IS ALCOHOL?

The term *alcohol* comes from the Arabic "alkohl," which means "finely divided spirit," a possible tribute to its intoxicating qualities. Scientifically, however, alcohol refers to a class of organic chemical compounds characterized by a hydroxyl, or -OH group, but more loosely to ethyl alcohol or ethanol, the active ingredient in fermented and distilled beverages.

Alcoholic beverages comprise three classes: beers, wines, and distilled alcohol products such as brandy and whiskey.

Beers are the fermented drink formed when germinated grain is brewed with yeast, a process which provides both alcohol content and carbonation. Many cereals or grains may be used, such as corn, wheat, rye, or rice. The final product has an alcohol content of 3 to 5 percent.

Wines, which are fermented grape juices with varying amounts of alcohol, come in an enormous variety due to the many subtle differences among strains of grapes. In the making of wine, the juice of grapes, with or without the color-producing skins, is fermented with yeast and attains an alcohol concentration of about 14 percent, a concentration at which the yeast itself dies and the process stops. Fortified wines such as sherry and port can be made by adding alcohol.

Distillation of wine produces brandy, while distillation of grain products makes whiskey. Brandies and whiskies usually contain between 40 and 50 percent of alcohol by volume. The measure of alcohol concentration in distilled spirits is popularly referred to as the "proof" and indicates twice the alcohol percentage. For example, "100" proof is 50 percent alcohol.

In addition to alcohol and water, distilled spirits contain small amounts of aromatic and flavoring chemicals called "congeners" that can exacerbate the intoxicating effects of alcohol and the resulting hangover.

Alcoholic beverages are high in calories (190 in an eight-ounce glass of wine) that are primarily in the form of fat-building carbohydrates. Except for beer, which contains small amounts of vitamin B, alcoholic beverages lack vitamin, mineral, and protein food values (see table 2.1). Excessive amounts of alcohol will give the drinker a "satisfied" feeling and a quick supply of energy.

Table 2.1
NUTRITIONAL VALUES OF
ALCOHOLIC AND NONALCOHOLIC BEVERAGES

Food Nutrient	Beer 12 oz.	Gin, Rum, Vodka, Whiskey (80 proof) 1½ oz.	Table Wine 3½ oz.	Ginger Ale 12 oz.	Milk 8 oz.	Orange Juice 8 oz.
Calories	150.0	100.0	85.0	113.0	160.0	117.0
Protein (grams)	1.0	—	trace	—	9.0	2.5
Fat (grams)	—	—	—	—	9.0	0.7
Carbohydrate (grams)	13.7	trace	4.3	29.3	12.0	26.0
Thiamine (milligrams)	0.01	—	trace	—	0.07	0.22
Riboflavin (milligrams)	0.11	—	0.01	—	0.41	0.07
Ascorbic acid (milligrams)	—	—	—	—	2.0	122.0
Calcium (milligrams)	18.0	—	9.0	—	288.0	27.0
Iron (milligrams)	trace	—	0.4	—	0.1	0.7

SOURCE: *Data adapted from Table 6.2, page 125,* Drugs And Alcohol, *2nd edition, Kenneth L. Jones, Louis W. Shainberg, Curtis O. Byer, 1969, 1973. Reprinted by permission of Harper & Row, Publishers, Inc., New York; and "Agricultural Handbook No. 456," Agricultural Research Service, U.S. Dept. of Agriculture, 1975.*

Thus, heavy drinkers often suffer malnutrition, filling up on empty calories instead of eating properly balanced foods.

WHAT HAPPENS WHEN YOU DRINK?

Alcohol, even in moderate amounts, has dramatic immediate effects on the body. Because it must be metabolized, alcohol affects various organ systems, and because it is a drug with psychoactive properties, alcohol affects feelings and behavior. As soon as it is drunk, alcohol is absorbed directly into the blood from the mouth, the stomach, and the small intestine, and is distributed throughout the body via the bloodstream. The presence of food in the stomach will slow down the absorption rate. Thus, drinking on an empty stomach can cause more rapid intoxication than when food has been consumed shortly before or during drinking.

Other circumstances that affect the rate or amount of intoxication include speed of drinking, type of beverage, body weight, body chemistry, drinking history and experience, and current mood. Concentrations of alcohol are found to be highest in organs rich in blood vessels (brain, liver, kidney, muscle), and lesser concentrations are found in tissues containing fewer blood vessels and little water (bone and connective tissue).

Most ingested alcohol is metabolized in the liver and becomes carbon dioxide and water. The rest, 5 percent, is eliminated in the breath, saliva, urine, and sweat. Alcohol is metabolized at the rate of about one gram per twenty-two pounds of body weight per hour. Thus, a man weighing 150 pounds can metabolize about seven grams of alcohol in an hour or the equivalent of about one shot of straight whiskey, eight ounces of beer, or one four-ounce glass of wine (Figure 2.1).

Alcohol exerts its primary effect on the brain. It depresses the central nervous system, particularly its controlling and integrative mechanisms. Depending on the blood alcohol concentration (BAC), alcohol may cause physical and psychological effects, the most common of which are shown in table 2.2.

The release of some higher brain function results in excitement, restlessness, and agitation in the early stages of intoxication. However, this phase is followed by general depression and a slowing down of body functions. The drinker may not be aware of what is happening, but it is apparent to onlookers. In addition, perception, balance, coordination, and judgment may be impaired, while the willingness to take risks may grow as the normal behavioral inhibitions are suppressed. Many crimes, accidents, and violent

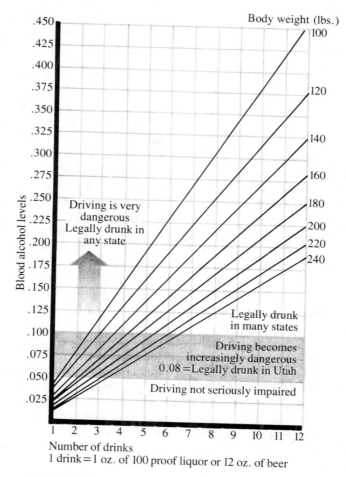

FIGURE 2.1

Blood alcohol levels
SOURCE: *adapted from Kenneth L. Jones, Louis W. Shainberg, and Curtis O. Byer,* Drugs and Alcohol. *New York: Harper & Row, 1973.*

Table 2.2
EFFECTS OF ALCOHOL IN THE BLOOD

Blood alcohol level	Effects
.05–.10%	Joviality, extra energy, release of inhibitions
.15–.20%	Slurred speech, staggering gait, gross intoxication
.20–.30%	Aggressive moodiness, emotional state of depression
.30–.40%	Sleepiness, unconsciousness, and coma
.50%	Death from respiratory failure

SOURCE: Data from "The Pharmaceutical Basis of Therapeutics," 3rd ed., Louis S. Goodman and Alfred G. Gilman, p. 150, Macmillan, New York, 1965.

deaths have occurred as the result of a single, isolated occasion of heavy drinking.

When combined with other depressant drugs such as sedatives and tranquilizers, alcohol may lead to depression, overdose, and coma (see chapter 3). This often happens when a heavy drinker is unable to fall asleep and takes a sleeping pill.

Alcohol's disastrous effects on driving ability is acknowledged in the criminal penalties against drunken drivers. In most states, a blood alcohol concentration level of .10 percent while driving is considered illegal. Figure 2.2 shows how to estimate blood alcohol levels. The age of the driver is also a factor here. The intoxicated adolescent who is inexperienced both as a driver and as a drinker may be a far greater menace than the older and more experienced driver with an equally elevated blood alcohol level.

These acute effects of alcohol do not necessarily constitute alcoholism. It is the chronic, repetitive consumption of alcohol in large amounts that leads to organic and functional changes characteristic of the disease of alcoholism.

AMERICAN DRINKING PATTERNS

On a per capita basis, every American drinks about 2.8 gallons of alcoholic beverages a year, a figure which has grown steadily over the past thirty years. Beer is the most popular drink, accounting for almost 50 percent of total alcohol consumption. One hundred years ago beer accounted for only about 20 percent of the total. Drinking of whiskey and other distilled spirits is presently about 40 percent, roughly half of the rate a century ago. Wine consumption has gone up from 5 to 12 percent and appears to be rising further.

Of course, not all Americans drink. Indeed, about one-third of them over the age of twenty-one are total abstainers or nearly so. Another third are light drinkers. About 22 percent are moderate drinkers. The heavy drinkers amount to 11 percent.

American men drink three times as much as women, and the highest proportion of heavy drinkers are men aged twenty-one to thirty-four and forty-five to forty-nine. While there are more drinkers among the higher socioeconomic groups, the proportion of heavy drinkers among those who drink at all is greater among lower socioeconomic groups. The problem of alcoholism, however, is found in all groups.

DRINKING AMONG ADOLESCENTS

Alcohol ranks as the leading psychoactive drug used by today's high school age population. According to a 1974 national survey, 60 to 70 percent of youth aged thirteen to eighteen have tried alcoholic beverages at least once. The survey also found that the frequency of alcohol consumption among American teenagers does not differ greatly from that of adults.

As adolescents grow older, they generally drink more. By the age of eighteen, about 20 percent of them drink heavily at least once a week. Boys drink more frequently than girls, but the difference narrows as they grow older. The 1974 survey found a higher proportion of abstainers among children with parents in semiskilled, manual, and farming occupations than among children of parents in managerial, professional, and clerical occupations. Black youths, particularly at junior and senior high school level, drink less than whites and other ethnic groups, and have fewer alcohol-related problems, whereas American Indian youths have the highest rates of problem drinking of all racial-ethnic groups.

Problem drinking affects an estimated 3.3 million youths between the ages of fourteen and seventeen. It not only involves frequent episodes of heavy drinking, but is accompanied by other deviant behavior, such as dropping out of school, drunken driving, and the use of other drugs, which can be dangerous, even fatal, when taken with alcohol.

TYPE OF DRINK			BAC per drink
Regular beer	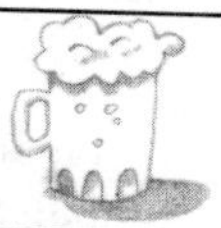	12 oz. serving 4% alcohol	.02
Red/white wine (champagne)	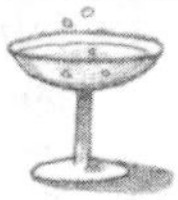	3 oz. serving 12% alcohol	.02
Hard liquors (whiskey, vodka, etc.)	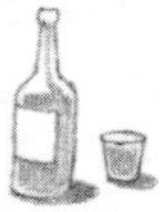	1 oz. serving 45% alcohol	.02
Martini, Manhattan	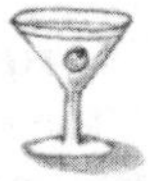	3½ oz. serving 30% alcohol	.04
Old-fashioned, Daiquiri, Alexander	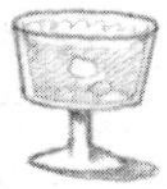	4 oz. serving 15% alcohol	.03
Highballs	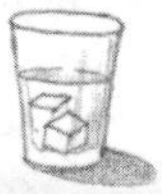	8 oz. serving 7% alcohol	.03

FIGURE 2.2

Blood alcohol content
(for person weighing 150 pounds)
SOURCE: *adapted from* ABCs of Drinking and Driving.
Greenfield, Mass: Channing L. Bate, Inc., 1978.

Alcohol is involved in at least one quarter of all deaths of Americans between the ages of fifteen and twenty-four; 8,000 of these occur yearly from alcohol-related highway accidents. Another 40,000 highway injuries among youth are also linked to alcohol.

The teenaged children of drinking parents are twice as likely to be moderate or heavy drinkers as are the children of abstaining parents. Studies found that it is the parents' general attitudes toward their children rather than specifically toward alcohol use that primarily affects children's drinking behavior.

Alcohol use has become a fact of adolescent life, which suggests that developing responsible drinking patterns in the young would yield better results than trying to impose abstinence on them.

The Many Costs of Long-Term Alcohol Abuse

ALCOHOLISM

The World Health Organization (WHO) defines alcoholics as being "excessive drinkers whose dependence on alcohol has attained such a degree that it shows a noticeable mental disturbance or an interference with their bodily or mental health, their personal relations and their smooth social and economic functioning or who show the prodromal (early) signs of such development."

Alcoholism is defined by the National Council on Alcoholism as "a chronic relapsing disease ending in death, characterized by tolerance for alcohol, the presence of an alcohol withdrawal syndrome on the cessation or diminution of alcohol intake, and/or physical diseases consequent to alcohol ingestion."

The concept of *tolerance for alcohol* is central to an understanding of alcoholism. Over a period of time the heavy drinkers' tolerance grows

because their bodies oxidize alcohol more readily. In other words, more alcohol is required to produce an effect equal to that previously produced by the lesser amount of alcohol. This phenomenon of tolerance enables persons to increase their capacity for alcohol gradually until they become alcoholics. When a significant tolerance develops, heavy drinkers continue to act sober, when in fact their blood alcohol levels would make other drinkers appear extremely intoxicated. Should such a person then rapidly decrease or refrain altogether from alcohol intake, a set of symptoms characteristic of the *alcohol withdrawal syndrome* ensues.

> Alcohol withdrawal symptoms include: abnormalities of temperature and pulse, nausea and vomiting, anxiety, wakefulness, abnormal eye movements, tremor, epileptic seizures, hallucinations; in its severe form, this condition is called *delirium tremens*, which is fatal in about 15 percent of the cases.

Causes of alcoholism

The most widely held view is that the interplay of many factors—biological, psychological, and social—predispose certain persons to the development of alcoholic disease.

There is evidence that alcoholism runs in families; the prevalence of alcoholism in certain cultural groups supports the notion of the importance of biological factors. This should not be taken to mean, however, that those with a strong family history of alcoholism are fated to succumb and therefore might as well give in. It does imply that such people should be vigilant in regulating their alcohol consumption. It is also widely agreed that psychological or psychopathological factors may precipitate alcoholism. Efforts to de-

Table 2.3
COMMON DRINKING PRACTICES
AMONG SOME ETHNIC GROUPS

Certain groups—Italians, Orthodox Jews, Greeks, Spaniards, Chinese, and Lebanese—regularly drink alcohol, yet have few problems of abuse. These cultures have long histories of relatively safe drinking, and share certain common drinking practices:

- Children are exposed to alcohol early in life, within a strong family or religious group.

- Parents present a consistent example of moderate drinking.

- The beverage, normally wine or beer, is viewed mainly as an accompaniment to food.

- Drinking is considered neither a virtue nor a sin and is not viewed as proof of adulthood or virility.

- Abstinence is socially acceptable; excessive drinking or drunkenness is not.

- Alcohol use is not the prime focus for an activity.

- These "ground rules" of drinking are widely agreed upon by members of the group.

SOURCE: Adapted from "Drinking Etiquette," National Institute on Alcohol Abuse and Alcoholism, U.S. Department of Health, Education, and Welfare.

lineate the relationship are complicated by the fact that most alcoholic patients are evaluated only after prolonged alcohol abuse. No single psychological factor or set of factors has been identified as predictive of alcoholism.

In some cases, social or cultural forces can be the most important in mitigating the possibility of alcoholism, as shown in table 2.3. The isolated, unemployed, and depressed ghetto derelict is generally the victim of social, rather than biological or psychological, forces. Although difficult to measure, highly permissive social attitudes toward drinking and drunkenness can contribute to alcoholism. For example, the rate of alcoholism is highest in France, a country in which imbibing wine in quantity is commonplace, even among children.

The progression toward alcoholism

In most individuals, the development of alcoholism is initially gradual, its progression often being imperceptible, easily deniable by the drinker and by those around him. Most often, it is only after several years of consistently heavy drinking that the disease becomes apparent, at which point psychological, social, and eventually physical deterioration rapidly set in (table 2.4).

Given the presence of predisposing factors, the disease requires only exposure to the critical element, alcohol, for progression to begin. The first stage is the social drinker, who has perhaps two drinks a day; this rate can gradually rise to about six or seven drinks a day, by which time the designation "heavy drinker" has been earned. Consistent, heavy drinking results in the development of tolerance. As the central nervous system is repeatedly bathed in high concentrations of the drug, physical dependence begins, accompanied by withdrawal symptoms that act both

Table 2.4
PROGRESSION TOWARD ALCOHOLISM

Social drinker:
  drinks moderately
    enjoys it
      can control it

    Heavy drinker:
      has trouble controlling it
        drinks heavily and regularly (with increased tolerance)
          drives while drunk
            gets drunk alone
              feels guilty about drinking

        Problem drinker:
          makes excuses to drink
            drinks surreptitiously
              drinks during the morning
                has blackouts and tremors
                  has driving accidents and arrests for drunken driving
                    loses interest in other activities
                      avoids family and friends
                        experiences work and money troubles
                          eats poorly
                            feels guilty and remorseful about drinking
                          acts hostile and resentful
                            develops *decreased* tolerance
                              fails repeatedly at efforts to control drinking

          Alcoholic:
            all of the above intensified
              drinking is an obsession
                gives up trying to control drinking
                  feels depressed and isolated
                    deteriorates physically

directly and indirectly to perpetuate alcohol-seeking behavior. Ability to control or to abstain from drinking becomes increasingly elusive. At this point, it may be said that dependence has become well established. With the onset of physical and psychological dependence on alcohol, the disease state of chronic alcoholism has been reached.

Psychological consequences

Chronic, heavy drinking causes serious alterations and disturbances in personality. These consequences may be organic, due to impairment of brain functioning, or functional, resulting from deterioration in personal and social relationships.

As drinkers lose control over their drinking, they experience powerful feelings of shame and guilt that are difficult to tolerate. To ward off these painful feelings, alcoholics divorce themselves from reality, most often with the help of more alcohol. They distance themselves from friends, coworkers, and family. Friendships are lost, performance at work diminishes, marital and other family relationships deteriorate. Job loss, separation or divorce, and accumulation of financial debts often rapidly follow. When such events occur, feelings of anxiety become even more acute; the alcoholic loses all sense of self-worth and progressively retreats into a state of psychological isolation and alienation. The depressive feelings that may have existed at the outset and may have prompted the search for euphoria now become exacerbated through drinking. As this mood-altering drug exerts its pharmacologic effects, acute depression sets in. To the alcoholic, this sequence appears to have but one antidote—more alcohol—which, in turn, only perpetuates the addictive cycle.

Social consequences

In addition to its effects on the individual alcoholic, alcoholism can cause serious psychological disturbances in those whose lives are connected with the alcoholic, such as spouses, children, close friends, and coworkers, even employers. People in this position are forced to make adjustments in their own lives to accommodate to the alcoholic's behavior. They may identify with the alcoholic and attempt to deny that there is a problem. Their own behavior may mimic the alcoholic's behavior with feelings of depression and helplessness. At the same time, the alcoholic can be the cause of powerful feelings of guilt, anger, or resentment in those who are intimately affected by his or her illness.

Not surprisingly, alcoholism is frequently named as the cause of a large proportion of divorces. It is found to underlie many cases of child neglect and child abuse and is thought to engender psychological disorders in the children of alcoholics. *It is said that every alcoholic individual directly affects at least four or five other persons.* Thus, while there are estimated to be about 11 million alcoholics in the U.S., there may in fact be 66 million lives intimately affected by the disease.

A family disease

The majority of alcoholics in the U.S. are married and living with their families. The impact of their progressive alcoholic behavior is that of a shared family disease. During the early phase of the illness, telltale signs are ignored and the consequences of irresponsible acts are covered up by the alcoholic's spouse and, sometimes, by the older children. This inspires resentments which, in turn, are felt by the alcoholic, causing further deterioration in family relationships. As the alcoholic continues to act in unpredictable and unacceptable ways, the family members accelerate their efforts to adjust. Arguments and drinking episodes are witnessed by the children. The family members, both adults and children, withdraw from friends. The alcoholic's spouse may feel lowered self-esteem, intense confusion, and anxiety. A frequent sign of alcoholism in the home is behavioral problems or lowered achievement at school. Children may have feelings of rejection, worthlessness, repressed rage, and a loss of the sense of trust necessary to maintain close, enduring relationships. Because alcoholism affects the whole family, treatment is often geared to the whole family as well (see Secondary Prevention, p. 206).

Alcoholism in special groups

Because of the severe stigma attached to alcoholism, society has tended to deny its occurrence in certain segments of the population, such as women and the elderly.

Few studies have been done on problem drinking in women. Thus, there is a widespread tendency to assume that female alcohol abuse barely exists. In fact, as the number of women drinkers has risen sharply since World War II, so has the number of women who are problem drinkers or alcoholics. Results of a Gallup Poll showed that between 1939 and 1978 the rate of female drinkers rose from 45 to 66 percent whereas in men there was only a slight increase of 70 to 77 percent within the same period.

As in men, no type of female alcoholic predominates. They are found in every age bracket, socioeconomic class, occupational category, and social or ethnic group. The highest rates of alcohol problems were reported by the divorced or separated, with single women next, followed by married women and widows.

Women without a previous history of alcohol abuse appear to be more likely than men to begin problem drinking following a major traumatic event, such as divorce or the death of a family member. Alcoholic men frequently slide into alcohol dependence after years of hard drinking with or without the impetus of a critical event.

Cross-addiction, or dependence on other mood-altering drugs besides alcohol, is more common in women, partly because doctors more readily prescribe medications including sedatives to women.

A major problem for alcoholic women is the scarcity of treatment resources. Because alcoholism is traditionally viewed as a "male" disease, treatment facilities available to women are limited and are not geared to meet women's practical and psychological needs. Also, since husbands of alcoholic women frequently divorce or leave their wives, these women carry the difficult burden of rehabilitation along with feelings of loneliness, abandonment, and the care and financial support of children.

In general, people drink less as they get older, partly because of their reduced ability to metabolize alcohol. Still, alcoholism afflicts a substantial number of people sixty years or older. The stresses of aging—loneliness, loss of spouse, lack of employment, or other meaningful activity,

and reduced physical abilities—can lead to alcohol abuse.

Alcoholism in the elderly often goes untreated because their alcohol-related behavior is perceived as due to the frailties of old age. The physical and mental disabilities resulting from years of heavy drinking often require acute medical attention, as shown by the high proportion of alcoholics among elderly hospital patients.

Economic costs

In 1976, the annual cost to society of alcoholism and alcohol abuse was estimated at 43 billion dollars (table 2.5). The largest area of economic cost—lost production of goods and services attributable to reduced productivity of employed alcoholics—amounted to almost 20 billion dollars. This figure represents the effects of inefficiency, absenteeism, faulty decision making, accidents, impaired morale of coworkers, and the cost of rehabilitation programs.

Health and medical costs of about 13 billion dollars represent expenditures for treatment of alcohol-related conditions. A further 5 billion dollars was spent for medical expenses and property damage due to auto accidents in which blood alcohol concentrations of at least .05 percent were found in the driver or pedestrian. Costs related to violent crime amounted to almost 3 billion dollars. Social service costs amounting to almost 2 billion dollars represent expenditures in the areas of child welfare and special welfare.

Losses due to fires caused by intoxicated persons total almost half a billion dollars in property damage or loss and costs spent to fight fires. These estimates do not assume that alcohol is always the direct cause, but they reflect the frequent involvement of alcohol in violence to persons and property.

Table 2.5

ESTIMATED ANNUAL COSTS DUE TO
ALCOHOL ABUSE AND ALCOHOLISM

Economic Cost	1976 Billions of Dollars
Lost production	$19.64
Treatment of alcohol-related conditions	12.74
Motor vehicle accidents	5.14
Violent crime	2.86
Social service costs	1.94
Fire losses	.43
Total	$42.75*

*Estimated $60 billion in 1980, adjusted for inflation
SOURCE: Data from The Third Special Report to Congress on Alcohol and Health, National Institute of Alcohol Abuse and Alcoholism, U.S. Dept. of HEW, 1978.

HEALTH EFFECTS

When ingested, alcohol affects the entire body; heavy drinking over a prolonged period will produce a number of diseases, some of them fatal. Some physical effects of alcohol result from its direct toxicity; others occur because the drug alters the metabolic process or the enzyme systems within certain cells.

The central nervous system

Sustained heavy drinking damages the brain and practically all parts of the nervous system. This may be due to the direct effects of alcohol on tissue or to the consequent depletion of the B vitamins, which represent an essential coenzyme in the nervous system.

Brain damage accelerates the aging process and impairs mental function, resulting in faulty judgment, marked instability in mood, difficulty in concentration, forgetfulness, and a "scatter-brained" state.

Peripheral neuropathy involves a degeneration of peripheral nerves that produces sensory changes. Pain may be produced by light stroking of the skin, whereas sticking the person with a sharp object such as a needle causes little reaction. Other symptoms include weakness and pain that are most pronounced in the legs, and then the arms.

Wernicke syndrome and *Korsakoff's psychosis* usually occur together. The former is characterized by global confusion (not knowing where one is or the people around one or what time it is), paralysis of the eye muscles causing double vision, and peripheral neuritis. B vitamins, especially thiamin, reverse some symptoms of Wernicke's disease in a few days. However, the patient is left with some degree of Korsakoff's psychosis, a condition characterized by short-term memory gaps. Because brain tissue is destroyed, the memory defect is often severe enough to make living alone impossible. The chances for recovery are poor—between 15 and 20 percent.

Other rare conditions associated with alcohol-induced nutritional deficiencies are:

Alcoholic cerebellar degeneration, which may exist alone or in combination with Korsakoff's psychosis; affects balance, gait, and coordination.

Central pontine myelinolysis and Marchiafava-Bignami's disease, which are thought to have an immunologic origin; cause the protective covering of brain cells to be destroyed.

Alcoholic amblyopia causes impairment of vision, but is reversible in time with large doses of vitamin B_{12}. (See Tobacco chapter.)

The digestive system

Since alcohol is swallowed and ultimately metabolized primarily in the liver, the organs of the digestive tract show many of its harmful effects.

Liver   The liver is the great chemical factory of the body. Within it food, alcohol, and other drugs are transformed into products ready for assimilation and elimination. The metabolism of the vast quantity of alcohol in an alcoholic's liver puts a great burden on its chemical resources and results directly in the pronounced liver damage that characterizes alcoholics.

Only 5 percent of the alcohol consumed is transformed or eliminated elsewhere in the body; 95 percent is burned, or oxidized, in the liver. In the oxidation of alcohol the removal of hydrogen ions takes place; the buildup of these hydrogen ions results in structural changes in the liver posing the metabolic problem of alcohol. Three main reactions frequently occur in progression as liver damage is increased: fatty liver, hepatitis, and cirrhosis of the liver.

Fatty liver, in which globules of fat displace the material of individual liver cells, is the initial change associated with alcoholism and is the most common abnormality seen in hospitalized alcoholics. In this condition the liver becomes enlarged, shiny, and greasy. Fatty liver occurs when at least 30 percent of caloric intake within a two-week period comes from alcohol; it disappears rapidly when alcoholic intake is stopped.

Hepatitis, or inflammation of the liver, is a second response of this organ to the metabolic insult of chronic drinking. This can be very severe and painful, with resulting enlargement of the liver, jaundice, weakness, and lethargy, fever, decrease or loss of appetite, and finally death. Alcoholic hepatitis, when fulminant, has a high mortality rate. There is no specific medication that can help it. Adrenal cortical hormones have been used for their anti-inflammatory effect, and in some cases may help increase appetite, but they have not reduced fatalities. More recently, antithyroid drugs have had a promising trial. Alcoholic hepatitis may subside with good nursing care and the discontinuation of drinking, although some degree of cirrhosis may remain.

Cirrhosis of the liver, the laying down of scar tissue, is the inevitable result of inflammation. The scar tissue replaces healthy cells, causing decreased liver function both in creating new body materials and in eliminating waste products. Symptoms of cirrhosis such as jaundice, fluid retention, and bodily wasting result from the accumulation of wastes and the inability to manufacture needed chemicals. The liver structure is deformed, which dams up the blood at its entrance and further decreases its function. The increased pressure may lead to internal hemorrhage, anemia, and poor blood clotting. Death can result from any one or a combination of these conditions.

Liver cirrhosis is the fourth leading cause of death in the United States among persons forty-five to sixty-five years of age, after heart disease, cancer, and stroke. It occurs more frequently in men than in women, reflecting the higher ratio of men among alcoholics. Although not all cases of cirrhosis are alcohol-related, and not all alcoholics develop the disease, about 85 percent of deaths due to cirrhosis are associated with alcohol. This link is so close that the extent of alcoholism in a population can be determined by the prevalence of cirrhosis of the liver (figure 2.3). Heredity and immunological factors, though they may play a role, are secondary to the effect of excessive alcohol consumption.

Although damage to the liver due to cirrhosis is irreversible, the outlook can be improved with total abstinence and a nutritious diet supplemented with multivitamins. In the United States, a nationwide acceleration of education and treatment for alcoholism has occurred during the late 1970s. Coincidentally, as of 1979, deaths from cirrhosis, previously climbing rapidly for twenty years, have levelled off and have begun to drop.

Pancreas   This organ is extremely important in the digestive processes, for it produces the enzymes that help digest meats, carbohydrates, and proteins; the pancreas also produces insulin.

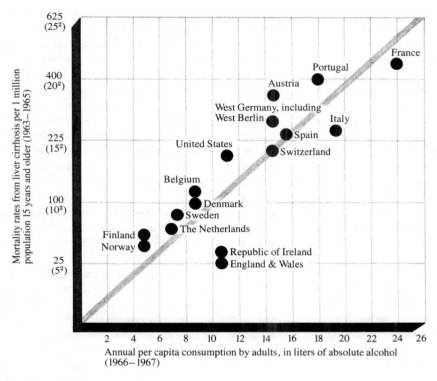

Y-axis: Mortality rates from liver cirrhosis per 1 million population 15 years and older (1963–1965)

625 (25²), 400 (20²), 225 (15²), 100 (10²), 25 (5²)

X-axis: Annual per capita consumption by adults, in liters of absolute alcohol (1966–1967)

2 4 6 8 10 12 14 16 18 20 22 24 26

Data points: France, Portugal, Austria, West Germany, including West Berlin, Italy, Spain, United States, Switzerland, Belgium, Denmark, Sweden, The Netherlands, Finland, Norway, Republic of Ireland, England & Wales

FIGURE 2.3

*Relationship between per capita consumption of absolute alcohol
and number of deaths from liver cirrhosis in fifteen Western European countries
and the United States*
SOURCE: *adapted from Hugo Solms, "Alcoholism in Europe," in "Work in Progress in
Alcoholism."* Annals of the New York Academy of Science, *Vol. 273, pp. 24–32,
1976.*

Excessive use of alcohol may result in pancreatitis—the inflammation of the pancreas and disturbance of its functioning. Pancreatitis occurs in acute or recurring form.

Acute pancreatitis appears most often in men thirty to forty years of age. In its mildest form, it may be dismissed as transient gastritis. However, it can also present itself as an acute emergency involving intense abdominal pain, a rapid pulse rate, and a drop in blood pressure similar to the abdominal crisis arising from a ruptured ulcer or appendix.

The patient with chronic pancreatitis, deprived of the enzymes that help digest food, becomes thin and malnourished. Stools that contain much undigested fat and protein become bulky and odorous. When enough pancreatic tissue is destroyed, the production of insulin is reduced and diabetes develops. The acute pain is replaced by chronic pain. When this occurs, the sufferer may take to pain-killing drugs, which may lead to addiction to other drugs as well as alcohol (see chapter 3).

Although there are other causes of pancreatitis, alcoholism is present in about 50 percent of all cases. The mechanism by which alcohol produces this disease is not yet fully known, although it is known that when ingested in large quantities over a long period of time, alcohol does cause chronic pancreatitis.

Mouth Chronic alcoholism is associated with gingivitis (swelling and bleeding gums) and other dental problems that can lead alert dentists to the discovery of alcoholism in their patients. Alcohol also affects the salivary glands by increasing stickiness of the saliva causing blockage of the salivary duct. This condition may lead to a mumps-like appearance due to swelling of the parotid glands.

Stomach Gastric hemorrhage from erosive gastritis is frequently observed in alcoholic patients, particularly those who also take aspirin routinely (see chapter 3). Peptic ulcers also have been associated with drinking, presumably due to increased gastric acid secretions caused by alcohol, leading to damage to the stomach lining. Alcohol is also known to retard the healing of ulcers.

Cardiovascular disease

Chronic consumption of alcoholic beverages in large doses damages the heart and cardiovascular system.

Heart attack Current evidence suggests that heavy drinkers—six or more drinks a day—have a high risk of dying from a heart attack. However, some studies show that moderate drinkers—one or two drinks a day—are less likely to suffer a heart attack than either abstainers or heavy drinkers. One of the explanations advanced for this apparent protection from heart attack is the presence of more high-density lipoproteins in the blood plasma of moderate drinkers. It is known that the more high-density lipoprotein in the plasma, the lower the risk of heart attack. However, not enough is known about this effect in moderate drinkers to justify the intake of alcohol for the purpose of raising high-density lipoprotein levels, particularly because of alcohol's known adverse effects. The safest and healthiest ways to protect against the risk of heart attack are moderate regular exercise and avoidance of obesity (see chapters 1 and 5).

Heart damage Once a person has suffered a heart attack, alcohol in doses over five drinks a day decreases one's life expectancy.

Heartbeat irregularities (Arrhythmias) Heavy drinkers have an increased frequency of heartbeat irregularities that can lead to death. In a large study, where over 95 percent of the sudden deaths were due to arrhythmias, 30 percent occurred among heavy drinkers, although they made up only 10 percent of the total sample studied. However, other factors such as cigarette smoking also affect the rate of sudden death (see chapter 4). Heavy smoking and drinking often go together.

Beriberi heart Alcoholics often become malnourished because heavy drinking reduces appetite. One type of malnutrition seen in alcoholics is lack of thiamine (vitamin B_1), which can lead to beriberi, a disease well known in Asia. It is accompanied by swelling of the ankles due to fluid retention, enlarged heart, and heart failure. The heart fails because blood vessels throughout the body dilate, expanding the space that the heart is required to fill continuously with fluid. The condition responds rapidly to the administration of a small amount of thiamine. Beriberi is rare in the U.S. today because thiamine is added to many food products.

Cardiomyopathy In some chronic alcoholics heart disease is due to a toxic effect on the heart muscle resulting from the laying down of scar tissue between the small fibers of the heart muscle, making it less flexible. This condition responds to prolonged medication if accompanied by abstinence from alcohol. The gravest cases are those in which the condition extends to muscles of the legs, arms, and trunk in an acutely painful inflammation.

High blood pressure There is evidence that use of substantial amounts of alcohol increases blood pressure. Even in nonintoxicating doses, alcohol results in an immediate, albeit slight, rise in blood pressure. Evidence of the long-term effects of heavy drinking comes from studies that have found that high blood pressure is more prevalent among heavy drinkers than either abstainers or moderate drinkers. The effect of alcohol on blood pressure increases with higher doses but levels off at about nine drinks a day. Stress and specific personality factors are thought to relate to this effect, but the mechanism of the relationship has not yet been explained.

Cancer

There is no doubt that heavy consumption of alcohol significantly increases the risk of cancers of the *mouth, esophagus, pharynx,* and *larynx* (figures 2.4 and 2.5) principally, if not exclusively, among those who smoke or chew tobacco. Whether alcohol increases the risk for these cancers in the absence of tobacco usage has not been firmly established. Alcohol, therefore, presumably acts essentially as a promoter of tumor growth.

Those who drink hard liquor (scotch, whiskey, vodka, gin, etc.) in heavy quantities run an increased risk of cancer of the oral cavity (except lip), the larynx, and the esophagus, although there is no evidence that the social drinker who consumes one or two drinks a day has an increased risk. When beverages with lower alcoholic con-

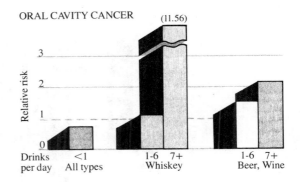

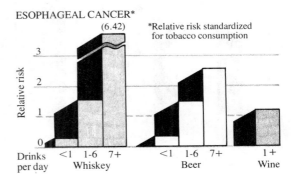

FIGURE 2.4

Relative risks of developing cancers of the oral cavity and esophagus by alcohol consumption
SOURCE: *adapted from E. L. Wynder and K. Mabuchi, "Etiological and preventive aspects of human cancer."* Preventive Medicine *1, pp. 300–324, 1972.*

tent such as wine and beer are drunk in great excess, some increased risk is also found. Those consuming heavy amounts of wine over a long period of time run an increased risk of cancer of the above sites. It is not surprising, therefore, that France, the country with the highest wine consumption, also has the highest rate of cancer of the upper alimentary tract in the Western world.

The risk of cancer is the same whether the liquor is drunk straight or diluted. Thus, the amount of alcohol consumed rather than the type of beverage is significant. Higher rates of cancers

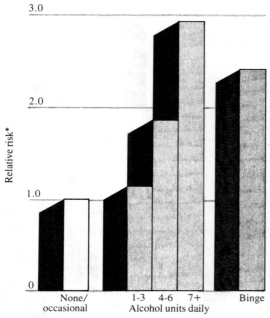

*Risk relative to 1.0 for none/occasional drinkers.
Patients=224; controls=414

FIGURE 2.5

*Relative risk of laryngeal cancer for males
by amount of alcohol consumed*
SOURCE: *adapted from E. L. Wynder, L. S. Covey, K.
Mabuchi,and M. Mushkinski, "Environmental factors in
cancer of the larynx." Cancer, Vol. 38, No. 4, p. 1596,
1976.*

of the upper alimentary tract occur in drinkers in lower socioeconomic groups—perhaps because the nutritional deficiencies that accompany alcoholism are more pronounced in these groups.

Minute amounts of nitrosamines have been found in beers and in a number of brands of Scotch whisky. Nitrosamines are chemical compounds that have been found to cause cancer in laboratory animals. Even if nitrosamines cause cancer in humans, the concentrations found in alcoholic beverages suggest no health hazard.

Liver cancer is also related to alcohol. Cirrhotics have a greatly increased frequency of liver cancer, although the relation between alcohol and liver cancer is unclear since the number of alcoholics is very large, while the incidence of liver cancer in the United States is relatively small. Nevertheless, it has been estimated that 30 percent of all liver cancers occurring in Western populations are due to alcohol.

Fetal alcohol syndrome

Birth defects found in the children of women who drink unusually heavily during pregnancy are collectively called the *Fetal Alcohol Syndrome* (FAS) (see chapter 6). FAS affects approximately two infants per 1,000 births; it includes mental deficiency, facial abnormalities, birthmarks, and defects of the heart, lungs, joints, and sexual organs.

FAS is the most frequent type of preventable mental deficiency. Its occurrence is unpredictable, twins having been born with one affected and the other apparently normal. The cessation of drinking as late as the second trimester of pregnancy decreases the number of defects. The most serious defects seem to be found in the offspring of the mothers who drink most heavily. No definite lower limit to the amount of drinking that can harm the fetus has been found. Therefore, women are advised to drink very lightly or not at all during pregnancy. Fortunately, most women appear to decrease or stop drinking spontaneously during pregnancy.

Miscellaneous effects of alcohol

Overweight When alcohol is metabolized, it provides almost twice as many calories as sugar or starch. Consumed in modest amounts, it may stimulate the appetite too, thus causing overweight. Overweight people are at risk of many illnesses, among them high blood pressure and diabetes, which, in turn, can damage the heart. Severe obesity increases the risk of heart attack (see chapter 1).

Other effects Alcoholism is associated with many types of *anemia* or decreases in the amount of red blood cells. Since the red blood cells are necessary to provide oxygen to the tissues, anemia brings with it fatigue and poor health. Most anemias of alcoholics are reversed just by stopping drinking. Other effects on the blood include interference with the scavenger action of white blood cells against invading bacteria and with chemical agents in the blood related to the immune system that help fight infection. All these make infections more frequent and harder to overcome for the alcoholic.

Alcohol can made the bones weaker (*osteoporosis*) and thus predisposed to fractures (see chapter 1).

Atrophy of the testicles is a direct result of alcohol consumption and a side effect of cirrhosis of the liver.

Drug interactions The combination of alcohol with other drugs is dangerous (see chapter 3, Drugs, under Depressants, page 220).

ACCIDENTS, CRIMES, AND VIOLENT DEATHS

Accidents

The sixth largest cause of death in the United States is accidents, with alcohol figuring significantly in a large proportion of them.

Alcohol is involved in about half of all fatal highway crashes and in about one-third of those where only injury is involved (see chapter 10). As many as 70 percent of single car fatalities involve alcohol, and where more than one vehicle is involved, the driver judged responsible for the incident usually has a markedly higher blood alcohol level than the others involved.

In fatalities involving pedestrians, 80 percent are attributable to alcohol.

Marked increases in rates of fatal highway crashes involving teenagers occurred within a few months after the lowering of the legal drinking age from twenty-one to eighteen.

Labor unions report that at least 18,000 deaths per year occur in the U.S. as a result of industrial accidents, and of these, 40 percent are alcohol-related, problem drinkers being three times as likely as others to be involved in these accidents. Alcohol is also involved in about 70 percent of drownings and about 80 percent of fire fatalities.

> In the ten years of the Vietnam War (1961–1971), 45,000 U.S. soldiers were killed. During the same ten years, 274,000 U.S. citizens died in crashes involving alcohol.

Crimes and violent deaths

Alcohol can release inhibitions, promote aggressive behavior, and thus precipitate crime in certain individuals. Police records show that in homicide cases, 80 percent of the offenders were under the influence of alcohol, as were about 50 percent of the victims. Alcohol has also been reported in one-third of all suicides and two-thirds of suicide attempts. More than 80 percent of all incarcerations, over 70 percent of assaults, 70 percent of robberies, and 50 percent of rapes are related to alcohol.

Prevention

PRIMARY PREVENTION

Primary prevention—averting the onset of a disease—is highly problematic in the case of alcoholism. We are dealing with a drug that is readily available and against which there are few social, or even legal, sanctions when abused by adults. Alcohol is an integral part of our social life— from the two-martini lunch, to the beer at the bar and grill, to the afternoon cocktail party, to the highball in the commuter train bar car, to the predinner cocktail, to the nightcap.

The fact is that alcohol can be experienced with enjoyment when taken in moderate amounts. The problem begins when drinkers consume more alcohol than their metabolic systems can tolerate. The immediate unpleasant effects of heavy drinking (nausea, dizziness, headache) may deter some from further indulgence. However, when the practice of excessive drinking is prolonged, tolerance develops, leading to alcoholic dependence. This sets in motion the development of the disease.

Drinking or not drinking alcohol, even in the company of others, is an act of personal choice, as is the decision that one has had enough. Every person who chooses to drink must assume the responsibility for preventing the onset of problem drinking in oneself. This requires drinkers to examine their own drinking patterns and exercise strict self-control. Moreover, they should consciously develop alternatives to drinking as a means of coping with stress. The vast majority of alcohol users do not become problem drinkers; for many, personal vigilance in monitoring their alcohol habit is a sufficient preventive measure.

Ways To Meet The Demands Of Social Drinking While Avoiding Drunkenness:*

- Know your limit.
- Eat while you drink.
- Don't drink fast. Sip for enjoyment; don't gulp for effect.
- Accept a drink only when you really want it.
- Cultivate taste. Choose quality rather than quantity.
- Skip a drink now and then.
- When dining out, if you must drive home, have your drinks with dinner, not afterward. Avoid the "one for the road."
- Beware of unfamiliar drinks.
- Don't drink to relax when what you really need is a change of pace or some sleep.
- Remember that the purpose of a party is socializing, not intoxication.

But primary prevention through individual responsibility does not work for everybody. Many drinkers need help from the institutions around them: the home, the school, the mass media, and the law.

The home

Young people's orientation to alcohol begins at home. Parents can teach responsible attitudes toward alcohol by clearly telling their children whether and when they approve of any drinking and by explicitly disapproving of excessive drink-

*Adapted from "Drinking Etiquette," National Institute on Alcohol Abuse and Alcoholism, U.S. Dept. of Health, Education, and Welfare.

ing. It is important that parents not confuse children by prohibiting alcohol or other drugs, while at the same time showing that they themselves "need" a drink. In homes where alcoholic beverages are present, parents should set an example of moderate use on appropriate occasions and also provide nonalcoholic alternatives. By managing life's problems without resorting to alcohol, parents can be positive models for their children (see chapter 3).

The evidence pointing to familial factors in alcoholism puts a particular burden on alcoholic parents. Children from alcoholic homes need to know that they are at higher risk for alcohol problems.

School

Peer pressure on teenagers to try alcohol and other drugs makes the schools logical places to deal with the problem. Although long-term effects of school education programs on drinking behavior are not yet known, there is enough experience with school programs to provide some guidelines.

Simple awareness of facts about alcohol and its consequences is not enough to deter the adolescent in the face of the desire to be "with it." Warnings about the negative consequences of alcohol often fail because they are confined to future effects that seem remote from the enjoyable, immediate effects experienced with alcohol.

School programs must take into consideration the fact that most problems related to alcohol abuse exist outside of school and therefore what is learned in school should be readily applicable to other life experiences. As the social milieus of school children are many and varied, approaches to alcohol must be adapted to the different norms and practices they may encounter regarding alcohol.

Curricula for alcohol education programs in schools should include opportunities for young people to develop personal and social skills that will increase their ability to make responsible decisions about whether or not to drink in a variety of situations. Those opportunities can be found in group discussions or role-playing in which the participants act out occasions where the invitation to drink is likely to arise. This requires positive attitudes toward the program on the part of the teachers.

The limited information available about problem drinking in youth indicates that, although the student who participates in school activities is more likely to be a drinker, the student who is a nonparticipant is more likely to be a *problem* drinker. The latter is also more likely to show disruptive social behavior than is the moderate teenage drinker.

Occasional alcohol abuse in the experimental years of high school, when many adult patterns are being imitated, does not necessarily mean a youngster will grow up to be an alcoholic. Youthful abuse of alcohol seems to be an expression of a general pattern of antisocial behavior. Thus, a further goal of alcohol education programs should be to foster a positive self-image. Adolescents can be encouraged to discover and pursue their own special interests—whether studies, hobbies, or sports—that will allow them to develop a sense of accomplishment and of their own worth. Such activities would also give them experience in coping with stress by means other than the use of alcohol.

The mass media

Television, radio, and the print media could be the most effective means of creating a mass understanding of the individual and social costs of alcohol abuse. Unfortunately, however, they are most often used heavily and effectively to glamorize and sell liquor products.

In 1978, the American people spent over $38 billion at the retail level for alcoholic beverages, including wine and beer. Of this, over

$688 million, or 1.8 percent, represents advertising expenditures by the liquor industry, and over $10 million, or .27 percent, went for federal, state, and local taxes. In that year, the various agencies of the federal government, including the military services, spent an estimated $350 million on the problem of alcohol abuse.

There are no legal restrictions on liquor advertising and the government does not require warnings against the harmful effects of alcohol, as it does in the case of tobacco. However, some sections of the mass media have voluntarily imposed restrictions on alcohol advertising. The liquor industry also attempts a certain amount of self-regulation, as well as public education about drunken driving and other hazards of alcohol abuse.

In addition to paid commercials, television programming often offers free exposure to the liquor industry. The casual use of alcohol in entertainment shows serves to support the notion that it is an unexceptionable part of American life. In 1975, a study surveying a two-day period found that over 80 percent of daytime soap operas and prime time programs mentioned alcohol or showed it being consumed. The lovable comedian and the sophisticated entertainer are frequently intoxicated on the home viewing screen. The effect of this kind of programming on attitudes toward alcohol drinking is not fully known, but it is certainly detrimental to alcohol education.

The law

The problem in alcohol legislation is how to avoid laws that are ultimately counterproductive. Our experience with the prohibition amendment provides a classic lesson in the ineffectiveness of a total ban. National prohibition outlawed the manufacture and sale of alcohol, but those who wanted to drink easily found illegal means of obtaining illegal liquor. Precisely because it was banned, drinking became the "smart" thing to do,

lending an unfortunate aura of sophisticated glamor to the custom. A further result of the ban was to increase general disrespect for law in the country, and eventually the amendment was repealed.

Laws aimed directly at the problem drinker have proved to be of limited effectiveness. Persons arrested for drunkenness become "revolving door" offenders, frequently reappearing in the courts on the same "vagrant" or "drunk and disorderly" charges that led to their initial arrest.

The newer view that alcoholism is a sickness rather than a crime is reflected in the law's changed emphasis, which now relies less on punishment and more on treatment. Federal laws such as the Alcoholic Rehabilitation Act of 1968 and the Comprehensive Alcohol Abuse and Alcoholism Prevention Treatment and Rehabilitation Act of 1970, have decriminalized drunkenness. Most importantly, these acts provide financial support for the planning, establishment, and maintenance of prevention, treatment, and rehabilitation programs.

Regulation of the alcohol industry Alcohol is a legally and socially acceptable drug in our culture. Every aspect of its manufacturing, transporting, wholesaling, and retailing in the United States is regulated by various governments: federal, state, and local. The U.S. federal government, through the Treasury Department's Bureau of Alcohol, Tobacco, and Firearms, collects taxes on alcohol amounting to approximately $10 billion yearly. This department suppresses traffic of illicit spirits, determines the size and shape of bottles, and oversees the content and purity of both domestic and imported beverages. It holds the power to inspect and, where necessary, fine or shut down wineries, breweries, and distilleries where contamination or illegalities occur.

Everything else is left to the states and local governments to regulate, which they do in widely differing ways. Table 2.6 shows the drinking ages on a state-by-state basis. Other aspects controlled

Table 2.6
U.S. DRINKING AGE, BY STATE*

Alabama	19	Montana	18
Alaska	19	Nebraska	19
Arizona	19	Nevada	21
Arkansas	21	New Hampshire	18
California	21 (18, 3.2% beer)	New Jersey	18
Colorado	21	New Mexico	21
Connecticut	18	New York	18
Delaware	20	North Carolina	21 (18, wine and beer)
District of Columbia	21 (18, wine and beer)	North Dakota	21
Florida	18	Ohio	21 (18, 3.2% beer)
Georgia	18	Oklahoma	21
Hawaii	18	Oregon	21
Idaho	19 (18, wine and beer)	Pennsylvania	21
Illinois	21 (19, wine and beer)	Rhode Island	18
Indiana	21	South Carolina	21 (18, wine and beer)
Iowa	19	South Dakota	21 (18, 3.2% beer)
Kansas	21 (18, for 3.2% beer)	Tennessee	18
Kentucky	21	Texas	18
Louisiana	18	Utah	21
Maine	20	Vermont	18
Maryland	20 (18, wine and beer)	Virginia	21 (18, beer)
Massachusetts	18	Washington	21
Michigan	19	West Virginia	18
Minnesota	19	Wisconsin	18
Mississippi	21 (18, beer)	Wyoming	19
Missouri	21		

*As of July 1978

by states and local governments include taxes, days and hours during which alcohol may be sold, number and location of places where it may be sold, who it may be sold by and to, and conditions under which it may be consumed in public.

The consumption of alcohol is also regulated by drinking and driving laws that limit the blood alcohol content of the driver to .10 percent in most states in the U.S. In Scandinavian countries, more stringent drinking and driving laws are in force. There, a blood alcohol level of .05 percent

is considered legal intoxication. Probably as a result, the proportion of fatal accidents where alcohol is involved is considerably lower there than in other countries (see chapter 10).

As with all laws, but especially those regulating alcohol, enforcement is crucial. Moderate laws that are uniformly and regularly enforced are much more effective than strict laws unevenly enforced.

SECONDARY PREVENTION

Alcoholism is a progressive, incurable disease that can lead to death. But its progress can be reversed and the alcoholic rehabilitated with appropriate treatment. The earlier this intervention or secondary prevention occurs, the easier it is to manage the psychological, social, and medical problems that accompany alcoholism. Treatment can vary greatly, depending upon the severity of the case, its underlying factors, and the therapeutic resources available.

The alcoholic's ability to acknowledge and feel the need for help is crucial to success in treatment. Denial of the condition to self and to others is the primary defense mechanism of the alcoholic, an obstacle that must be eliminated before treatment can begin. Often a progression of unfortunate events has to occur before the alcoholic will face up to his or her condition: e.g., severe difficulties on the job, family disruption, confrontations with friends, the onset of medical problems, a crisis such as a highway accident, or an arrest due to drunken driving. Education about the dangers of alcoholism is essential in motivating the alcoholic to accept professional help in good time.

The treatment process

Detoxification, or the cessation of alcohol intake, is the first step in the alcoholic's treatment. After prolonged use of alcohol, abstinence is usually accompanied by acute withdrawal symptoms lasting for three to seven days. Sedatives are frequently administered to reduce the severity of withdrawal symptoms. Vitamins and other nutritional supplements are also used during this period. Withdrawal symptoms are best treated in a hospital or clinic. When treatment is on an outpatient basis, ready access to a hospital should be available because acute problems can arise during detoxification. In general, when carried out under adequate supervision, detoxification is a safe, effective, and comfortable process.

The real measure of therapeutic success lies in long-term *rehabilitation*. The detoxified alcoholic must learn to cope with the problems and stresses of daily living that he or she sought to avoid by drinking. Thus, after abstinence comes the development of self-reliance, responsibility, and maturity, and the rediscovery of values and goals that can lead to a new and more productive way of life. For rehabilitation to be successful, the alcoholic must seek out and participate in it, along with close friends and family members who may be affected.

Treatment programs

Alcoholics Anonymous Alcoholics Anonymous (AA) is generally recognized around the world as one of the most effective treatment resources for alcoholics. AA is a voluntary network of recovering alcoholics who provide mutual support to anyone who desires to attain and maintain sobriety. In the words of AA, "The only requirement for membership is a desire to stop drinking." No membership dues are required. AA, which was started in the United States in 1935, today has a membership of one million men and women in ninety-two countries.

AA members maintain sobriety by staying away from the first drink, one day at a time. The commitment to total abstinence is strengthened by sharing experiences and struggles with fellow members at regular group meetings, and by helping others recover from alcoholism. The "Twelve Steps" program provides a basis for living that includes not only abstinence and the resulting physical and emotional rehabilitation, but also a total philosophy of life.

Anonymity in the public media is a tradition for all AA members. Anyone, including nonalcoholics, may attend open meetings, but there are discussion meetings for alcoholics only. An AA referral center can be found in virtually any telephone directory and is usually staffed by volunteer AA members. Whatever other treatment may be employed, AA remains a key element.

Al-Anon A parallel organization based on the AA model, Al-Anon is designed to help the nonalcoholic family members, friends, or associates maintain or regain their own emotional health. Al-Anon groups use the same "Twelve Steps" program and apply the same method of open and free exchange of experience and attitudes of hope within the context of positive peer pressure as occurs in AA meetings.

Alateen Also part of the AA movement, Alateen is for teen-aged children of alcoholics. These groups are not as numerous as AA but have been found to be quite effective in helping children work out their problems through a group.

Employee Alcoholism Programs Many companies have programs for employees with alcohol problems. Although a company has no right to interfere with an employee's drinking, it may discipline an employee who cannot manage his or her job. The concept that alcoholism is a disease has become widely accepted by management and labor. Employees who might otherwise be penalized for decreased work performance, frequent absence, or other signs of disturbed work relationships are usually referred to a company's medical department or counseling service. If alcoholism is found to be the cause, treatment is offered as an alternative to dismissal. Defining success as the ability to return to normal work performance rather than simply turning up every day, company programs report success rates of between 50 and 80 percent.

The cornerstone of a successful company program is clear, well-publicized, and unanimous support by management. Supervisors and foremen are key personnel in implementing this program, and should be trained and motivated for the function of identifying "problem employees" who ought to be referred to the alcohol program. If a union is involved, the program will be strengthened if union representatives are included in planning. Although most company alcohol programs have been confined to large companies, some small companies can easily institute similar programs using community facilities such as AA, rehabilitation centers, or detoxification centers.

Treatment aids and techniques

Individual Therapy by a trained psychotherapist goes beyond counseling to increase self-awareness, change self-destructive behavior, and, if it exists, treat underlying psychopathology.

Group Therapy can break through the defensive mechanisms that enable alcoholics to deny their drinking and avoid responsibility for managing their own lives. In addition, because these groups are composed of fellow alcoholics, they offer empathetic support and acceptance.

Family Therapy deals primarily with the damage done within the family of an alcoholic. Family members and alcoholics work with the same therapist. Nonalcoholic family members come to understand how they might have participated in destructive patterns of behavior in their attempts to cope with the effects of alcoholism. They learn how to break those patterns, confront their own problems of denial and depression, and make changes that will contribute to their own well-being and, frequently, to the alcoholic's recovery.

Deterrent Drugs. Disulfiram (Antabuse)® is a drug which, when taken by itself, is relatively harmless, but causes a pronounced unpleasant reaction when alcohol is consumed. Disulfiram slows down the metabolism of alcohol and gives rise to several toxic symptoms: headache, nausea, retching, and shock. It provides helpful "insurance" against drinking for those who feel they need external support.

Psychoactive Drugs. Sedatives are frequently prescribed during detoxification to alleviate severe withdrawal symptoms. However, these medications must not be used on a regular basis in after-care or long-term treatment since they may cause further drug dependence, or even perpetuate the alcoholic's dependence on alcohol. When they are prescribed (for example, in the treatment of an underlying psychiatric disorder that emerges once the patient stops drinking), it is only with a clear understanding of the problems for which they are used and the dangers they present. They should therefore be prescribed in the lowest dose and for the shortest duration possible.

Can the recovered alcoholic drink again?

Can a recovered alcoholic return to normal drinking? Many researchers have tested this idea by following up groups of recovered alcoholics. While some reports may be found that appear to indicate such a possibility, the overwhelming opinion of experts in the field of alcoholism treatment, based on clinical experience and research, is that total and permanent abstinence is the only method of arresting the illness. Sooner or later, sober alcoholics who attempt to return to normal drinking will find once again that they cannot control their drinking.

SOURCES OF INFORMATION ON ALCOHOL AND ALCOHOL ABUSE

National Clearing House on
Alcohol Information
P.O. Box 2345
Rockville, MD. 20852
(301) 468-2600

National Council on Alcoholism
733 Third Avenue
New York, N.Y. 10017
(212) 986-4433

Rutgers Center of Alcohol Studies
Publications Division
New Brunswick, N.J. 08903

Alcoholics Anonymous
General Services Office
Public Information Dept.
468 Park Avenue South
New York, N.Y. 10016
(212) 686-1100

Alateen Information Center
Alanon Family Groups
200 Park Avenue South
New York, N.Y.
(212) 254-7230

Women for Sobriety, Inc.
P.O. Box 618
Quakertown, PA. 18951

CHAPTER

3

Drugs

With the discovery in 1928 of the drug penicillin an enormous advance took place in medicine. For the first time, a large number of infectious diseases could be cured, diseases that through the ages had normally killed many people. Today, there are dozens more so-called miracle drugs, which, when properly used, have a legitimate place in medical practice. The increasing reliance upon drugs today, however, and especially their application to mental stresses and illnesses, has expanded their use far beyond any anticipation. The psychoactive drugs—from heroin to cocaine, from "uppers" to "downers," bennies to "poppers," Valium®, Darvon®, aspirin, and so forth— are being consumed by the ton: for "kicks," sleeplessness, lessening stress, altering moods, alleviating general dissatisfaction with life, and relieving anxiety. Americans have come to place an enormous reliance on the promised benefits of a pill. Doctors have often accepted the quick solution to a problem offered by drugs, sometimes inadvertently starting patients on a cycle of drug dependency.

The users of many of these drugs often find themselves paying a high price for their dependency. Legitimate drugs, both prescription and nonprescription, are being used improperly with often fatal results from overdosage or from mixing with other potent substances such as alcohol. Most people are not aware of the risks they take in habitually swallowing pills or of the interactions possible between several types of medicine.

What is clearly true is that most of us don't need medicines most of the time. Yet most of our medicine cabinets are stocked with excess, overage drugs that constitute a continuing hazard to ourselves and to our children. Drugs, a symbol of the modern medical progress we are benefactors of, remain still a means to an end, not an end in themselves. The truly healthy body and mind does not need them.

Glossary

ADDICT   A compulsive drug user preoccupied with the procuring and use of many drugs, who reverts to drug use even after withdrawal.

BEHAVIORAL TOXICITY   Adverse and often long-term effects of psychoactive drugs, such as impairment of judgment, memory, or learning ability, and the loss of motivation, coordination, or motor skills.

DEPENDENCE   Physical or psychological need for a drug. Tolerance may or may not be present.

HALF LIFE   The time, in a chemical reaction, for half of the substance to disappear or be converted.

TOLERANCE   Capacity to consume increasing amounts of a drug without effect.

TOXICITY   Health-threatening effect of a drug, sometimes the result of interactions with other drugs.

WITHDRAWAL   The symptoms, often painful and sometimes life-threatening, that accompany discontinued use of a habit-forming substance.

History and Definitions

Drugs are chemical agents that affect body processes. Their use predates recorded history. However, not until 150 years ago, when chemists were able to isolate and purify the active constituents in therapeutic substances, was the way made clear for the pharmacological progress that has made modern medicine possible. By 1979, pharmacists in the U.S. were filling well over one billion prescriptions a year.

Among the powders, extracts, and infusions that constituted our earliest pharmacopoeia were a good many that affected the central nervous system. Indeed, mood- and mind-altering substances were among the first drugs to become widely used.

Alcohol, a potent central nervous system depressant, is probably the most common and oldest psychoactive drug. We know that the Egyptians were making beer in commercial breweries more than 4,000 years ago. Sumerians probably had recognized the benefits of opium at about that time too, since their symbol for the poppy was a combination of the signs for "joy" and "plant." Certainly, the Greeks and Arabs were

prescribing poppy juice and poppy infusions some three hundred years before the Christian era.

In the Western hemisphere, the Andean Indians of Peru and Bolivia found that chewing on leaves of the coca plant (from which cocaine is derived) helped them to resist both cold and hunger and to overcome fatigue. They have been using this stimulant since the days of the Incas. Further north, Mexican and Central American Indians were well acquainted with the hallucinogenic properties of peyote long before the Spanish arrived.

Cannabis, from the hemp plant, the source of hashish and marijuana, has been cultivated since at least 800 B.C., when its mind-altering derivatives were used in India for medical and religious purposes. There is some evidence that the Chinese may also have been familiar with cannabis as early as 2500 B.C.

Modern pharmacology has added far more potent psychoactive substances to the medicine chest. Opium, for example, was converted to morphine and codeine when chemists were able to isolate its alkaloids. In 1874, acetylated morphine was developed. This most powerful narcotic was called heroin; it was used initially as a cure for morphine addiction. At the beginning of the twentieth century, barbiturates (depressants) and amphetamines (stimulants) became available.

The age of psychopharmacology can truly be said to have begun after World War II, with the discovery and development of drugs that control or modify the symptoms of mental disorder. These drugs include lithium, chlorpromazine, Thorazine®, and Stelazine®. Psychiatrists were equipped now with agents that could not only relieve the anxiety and agitation of mental patients but also actually reduce psychotic behavior. Tricyclic antidepressants, like Tofranil® and Elavil®, and monoamine oxidase (MAO) inhibitors, known as mood elevators, followed soon after and proved invaluable in relieving depression. In 1957 came the benzodiazepine tranquilizers; these antianxiety drugs like Valium® and Dalmane® are today's most widely prescribed psychoactives.

DEFINING DRUG ABUSE

Drug abuse is not a static concept. What is considered drug abuse today may not be considered drug abuse tomorrow, for the term does not describe a condition so much as it renders a judgment about the use of a specific substance by specific individuals or groups.

Most mood-changing and mind-altering drugs can be used for a number of different purposes. Substances that relieve pain or anxiety, overcome fatigue or depression, and induce sleep, euphoria, or hallucinations may have religious and recreational as well as medical applications, and these nonmedical applications have often been sanctioned by society. Indeed, there is considerable tolerance, if not outright approval, of the recreational use of certain drugs in the United States, while religious use has been highly regarded in other cultures.

What constitutes drug abuse, then, is determined largely by the attitudes and prejudices, the moral and religious convictions of a particular culture at a particular time. These same factors are reflected in laws to control or eliminate the use of certain drugs; these laws are also influenced as much by the nature of drug-using populations as by the nature of the drugs themselves or the extent of their misuse. The first antidrug measures in the United States, for example, almost invariably singled out opium—usually opium for smoking—and the population most affected was composed almost entirely of Asian immigrants.

When San Francisco passed an anti-opium ordinance in 1875 aimed at the city's Chinese residents, no similar laws were being passed affecting the sizable segment of Americans who were then hooked on patent medicines liberally laced with morphine, laudanum, or cocaine. A few states subsequently moved to ban the use of all narcotics, but not until 1914 was there a national law on the books.

Drug laws are heavily influenced by popular beliefs about drugs that are quite often ill-founded. Yet we tend to cling to our "drug myths." For example, very little of what "everybody knows" about marijuana has ever been true. Early in this century, the public seemed convinced that marijuana produced erratic and even psychotic behavior. The notion of marijuana-crazed rapists and murderers persisted, unaffected by the absence of any such persons. When this particular myth faded, it gave way to the belief that marijuana use almost invariably led to heroin addiction. In time, and after several million pot smokers had failed to become addicts, this myth, too, dissolved and was replaced by the comfortable illusion that marijuana is really a pretty harmless recreational substance with very little risk to the users. However, this belief is no more valid than the vision of marijuana-crazed killers or the conviction that pot-smoking leads inexorably to mainlining heroin.

Despite these changing attitudes, it was generally accepted until quite recently that drug abuse was the use of any mind- or mood-altering drug for purposes other than medical. Excluded from this definition by many, but certainly not all, Americans was the use of alcohol. Today, a good part of the nation, including most mental health professionals and drug abuse workers, still holds to that strict standard of drug abuse. But a sizable portion of the population, perhaps a majority, has moved to a far less restrictive position. Their notion is that recreational or social drug use and self-medication is acceptable unless it diminishes or endangers the physical or mental health of the user.

This more flexible attitude fails to take account of three shortcomings. First, most drug users either do not know or refuse to recognize the physial or psychological risks they run. Nor is it possible for them to assess all the risks, since there has not yet been sufficient study of most psychoactive drugs. Secondly, there is, in addition to the physical and mental effects of drug use, a well-documented social effect. Finally, the newer, looser standard sanctions behavior that is in fact illegal, placing public attitudes and the practices of several million Americans in clear conflict with the law.

It is also true that drugs taken on doctors' orders or procured by prescription are also often abused. Indeed, the amount of "prescription drug abuse" is increasing. By far the most frequently misused psychoactive drugs today are tranquilizers, almost all of which are physician prescribed. In 1979, 168.2 million prescriptions were written for psychoactive drugs, of which 81.5 million were for tranquilizers alone.

Few families consciously sit down and work out their own definitions of drug abuse; most of them simply go along with current opinions and attitudes. Yet young people growing up in a society in which psychoactive drugs are often readily available and widely used should be prepared to make individual judgments about what are abusive uses.

To make reasonable judgments, they need accurate information. They cannot depend upon the latest drug myths. They need to know about the effects and side effects of drugs, about toxic reactions and interactions with other drugs, including alcohol. It is important for them to understand dependence, drug tolerance, and addiction and recognize as well the impact of sustained drug use on their physical, mental, and emotional development.

TOXICITY

The nonmedical use of drugs is a common cause of drug poisoning and acute drug reaction; it is often the result of overdose. Almost all drugs have toxic effects, and physicians routinely monitor their patients to minimize the danger of toxic reactions by the combination of medications or the dosage they prescribe. Self-medicators, however, are rarely able to protect themselves in this way. They are also frequently the victims of toxic drug interactions such as the poisonous and sometimes fatal results of combining alcohol with tranquilizers or barbiturates (see table 3.1).

BEHAVIORAL TOXICITY

Physicians use this term to describe such adverse and often long-term effects of psychoactive drugs as the impairment of judgment, memory, or learning ability, and the loss of motivation, muscular coordination, or motor skills. The regular use of marijuana, for example, is likely to result in diminished attention span and the loss of short-term memory. It can cause users to become increasingly self-absorbed and incapable of dealing with more than short-term goals. A particularly serious effect of marijuana's behavioral toxicity is its impact on driving: the drug's effect on motor skills, judgment, and perception has made it a factor in 16 percent of all highway fatalities.

ADDICTION AND DRUG DEPENDENCE

At one time, *addiction* referred specifically to *physical dependence on* a psychoactive drug as it was first observed among users of narcotics—opium and opium products like morphine, codeine, and heroin. Soon after the development of morphine, doctors noted that patients developed a *tolerance* for it, and increasingly larger doses were needed to achieve the same effects. As tolerance built, patients became physically dependent upon morphine and required it on a regular basis in order to function normally. When deprived of morphine, they experienced an extreme abstinence syndrome called *withdrawal*. During withdrawal, patients became irritable, weak, and depressed; they experienced nausea and vomiting, intestinal spasms, and diarrhea. As withdrawal progressed, and it could last from seven to ten days, patients would alternately shiver and sweat; they suffered cramps and pains in the back and extremities. Since they were able to take little food or fluid during withdrawal, weight loss and dehydration were often extreme.

As other psychoactive drugs were developed, used, abused, and studied, it became clear that other patterns of compulsive drug use existed, and the old definition of addiction was scrapped. Today, an addict is generally perceived as a compulsive drug user preoccupied with the procurement and use of many drugs and likely to resume use even after withdrawal.

The new concept of *drug dependence* evolved as researchers discovered that users could become physically dependent on a number of different drugs even when no tolerance was created. It was possible for users to become physically dependent on alcohol, nicotine, caffeine, amphetamines, barbiturates, and tranquilizers, and to suffer withdrawal when deprived of them. Heavy coffee drinkers, for instance, may suffer headache when they stop drinking coffee and their caffeine supply is cut off (see Chapter 1). Withdrawal from most of these drugs was less severe than narcotic withdrawal, although barbiturate withdrawal could be even more severe, causing convulsions and sometimes death.

It was also discovered that drug dependencies could exist even when neither tolerance nor physical dependence was created. Some drugs produced a *psychological dependency*, a craving so strong as to be practically irresistible. Basic to psychological dependency is the reinforcing power of pleasure-providing drugs. One measure of a drug's reinforcing power is the amount of effort subjects in animal studies will expend in order to self-administer a single dose. For example, to obtain cocaine animals will press a lever more than 4,000 times, and will often continue to self-administer the drug until they die of its toxic effects.

Cigarette smokers are a classic example. Most will acknowledge the health risks of smoking, yet they will continue to smoke because of their psychological dependence on cigarettes (see chapter 4).

PATTERNS OF ABUSE

During the early part of the twentieth century, the drugs most often abused were narcotics, and the abusers were generally white, adult, and rural, as likely to be female as male. Most of these drug-dependent Americans had stumbled into addiction by mischance, hooked by patent medicines or by heavy-handed doctoring before synthetic analgesics were available to replace morphine as a pain reliever.

Narcotics became an urban rather than a rural problem after the 1930s. But there was little cause for general alarm until the late 1960s, when heroin use increased rapidly in large urban centers, particularly among low-income members of racial and ethnic minorities. Heroin, however, did not remain restricted to low-income areas. Its use in the middle class, particularly by adolescents, grew rapidly until it peaked sometime between 1970 and 1972.

While the heroin danger seemed to abate after this time, estimates fluctuate, and it is possible that there has been little real reduction in abuse. Meantime, there has been an increase in *polydrug abuse*, the use of different drugs, including both heroin and cocaine, in combination with each other and with alcohol.

Drug problems can often be identified in terms of specific drugs and specific groups of drug users. For example, the use of hallucinogens—lysergic acid diethylamide (LSD) and such related drugs as psilocybin, dimethyltryptamine (DMT), and mescaline—was associated with the rise of a psychedelic subculture during the late 1960s. After this, the use of hallucinogens declined. During 1976, one of the more dangerous and initially least popular of the hallucinogens, phenocyclidine (PCP, commonly known as "angel dust") suddenly reappeared on the drug scene. In spite of its capacity to induce psychotic behavior, coma, and even death, PCP quickly became a popular drug of abuse among adolescents. Researchers have found that a "bad trip" from PCP mimics the mental nightmare of schizophrenia.

Among older adults, especially women, considerable prescription drug abuse exists, particularly of tranquilizers. However, physicians are more cautious about barbiturates and the amount of amphetamine being prescribed, and abuse has been greatly reduced as doctors have come to recognize its dangers.

In recent years public attitudes toward drug use have softened as have our attitudes toward drug laws and enforcement. Thus, it is hardly surprising that between 1972 and 1977, the use of marijuana and cocaine increased significantly. Young adults today between eighteen and twenty-five are the heaviest users of drugs for recreational and social purposes.

But recreational drug use is not confined to young adults. It has increased dramatically among adolescents and preadolescents as well. Between 1975 and 1978, the daily use of marijuana by high school seniors nearly doubled. Studies in Maine and Maryland found that one high school student in six was getting high every day. In New York State, one quarter of a million school-age children started using marijuana in 1977, and one-third of the state's seventh and eighth graders had already tried the drug. The same study also revealed that youngsters are not likely to stop at pot, for 118,000 students had begun using cocaine and 125,000 had started on PCP. Among public and private school students in the New York metropolitan area surveyed by Phoenix House, more than 30 percent were using at least two different psychoactive drugs in 1978.

Drugs of Abuse and Their Effects

NARCOTICS

The narcotics (from the Greek *narco*, to "deaden" or "benumb") are pain-killing and sleep-inducing substances that have been known to man for millennia. They include not only opium and its derivatives—morphine, codeine, and heroin—but also synthetic opioids like meperidine (Demerol®) and methadone.

Raw opium, extracted from the seed capsules of the poppy plant, cultivated in the Middle East, Far East, and recently in Mexico, forms a brownish gummy mass from which morphine and codeine are extracted. Heroin is subsequently produced from morphine.

Opium itself, which is usually smoked, is rarely seen in the United States today. *Codeine* is used primarily as a pain killer and cough suppressant. Since it is almost invariably taken by mouth, a most ineffective way of administering a natural opioid, its effects are generally so mild that it is rarely considered a drug of abuse.

Meperidine was introduced as a morphine substitute that could effectively be administered orally and would not create a physical dependency, but it proved less potent and more addictive than expected. Abusers of meperidine are frequently found in the health professions.

Although *morphine* is favored by some narcotic abusers, *heroin* is overwhelmingly the addict's drug of choice. There is no significant difference in the ways the two drugs act. However, heroin is two to four times more potent by weight and its effects when injected are felt somewhat sooner than when morphine is injected. Three milligrams of heroin injected beneath the skin will have the same effect as 10 mg. of morphine, and both are equivalent to between 80 and 100 mg. of meperidine.

Pure heroin is white and crystalline and has an alkaloid's bitter taste. Since it loses almost all of its impact when taken orally, heroin is usually administered by other means. It can be smoked and is often inhaled, but the route preferred by most users is injection, either beneath the skin or directly into a vein. Intravenous injection not only produces the most immediate effects but also provides a "rush," an initial sensation that is extremely pleasurable and frequently compared to orgasm.

The intensity of the drug's effects also depends upon quantity and purity, for the drug is routinely adulterated or "cut" so that illicitly purchased heroin is less than 5 percent pure. Other factors affecting reaction are the interval since the user's last dose and the extent of his or her tolerance to the drug.

Generally, the effects of heroin include drowsiness, mental clouding, and a heavy feeling in the extremities. Users may fall into a light sleep with vivid dreams. During this period of heavy

sedation, they may experience euphoria characterized by a feeling of overall contentment, and the absence of anxiety, appetite, and even sexual desire. Not all users experience euphoria. For many, particularly inexperienced users, the immediate effects of heroin can be decidedly unpleasant and include nausea and vomiting.

Although the drug has other unattractive side effects, such as constipation, heroin apparently does little long-term physical damage. However, since users rarely inject the drug under hygienic conditions, they are prey to infections. They often develop skin abscesses or contract hepatitis and even endocarditis (an inflammation of the heart lining and valves).

Heroin addicts can overdose, but it is difficult to determine just how often an overdose proves fatal. Frequently, long-term heroin abusers will collapse and die within minutes or even seconds of injection. For many years, these deaths were routinely recorded as fatal overdoses, for their most striking feature was a sudden and massive flooding of the lungs (pulmonary edema), which is similar to what was described in cases of accidental overdoses of morphine. What was not determined was whether or not the victims had injected more heroin than their systems could handle. Considering the low potency of most illicit heroin and the tolerance of most long-term abusers, medical authorities now question the cause of these deaths, and there is some speculation that the presence of quinine, used to cut heroin, or the drinking of alcohol at the time of the injection might be factors in these fatalities.

Although a physical dependence is created by heroin, withdrawal is today much less severe than that described earlier in this section. While long-term users of the drug require as many as four to eight doses a day to avoid discomfort, their tolerance is far less than the tolerance of addicts ten years ago. Because, until quite recently, the quality of illicit heroin has been poor and the cost so high, physical dependency was rarely pronounced, and withdrawal for most addicts was no more severe than a mild case of flu.

However, the current influx of low cost and potent heroin from the Middle East now threatens users with far more severe consequences.

During the time heroin was costly and difficult to obtain, many heroin users turned to "T's and Blues". These are a combination of two relatively safe drugs—Talwin, a pain killer, and Pyribenzamine, an antihistamine. Drug users dissolve the pain reliever with the blue antihistamine tablet in water, and then inject the mixture. The "rush" received from this mixture is similar to that experienced from heroin. The long-term effects are as yet unknown but this combination has the potential for becoming a major addictive problem.

Methadone, a synthetic narcotic used in the treatment of drug abuse, is itself a drug of abuse. It is less desirable to most abusers, having been designed for oral administration, which denies users the pleasurable "rush" of injection, though permitting them to self-medicate without danger of infection. Methadone is readily available through illicit channels, since so much of it is diverted to the illegal market by clients of treatment programs. Long-term heroin abusers will often switch to methadone to meet the needs of a physical dependency at times when their drug of choice is hard to find or too costly.

STIMULANTS

Many drugs are considered central nervous system (CNS) stimulants, including the xanthines (caffeine and two other naturally occurring alkaloids). Those with the greatest potential for abuse, however, are cocaine, amphetamines, and similar stimulators of the CNS like phenmetrazine (Preludin®) and methylphenidate (Ritalin®).

Cocaine

As a drug of abuse, cocaine has a long and not unglamorous history. In pre-Colombian times, South American Indians discovered the restorative powers of coca leaves long before they were used to produce flavoring for soft drinks. (The coca leaves that produce cocaine should not be confused with such similar-sounding flavoring sources as the cocoa bean, from which chocolate is made, or the kola nut.)

The cocaine alkaloid, first isolated in 1858, was the first local anesthetic available to physicians. But the drug's psychic effects were soon recognized, and it was prescribed during the latter part of the nineteenth century as treatment for complaints as varied as irritability and inadequate sexual drive.

Its nonmedical use also dates from this period. Known as "the king of drugs" because of its scarcity and cost, cocaine was never a common drug of abuse in the United States until the 1970s, when its use escalated sharply. Still regarded as a glamorous substance, because of its identification with celebrated entertainment figures, cocaine has acquired a heterogenous clientele covering most social and economic classes and age groups. Particularly significant is the great increase in youthful abuse of cocaine. The notion that "smoke and dope are okay" is widespread; cocaine and marijuana are mistakenly perceived by young people as "safe" drugs that can be used for recreational purposes with little danger.

The initial effects of cocaine are usually highly pleasurable. The drug produces euphoria, feelings of well-being, and increased self-confidence. Users have a sense of being more energetic and alert. They are often talkative and restless and may become stimulated sensually. There are also less attractive effects—irritability, delusions of persecution, and even hallucinations. Some users may become psychotic, and outbursts of violent behavior are not uncommon.

Effects of cocaine, however, are generally short-lived, particularly today when the drug is usually adulterated in much the same manner as heroin. But it is powerfully reinforcing. Users become depressed as the effects diminish and the urge to continue administering the drug is strong. Often, users consume large amounts in a spree that lasts an entire evening. In the attempt to sustain euphoria, the interval between doses may become as brief as 20 minutes, and intakes as high as 10,000 mg. in a single day have been reported.

Cocaine usually is inhaled, a practice that exposes regular users to a significant risk of damage to the nasal passages. Inflammation and ulceration are common. However, the danger of a perforated septum because of chronic cocaine use is apparently much less than doctors once imagined. Few cases have actually been observed.

A far greater danger to cocaine users is death from cardiac arrest or, more frequently, from respiratory arrest. The number of cocaine fatalities has kept pace with the growing use of the drug. In many fatalities where cocaine is a factor, other drug use is involved as well, for cocaine users are the drug abusers most likely to be involved with more than one psychoactive substance. Indeed, the use of cocaine and heroin in a combination known as a "speedball" is popular with some young users.

The method of administration in most cocaine-related deaths in the United States is intravenous injection. Since concentrations of the drug build up more rapidly in the bloodstream, the effects of injected cocaine are more pronounced than effects of inhaled cocaine.

Smoking cocaine, a new and even more risky means of administering it, has recently become popular. Since it is not easy or very rewarding to smoke the compound known as cocaine hydrochloride present in street cocaine, sophisticated users convert this substance to an alkaloid known as "free base." The conversion is accomplished with kits available through drug paraphernalia dealers.

The danger of smoking cocaine is extreme. Smokers cannot control the dosage and they usually increase their intake rapidly. The impact of this increased intake is evident in studies of long-time smokers in Peru. They have developed dependencies far more severe than any previously observed in cocaine users and run a far greater risk of administering a toxic or fatal dose.

Amphetamines

Abuse of amphetamines increased rapidly after World War II and peaked during the late 1960s when between eight and ten billion doses were being produced annually by the American pharmaceutical industry. Since then, because of the drug's well-publicized dangers, its reclassification as a dangerous substance, and the reluctance of most physicians to prescribe it, amphetamine abuse has declined considerably.

During the drug's most popular period, it was widely prescribed as an aid to both weight reduction and to relief of depression. Amphetamines were also used by students to ward off sleep when preparing for exams and by truckers driving through the night. Many users also learned that amphetamines made them feel good. They experienced a euphoria similar to that induced by cocaine, along with a sense of well-being and enhanced self-confidence. They seemed to think more clearly and sharply. Some doctors still prescribe amphetamines for dieters despite the scientific evidence showing that the pills are not effective in the long run for weight control.

Most amphetamine users administer the drug orally at first, using amphetamine sulfate (Benzedrine®) or dextroamphetamine sulfate (Dexedrine®). Tolerance develops quickly, and the feeling of depression that accompanies the waning effects may cause users to continue drug-taking and increase the doses.

To maximize the impact of amphetamine, many users inject the drug (using crystalline methamphetamine). Not only are the effects more potent, but users experience an extremely pleasurable "rush"—similar to the sensation created by "mainlined" heroin. Initially, an amphetamine abuser or "speed freak" may inject doses of 20 to 40 mg. several times a day. During a run, however, doses as high as 300 mg. are common and have even reached 3,000 mg. The intervals between injections may contract to as short a period as two hours. Total daily intake of orally administered amphetamine runs about 200 mg. for regular users and may be as high as 1,000 mg. during a drug-taking spree.

Along with the feelings of power and expanded capacities, reduction of hunger, and fatigue, some amphetamine users may experience enhanced and prolonged sexual capacity. Less desirable sensations appear as the run continues. Users become irritable, see frightening visions, and even true hallucinations. They develop the same paranoid feelings that cocaine users do, but for longer periods of time, and may react with outbursts of extreme violence.

The run ends when the user has exhausted the drug supply or is too disorganized or paranoid to continue. Then comes the "crash," a prolonged period of heavy sleep followed by lethargy and a depression so profound that many users become suicidal and most feel a need to immediately resume drug use.

The thought processes of heavy users may become psychotically disorganized as a result of the paranoia and hallucinations they experience. This amphetamine psychosis, which closely resembles paranoid schizophrenia, can last for as long as one week after a run of drug-using, or until all the amphetamine in the body is excreted. For sensitive users, single doses of Dexedrine as low as 55 to 75 mg. have produced psychosis.

Chronic users generally experience weight loss and may suffer from ulcers and abscesses. They risk the dangers of infection through injections that are rarely hygienic. But more frightening is the evidence of long-term mental impairment and memory loss that has been observed in "burned-out" speed freaks, long-term users who apparently waited too long to quit.

Multiple drug use among amphetamine abusers is common. Many experienced users attempt to control the stimulating effects of the drug by administering it in combination with a depressant, often a narcotic (in an "amphetamine speedball") or alcohol. But these experiments are rarely successful.

Methyphenidate (Ritalin), related to amphetamine, is a milder stimulant with similar effects and abuse potential. *Phenmetrazine* (Preludin) is the stimulant of choice among abusers in Sweden, where the problem of stimulant abuse is severe. Violence under the influence of the drug is not unusual, and suicide attempts have followed periods of prolonged use.

DEPRESSANTS

A wide variety of drugs fall into the category of CNS depressants, most often employed as calming agents (sedatives) and sleep inducers (hypnotics). By far the oldest, most common and most abused CNS depressant is alcohol. Other drugs of abuse in this category include barbiturates and such nonbarbiturate sedatives and hypnotics as glutethimide (Doriden®), methyprylon (Noludar®), and methaqualone (Quaalude®, Sopor®). They also include tranquilizers, the most widely prescribed of all psychoactive drugs.

Since the development of the newer nonbarbiturate hypnotics, the abuse of older barbiturate substitutes such as chloral hydrate and paraldehyde, which are volatile solvents found in certain household products, has diminished.

Today, the most often abused barbiturates are such short-acting agents as pentobarbital (Nembutal®), secobarbital (Seconal®), and amobarbital (Amytal®), as well as the combination of secobarbital and amobarbital (Tuinal®). All are usually taken orally, though barbiturates can also be injected. Youthful abusers identify these drugs by their distinctively colored capsules, specifying "red devils" for pentobarbital and "yellow jackets" for secobarbital.

Nonmedical and compulsive barbiturate use can be iatrogenic, inadvertently induced by a physician. For example, a temporarily abstinent alcoholic, given barbiturates to overcome insomnia, might subsequently adopt a pattern of use that will produce intoxication rather than sleep. Other patients can become abusers of barbiturates after prolonged use for insomnia. They start by increasing their nighttime dosage, then begin taking a few capsules for sedation in the morning. In time, the drug becomes a basic part of their lives, and if no physician will prescribe a sufficient amount, they will turn to the illicit market in barbiturates that exists in every major city.

Intoxication, whether induced by barbiturates, alcohol, or other CNS depressants, presents a similar pattern. There can be a feeling of euphoria and self-confidence accompanied by a slowdown in speech and thought, a loss of coordination and memory. Basic personality traits are exaggerated. Users frequently become irritable, quarrelsome, and sloppy. They may also become hostile, paranoid, and suicidal. The suicidal inclinations of depressant abusers emerge in the statistics of suicides involving "sleeping pills."

Physical dependencies are created by all CNS depressants, but significant tolerance for barbiturates does not normally develop until use becomes almost continuous. The daily use of 400 mg. for three months will produce a tolerance strong enough to result in withdrawal symptoms for one-third of the users who take that much of the drug. Withdrawal symptoms are similar for all CNS depressants including alcohol and range from tremors, weakness, and insomnia to convulsions and delirium. Long-term barbiturate users risk accidents and injuries during intoxi-

cation. However, they are not likely to suffer the nutritional deficiencies that alcoholics do. In extreme cases, death has resulted from exhaustion and cardiovascular collapse during depressant withdrawal.

Both *glutethimide* (Doriden) and *methyprylon* (Noludar), nonbarbiturate hypnotics, were developed during the 1950s to provide the benefits of barbiturates without their ill-effects. However, both will cause intoxication and create physical dependencies. Withdrawal from these drugs is no different than withdrawal from any other depressant.

A far more frequently abused drug is *methaqualone* (Quaalude, Sopor), which is not only a sedative-hypnotic but also has anticonvulsant, antispasmodic, and local anesthetic properties as well. The half-life of methaqualone is considerably shorter than the half-life of barbiturates, but use of the drug frequently results in hangover. A mild overdose will cause extreme CNS depression; a severe overdose can result in delirium and convulsions. When used as a sedative, doses of 74 mg. three or four times a day may be prescribed. To induce sleep, the dosage usually ranges between 150 and 500 mg. Methaqualone abusers, however, average a daily intake of 725 mg. and have been known to take as much as 2,000 mg. in a day.

The popularity of this drug is based in part on the perceptions of abusers, who maintain the drug produces a dissociative "high" without the drowsiness barbiturates induce. Another reason for its popularity is an undeserved reputation as an aphrodisiac.

It should be noted that certain users respond to both barbiturates and nonbarbiturate hypnotics in an idiosyncratic manner: they become excited rather than calmed. This reaction occurs most frequently among young and elderly users.

The National Academy of Sciences Institute of Medicine criticized the use of sleeping pills in 1979, saying they were often ineffective and potentially dangerous. However, doctors that same year wrote 23,500,000 prescriptions for sleeping drugs. The institute reported that "the consensus among specialists in sleep disorders seems to be that hypnotic drugs (sleeping pills) should not be the principal form of treatment for most patients with persistent insomnia."

Tranquilizers, primarily the benzodiazepines (Librium®, Libritabs®, Tranxene®, Valium®) are prescribed frequently for anxiety and can be used effectively as hypnotics. Valium®, for instance, is the most frequently prescribed of all prescription drugs in the U.S. However, abuse is frequent, dependence is common, and when high doses are used, severe withdrawal, including seizures, can result. Also, the toxic interaction of tranquilizers and other CNS depressants is far from rare. Indeed, the additive effect of alcohol in combination with either tranquilizers or barbiturates is responsible for one of today's most common medical emergencies: drug overdose.

U.S. Federal Drug Administration officials are concerned that tranquilizers are grossly overprescribed, and they are asking all drug companies who manufacture these chemicals to post this warning on all labels: "Anxiety or tension associated with the stress of everyday life usually does not require treatment with an anxiolytic (anti-anxiety) drug."

HALLUCINOGENS

Few hallucinogens induce true hallucinations. Most create hallucinatory impressions by distorting perceptions, altering the ways we see, hear, feel, and smell. In this regard, they resemble such nonhallucinogens as cocaine and amphetamine. Hallucinogens, something of a grabbag classification, include marijuana and hashish, lysergic acid diethylamide (LSD), and other adrenalin-related hallucinogens—mescaline, psilocybin, and dimethyltryptamine (DMT)—and phencyclidine (PCP).

The oldest known hallucinogens come from the hemp plant, *Cannabis sativa*, which can be grown practically anywhere in the world. The active components in cannabis, called cannabinoids, are concentrated in the flowering tops of the plants. *Hashish* is produced from the dried, resinous exudate of these tops. *Marijuana* is normally made from the entire plant, which is cut, dried, and chopped for use in cigarettes.

There are some sixty different cannabinoids, of which THC (delta-nine-tetrahydrocannabinol) is the most prevalent psychoactive. Hashish usually has a THC content of between 5 and 12 percent, while marijuana's THC content can vary from .01 percent in some American-grown hemp to as high as 8 percent in Jamaican *ganja*. In recent years, the potency of marijuana used in the U.S. has risen from about 0.2 percent to almost 2 percent THC. A marijuana cigarette that is 2 percent THC contains about 1,000 mg., of which half is delivered when the cigarette is smoked.

Marijuana

The effects of marijuana are felt relatively soon after smoking and usually peak within 70 minutes, remaining at that level for the next hour before diminishing. Three to four hours later, smokers are rarely aware of any lingering effects. But most of the THC will linger in their bodies for some time. Five days after a marijuana cigarette has been smoked, 20 percent of its THC still remains in the body's fatty tissues. Obviously, marijuana users who smoke several times a week keep building up the amount of THC in their bodies.

Users claim to feel more relaxed soon after inhaling marijuana smoke, a little sleepy or "dreamy." They have a sense of well-being and believe they see things and hear things more clearly. They laugh readily; their perception of time becomes distorted; their mouths feel dry and they often have a craving for sweets. Some marijuana users maintain that the drug enhances sexual relations.

High doses of THC can induce greater sensory distortions and even hallucinations, delusions, and paranoia. The user's feeling of well-being evaporates and is replaced by anxiety that comes close to panic.

Studies of long-term effects during the late 1970s showed that marijuana is far more physically dangerous than earlier research had indicated.

- Marijuana smoking has been shown to be potentially more damaging to lungs than cigarette smoking. In a study of vital capacity (the amount of air the lungs can move following a deep breath), subjects who smoked an average of four marijuana cigarettes a week showed less capacity than subjects who smoked a pack of cigarettes daily.

- There is evidence that marijuana reduces the amount and mobility of sperm in male users and also increases the amount of abnormal sperm.

- A study of female users found they had three times as many defective monthly cycles as nonusers.

- Marijuana administered to pregnant rats resulted in early death of embryos. A sample of rhesus monkeys exposed to the human equivalent of one to three marijuana cigarettes a day lost 44 percent of their offspring.

- A consistent finding in marijuana-treated animals has been a diminished capacity of the immune system to respond and combat infection.

- Short-term changes in the brain have been demonstrated by several studies, and one that used electrodes deeply implanted in animal subjects found convincing evidence of structural changes in brain cells.

While the evidence of physical damage mounts, our understanding of the psychological damage to young users is also increasing. There is considerable clinical evidence of marijuana's ability to reduce attention span and concentration and cause severe memory loss.

This short-term decline in mental capacity is one aspect of marijuana's behavioral toxicity. Another is the loss of coordination, judgment, and perception that has made marijuana a leading cause of automobile fatalities.

It is the long-term impact of marijuana, however, that makes its use by adolescents so risky, for the behavioral changes that result from prolonged use inhibit and may even prevent the intellectual and emotional growth required during adolescent years. This is the period when persons mature and begin developing adult means of coping with their own needs and the needs of others. But the overwhelming tendency of young marijuana users is to become increasingly self-absorbed. Instead of acquiring the discipline that allows them to defer pleasure, they return to an almost infantile expectation of immediate gratification. When they most need to consider long-term goals, they generally operate with a time frame of days and weeks. Finally, because young marijuana users are able to avoid many emotional storms of the troubled teenage years by ducking out on reality with drugs, they sometimes fail to develop the coping skills they need as adults.

Although a physical dependency on marijuana is not created, users do develop a tolerance for the drug. Often they will try elaborate devices, now supplied by a thriving drug paraphernalia industry, to enhance the effects of marijuana. Some users attempt to increase potency with additives, using roach powder, rat poison or other drugs, most often phencyclidine (PCP).

LSD

LSD (lysergic acid diethylamide), first prepared by Swiss chemists in 1939, became a leading drug of abuse in the United States during the mid-1960s. Its popularity waned considerably during the 1970s, as did the popularity of other adrenalin hallucinogens. Recently, however, LSD and other hallucinogens have made a comeback, and their use by adolescents increased sharply between 1977 and 1979.

Sold illicitly as a powder, solution, capsule, or pill, LSD is most often taken orally (although tobacco soaked in an LSD solution can be smoked) and sometimes used in combination with other hallucinogens. A potent psychoactive, LSD in doses as low as 20 mg. has a pronounced effect on the central nervous system. Rarely are frequent doses taken on a regular basis.

Soon after taking 50 to 100 mg. of the drug, users lose touch with reality, feel disconnected from their bodies, and lose their sense of body image. Perceptions of time, distance, form, and color are altered. Fixed objects seem to change and move about. Emotional changes are extreme. Although users find it difficult to concentrate, they often believe they are having profound insights, making earth-shaking discoveries.

Perceptual distortions, however, may create anxieties in users and frightening delusions can result in what is called a "bad trip." As the trip goes on—and the effects of LSD last as long as twelve hours—the sense of not being in control of themselves can push terrified users into an acute state of panic often accompanied by fears of imminent insanity.

The LSD trip can result in a toxic psychosis. Megalomania or paranoia developed under the influence of the drug have had both suicidal and homicidal outcomes. Although some users have suffered psychotic reactions lasting several years, there is reason to believe that these cases involve factors other than drug use. There are instances where the effects of a single dose have persisted for up to three weeks, and some users suffer recurrences of the LSD experience more than a year after using the drug. These recurrences, called "flashbacks," most often involve visual or auditory images. They may be triggered by the use

of another drug, like marijuana or barbiturates, or can occur when the victim is tired or anxious.

Users rapidly develop a tolerance for LSD and for all adrenergic hallucinogens—mescaline, psilocybin, and dimethyltryptamine (DMT). But none of these drugs creates a physical dependency.

Adrenalin-related hallucinogens

Peyote is what the buttons of the mescal cactus, *Lophophora Williamsii*, are called, and they were used as hallucinogens by the Aztecs and other Mexican Indians long before the Spanish reached the New World. Late in the nineteenth century, peyote cults spread among such Great Plains Indian tribes as the Kiowa and Comanche. *Mescaline*, the principal hallucinogen in peyote, was isolated from mescal buttons in 1918. The effects of both peyote and mescaline resemble the effects of LSD, although these drugs are considerably less potent.

Psilocybin was isolated in 1954 from a species of Mexican mushroom (*Psilocybe mexicana*) with hallucinogenic properties. The effects of psilocybin, which is a more powerful hallucinogen than either peyote or mescaline but far less potent than LSD, are evident ten to fifteen minutes after the drug has been taken and last from five to six hours. Users often report much anxiety during the early stages of a psilocybin trip.

The effects of *DMT* (*dimethyltryptamine*) last for less than an hour and closely resemble the effects of other adrenergic hallucinogens, although they are believed to induce a state of panic more frequently. This may be the result of DMT's rapid action, which allows little time for users to adjust to changes in sensory perceptions.

Phencyclidine (*PCP*), most commonly known as "angel dust," was first synthesized for use as a general anesthetic, but revealed erratic side effects and subsequently was used legally only by veterinarians as an immobilizing agent for primates. The drug's illicit use as a hallucinogen began in 1965 on the West Coast. Its popularity was limited by the extreme reactions of users. For reasons that are not easy to understand, PCP reappeared on the West Coast during the early 1970s and spread quickly across the country. By 1977, nearly 6 percent of the nation's youngsters between twelve and seventeen had used the drug, as had nearly 14 percent of young adults between eighteen and twenty-five.

A white powder, easily dissolved in water, PCP was originally administered orally. It can be injected or inhaled, but the most popular mode of use is smoking, after the drug has been sprinkled on a marijuana cigarette.

Effects of phencyclidine usually last from four to six hours. There is the sense of being disconnected from one's body and loss of body image. Users feel separated from their surroundings. Time expands. Sense of touch is dulled. Coordination diminishes. Yet there are feelings of increased strength and power. Hallucinations may occur and sometimes feelings of anxiety. But the most frightening aspect of the drug is the bizarre behavior it can induce. Studies show that PCP can make some people violent although they have had no previous history of violence. Users have attacked, injured, and killed close friends. One killed his mother. Another stepped off the roof of a building.

PCP overdose has become a frequent medical emergency that can involve respiratory depression, convulsions, and coma. At high doses, phencyclidine has induced comas lasting several days.

Often the aftermath of PCP abuse is phencyclidine-induced psychosis, and it can result from a single dose. Lasting up to three weeks, PCP psychosis is characterized by violent behavior in its initial stage and can easily be misdiagnosed as schizophrenia.

Persistent use of phencyclidine may result in loss of reasoning skills and memory. Speech is affected, and chronic users may also experience mood disorders and become more depressed, anxious, or violent.

VOLATILE NITRITES

These vasodilators relax smooth muscles of the body's small blood vessels. The best known of volatile nitrites, *amyl nitrite*, has been used to provide relief for victims of angina pectoris since 1867. Packaged in fragile glass covered with cloth webbing, amyl capsules can be easily crushed beneath the nostrils and inhaled to relieve anginal pain.

During the late 1960s, amyl nitrite developed a reputation as an aphrodisiac, and amyl capsules, or "poppers," were in great demand to provide an expanded orgasmic experience during sexual intercourse. Sales of the drug rose sharply, but were brought under control in 1968 when amyl nitrite became available only by prescription.

However, other volatile nitrites, including *butyl nitrite*, which has essentially the same effects as amyl nitrite but lacks its history of medical use, have since become available to abusers through the drug paraphernalia market. Under such trade names as Rush, Bullet, and Locker Room, these substances are sold ostensibly for use as room deodorizers.

In addition to a sensation of light-headedness as blood rushes through the veins, abusers of volatile nitrites experience headaches, nausea, and dizziness. There is considerable strain on the heart and some indication that long-term effects may include anemia and irritation of the lungs.

Prevention, Intervention, and Treatment

To understand what it is that drug abuse prevention prevents and drug abuse treatment treats, it is necessary to recall society's changing perception of what constitutes drug abuse. The older and stricter definition was the use of any mind- or mood-altering drug for purposes other than medical. But today's far less restrictive position is generally more tolerant of what is considered social or recreational use of certain drugs. It holds drug abuse to be only the nonmedical use of a psychoactive substance that diminishes or endangers the physical or mental health of the user.

The shortcomings of this more flexible notion of drug abuse, mentioned earlier, include the unwillingness of most users to recognize the risks they run, the limited research available on the effects of most psychoactive drugs, and the sanctioning of behavior that is clearly in conflict with the law.

A tragic flaw in this current, popular definition is its focus on specific physical and mental hazards. While many psychoactive drugs—though not all—are physically and mentally harmful, preoccupation with physical and mental risks detracts from the more serious chronic effects of drug abuse—the effects that are primarily emotional and social. When the use of a mood- or a mind-changing substance is a recurring or predictable part of behavior, it produces changes in attitudes, habits, and concepts of self that are pronounced and distinctive enough to be readily recognizable as symptoms of a disability. It is this disability, this pattern of behavior and frame of mind, that is the target of drug abuse prevention, intervention, and treatment.

The misuse of drugs can begin for many reasons. Often these reasons reflect attempts to enhance aspects of everyday life—to be sharper in school or at work, to be more relaxed during leisure hours, to overcome shyness or self-consciousness in social or sexual situations. Many users maintain they simply want to "feel good," although their drug-taking may actually be a way to avoid feeling bad, to escape an emotional conflict or problem. But it doesn't matter what the initial motivation is. Once drug-taking is a regular or predictable activity, no further reason is needed. Drug use is self-reinforcing, and it becomes an integral part of the user's life.

Today, not only does drug abuse reinforce itself, but it is often socially reinforced. With the growing number of drug-using youngsters, increasingly strong pressures are brought to bear on individual young people to share drugs with their friends. Indeed, it can be difficult for teenagers to keep friends who use drugs when they do not. What many adolescents and preadolescents fail to realize is that keeping such friends by sharing their drugs means sharing what soon becomes a way of life.

While it is true that using psychoactive drugs is a matter of choice, choices become progressively harder to make once use begins. Drug use quickly produces pronounced changes not only in social patterns but also in the way drug users think, the way they deal with others, and the way they regard themselves. The goal of drug abuse prevention, therefore, is not only to reduce the likelihood of youngsters becoming involved with drugs, by informing them of drug dangers, but also to foster attitudes and habits that provide young people with positive values and that make them less likely to adopt drug-abusing patterns of behavior. Intervention attempts to change behavior once drug abuse has begun, while treatment involves the far more difficult process of breaking habits and entrenched patterns of behavior, and of encouraging and supporting an altered way of living.

The division of prevention, intervention, and treatment are nowhere near as neat as they may seem. They are, in reality, part of a continuum, and it is almost impossible to say where one leaves off and the next begins. At what point does a youngster become a candidate for intervention—after one marijuana cigarette, or two, or ten? When is treatment necessary—when a teenager starts staying away from home, starts missing school, or drops out completely? These decisions must be made based on the individual youngsters involved, their homes, and families, and the prevention, intervention, or treatment services available in or through the school and in the community.

PREVENTION

In the home

Drug abuse prevention starts at home, for parents are by far the most effective preventers. They are able to encourage positive attitudes about drugs by example, by the way they use tobacco and alcohol, and by the way they use medication. Parents who frequently drink excessively or self-medicate when they feel tense or overwrought are giving their children a damaging set of signals.

Equally important is the way parents dispense medication to their children when they are small. The mother who gives a fretful baby aspirin to quiet the child's crying is establishing a dangerous pattern. Parents who treat imaginary complaints, like the mythical tummy ache that keeps a youngster home from school, by providing medication instead of the attention the child needs are teaching that youngster to misuse drugs. Many children develop bizarre notions about the magical properties of drugs. Unless they see clearly how drugs are properly used, these notions can be reinforced along with other inappropriate ideas of drug use.

Another area where parental example can be dangerous is in the handling of anger or frustration. Not only is it terrifying for children to see adults out of control, it also gives them little idea of how to deal with the powerful emotions they themselves feel. Parents who give way to rage or despair leave the way open for their youngsters to turn to drugs as a means of coping with feelings that frighten or depress them.

As youngsters grow and begin to develop their own ideas and attitudes, it's important for parents to make clear where they stand on the nonmedical use of drugs. This is rarely effective when presented simply as "No drugs, and no discussion." Parents should be willing to discuss drug use and should bring to that discussion at least as much information as their children pos-

sess. They should be prepared to make distinctions between the use of alcohol and marijuana and between the use of both these substances by adults and by adolescents.

Drugs should not be discussed in a vacuum, but in the context of a youngster's other attitudes and feelings. It is not always easy for parents to develop the kind of open communication that allows adolescent children to talk comfortably about what they feel. They try to mask their fears and uncertainties. For parents, it takes patience and some recollection of their own adolescent years to hear some of the things their teenagers worry about.

In school

Drug education in the schools has not always proven a productive means of prevention. Until the mid-1970s, most school drug education programs took an ostensibly factual approach, stressing dire consequences, usually in moralistic tones and almost invariably in a traditional classroom setting. Prevention professionals found that the facts were often incorrect and that "scare tactics" tended to increase curiosity and experimentation.

Since that time, drug education programs have tended to avoid simplistic presentations. They use more accurate information and a variety of different forms—rap sessions, student information tables, student peer leaders—and involve other teachers as well as parents. Drug educators have devised special programs for children whose truancy or classroom behavior indicates a greater vulnerability to drug abuse. These programs not only deal with drug facts and drug dangers but also help youngsters to develop more positive value systems, build self-esteem, and find new areas of interest.

In the community

Community drug abuse prevention activities include special recreation programs for adolescents, after-school and evening programs, and teen centers. There may also be local information programs disseminating information about drugs and drug abuse services on radio, in newspapers, and on billboards. In many communities a "hot line" provides information and referral to drug abuse agencies.

In a growing number of communities today, parent groups are being formed. Usually, these groups are started after some incident or series of incidents has focused attention on the extent of youthful drug abuse. Often, parents will draw together for mutual support, to resolve questions of adolescent behavior like curfews, chaperones, and party crashing. Many of these groups have been able to confront youthful drug abuse and to change it dramatically.

Through legislation

Harsh drug laws, as a means of preventing drug abuse, no longer have popular support. Indeed, the pendulum has swung the other way. The decriminalization of possession of small amounts of marijuana in some states and the nonenforcement of antipot laws in others are a reflection of more tolerant public attitudes toward what is now called "social" drug use.

These new laws, however, have contributed significantly to the increase in youthful drug abuse, for they have delivered to young people the very clear message that getting high is okay—it has society's approval and is sanctioned by law. Amplifying this message is the presence of "head shops" selling drug paraphernalia in neighborhood shopping malls and suburban shopping centers across the nation. Several communities and a number of states have moved to control head shops, recognizing that these shops, which distribute literature, materials, and some very sophisticated equipment that make it possible or more enjoyable to use illicit drugs, sell to children, attract children, and attract drug dealers as well. They are, in fact, small learning centers and supply posts for young abusers. The U.S. Department of Justice has prepared model legislation, which several state legislatures have adopted,

to control the sale of drug paraphernalia, and parent groups in many different parts of the country are urging that this legislation be passed.

INTERVENTION

In the home

As parents are the most effective drug abuse preventers, so are they best able to intervene early in the drug abuse process. Youngsters who have been experimenting with drugs often develop feelings of guilt or anxiety and may well raise the matter with parents if they feel secure enough to be sure their parents won't respond with anger.

When this happens, parents can frequently help their children to deal with guilts and anxieties, find ways to break social patterns, and cope with feelings that may have contributed to drug use. While parents should approach the question of experimentation with understanding, this understanding cannot extend to condoning the use of drugs. Indeed, as a bottom line, parents must make clear their "no drugs" position and be prepared to enforce it. Often, such a hard line strains parent-child relationships.

Few parents today want to think of themselves as authoritarian. They do not enjoy defining the parent-child relationship in terms of compulsion. They would prefer to stress its emotional rewards, the satisfactions that come from loving and sharing and trusting. As a result, some parents seek to create and sustain this kind of rewarding relationship by retreating from the exercise of parental authority. Yet, while it is useful to seek communication instead of simple compliance, to favor reason over commands, parents cannot throw up their hands when these methods fail.

Children will test their parents, always seeking more control over their own lives. They will demand freedoms before they are able to deal with them, and many youngsters today are winning their fight for premature freedoms only to lose something far more valuable—the sense of security of a neat and orderly environment that they need to mature comfortably.

When dealing with experimentation or the beginnings of regular drug use, parents must recognize that they can exercise considerable control over their children's lives if they are willing to risk their offsprings' displeasure. It is equally important for parents to realize that no matter how much youngsters may resent and protest restrictions, they will usually find a great deal of comfort in this demanding expression of parental love and concern.

In schools and communities

School programs to halt the drug abuse process once it has begun involve individual counseling and group counseling, with the use of student peer group leaders. Schools also refer youngsters to outside agencies, like the Step One program operated by Phoenix House in New York City, which is staffed by both licensed teachers and drug counselors.

What is important in intervention is ensuring that a youngster gets all the help he or she needs to begin changing behavior and goals. This may be weekly or semiweekly counseling sessions or even daily participation in an afterschool program or an alternative educational program like Step One. Should this prove ineffective, however, the youngster may well need the more demanding structure of a treatment program.

TREATMENT

Young people with serious drug abuse problems often respond well to treatment in a residential community that uses the therapeutic concept originated by Synanon and developed subsequently by programs like Phoenix House. Vital to this brand of therapy is interrupting the drug abuse cycle, a way of life that is protected by attitudes, habits, and a circle of fellow drug abusers. In such a residential facility, the break with both the past and the outside world is complete. Residents start relearning attitudes and habits, living in the artificial world of the community with its rigid behavioral demands and emotional safeguards. Helped by staff counseling and peer support, using the group encounter as a means to discover themselves, they are most often able to end drug dependency and acquire new values and goals, within a period of twelve to eighteen months.

Resources

The latest information on drug abuse prevention and treatment is available on request from:

National Clearinghouse for Drug Abuse
Information
Room 10A–56
5600 Fishers Lane
Rockville, MD. 20857
(301) 443-6500

To learn about prevention programs and activities of the National Institute of Drug Abuse, write to:

Prevention Branch
Division of Resource Development
National Institute on Drug Abuse
Room 10A–30
5600 Fishers Lane
Rockville, MD. 20857

Each state has a single agency responsible for drug abuse prevention, intervention, and treatment. These agencies are usually the best sources of information about local problems.

Although this chapter is primarily about drug abuse, it is important to know how everyday medications can interact dangerously with other medications, foods, or drink. For this reason, the following table (table 3.1) is included. It lists the fifty most commonly prescribed medications, whether they are habit-forming, what other substances may cause harmful interactions, and when to avoid taking them.

Table 3.1
MOST COMMONLY PRESCRIBED DRUGS AND THEIR INTERACTIONS

Drug Category and Generic Contents	Brand Names	Habit Forming	Possible Harmful Interactions
			(P) = Avoid during pregnancy (L) = Avoid during lactation (D) = Avoid driving
1. Analgesics (pain relievers)			
Propoxyphene	Darvon® (propoxyphene), Darvocet-N® (propoxyphene and acetominophen), Darvon Compound 65® (propoxyphene, aspirin, caffeine, and phenacetin)	Yes	Alcohol, cigarettes, muscle-relaxing drugs, tranquilizers, narcotics, sedatives, antihistamines, anti-inflammatory medications, anticoagulants, probenecid (P + L) (D)
Acetaminophen	Tylenol®, Phenaphen®, Tempra®, and others	No	May increase effects of anticoagulant drugs, such as Coumadin® (Warfarin).
Acetylsalicylic acid	Aspirins and other drugs having aspirin as main pain reliever (Alka-Seltzer®, Bufferin®, Emperin®)	No	Probenecid, spironolactone, sulfinpyrazone, propranolol, antacids, phenobarbital, reserpine, PAS (para-asninosalicylic acid), cortisone, furosomide, indomethocin, phenylbutazone, anticoagulants
Butalbital, aspirin, codeine, caffeine, phenacetin	Fiorinal®	Yes	Alcohol, other sedatives, general anesthetics, anti-inflammatory medications, oral anticoagulants, tricyclic antidepressants, digitalis preparations, phenytoin sodium methotrexate, oral drugs to treat diabetes (P+L) (D)
Oxycodone HC1, oxycodone terephthlate, aspirin, phenacetin, and caffeine	Percodan®	Yes	Alcohol, sedatives (including antihistamines), oral drugs for diabetes, methotrexate, probenecid, sulfinpyrazone, muscle relaxants (P+L)

Drug Category and Generic Contents	Brand Names	Habit Forming	Possible Harmful Interactions
2. Anorexics (appetite suppressants)			
Amphetamines*	Biphetamine®, Bamadex®, Dexedrine®, Desoxyn®, Benzedrine®, Obotan®	Yes	Tricyclic antidepressants; guanethidine; MAO inhibitors, phenothiazines, sodium bicarbonate, strong pain killers, hydralizine, methyldopa, reserpine, thiazide diuretics, amantadine, vitamin C. Avoid beer, Chianti wine, and vermouth (P+L)
Phentermine, mazindol, diethylproprion, clortermine, fengluramine (nonamphetamines)**	Fastin®, Pre-Sate®, Xoranil®, Tenuate®, Pondimin®, Sanorex®, Ionamin®	Yes	
3. Antiarthritics			
Allopurinol	Zyloprim®	No	Diuretics (mainly thiazides) may decrease effectiveness of allopurinol® (L)
Indomethocin	Indocin® (no generics available)	No	Steroids, aspirin, oral anticoagulants, probenecid, phenylbutazone (P+L) (D)
4. Antibacterials and Antiseptics			
Sulfanomides	Sulfamethoxaxole, Sulfamethoxale & Trimethoprim, Sulfisoxazole, Bactrim®, Gantanol®, Septra®, Azo-Gantrisin®	No	Amino benzoic acid, baking soda, Methenamine, Methotrexate, oral anticoagulants, Phenytoin, probenecid, Sulfinpyrazone, Isoniazide, aspirin, Phenylbutazone, Trimethoprim, penicillin, paraldehyde (P+L)

*Avoid sour cream.
**Avoid chocolate drinks and cheese.

Table 3.1
MOST COMMONLY PRESCRIBED DRUGS AND THEIR INTERACTIONS

Drug Category and Generic Contents	Brand Names	Habit Forming	Possible Harmful Interactions
			(P) = Avoid during pregnancy (L) = Avoid during lactation (D) = Avoid driving
5. Antibiotics			
Cephalosporins	Cephalothin, cephaloradine, cephalexin, cephaloglycin, cephalozin, cephapirin, cephradine, Anspor®, Keflex®, Kafocin®, Velocef®	No	Oral anticoagulants, probenecid (may prolong its action in the body) (P+L)
Tetracyclines	Achromycin V®, Panmycin®, Robitet®, Sumycin®	No	Oral anticoagulants may have effects increased. Penicillins may have their effectiveness decreased. Antacids, iron and minerals may reduce absorption. Avoid alcohol. Avoid milk until 1 hour after dose (P+L)
Erythromycin	Ilosone®, E.E.S.®, E-Mycin®, Erythrocin®, Ilotysin®	No	Clindamycin, Lincomycin, Penicillins, aminophylline, oxytriphylline, theophyllin, alcohol. (P+L) with estolate forms (Ilosone)
Penicillins (penicillinase resistant)	Methicillin, nafcillin, oxacillin, cloxacillin, dicloxacillin, Amcil®, Omniphen®	No	Tetracyclines, chloramphenicol, erythromycin, troleandromycin, antacids
Penicillins (nonpenicillinase resistant)	Penicillin G, Penicillin V., Pentids®, Pen-Vee-K®	No	

Drug Category and Generic Contents	Brand Names	Habit Forming	Possible Harmful Interactions
Aminoglycocides	Streptomycin, Neomycin, Kanamycin, Gentamycin, Tebramycin, Amiracin, Garamycin®, Nebrin®, Kantrex®, Amikin®	No	Potent diuretics. Avoid taking two drugs from this same family concurrently. (P+L)
Ampicillin	Amcill®, Omnipen®, Polycillin®, Principen®	No	Erythromycin, chloramphenicol, tetracyclines, antacids. (P)
Ampicillin and probenecid	Polycillin-PRB®	No	
6. Antidepressants			
Amitriptyline (tricyclic antidepressant)	Elavil®, Triavil®	No	Amphetamines, atropine, Levodopa, anticoagulants, sedatives, tranquilizers, antihistamines all have increased effects. Do not take with other antidepressants with monamine oxidase inhibitors. (P+L) unknown.
7. Antidiarrheals			
Diphenoxylate, atropine	Lomotil®	Yes	Other addictive drugs, alcohol, anesthetics, anti-depressants, sedatives, haloperidol, phenothiazines, quinidine. (P+L) unknown.

Table 3.1
MOST COMMONLY PRESCRIBED DRUGS AND THEIR INTERACTIONS

Drug Category and Generic Contents	Brand Names	Habit Forming	Possible Harmful Interactions
			(P) = Avoid during pregnancy (L) = Avoid during lactation (D) = Avoid driving
8. Antihistamines/Decongestants			
Brompheniramine, phenylephrine, phenyl-propranolamine	Dimetapp®	No	Alcohol, other central nervous system depressants, beta-blocking agents like propranolol, digitalis, MAO and tricyclic antidepressants. Avoid coffee, tea. (L) (D)
Brompheniramine, Pseudoephedrine	Drixoral®	No	Sedatives, medicines for seizures, strong pain killers, antidepressants, MAO inhibitors, oral anticoagulants, alcohol
Pseudoephidrine, tripolidine hydrochloride	Actifed®	No	Alcohol, central nervous system depressants, beta-blocking agents (like propanolol), digitalis, MAO and tricyclic antidepressants. Avoid coffee, tea. (D) (L)
9. Antihypertensives (for high blood pressure) Methyldopa	Aldomet®	No.	Amphetamines, oral anticoagulants, L-Dopa, antidepressants, alcohol. Cough, cold, or sinus remedies only under physician's supervision.
10. Anti-inflammatory Agents Ibuprofen (for arthritis)	Motrin®	No	Alcohol, anticoagulants, oral antidiabetic drugs, phenytoin, sulfa drugs (P)

Drug Category and Generic Contents	Brand Names	Habit Forming	Possible Harmful Interactions
Corticosteroids	Beclomethasone, dexamethasone	No	Aspirin, barbiturates, diuretics, estrogens, indomethocin, phenytoin, drugs for glaucoma, digitalis, antihistamines, insulin, and oral diabetic drugs. Avoid tobacco. (P+L)
Prednisone and other corticosteroids	Prednisone as generic. Meticorten, Orasone, Deltasone, Fernisone, Lisocort, and others	over long period	Aspirin, barbiturates, estrogens, oral anticoagulants, Indocin®, phenytoin, oral antidiabetic drugs. Avoid heavy smoking.
Phenylbutazone/oxyphenbutazone	Butazolidine, Butazolidine Alka	No	Anticoagulants, oral drugs for diabetics, aspirin, penicillins, sulfa drugs, antihistamines, heart medicines, griseofulvin, desatives, tricyclic antidepressants, indomethocin, phenytoin. Avoid alcohol. (D)
11. Antispasmodics and Anticholinergics			
Atropine Butabarbital, belladonna	Belladonna Barbidonna®	No	Pilocarpine eye drops, MAO inhibitors, haloperidol, antidepressants, antihistamines, strong pain killers, vitamin C, mood elevators, phenodiazines, alcohol (D)
Phenobarbital belladonna	Bellergal®		
Phenobarbital	Donnatal®	Yes	Alcohol, antihistamines, haloperidol, phenothiazines, anticoagulants, digitalis, tetracyclines, anticonvulsants, antacids, MAO inhibitors, tricyclic antidepressants, other sedatives, and tranquilizers (P+L) (D)

Table 3.1
MOST COMMONLY PRESCRIBED DRUGS AND THEIR INTERACTIONS

Drug Category and Generic Contents	Brand Names	Habit Forming	Possible Harmful Interactions
			(P) = Avoid during pregnancy (L) = Avoid during lactation (D) = Avoid driving
12. Antivertigo Agents			
Meclizine HCl	Antivert®	No	Alcohol, sedatives, antihistamines, some antibiotics that may affect hearing such as streptomycin, narcotics, drugs with atropinelike actions, MAO inhibitors (P+L) (D)
13. Bronchial Dilators (for asthma)			
Aminophyllin (xanthine derivative) other xanthines: Theophylline, Dyphylline, Oxtraphylline	Amesec® (aminophylline plus secobarbital), Brondecon® (oxtriphylline and gniaifensin), Choledye®, Elixophyllin®, Isuprel Compound Elixir® (phenobarbital, isoproterenol, ephedrine, theophylline, potassium iodide)	No	Xanthine derivatives may increase action of other drugs used to treat asthma. However, the combined effect may be beneficial. Can decrease effect of drugs for gout and effect of lithium for depression. (P) unknown.
14. Cardiovascular Preparations			
Nitroglycerine and other nitrates (for angina)	Usually prescribed as generic although there are many trade names, including Etrytritzl Etranitrate, Isosorbide, Pentaerythrito Tetranitrate	No	Propranolol, alcohol, drugs for high blood pressure, phenylephrine, epinephrine, ephedrine (many cough and cold remedies available without prescription contain these). Avoid tobacco and caffeine.

Drug Category and Generic Contents	Brand Names	Habit Forming	Possible Harmful Interactions
Propranolol (for angina, rhythm disturbances, high blood pressure)	Inderal®	No	Aminophylline, epinephrine, Isuprel, oral antidiabetic drugs, phenytoin, digitalis, alcohol. Avoid tobacco. (D)
Digoxin (a form of digitalis) (for congestive heart failure and rhythm disturbances)	Lanoxin®, or available as generic	No	Ephedrine, cortisonelike drugs, diuretics, quinidine, reserpine, phenylbutazone, antacids, and laxatives, phenobarbitals, guanethidine. Avoid caffeine (coffee, cola, tea) and tobacco. (P) early months, (L)
Quinidine salts (for rhythm disturbances)	Quinidine sulfate (Cin-Quin®), Quinidex®, quinidine gluconate (Duraguin®), quinidine poly glactouronate (Cardioquin®)	No	Diamox, antacids, anticoagulants, sodium bicarbonate, antihypertensive drugs, atropinelike drugs, drugs for glaucoma and myasthenia gravis, reserpine, digitalis, propranolol, phenytoin. Avoid over-the-counter cough, cold, and sinus medicines.
15. Dermatologicals			
Selenium sulfide (for dandruff)	Selsun	No	None known
Anti-fungal, anti-bacterial	Triamcinolone, Neomycin, Gramicidin, Nystatin. Mycolog (cream, ointment)	No	None unless used for a long time in large amounts
16. Diuretics			
Chlorthalidone (for high blood pressure, congestive heart failure, hepatic cirrhosis, corticosteroid and estrogen therapy, certain kidney problems)	Hygroton®	No	Alcohol, anesthetics, sedatives including antihistamines, antidepressants. Increase foods with potassium. (P+L)

Table 3.1
MOST COMMONLY PRESCRIBED DRUGS AND THEIR INTERACTIONS

Drug Category and Generic Contents	Brand Names	Habit Forming	Possible Harmful Interactions
			(P) = Avoid during pregnancy (L) = Avoid during lactation (D) = Avoid driving
Furosemide (for high blood pressure, excess fluid in body)	Lasix® (no generic equivalants)	No	Alcohol, other antihypertensive drugs, phenothiazines, drugs for gout (allopurinol and probenecid), aspirin, other potassium-depleting drugs, lithium. Increase foods with potassium. (P)
Thiazide (for high blood pressure)	Esidrix®, Hydro Diuril® (hydrochlorothiazide), Diuril® (chlorothiazide), Aldactazide® (spironolactone with hydrochlorothiazide), Diupres® (chlorothiazide and reserpine), Hydropres® (hydrochlorothiazide and reserpine), Ser-Ap-Es® (hydrochlorothiazide, hydralizine, reserpine), many others.	Not unless in combination with a habit-forming drug	Alcohol, lithium, steroids, oral antidiabetics, tricyclic antidepressants, narcotic pain relievers, MAO inhibitors, drugs to lower uric acid (probenecid, allopurinol), phenothiazines. Increase foods with potassium. (D) (P+L)
17. Histamine H₂ Antagonist (for peptic ulcers) Cimetidine	Tagamet®	No	Penicillin G, oral anticoagulants, Bethanacol, propanotheline. Avoid alcohol, tobacco, caffeine. (D)
18. Hormones Androgens (therapy for certain breast cancer, hypogonadism in males)	Fluoxymesterol, Halotestin®, Methyltestosterone, Metandren®, Oreton®, testosterone, enanthate, Delatestryl®	No	May increase response to anticoagulants. Adrenal steroids may add to edema. (P+L)

Drug Category and Generic Contents	Brand Names	Habit Forming	Possible Harmful Interactions (P) = Avoid during pregnancy (L) = Avoid during lactation (D) = Avoid driving
Estrogens (for estrogen deficiency, osteoporosis, prostate cancer, uterine bleeding)	Premarin®, Amnestrogen®, and many others. Also made as estrogenic substances with many different trade names, conjugated estrogens, and esterified estrogens. When combined with another hormone, they prevent pregnancy (see oral contraceptives).	No	Clofibrate, phenobarbital, meprobamate, oral antidiabetic drugs. Avoid tobacco. (P)
Oral contraceptives: most contain estrogen plus a progestational hormone.	Lo-Ovral®, Norinyl®, Norlestestrin®, Ortho-Novum®, Ovral®, Ovulen®, among others	No	Anticoagulants, oral antidiabetic drugs, clofibrate, guanethidine, antihistamines. *Do not smoke.* (L) (See Chapter 6.)
19. Mineral Supplement			
Potassium Chloride	Slow-K®, Klorvess®, Kaon®, Kay Ciel®	No	Digitalis, thiazide diuretics, spironolactone, Triamterene. Limit alcohol.
20. Sedatives/Barbiturates			
Phenobarbital	Usually generic. Also Eskabarb®, Donnatal® (phenobarbital and atropine)	Yes	Alcohol, anesthetics, other sedatives, antidepressants, oral anticoagulants, phenytoin, griseofluvin, steroids, digitalis preparations, antihistamines, oral drugs to treat diabetes. (P+L) (D)

Table 3.1
MOST COMMONLY PRESCRIBED DRUGS AND THEIR INTERACTIONS

Drug Category and Generic Contents	Brand Names	Habit Forming	Possible Harmful Interactions
			(P) = Avoid during pregnancy (L) = Avoid during lactation (D) = Avoid driving
Flurazepam hydrochloride	Dalmane® (no generics available)	Yes	Alcohol, anti-convulsants, other sedatives, narcotic drugs. Avoid tobacco. Avoid caffeine for 6 hrs. before retiring. (P+L) (D)
21. Thyroid Preparations	Proloid®, Armour Thyroid®; Most likely prescribed under generic name of levothyroxine, (Synthroid®) liothyronin (Cytomel®) Thyroglobulin, Thyroid	No	Anticoagulants, Cholestyramine, cough and cold medicines, oral antidiabetic medicine, phenytoin, tricyclic antidepressants, digitalis, sedatives, stimulants, some appetite suppressants.
22. Tranquilizers Clorazepate (a benzodiazepine). Other similar drugs include: chlordiazepoxide diazepam lorazepam oxazepam prazepam.	Tranxene®, Azene®	Yes	Alcohol, antihistamines, sedatives, narcotics, other tranquilizers, strong pain medicine, medicine for seizures, tricyclic antidepressants, MAO inhibitors, antacids. Avoid caffeine and tobacco. (P+L)

Drug Category and Generic Contents	Brand Names	Habit Forming	Possible Harmful Interactions
			(P) = Avoid during pregnancy (L) = Avoid during lactation (D) = Avoid driving
Chlordiazepoxide hydrochloride	Librium®	Yes	Other depressants of central nervous system like sedatives, antihistamines, strong pain killers, anticonvulsants. Oral anticoagulants, antihypertensives, tricyclic antidepressants, alcohol. (P + L) (D)
Chlordiazepoxide hydrochloride and clinidium bromide (anticholinergic/antispasmodic)	Librax®	Yes	Alcohol, other central nervous system depressants, anesthetics, antacids or antidiarrheal medicines, narcotics, sedatives, pain killers. Avoid caffeine and tobacco. (P + L) (D)
Diazepam	Valium®	Yes	Alcohol, other depressants, anticonvulsants, antidepressants, antihistamines, strong pain killers, oral anticoagulants, antihypertensives (P + L) (D)

SOURCE: H. Winter Griffith, M.D.

CHAPTER

4

Tobacco

Three decades ago, medical science came up with the first evidence directly linking cigarette smoking to lung cancer. Today we know as well that many diseases of the cardiovascular system have their roots in the relatively recent American habit of inhaling tobacco smoke.

Though the U.S. government has repeatedly warned of the health effects of smoking, for many reasons it has been unable to legislate a curb of the habit. The government does require, however, that a warning label be attached to every cigarette package and be displayed in all advertising. Cigarette advertising has also been banned from television. Fortunately, thousands of Americans are quitting the habit, and smoking has become less chic. Unfortunately, however, it is still used as an evidence of maturity among teenagers.

Self-discipline is evidently the key to slashing the enormous costs spent each year in caring for those who smoke. We must, by our example, set an example for the next generation and discourage their smoking. We have already made great strides toward developing a less harmful "smoke" for those who can't break the habit, but we should continue our efforts toward a smokeless society.

Glossary

CARCINOGEN Any substance that produces cancer.

CATECHOLAMINES Biologically active organic compounds, such as epinephrine and norepinephrine.

MAINSTREAM SMOKE That portion of the smoke drawn from the mouthpiece of a tobacco product during puffing.

NICOTINE A colorless alkaloid present in tobacco. It exerts a stimulating effect if tobacco is inhaled or chewed or snuffed. The nicotine effect is thought to be the major incentive for tobacco users.

PASSIVE INHALATION Involuntary exposure to tobacco smoke by a nonsmoker in the presence of smokers.

SIDESTREAM SMOKE Emits from the smoldering tobacco product in a steady stream. Smoke particles and selected smoke constituents are found in sidestream and in even greater concentrations than in mainstream smoke.

TAR More properly called "particulate matter" or "smoke condensate." It consists of aerosol particles that are the dark brown residue present in tobacco smoke. The cancer-inducing potential of tobacco smoke lies mainly in its "tar." This condensate, not nicotine, causes the yellow/brown stain on the fingers and teeth of some cigarette smokers.

TOBACCO The origin of the word probably comes from the name of the hollow tube, *toboca* or *tobago*, through which the Carib Indians of the West Indies inhaled or snuffed a mixture of dried leaves.

MACROPHAGES A type of phagocyte, or scavenger cell, that ingests dead tissue and degenerated cells.

History and Definitions

The tobacco habit is one of our most hazardous afflictions. It is also one of our most prevalent. We smoke cigarettes, cigars, and pipes, chew tobacco, and even sniff it, which suggests its powerful appeal. The fact that so many people continue to smoke, even though they know very well it may affect their health, is difficult for nonsmokers and health educators to understand, but it is clear that some deep-seated satisfaction is involved.

Our use of tobacco is centuries old. When Columbus landed on the island of San Salvador in 1492, he was given "certain dried leaves" as gifts. A century later, Sir Walter Raleigh brought tobacco back from the New World and popularized its use in England. From the beginning, to-bacco use was accompanied by warnings, the most famous of which was James I of England's *Counter-Blaste to Tobacco*. Pope Urban VII prohibited its use in Catholic churches in 1642. In 1699 a report from the court of Louis XIV asked "Whether the Frequent Use of Tobacco Shortened the Life." The conclusion: it did.

Others, however, saw tobacco as a boon. Dr. Jean Nicot de Villemain, the sixteenth century French ambassador to Lisbon who gave his name to nicotine, introduced snuff to Catherine de Medici and her court to alleviate migraine headaches. Tobacco use was also thought to cure colds and fever and protect from the plague.

While pipe smoking and, later, cigar smoking began centuries ago, cigarette smoking is much more recent. Paper-wrapped cigarettes were first used in Turkey and parts of Russia. The practice of rolling "papyrosi" spread westward by way of the migration that accompanied European wars. Cigarettes became popular in Europe, particularly in Spain, England, and Finland, around 1900.

In the United States, cigarettes were still little used in the early 1900s. While their per capita annual consumption was slightly under 100 as late as 1910, it increased to almost 400 a year in 1920, and to almost 1,000 a year in 1930. During World War II, cigarette smoking became popular, particularly among men, as automated manufacturing lowered the price. By the 1970s, men and women together smoked an average of 4,100 cigarettes a year. Since then, many male smokers have stopped smoking cigarettes while many women have started. Thus, today the proportion of adult smokers is about the same in both sexes—about 36 percent.

Although tobacco is not addictive in the true sense of the word, its use is deeply ingrained and hard to stop for millions of people. Many of its symptoms and side effects, including withdrawal effects, continue to afflict those who were heavy smokers, long after they stop smoking.

Doctors have known for two centuries that smoking causes various diseases. As early as 1775, medical literature described a case of mouth cancer believed caused by pipe smoking. In the 1830s, a Harvard University surgeon reported that chewing tobacco could lead to tongue cancer. Sigmund Freud was repeatedly urged to give up cigars in an effort to stop the spread of the mouth cancer that in 1939 took his life.

In the late 1930s, a study of patients in Cologne, Germany was among the first to show that lung cancer patients smoked more than other people. By the 1950s, more and more studies in the United States and Great Britain associated tobacco use with lung cancer. At the same time, strong scientific evidence was accumulating that related smoking to other diseases. Epidemiological, biological, and chemical studies linked smoking with heart and lung disease (emphysema and chronic bronchitis) and strokes, as well as cancer. This relationship was clearly shown in studies by a group of British physicians published in 1954, in a population study conducted by the American Cancer Society also published in 1954, and in a study of men in Framingham, Massachusetts, published in 1960.

In 1953, the first definitive experimental evidence showed tobacco "tar" caused cancer when applied to the skin of test mice. In 1957, the first specific cancer-causing elements, or carcinogens, in tobacco smoke were discovered and classified. Over the years, additional carcinogens and cancer-promoting elements have been identified in tobacco smoke.

At the government level, the Royal College of Physicians published its "Report on Smoking and Health" in London in 1962. In the United States, the Surgeon General's first report on smoking and cancer was issued in 1964. These reports were followed by others from many nations, all describing smoking's many ill effects. In graphic illustration, table 4.1 shows the higher rates of deaths from various diseases for smokers compared with nonsmokers.

Apart from scientific studies, simple dictates of logic and common sense tell us that smoking is unhealthy. Our respiratory tract has adapted itself to normal pollution—the dust of flowers, plants, sands, and rocks. But evolution has not prepared our lungs to withstand deeply inhaled cigarette smoke or, for that matter, the dusts of the industrial workplace. Tobacco smoking overloads our metabolic system with foreign substances the body cannot easily metabolize or eliminate.

Table 4.1
RATIO OF DEATH RATES AMONG MEN WHO SMOKED
COMPARED WITH DEATH RATES OF MEN WHO NEVER SMOKED*

	Age 45–64	Age 65–79
Cancer (total)	2.14:1	1.76:1
Lung (excl. trachea, pleura)	7.84:1	11.59:1
Buccal cavity, pharynx	9.90:1	2.93:1
Larynx	6.09:1	8.99:1
Esophagus	4.17:1	1.74:1
Bladder and other urinary	2.00:1	2.96:1
Kidney	1.42:1	1.57:1
Prostate	1.04:1	1.01:1
Pancreas	2.69:1	2.17:1
Liver, biliary passages	2.84:1	1.34:1
Stomach	1.42:1	1.26:1
Colon, rectum	1.01:1	1.17:1
Leukemia	1.40:1	1.68:1
Other specified sites	1.64:1	1.14:1
Cancer—site not specified	2.23:1	1.78:1
Heart and circulatory		
Coronary heart disease	2.03:1	1.36:1
Rheumatic heart disease	0.99:1	0.85:1
Hypertensive heart disease	1.40:1	1.42:1
Other heart disease	2.71:1	1.09:1
Aortic aneurysm (nonsyphilitic)	2.62:1	4.92:1
Cerebral vascular lesions	1.38:1	1.06:1
Other circulatory diseases	1.80:1	1.18:1
Other diseases		
Emphysema	6.55:1	11.41:1
Pneumonia, influenza	1.86:1	1.72:1
Other pulmonary diseases	2.68:1	2.26:1
Gastric ulcer	2.95:1	4.06:1
Duodenal ulcer	2.86:1	1.50:1
Cirrhosis of liver	2.06:1	1.97:1
Nephritis & other kidney diseases	1.08:1	1.05:1
Diabetes	1.11:1	1.05:1
Other specified diseases	1.28:1	1.28:1
Ill-defined diseases	1.66:1	1.18:1

Adapted from American Cancer Society, 1966
*For those who never smoked, the number is 1.

Health Effects

CANCER

General principles

It is estimated that in the U.S. in 1980 about 33 percent of all cancer deaths in men and about 10 percent in women were related to smoking. The death rate is lower for women because until recently they smoked less than men. The degree to which tobacco contributes to cancer varies by the location of the cancer. It also depends on how intensely you smoke. The more you inhale and the longer you have smoked, or used another tobacco product, the greater your risk.

Furthermore, different parts of the body are more susceptible to tobacco smoke than others. Particularly affected are those with which the smoke comes in direct contact, like the lungs, the mouth, the larynx, and the esophagus. Chewing tobacco and inhaling snuff can also cause cancer of the larynx and esophagus, particularly when the tobacco juice is swallowed. Other organs such as the pancreas, the kidney, and the bladder, although not in direct contact with tobacco smoke, are affected by the substances that the body absorbs or metabolizes from tobacco components.

On stopping smoking, the degree to which the risk of cancer is reduced depends not only on the amount smoked but also on the habit's duration (see figure 4.1). If a person quits after smoking heavily for at least twenty years, there is usually no decrease in risk for three years. This is because of the long, latent period between cancer's first unobservable start in the body and the time it begins to cause noticeable symptoms.

At the same time, stopping smoking usually has some immediate health benefits—even if they are only a reduction in coughing and an increase in the senses of smell and taste. And soon the chances of a longer life begin improving.

Lung cancer

In 1912 lung cancer was so rare that the author of a scientific treatise on the subject apologized for writing about it. Sadly, today lung cancer kills more men aged thirty-five to fifty-four than any other form of cancer. Among women of the same age group, it is the second leading killer (after breast cancer). This female death rate is expected to increase, for although tobacco use is declining among men, it is increasing among women.

Smoking is the major cause of lung cancer. The evidence for this is consistent and decisive:

- Lung cancer (especially the most common type) occurs rarely in nonsmokers.
- The risk of lung cancer increases in proportion to the number of cigarettes smoked, their tar content, and the depth of inhalation.
- Carcinogens and co-carcinogens (substances that help other substances cause cancer) have been positively identified in tobacco smoke.
- Cigar and pipe smokers die of lung cancer more often than nonsmokers, but much less often than cigarette smokers. Cigar or pipe smokers who get lung cancer usually smoke more than seven cigars or pipefuls a day.
- Genetic factors do not appear to affect lung cancer incidence.
- Breathing air in a smoke-filled room has not been shown to increase the risk of lung cancer or any other tobacco-related cancer.
- Air pollution does not seem to measurably increase the risk of lung cancer among either smokers or nonsmokers. Seventh Day Adventists, whose religion prohibits smoking, have very low rates of lung cancer, even if they live in large cities.
- Where occupational exposure increases the risk of lung cancer (see chapter 16), it occurs primarily among smokers.
- Chronic coughs, independent of the amount of smoking, have not been shown to increase lung cancer risk.

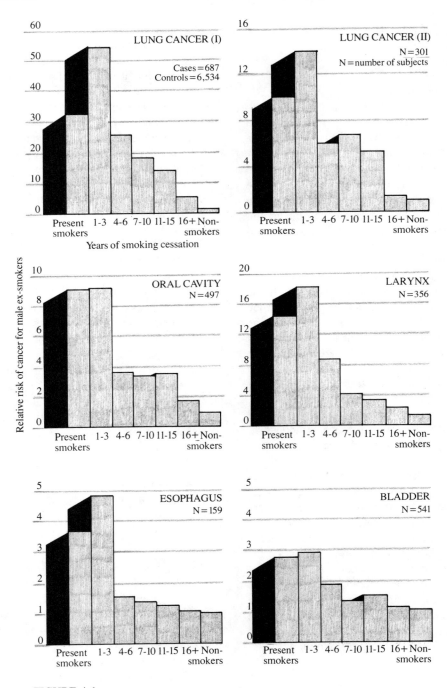

FIGURE 4.1

Relative risk of male ex-smokers for cancer by years since quitting smoking
SOURCE: *American Health Foundation, 1977.*

Clearly, then, there is no particular type of individual, regardless of activity, whose risk of lung cancer is innately greater or lesser than another's. Increased risk of lung cancer depends principally on cigarette smoking and its intensity.

If you smoke at least twenty cigarettes a day for more than twenty years, your chances of getting lung cancer won't change for the first three years after you stop smoking. It will take ten years of nonsmoking before your chances of getting lung cancer approach those of people who have never smoked.

Mouth cancer

The mouth and oral cavity are subject to cancer of the tongue, cheek lining, floor of the mouth, tonsils, soft and hard palate, and pharynx, as well as of the lip. By the time these mouth cancers are diagnosed, more than 50 percent of them spread to the lymph nodes. More than twice as many men as women die from cancer of the oral cavity, and it ranks as the seventh most common cancer death in men, the twelfth in women. Any use of tobacco—cigars, pipes, cigarettes, chewing tobacco, and snuff—increases the risk of cancer of the mouth. Chewing betel nuts that contain tobacco, a habit widespread in Asia, is also associated with this type of cancer.

Whether you will develop mouth cancer depends principally on tobacco use, but your risk is greatly increased when smoking is accompanied by excessive drinking (see chapter 2). The fact that men smoke and drink more than women do causes their substantially greater susceptibility. As women smoke and drink more, their mouth cancer rates can be expected to increase.

Among pipe smokers, cancer often develops where the pipe is held. Concentration of smoke, not heat, is the reason. Similarly, snuff and chewing tobacco cause more mouth cancers at the spot where the tobacco is held. This indicates that carcinogens are present in cured tobacco as well

as in the smoke. Although an increased risk of lip cancer is associated with pipe and cigar smoking, the main cause of lip cancer is exposure to the ultraviolet rays in sunlight (see chapter 13). Syphilis increases the risk for cancers of the front two-thirds of the tongue.

When nonsmokers develop cancer of the mouth, it is most likely to appear in the tongue or in the lining of the cheek. Among nonsmokers, it is more likely to occur in women than men, perhaps because women are more susceptible to iron deficiencies (see chapter 1).

If you have quit smoking, your chances of getting mouth cancer decrease with each successive year. After sixteen years of not smoking, your risk approaches that of people who have never smoked. If no one used tobacco, the incidence of cancer of the oral cavity would be cut by about 80 percent in men and 40 percent in women.

Larynx Cancer

Cancer of the larynx ranks as the thirteenth most common cause of cancer death among men and the nineteenth among women. Almost three-quarters of larynx cancers occur in the vocal cords. One of the consequences of this disease is obvious and socially debilitating—loss of speech. On the average, larynx cancer appears at around age sixty.

As with lung cancer, cigarette smokers run the greatest risk of getting cancer of the larynx. Their risk increases with the amount of cigarettes smoked and the depth of inhalation. Cigar and pipe smokers also run a substantial risk of getting larynx cancer. Risk among smokers is significantly enhanced by drinking (see chapter 2).

Men are about six times more likely to develop larynx cancer than women, because at the age when cancer is likely to appear, they have smoked more tobacco and consumed more alcohol. Among ex-smokers, the risk of larynx cancer decreases gradually and approaches that of a nonsmoker ten years after quitting. Where a job increases the risk of larynx cancer, it is usually only among smokers (see chapter 16).

If no one used tobacco, larynx cancers would be reduced by about 90 percent in men and 70 percent in women. These differences reflect the fact that men smoke more at the age when most people develop larynx cancer.

Cancer of the Esophagus

Cancer of the esophagus (the tube that connects the mouth with the stomach) occurs more than twice as frequently among men than women. This disease ranks fifteenth in cancer deaths among men and eighteenth among women. Incidence and mortality rates are higher among non-whites than whites. On the average, esophageal cancer is diagnosed at age sixty, and the five-year survival rate is very poor—only about 4 percent.

Cigar and pipe smoking appear as much as cigarette smoking to contribute to the development of esophageal cancer. Heavy drinking combined with smoking raises the risk of cancer of the esophagus (see chapter 2). Alcohol and tobacco act together to increase the risk of esophageal cancer beyond that of the two alone.

The risk is increased by the number and type of cigarettes smoked each day.

If no one used tobacco, the death rate from esophageal cancer in developed countries would probably drop by about 50 percent among men and 20 percent among women, again reflecting their different long-term smoking habits.

Kidney cancer

Cancer of the kidney or other urinary organs (excluding the bladder) occurs approximately 60 percent more frequently in males than in females and is the twelfth most common cancer death among men and the fifteenth among women. The sex difference is partly explained by different smoking habits. The risk in women appears to be affected by obesity (see chapter 1). On average, the disease occurs principally around fifty-eight years of age.

The increased risk of kidney cancer among tobacco users is most strongly noted among cigarette smokers, indicating that inhalation of the smoke is required. As with other tobacco-related cancers, the more cigarettes smoked per day, the greater the risk. In the absence of cigarette smoking, the incidence of kidney cancer would be reduced by about one-third in men and 10 percent in women.

Bladder cancer

Bladder cancer is the fifth most common cancer death in men and the eleventh in women. It is three times more common in males, largely because men smoke more and are exposed more frequently to carcinogens in the workplace. (see chapter 16). The average age at which the disease develops is sixty-two.

Cigarette smokers are more likely to develop bladder cancer and about twice as likely to die from it than nonsmokers. Other forms of tobacco use do not appear to be associated with this disease, which indicates that inhalation is an important factor. The exact carcinogen in tobacco smoke, which is responsible for this risk and which is likely to be detected in the urine of smokers, remains to be identified.

An estimated 33 percent of male and 10 percent of female bladder cancer cases would not occur if people didn't smoke.

Cancer of the pancreas

This type of cancer is the fourth most common cancer death in men and the eighth in women. Cancer of the pancreas appears to be increasing in incidence in both sexes. Most victims develop pancreatic cancer in their early sixties and most die from it.

As in lung cancer, the risk of pancreatic cancer increases with the number of cigarettes smoked. The mechanism by which this happens, however, is unknown. It is suspected that a tobacco carcinogen may enter the pancreatic fluid and thus affect the duct epithelium from which most pancreatic cancers originate. The disease is not associated with pipe smoking, although heavy cigar smoking may increase risk. Pancreatic cancer has been shown to be related to a diet high in fat (see chapter 1). If no one smoked, pancreatic cancer would kill about 40 percent fewer men and 10 percent fewer women.

CARDIOVASCULAR DISEASE

General principles

Cardiovascular diseases are those which affect the heart and blood vessels. One million Americans each year die of cardiovascular diseases, slightly more than half of all reported deaths. In most developed nations, with the notable exception of Japan, these diseases are the leading cause of death after age forty. With the possible exception of cerebral hemorrhage—stroke—cardiovascular diseases are principally caused by eating too much saturated fats and cholesterol (see chapter 1). Nevertheless, tobacco contributes significantly to cardiovascular disease, particularly when it occurs before age sixty. (see figure 4.2).

The damaging effect of tobacco on the cardiovascular system is caused by inhaling cigarette smoke deeply. Cigar and pipe smokers have a lower risk of cardiovascular disease, apparently because they inhale less. When tobacco smoke and chewing tobacco or snuff is only held in the mouth, nicotine is absorbed into the blood slowly. But when it is inhaled deeply, the nicotine is rapidly absorbed. Nicotine stimulates the release of organic compounds that may cause the heart to speed up or to beat irregularly thereby increasing the blood pressure. Such a chemical reaction may also enhance the formation of blood clots.

There is no general agreement on precisely how the by-products of smoke actually cause heart attacks, arteriosclerosis, or other cardiovascular diseases. More research is needed.

Atherosclerosis

Arteriosclerosis, or hardening of the arteries, results from the thickening and loss of elasticity in the walls of the arteries. Atherosclerosis, its most common form, consists of a gradual development of plaques or localized thickenings of tissues that line large arteries. The plaques or thickness cause an irregular narrowing of the arteries, which may eventually reduce and even block blood flow. This can lead to a heart attack, stroke, gangrene, or damage to some other tissue or organ.

Atherosclerosis is more common and more severe in older than in younger people, but is not merely an effect of aging. In affluent societies, it can develop in those under thirty. Heart attacks frequently strike people in their forties, sometimes even younger. Atherosclerosis is principally associated with elevated blood cholesterol and abnormal levels of blood fats (lipoproteins). High blood pressure also helps cause it.

Autopsies performed on men who died from heart attacks have shown that smoking cigarettes raises the risk of getting atherosclerosis. They indicate that smoking cigarettes, and the amount smoked per day, are linked with the severity of atherosclerosis in the aorta—the main artery of the body—and those that supply the heart. There is, as yet, little information about women, and none on children, but there is no reason to suppose that they run less risk than men if they smoke.

Heart attack

The term *heart attack* (also known as myocardial infarction) includes nonfatal and fatal heart attacks. Heart attacks kill some 650,000 Americans each year—two-thirds of all those who die of cardiovascular diseases. These attacks result from a restriction or obstruction of the arteries that supply blood to the heart.

Heart attacks occur when the blood supply received by the heart is so limited that part of the heart muscle dies from lack of oxygen. The prin-

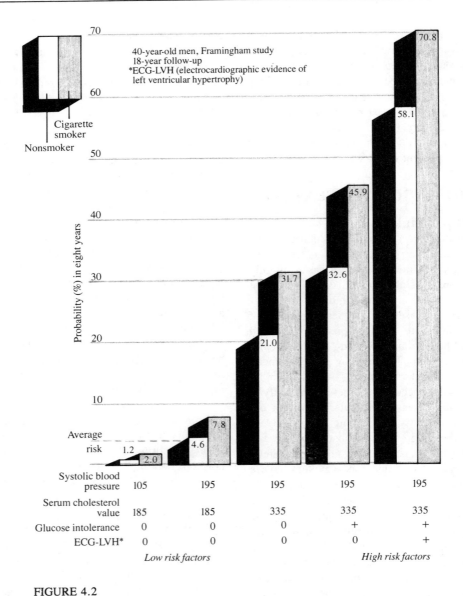

FIGURE 4.2

Probability of development of cardiovascular disease in eight years for cigarette smokers and nonsmokers according to level of other risk factors
SOURCE: *adapted from W.B. Kannel, "Prevention of Cardiovascular Disease,"* Current Problems in Cardiology, *Vol. 1, pages 5–68, 1976*

cipal underlying cause is a high amount of cholesterol in the blood (see chapter 1).

If you smoke, your chances of a heart attack are three times greater than those of nonsmokers. Sudden cardiac deaths account for more than half of all heart attack deaths. Sometimes the heart is so severely damaged that it simply ceases to contract. More often, sudden death occurs because the normal electrical currents that induce the heart to beat in a synchronized way become disorganized, causing erratic, ineffectual contractions known as ventricular fibrillation. A heart attack can kill you within minutes or a few hours after the onset of symptoms unless you are treated quickly.

Combined with other risk factors like high blood pressure or elevated blood cholesterol, smoking increases the risk of sudden death beyond that of merely adding up individual factors. The risk is greater in young adults. Your chance of suffering a heart attack increases as you smoke more cigarettes, inhale deeper, and smoke longer. Some studies suggest that the increased risk applies mainly to cigarette smoking. If you quit smoking, your chance of a heart attack drops to that of a nonsmoker after about a year.

Although most studies have concentrated on the effects of smoking on men, some studies show that women who smoke a lot significantly increase their risk of heart attack. Women who use oral contraceptives double their risk of heart attack; for those who also smoke, the risk is multiplied tenfold (see chapter 6).

Angina pectoris

Angina pectoris is often marked by pain, a sense of pressure, or a strangling feeling in the center of the chest. Angina pectoris is usually brought on by physical exertion and is a sign that the heart is not getting enough blood. Its symptoms subside when you rest.

Doctors don't know for sure whether smoking causes or contributes to angina pectoris. However, among patients who already have angina, smoking will reduce the amount of exercise required to induce pain. The effect is thought to be caused by elevated carboxyhemoglobin levels—levels of hemoglobin affected by carbon monoxide—in smokers' blood.

Peripheral vascular disease

Peripheral vascular disease (PVD) includes several different diseases of the blood vessels in the arms and legs. PVD most commonly strikes the legs. It results from atherosclerosis of the arteries that supply blood to the legs. Reduced blood supply causes pains in the calf muscles and thigh, often brought on by exercising. The medical term for this condition is intermittent claudication. The symptoms disappear after a short rest. Among the elderly and among diabetics, the blood supply may be so reduced as to cause the tissues to wither or even die.

About 90 percent of PVD patients smoke. If you smoke a lot, whether male or female, your chances of getting peripheral vascular disease are three times that of a nonsmoker. Surgeons operating on diseased limbs report that continuing to smoke worsens the patient's outlook. Among diabetics, those who smoke have a 50 percent higher risk of developing PVD than those who don't.

Buerger's disease

Buerger's disease is an uncommon inflammation of leg arteries and veins. It chiefly affects men twenty to forty years old, particularly those who smoke heavily. It rarely occurs among nonsmokers. Smoking affects both its occurrence and progression. Buerger's disease scars and clots vessels, which reduces blood supply to the leg.

While the cause of Buerger's disease is unknown, some medical researchers think it may be due to sensitivity to tobacco protein.

Atherosclerotic aneurysms of the aorta

Atherosclerotic aneurysms—or swellings—of the aorta are a form of peripheral vascular disease causing 10,000 deaths per year. An aneurysm is an outpouching or sac filled with blood caused by a local swelling of an artery. Atherosclerosis, particularly of the abdominal aorta, becomes so severe in some individuals that the artery leaks or ruptures, leading to massive hemorrhage. It is responsible for up to 3 percent of all cardiovascular deaths.

Although the cause of atherosclerotic aneurysms is not known, smoking increases your risk of death. Studies show that smokers of one pack a day have four to five times the risk of nonsmokers, and two-pack a day smokers have seven to eight times the risk. Aneurysms become apparent after age fifty, and their incidence increases with age. They are five times more common in men than in women.

High blood pressure

Hypertension or high blood pressure is a condition in which blood pressure rises to dangerous levels affecting health. High blood pressure is associated with increased risk of heart attack and is a major cause of stroke. Most epidemiological studies find that cigarette smoking by itself does not increase high blood pressure incidence. Studies of multiple risk factors, however, show that smoking aggravates the condition of individuals who already have hypertension or high cholesterol levels in the blood.

Malignant hypertension, although rare, is a rapidly progressive and very severe form of high blood pressure, especially when diagnosed late. Some studies show that about three-fourths of those with malignant hypertension were smokers, a significantly higher proportion than is usually found in people with less severe high blood pressure.

Cigarette smoking has not been shown to chronically raise the blood pressure of persons with essential hypertension, the most common variety. If you have hypertension, however, you can reduce your risk of a heart attack by half by quitting smoking.

Stroke

Although we know that smoking plays a major role in heart disease, the evidence for its role in strokes is inconclusive. In men, studies show a small but increased risk of stroke among cigarette smokers compared with nonsmokers. The risk increases with age. However, the association may be due more to the aging process than to smoking.

On the other hand, women who both smoke and take oral contraceptives have been found to have significantly more strokes than those who neither smoke nor use birth control pills. Using oral contraceptives alone increases the risk about six times. When cigarette smoking is added, the risk is increased to twenty times (see chapter 6).

CHRONIC OBSTRUCTIVE PULMONARY DISEASE

Smoking is the most important cause of chronic obstructive pulmonary disease, which includes chronic bronchitis and emphysema. This disease accounts for about 2 percent of all deaths in the United States and, in older men, as many as 15 percent. Symptoms include coughing, wheezing, breathlessness, and recurring respiratory infections.

Cigarette smokers of half a pack a day are five times as likely to die of chronic obstructive pulmonary disease as nonsmokers. Smokers of a pack a day face a risk ten times greater than nonsmokers, and smokers of two packs a day are twenty times as likely to die of chronic, obstructive pulmonary disease. Inhaling the smoke significantly increases the risk. The risk also increases with age. By the time many middle aged or elderly smokers give up cigarettes, irreversible lung damage has already occurred.

Although the lung damage caused by these diseases is irreversible, you can usually reduce the frequency of symptoms, particularly the phlegm-producing cough, by stopping smoking.

The capacity to inhale and exhale air rapidly and easily is the most actively researched aspect of lung function. It can be evaluated simply by measuring the maximum volume of air that can be exhaled in one second after a deep inhalation of air. Cigarette smokers have been found to have a 10 to 15 percent lower lung function than nonsmokers of comparable age and height. Pipe and cigar smokers usually differ only slightly from nonsmokers. Ex-smokers tend to fall between smokers and nonsmokers. Certain lung changes, particularly those involving the alveoli, or air cells, appear to be irreversible. Research shows that the normal decline in lung function with age is greater for cigarette smokers than for nonsmokers, and is greater for heavy smokers than for light smokers.

Most authorities agree that the risk of chronic obstructive pulmonary disease assocated with cigarette smoking is much greater than that associated with air pollution (see chapter 11). The risk incurred by on-the-job exposure varies with the nature of the risk. But most authorities also agree that occupational exposure, with some notable exceptions, does not approach the risk posed by cigarette smoking (see chapter 16).

In summary, smoking, particularly of cigarettes, causes changes in the respiratory tract that produce excessive mucus, impaired clearance of mucus, obstruction of the smaller airways, and swelling and rupture of the lung's air cells. These changes result in chronic cough, difficult breathing, and easy tiring, among other symptoms. They subject an appreciable number of people to recurrent illness, disability, and even death from chronic, obstructive pulmonary disease.

The severity of the disease varies from person to person, depending on innate resistance, hered-ity, frequency of respiratory infections, exposure to dusts, fumes and gases, and general air pollution. But smoking is by far the most important general cause.

PEPTIC ULCER

The term *peptic ulcer* describes a mixed group of disorders sharing a common feature—a hole in the lining of the stomach or duodenum (the upper part of the small intestine). It is usually chronic because the ulcers continually heal and recur. Peptic ulcers are caused by diverse genetic and environmental factors, most of which have not yet been identified. About 300,000 new cases are diagnosed each year in the United States. Ten percent of all Americans can expect to suffer from ulcers during their lifetime. Ulcers are about twice as common in men as in women, and duodenal ulcers are about four times as common as stomach ulcers.

Cigarette smokers are about twice as likely to get peptic ulcers, both gastric and duodenal, and to die of them, as nonsmokers. Most studies also show that long-term smokers get significantly more ulcers than those with a short smoking history. Also, those who only smoke pipes or cigars and those who have quit smoking altogether get far fewer ulcers. Cigarette smoking also appears to retard ulcer healing.

ALLERGY

The relationship between tobacco and allergies is highly complex, though it is generally agreed that exposure to tobacco and tobacco smoke can make an allergy more severe. Whether tobacco causes or contributes to an allergic reaction remains to be determined.

A source of difficulty is the variety of substances used to manufacture tobacco and created by its combustion. For example, raw tobacco can be contaminated by foreign matter like insecticides, bacteria, fungi, or airborne allergens deposited on the leaf's surface. In addition, chemical reactions take place during preparation of the green leaves for commercial use, and various additives further alter their composition.

Tobacco smoke itself contains an estimated 2,500 components. Qualitative and quantitative differences exist between the smoke actively inhaled through the cigarette, and that which is discharged into the air, called *sidestream smoke*. Results of studies of true allergic reactions to either active smoking (deliberate inhalation) or passive smoking (exposure to air pollutants emitted in sidestream smoke) among healthy persons or those suffering from known allergies are not definitive.

Nevertheless, people with allergies, especially those with rhinitis (an inflammation of the nasal mucous membranes) or with asthma, may be more sensitive than nonallergic persons. Limitations in the technology of testing for allergies further complicate a clarification of the role of tobacco in allergies.

IMMUNE RESPONSE

When the body is invaded by a substance that it recognizes as "foreign," the body's immune system reacts by creating antibodies to attack the foreign substance. This response may occur locally (at a specific organ site) or systemically (throughout the body).

The body's respiratory system, for example, has a well-defined local defense system. First, there are two ciliated cells with tiny hairs that line the respiratory system. The cilia prevent accumulation of inhaled matter in the lungs by transporting the particles away from the lungs. If the ciliated cells are rendered ineffective by smoke or other irritants, cells called *macrophages* take up their work by engulfing and digesting hazardous substances such as bacteria.

Experiments have not yet been able to demonstrate clearly a decrease of the cilia action due to cigarette smoking. However, it has been determined that smokers have more macrophages in their lungs than nonsmokers, which may indicate the irritation of the cilia, perhaps in response to the toxic ingredients of cigarette smoke.

Studies of systemic immunological responses have shown that cigarette smoking may decrease the body's production of antibodies, thus increasing its susceptibility to infection. It is true that the incidence of flulike illnesses is greater among smokers of more than half a pack a day than among nonsmokers. In addition, pregnant women who smoke have more urinary tract infections than those who do not smoke.

Thus, exposure to tobacco smoke is known to alter components of the body's immune systems. But the mechanism by which these changes may contribute to or cause disease is still under investigation.

AMBLYOPIA

A form of dimness of vision called amblyopia is associated with tobacco use. Marked by a sight defect in a particular area of the visual field, amblyopia is thought to be related to a genetic or inherited vitamin B_{12} deficiency or to an error in the metabolism of cyanide. As smokers have lower levels of vitamin B_{12} in their blood and tissues—because this vitamin is used to detoxify cyanide present in cigarette smoke—they are at greater risk for amblyopia. Nutritional deficiencies associated with excessive alcohol consumption may also cause this condition.

PREGNANCY

Accumulative evidence shows that certain toxic substances in tobacco smoke pass through the placenta of a pregnant woman and reach her developing fetus, thus potentially harming the woman and her child, both before and after birth.

A pregnant woman needs an abundant supply of oxygen and nutrients both for herself and for the growing fetus. If she smokes, the carbon monoxide produced when tobacco is burned accumulates in the blood. There, it reduces the amount of oxygen present. Less oxygen is therefore available to her baby. In addition, nicotine from cigarettes constricts the blood vessels in the placenta and elsewhere in the woman's body, further decreasing the amount of oxygen and nutrients delivered to the fetus.

As a result, a smoking mother's placenta cannot promote fetal growth as effectively as a nonsmoker's. The placenta becomes abnormal in structure and function in direct ratio to how much a pregnant woman smokes.

Pregnant smokers are more prone to heavy bleeding from the placenta late in their pregnancy. This increases the need for hospitalization, blood transfusions, and cesarean sections to save the life of mother and baby. In a classic study involving 50,000 births, pregnant women who smoked a pack or more of cigarettes a day were 50 percent more likely to bleed than nonsmokers. Those who smoked one to twenty cigarettes a day were 20 percent more likely to bleed.

Babies born to pregnant smokers weigh an average of almost 7 ounces less than babies whose mothers do not smoke. Popular opinion holds that cigarettes depress appetites, and that this is responsible for the lessened growth of the smokers' infants. But this cannot be the only explanation. The babies of smokers who eat adequately are still frequently underweight. The more a woman smokes, the more likely it is that her baby will be underweight. Conversely, if she stops smoking by the fourth month of pregnancy, the risk of delivering a low birth-weight baby decreases.

Babies born to smoking mothers are also more likely to be premature. Studies show that up to 14 percent of premature deliveries may be caused by maternal smoking. Frequently, this complication is due to premature rupture of the membranes, or sac of amniotic fluid, surrounding the baby. When the "bag of waters" breaks prematurely, the mother's uterus can become infected if she does not go into labor promptly. Since there is also risk involved in giving birth to a premature infant, this condition requires hospitalization.

Mothers who smoke also experience a higher rate of miscarriages and stillbirths. These occur in direct relation to the level of smoking. Mothers who smoke have been shown to have close to a 30 percent greater chance of having a miscarriage than nonsmokers.

Infant deaths shortly after delivery are also more common among women who smoke. This is especially true in groups where infant deaths are high for other reasons—among the poor and in women with a history of premature births or babies of low birthweight. The sudden infant death syndrome—so-called crib deaths—also occurs more frequently among families in which the mother smoked during and after her pregnancy.

Smokers' infants also die more often at birth because of complications from maternal bleeding that endangers their blood supply. Maternal bleeding can cause respiratory distress at birth and pneumonia early in life. These problems occur more frequently in children of smoking mothers than nonsmokers.

As yet, there is only suggestive evidence that babies born to smokers are more likely to be born with malformations. Additional research is needed.

CHILD DEVELOPMENT

Since anything a nursing woman eats, drinks, or smokes can be found in her breast milk, it is not surprising that the milk from women who smoke contains nicotine metabolites that are passed on to the infant. Nicotine may decrease milk production and make successful breast feeding more difficult.

Whether babies are breast or formula fed, parents who smoke can damage their infants' health by exposing them to tobacco smoke. Hospital admission of infants with bronchitis and pneumonia show a 30 percent higher rate for children of mothers who smoke than for those of nonsmokers. Smoking thus increases the child's risk of infant death or of lung damage that may persist into adult life.

The children of mothers who smoke during pregnancy don't grow as fast as children of nonsmokers. A small average decrease in growth rate (one centimeter or .39 of an inch) was found in a group of eleven-year old British children whose mothers smoked ten or more cigarettes a day during pregnancy. Whether this decreased growth rate continues is yet to be determined.

Prevention

HOW TO PREVENT THE ONSET OF SMOKING

Most smokers begin as teenagers, a few starting before age twelve, most between twelve and eighteen, and some after eighteen. If you do not smoke by age twenty, you will probably never smoke. Parents need to know all they can about how children begin smoking, as well as how it can be stopped.

Although the smoking habit has decreased markedly among adults today, it is alarmingly high among teenagers and even children. About 12 percent of all adolescents between twelve and eighteen smoked regularly in 1979, a drop from the 15 percent recorded in 1974. But rates for women smokers aged seventeen to twenty-four have increased and now exceed those of men.

Cigarette smoking among the young is a source of special concern. Habits acquired early in life are hard to break. The longer you smoke, the greater your risk of developing a smoking-related disease. While these diseases do not gen-

erally develop until adulthood, teenagers who smoke also cough, produce phlegm, wheeze, and suffer other respiratory problems more than their nonsmoking contemporaries.

Most teenagers start smoking because their friends already do. In some cases, social pressure may be reinforced by a psychological predisposition to smoke.

Social pressures

Three major sources—family members, friends, and the advertising media—all transmit prosmoking attitudes and provide attractive models for young people to imitate.

Nevertheless, the earliest influences come from the family. Whether a child smokes is directly related to the number of family members who smoke. Children with two parents who smoke are more likely to smoke than those who have only one smoking parent. Children and adolescents whose brothers and sisters smoke are more likely to smoke themselves than those whose siblings do not.

Even stronger pressure to smoke comes from friends. The more friends you have who smoke, the more you are likely to smoke.

Finally, although cigarette advertising has been banned on television, ads still appear in magazines, newspapers, and billboards. Indeed, they have been increased to take up the slack and maintain a powerful commercial pressure to smoke.

Psychological predisposition

Studies show that smokers often feel their lives are controlled by forces external to themselves. They tend to be somewhat less independent and self-confident and more anxious, outgoing, and impulsive than nonsmokers.

Although curiosity and rebelliousness may lead some teenagers to start smoking, these factors are not as important as they might seem.

Teenagers who smoke are often impatient to grow up and achieve adult status, though at the same time they tend to keep peer values. Nonsmoking teenagers tend to hold more traditional adult values like long-range goals. They are more likely to participate in sports and community activities. Despite these differences, there seems to be no one characteristic that distinguishes teenage smokers from nonsmokers.

What parents can do

The best way to prevent your child from smoking is by not smoking yourself. If parents don't smoke and clearly disapprove of smoking, children are much less likely to smoke; if they do smoke, they tend to do so much less frequently. If you smoke, quit. As an example for your children, quitting is as effective as never having smoked.

Although parents can prohibit their children from smoking, it rarely works and may actually encourage smoking. A more effective strategy would be for parents to encourage a healthy lifestyle and behavior in every way. This avoids the forbidden fruit syndrome that makes conduct more appealing to some children just because it is prohibited.

If your teenagers are experimenting with cigarettes, you can at least require that they don't smoke at home. By so doing, you will be saying not only that smoking is bad, but that you have a right to be in a smokeless environment.

Parents should, of course, not make smoking easier by giving their teenagers cigarettes or the money to buy them. Here, as with other temptations, availability leads to submission. Some studies indicate that approximately 10 percent of smokers get their first cigarette at home from a family member.

Parents should also provide a sense of support and caring so children feel free to discuss problems with them. They can relate examples from their own childhood to help children anticipate similar experiences.

What schools can do

School attempts to dissuade teenagers from smoking have had rather disappointing results. With few exceptions, these programs mainly provide factual information on smoking's long-term hazards. Although they have increased students' knowledge about cigarette smoking and changed some attitudes, regrettably, the programs have not actually stopped teenagers from smoking. The prospect of getting a disease sometime in the distant future does not appear to override peer pressure to smoke. Even when kids have adopted negative views toward smoking, many still light up.

One puzzling disappointment has been the recruitment of older students to talk with younger ones to dissuade them from becoming smokers. This approach assumed that students would be more receptive to antismoking messages from peers than from teachers or other authority figures. But neither these programs nor those conducted by teachers have reduced the number of new smokers.

A more promising approach focuses on the psychological as well as social factors that promote smoking. A twelve-session program combines group discussions, demonstrations, and role playing where the students act out social situations including those related to smoking. The program teaches students the basic skills needed to resist direct social pressures to smoke, helps decrease their susceptibility to indirect social influences by promoting greater self-confidence, and helps them learn how to decrease the anxiety in social situations that often lead to smoking. Although this type of program has reduced the number of new smokers by about half, its long-term effectiveness has not yet been established.

What the community can do

The community, too, can help prevent the spread of cigarette smoking. In a sense, every member of society helps decide whether or not children and adolescents become smokers. This is particularly true of highly visible individuals like entertainers, athletes, politicians, and other public figures who serve as role models. Their strong and unequivocal opposition to smoking can show young people that smoking and success are not synonymous.

Since the tobacco industry wants to sell its products, it is unrealistic to expect it not to advertise. Although cigarette ads are not ostensibly targeted at teenagers, they make smokers appear to be sophisticated, successful, sexually appealing, mature, cool, masculine or feminine: in short, all the qualities that teenagers hope to acquire.

The community must counter these misleading images, not only by proclaiming smoking to be "hazardous to your health," but also by reinforcing the growing public perception that smoking is no longer socially acceptable. In the absence of bans on tobacco, the law prohibiting sale of cigarettes to minors should be strictly enforced. "Clean indoor air acts" should be passed and enforced. These prohibit smoking in certain public places or at least provide for nonsmoking areas.

Public service announcements on television and radio should warn young people about smoking's dangers, and continue to build a negative image. Similar announcements could appear in newspapers, magazines, and other publications.

HOW TO STOP SMOKING

If you smoke, the most important health decision you can make for the rest of your life will be to stop. The following may help you in making your decision to give up smoking for good. You can do it either on your own or with the help of an organized method. The crucial consideration is your motivation and commitment to quit. (See table 4.2 for a glossary of smoking terms.)

About 35 percent of adult men and 25 percent of adult women—some 60 million Americans—have quit for at least a year. Many techniques have been developed to help smokers who either have tried to quit on their own and failed, or are reluctant to try unless they get help.

Table 4.2
SMOKING CESSATION TERMS DEFINED

- *Quit*—to abstain from smoking for at least 24 hours.
- *Ex-smoker*—an individual who has quit smoking for one year or more.
- *Cold Turkey*—abrupt and immediate halt to smoking.
- *Tapering Off*—a gradual reduction in the number of cigarettes smoked, leading to quitting.
- *Withdrawal Symptoms*—psychological and physical changes that may accompany quitting.
- *Aversion*—a behavior modification technique that uses an unpleasant stimulus to get smokers to quit.
- *Self-Help*—a do-it-yourself approach to quitting.
- *Multiple Treatment Approach*—different techniques combined within the framework of one program.
- *Maintenance*—strategies that enable a quitter to stay off cigarettes.

Evaluating relative effectiveness of quitting methods

It is difficult to assess accurately the effectiveness of the various techniques designed to get smokers to quit. Reported success rates are often based on somewhat different definitions of "quitter" and "participant." Groups of smokers may not be comparable. For example, smokers who pay several hundred dollars for help in quitting or who allow themselves to be subjected to unpleasant psychological stimuli may be much more motivated to quit than those who attend free clinics or participate as volunteers in research studies.

Also, different approaches are sometimes grouped under the same category even though they share only a few common features. Frequently, results vary widely even when the same method is used because of diversity in the characteristics of the leader, the participants' motivations, or the program's format.

For all these reasons, comparisons between methods are often invalid. What is most important, however, is the desire to quit smoking. This desire is far more crucial to success than the specific method used.

Choosing a quitting method

No single technique works uniformly well for everyone. People differ in personality, emotions, personal needs, smoking habits, the strength of their addiction to cigarettes, and whether they have the motivation and commitment to quit.

Little is known about which method works best with which people. Some persons need the support of a group; others feel uncomfortable in groups and prefer an individual approach—either on their own or with the aid of a therapist. Many smokers may want a combined approach that provides a diversity of techniques from which to pick and choose. Do not hesitate to try a variety of approaches until you find the most effective one.

Self-help

Most people who quit (over 95 percent) of the 30 million ex-smokers in the United States) have done so on their own. Smokers may stop temporarily or only when they experience alarming symptoms like loss of breath or chest pains. Others simply decide to quit and do so.

What follows is a seven-day plan called the *Countdown to Quitting*. The first six days are designed to prepare you for the quitting process. The seventh day is QD (Quit Day). On that day, you will quit smoking and then practice proven techniques to prevent and eliminate all cigarette urge sensations. In this way your withdrawal discomfort will be minimized. Quitting is a lot easier when you know how to do it.

Each day of the *Countdown to Quitting* contains assignments and exercises. The more of them that you carry out, the easier quitting will be.

Six days until I become an ex-smoker

1. Mark on a calendar seven days from today, the letters QD. This date represents the day that you will become an ex-smoker. Reflect on this date throughout the week. It is the day you will become free of cigarettes for good.

2. On a separate sheet of paper make two lists. On the first one write down *all* the reasons why you want to quit smoking. On the second one write down your reasons for wanting to continue smoking. Compare the lists.

3. Starting today, record every cigarette you smoke from now until QD. Photocopy or cut out the cigarette pack wrap in figure 4.3. Join the edges of the "pack wrap" with scotch tape so that it forms a closed circle. Slip it over the pack of cigarettes you are smoking. Each time you smoke a cigarette, use a pen or pencil to place a slash in the pack wrap box that corresponds to the appropriate day and time. At the end of each day, add up the number of cigarettes you smoked and write this amount at the bottom of the appropriate column next to the letter "S" ("S" stands for Summary).

4. Over the next six days, make the following changes in the way you smoke:
   a. When you notice an urge to light up a cigarette, wait a *full five* minutes before doing so. During this delay, continue to do whatever you were doing.
   b. Do not smoke automatically; smoke only when you really want to. In this manner, you may be able to cut out some unnecessary cigarettes. Don't fight with yourself over the cigarettes you really want to smoke; go ahead and smoke them. Only cut out *unnecessary* cigarettes.

5. For the next six days, do not purchase cigarettes by the carton. Buy them one pack at a time.

6. Before you go to sleep tonight, repeat one quit reason ten times in front of a mirror.

AHF ✤ Stop Smoking System

PACK WRAP — Slip around pack and place a slash in the box which indicates the time each cigarette was smoked.

	Wednesday		Thursday		Friday		Saturday		Sunday		Monday	Total
4		4		4		4		4		4		
5		5		5		5		5		5		
6		6		6		6		6		6		
7		7		7		7		7		7		
8		8		8		8		8		8		
9		9		9		9		9		9		
10		10		10		10		10		10		
11		11		11		11		11		11		
Noon		Noon		Noon		Noon		Noon		Noon		
1		1		1		1		1		1		
2		2		2		2		2		2		
3		3		3		3		3		3		
4		4		4		4		4		4		
5		5		5		5		5		5		
6		6		6		6		6		6		
7		7		7		7		7		7		
8		8		8		8		8		8		
9		9		9		9		9		9		
10		10		10		10		10		10		
11		11		11		11		11		11		
Mdnt.		Mdnt.		Mdnt.		Mdnt.		Mdnt.		Mdnt.		
1		1		1		1		1		1		
2		2		2		2		2		2		
3		3		3		3		3		3		
S		S		S		S		S		S		

FIGURE 4.3

Cigarette pack wrap
SOURCE: American Health Foundation

Five days until I become an ex-smoker

1. Assignment review:
   a. Continue recording each cigarette you smoke on your pack wrap.
   b. Delay five minutes after an urge hits you.
   c. Try to cut out unnecessary cigarettes.
   d. Buy your cigarettes by the pack.
   e. Repeat a quit reason ten times in front of a mirror.
2. Stop using all smoking paraphernalia. This means no lighters or cigarette cases or containers. Use only matches to light your cigarettes.
3. What follows is the "Why Do You Smoke" questionnaire. For each statement, circle the number that describes how often you feel this way about smoking. After answering *all* the questions, you can score your results by reading "How to Score." Then learn the significance of your score by reading the descriptions under "What Your Score Means."

WHY DO YOU SMOKE?

	always	frequently	occasionally	seldom	never
A. I smoke cigarettes in order to keep myself from slowing down.	5	4	3	2	1
B. Handling a cigarette is part of the enjoyment of smoking it.	5	4	3	2	1
C. Smoking cigarettes is pleasant and relaxing.	5	4	3	2	1

		always	frequently	occasionally	seldom	never
D.	I light up a cigarette when I feel angry about something.	5	4	3	2	1
E.	When I have run out of cigarettes I find it almost unbearable until I can get them.	5	4	3	2	1
F.	I smoke cigarettes automatically without even being aware of it.	5	4	3	2	1
G.	I smoke cigarettes to stimulate me, to perk myself up.	5	4	3	2	1
H.	Part of the enjoyment of smoking a cigarette comes from the steps I take to light up.	5	4	3	2	1
I.	I find cigarettes pleasurable.	5	4	3	2	1
J.	When I feel uncomfortable or upset about something, I light up a cigarette.	5	4	3	2	1
K.	I am very much aware of the fact when I am not smoking a cigarette.	5	4	3	2	1
L.	I light up a cigarette without realizing I still have one burning in the ashtray.	5	4	3	2	1
M.	I smoke cigarettes to give me a "lift."	5	4	3	2	1
N.	When I smoke a cigarette, part of the enjoyment is watching the smoke as I exhale it.	5	4	3	2	1
O.	I want a cigarette most when I am comfortable and relaxed.	5	4	3	2	1
P.	When I feel "blue" or want to take my mind off cares and worries, I smoke cigarettes.	5	4	3	2	1
Q.	I get a real gnawing hunger for a cigarette when I haven't smoked for a while.	5	4	3	2	1
R.	I've found a cigarette in my mouth and didn't remember putting it there.	5	4	3	2	1

How to score:

1. Enter the numbers you have circled to the Test questions in the spaces provided on page 266, putting the number you have circled to Question A over line A, to Question B over line B, etc.
2. Total the 3 scores on each line to get your totals. For example, the sum of your scores over lines A, G, and M gives you your score on *Stimulation*—lines B, H, and N gives the score on *Handling*, etc.

This questionnaire is part of the "Smoker's Self-Testing Kit" published by the DHEW National Clearinghouse for Smoking and Health

Totals

_____ + _____ + _____ = _____
  A   G   M   Stimulation

_____ + _____ + _____ = _____
  B   H   N   Handling

_____ + _____ + _____ = _____
  C   I   O   Pleasurable Relaxation

_____ + _____ + _____ = _____
  D   J   P   Crutch: Tension Reduction

_____ + _____ + _____ = _____
  E   K   Q   Craving: Psychological Addiction

_____ + _____ + _____ = _____
  F   L   R   Habit

Scores can vary from 3 to 15.
Any score 11 and above is _high_; any score 7 and below is _low_.

What your score means

The higher your score in any given factor (e.g., stimulation), the more important the role that factor plays in your smoking habit. Below is a brief explanation of the significance of a high score in each factor.

1. _Stimulation_. You are one of those smokers who is stimulated by the cigarette. You feel that it helps to wake you up, channels your energies, and keeps you going.
2. _Handling_. You get a great deal of satisfaction from keeping your hands busy—lighting up the cigarette, holding it, flicking the ashes, etc.
3. _Pleasurable Relaxation_. Typically, this person uses the cigarette as a reward when he or she can sit down and take a break. It enhances the pleasure of situations such as parties or afterdinner relaxation.

4. _Crutch/Tension Reduction_. The cigarette is used as a crutch in moments of stress, discomfort, and pressure. It has the effect of a tranquilizer; you light up when you are tense or angry. When you anticipate stress, it is a way of putting things off and taking time to "collect your thoughts."
5. _Craving/Psychological Addiction_. The smoker here feels completely dependent on cigarettes. The craving for the next cigarette begins to build the moment he or she puts one out. This kind of smoker is constantly aware of the fact that he or she is not smoking and feels terrified at the prospect of being without cigarettes for an extended period of time.
6. _Habit_. This smoker is no longer getting much satisfaction from cigarettes. He or she lights them without realizing it or even really wanting one and frequently has more than one cigarette lit at the same time. The habit is truly automatic.

Four days until I become an ex-smoker

1. Assignment review:
   a. Continue recording each cigarette you smoke on your pack wrap.
   b. Delay five minutes after an urge hits.
   c. Try to cut out unnecessary cigarettes.
   d. Buy your cigarettes by the pack.
   e. Stop using all smoking paraphernalia.
   f. Repeat a quit reason ten times in front of a mirror.
2. Switch to a different brand of cigarettes from the ones you usually smoke. It doesn't have to be a brand you dislike, just a different one.
3. Save your cigarette butts and place them in a clear bottle or jar. Continue doing this until your "butt bottle" is filled to the top.
4. Change the place where you carry and store your cigarettes; keep them in a different pocket, a new drawer, on the opposite side of your desk, in your coat instead of your purse, etc.
5. Figure out the "Dollars and Sense" of quitting smoking by filling in the information below:

THE DOLLARS AND SENSE OF SMOKING CESSATION

Money You Have Already Spent on Cigarettes
1. Average number of packs smoked per day. _____

2. Average number of packs smoked per year. (Multiply figure in #1 by 365.) _____

3. Total number of years smoked. (Subtract the age at which you started smoking from your present age.) _____

4. Total number of packs smoked to date. (Multiply figure in #2 by figure in #3.) _____

5. Total amount spent on cigarettes to date. (Multiply figure in #4 by 40¢, which is the average cost of a cigarette pack over the last 20 years.) _____

Money That You Will Spend on Cigarettes
6. Average number of packs smoked per year. (Same as #2.) _____

7. Number of years of future smoking. (Subtract your present from 69 years; 69 is the average life expectancy for a smoker as compared to 76 years for a nonsmoker.) _____

8. Number of cigarette packs you will smoke over the rest of your life. (Multiply the figure in #6 by the figure in #7.) _____

9. Total amount of money you will spend on future smoking. (Multiply figure in #8 by $1.00, which will be the average future cost of a pack of cigarettes.) _____

10. Lifetime cost of smoking. (Add figures in #5 and #9.) _____

Three days until I become an ex-smoker

1. Assignment review:
   a. Continue recording each cigarette you smoke on your pack wrap.
   b. Delay *ten* minutes after an urge hits. (This represents a slight change from the five-minute delay).
   c. Try to cut out unnecessary cigarettes.

d. Buy your cigarettes by the pack.

e. Stop using all smoking paraphernalia.

f. Continue to smoke your new brand.

g. Place all your butts in the butt bottle until it is filled up.

h. Change the place where you carry and store your cigarettes.

i. Repeat a quit reason ten times in front of a mirror.

2. Observe the smokers around you. Study them to see whether they appear glamorous, sophisticated, debonair, happy, sad, attractive, nervous, relaxed, etc.

3. While smoking, hold your cigarette with the hand opposite the one that you usually smoke with.

Two days until I become an ex-smoker

1. Assignment review:

a. Continue recording each cigarette you smoke on your pack wrap.

b. Delay *ten* minutes after an urge hits.

c. Try to cut out unnecessary cigarettes.

d. Buy your cigarettes by the pack.

e. Stop using all smoking paraphernalia.

f. Continue to smoke your new brand.

g. Place all your butts in the butt bottle until it is filled up.

h. Change the place where you carry and store your cigarettes.

i. Continue to observe the smokers around you.

j. Repeat a quit reason ten times in front of a mirror.

k. Hold your cigarette with the opposite hand.

2. Increase your fluid intake by drinking six to eight glasses of water a day. This will prepare your body for flushing out the substances in tobacco smoke.

3. Take it easy today and get as much sleep as you need tonight so that you will be well rested for QD.

4. Check off the positive effects you expect will come with quitting.

_____ generally better health

_____ restoration of good breathing

_____ better circulation throughout the body

_____ easier, deeper, more satisfying sleep

_____ a younger, brighter, more alive look

_____ improved self-image and self-respect

_____ a greater sense of security

_____ a greater sense of responsibility toward goals and values

_____ more energy, strength, and endurance

_____ improved sense of taste, smell, vision, and hearing

_____ improved sexual response

_____ feeling refreshed upon awakening

_____ a longer life

_____ a healthier mental attitude

_____ a higher level of mental functioning (e.g., improved memory, better thought organization, etc.)

_____ restoration of the esteem and respect of loved ones

_____ complete freedom from an enslaving habit

_____ more money to save or spend

One day until I become an ex-smoker

1. Assignment review:

a. Continue recording each cigarette you smoke on your pack wrap.

b. Delay ten minutes after an urge hits.

c. Try to cut out unnecessary cigarettes.

d. Stop using all smoking paraphernalia.

e. Continue to smoke your new brand.

f. Place all your butts in the butt bottle until it is filled up.

g. Change the place where you carry and store your cigarettes.

h. Drink six to eight glasses of water per day.

i. Get enough rest.

j. Hold your cigarette with your opposite hand.

2. Do not linger at the table after each meal. Immediately get up and go for a walk.

3. Make up quit smoking slogan signs. Place one in a visible location at home and one at work. Examples are:

"Smokers Have Everything—Emphysema, Heart Disease, Lung Cancer"

"Little Orphan Annie's Parents Smoked"

"Smoking Pays—the Doctor, the Hospital, the Undertaker"

4. Develop a positive attitude about quitting. See it as a gain, rather than a loss. Commit yourself to the idea of *wanting* to quit rather than *having* to quit.

Quit day and beyond

Part I—Preventing the Urge

The following techniques have proven effective in *preventing* the desire to smoke. The more techniques you use, the easier it will be for you to quit. Keep doing these exercises until you feel comfortable as an ex-smoker.

1. Get rid of all smoking materials. Throw out *all* your cigarettes by breaking them in half and wetting them down. Clean out all ashtrays in your home, office, or car and put them away. Discard your matches and hide lighters.

2. Scramble up your day and do things differently. This will help eliminate triggers for wanting a cigarette. For example: change the order of your morning routine; don't sit in your "smoking" chair after dinner; drive a different route to work; eat lunch in a new place; spend more time in nonsmoking areas.

3. After each meal do not linger at the table, but rinse your mouth out with a mouthwash and go for a short walk.

4. Play with a manual substitute such as a key chain, worry beads, paper clip, or coin.

5. Avoid fatigue and get your normal sleep requirements.

6. Shower or bathe twice daily. You can't smoke while in the shower, and it'll help soothe your nerves.

7. Keep as busy as possible. Find things to do such as visiting a nonsmoking friend, going to a movie, fixing something around the house, working on a crossword puzzle, or knitting a sweater.

8. Try to avoid coffee, coca cola, and alcohol as much as possible.

9. Drink a lot of water and fruit juice throughout the day, especially when you are hungry or have a desire to smoke.

10. Eat plenty of fresh fruits and vegetables as they are low in calories.

11. Find some oral substitutes and use them to reward yourself in the same way you may have formerly used cigarettes. Good examples are sugarless gum and candy, diet soda, cinnamon sticks, toothpicks, and plastic cigarettes.

Part II—Dealing with the Urge

The following techniques have proven effective in *eliminating* any cigarette urge that may develop. Use them when an urge hits.

1. Smokeless inhalation
   a. Take a deep breath through your mouth.
   b. Hold the air in your lungs for three seconds.
   c. Exhale slowly through pursed lips.
   d. Repeat this procedure until the urge leaves (it may take two to ten deep breaths, depending upon the urge).
2. Ex-Smoker's ritual
   a. Choose a negative consequence of smoking that is particularly unpleasant for you (e.g., uncontrollable coughing, gasping for breath, having a heart attack, cancer surgery, being out of control).
   b. Write your negative consequences on a piece of paper.
   c. Mentally imagine this unpleasant scene for fifteen seconds.
   d. If the urge still persists, imagine the scene for another fifteen seconds.
   e. Repeat the ritual until you are no longer aware of the urge.
   f. When the urge has left, reward yourself by imagining a pleasant, positive scene for fifteen seconds (e.g., ocean, forest, mountain, favorite activity).
   g. Write your positive scene on a piece of paper.
3. Butt revival
   a. Keep your butt bottle in a conspicuous location.
   b. Look at your butt bottle.
   c. Open it up and take a smell.
   d. Add water to highlight the odor.
4. Leave the scene of an urge
   a. When possible, get away from a situation that triggers an urge.
   b. A short walk and/or new environment can do wonders.
5. Ex-Smoker's inspiration—"The urge for a cigarette will go away whether you smoke a cigarette or do not smoke a cigarette".

Part III—Other Helpful Techniques

1. Reward yourself with little things that make you feel good. Treat yourself to a bubble bath; buy the hardcover edition of a book rather than wait for the paperback to come out; get the game or puzzle you've been wanting; buy or pick a flower; picnic in the park during lunchtime; try a new perfume or cologne; give yourself some "me-time."
2. Make a ciggy bank. Find a clear jar or container and place it alongside your butt bottle. Each day deposit in it the amount of money you would have used to buy cigarettes. After the money has accumulated for a few months, use the money to pay for something special you would really like (e.g., a color television, a sewing machine, a food processor, or a weekend trip).
3. Place a rubber band on the wrist of your smoking hand. Give yourself a zap to get rid of a cigarette urge. You can also use the band as a device for keeping your hands busy.
4. Thought stopping—this procedure was developed by psychologists to help eliminate obsessive/compulsive thoughts. It works well for cigarette thoughts too. Whenever they occur, yell out the word STOP!!! as loud as you can. This will startle the thought away. Practice this technique at least ten times. There is also a silent version of thought stopping. For this technique, imagine yelling "STOP!!!", while trying to visualize the word in large capital letters, a flashing red light, or a STOP sign.
5. By saying positive statements to yourself, you will increase your strength and resolve to both quit and "stay quit." When you suddenly find yourself wanting to smoke, silently repeat one or two positive messages to yourself over and over.

Examples: "I *choose* not to smoke," "I am in control of myself," "One *will* hurt," "I shall not be a slave to tobacco," I shall kick the habit," "My cigarette urges will go away."

6. Profit from your difficult times. Having cigarette urges is a natural part of the quitting process; don't let it frustrate you. Every time you overcome the desire to smoke you are demonstrating your ability to be in control. Look upon urges and their elimination as a positive step in the quitting process.

7. One smoke, one smoker. Alcoholics Anonymous uses the phrase "One drink, one drunk." We believe the same concept applies to cigarettes. Ex-smokers simply can't handle that "just one" cigarette. The likelihood of going back to your former smoking habit is too great, even when you just borrow a few drags from a friend's cigarette.

Other Aids

Self-testing kits are another aid for the do-it-yourself quitter. The American Cancer Society kit includes instructions for quitting over a seven-day period, a quitting calendar, a phonograph record of quitting experience, a breathing exercise, songs and skits, a poster, tips on maintenance, and "I quit" buttons. Several million people have used this kit.

Many other aids are available to help smokers quit on their own. The most popular is a filter that progressively reduces tar and nicotine levels, permitting smokers to be gradually weaned from their physical dependence on cigarettes. Some systems employ reusable filters; others provide disposable filters, one to be used daily. There has been no evaluation of the filter method.

Group programs Voluntary organizations, commercial firms, lay persons, health institutions, and health professionals all conduct group programs to help smokers quit. Generally these are weekly sessions over a period of four to twenty weeks, with the average lasting about eight weeks. Some groups may meet two or three times a week or even daily. The groups, varying in size from eight to twenty, usually contain the same people throughout treatment and provide social pressure to abstain from smoking.

Group leaders give information about smoking and health, stimulate discussions, answer questions, offer support, and explain how to handle problems that come up when quitting. Exercise, role playing, or relaxation techniques may be used. Some groups use aversion methods, hypnosis, or drugs. Commercial clinics follow a specific format with targeted quitting dates or weekly goals. Participants generally keep records of their smoking. Some groups use special manuals.

An example of a widely attended group program is the Five-Day Plan of the Seventh Day Adventist Church. The Adventists say that more than 12 million smokers around the world have enrolled in their clinics, which started in the 1960s. The program has been much copied by others.

The program consists of five consecutive one and one-half to two-hour daily sessions with several weekly follow-up meetings. During the first session, a film of surgery on a cancerous lung is usually shown. Sometimes actual lung specimens are displayed. Participants are required to quit smoking at the beginning of the program, and coffee, tea, alcohol, and cola are prohibited for the week. Physical fitness, exercise, balanced diets, high fluid intake, warm baths, hot and cold showers, body rubs, deep breathing, and a "buddy system" are encouraged. Clergymen, psychologists, or physicians give spiritual, mental, or medical lectures and conduct counseling. A five-day, live-in program, an adaptation of the five-day plan, is also offered.

Individual counseling Varied approaches are used by individual counselors. Their results often reflect the counselor's abilities and commitment. The most intensive programs are conducted by psychologists and psychiatrists, who also handle personal problems that might hinder quitting.

The least intensive approach is often the advice that physicians pass on to their patients about quitting. Yet the role of the physician in helping patients stop smoking can be decisive. Because physicians have access to patients' medical records and exert authority and influence over patients, they are in a unique position to help patients quit.

If the physician cannot help, a patient can be referred to a voluntary or commercial program.

Other techniques for quitting

Here are a variety of quitting techniques, which can be employed along with self-help or group programs, most requiring supervision.

Medication Drugs have long been used to help smokers quit. Some drugs help smokers overcome their habit while others relieve withdrawal symptoms. The former are supposed to act as substitutes for tobacco or deterrents to its use. The most common of the smoking substitutes is lobeline sulphate, commonly found in tablet form. It is thought that lobeline satisfies the craving for nicotine and thus helps smokers quit. However, some studies show that it is no more successful than a placebo.

Smoking deterrents like astringent mouthwashes are prepared mainly from silver nitrate, copper sulphate, or potassium permanganate. They deter smoking by irritating the mucous membranes in the mouth and nose.

Upon examination, few tobacco substitutes or deterrents are effective. The only successes appear to be with the Swedish nicotine chewing gum and some of the mouthwashes. A deterrent may be useful, however, if combined with a support program and maintenance methods.

Certain drugs have also been used to reduce the physiological and psychological withdrawal symptoms related to quitting. Some have a relaxing effect, others aim to help the patient sleep or overcome nervousness, while still others try to prevent weight gain or fatigue. They include sedatives, tranquilizers, and anticonvulsants. Tranquilizers are ineffective and may have negative effects (see chapter 3). Since most drugs are used in combination with counseling or behavior modification, their contribution is difficult to assess.

Overall, well-controlled studies on the use of drugs to get people to stop smoking have shown that they are only marginally effective.

Hypnosis Hypnosis is used to heighten a smoker's suggestibility. Subjects respond more readily to commands or suggestions while in a hypnotic state, and will often attempt to carry out what they are told to do. Despite its former association with black magic and mysticism, hypnosis has helped many smokers quit.

Although one well-known technique has reportedly produced good results in a single session, most hypnotists require two to five sessions because hypnotic suggestions can wear off. In addition, many subjects are taught self-hypnosis so they can reinforce their own nonsmoking efforts whenever necessary.

Hypnotic suggestions are varied, depending on the individual practice of the hypnotist. Some may have you imagine yourself a nonsmoker; they may suggest that you breathe deeply whenever the urge to smoke occurs, lifting your arm, or rolling your eyes. Others encourage you to concentrate on how dreadful cigarettes taste and smell. Others ask you to develop positive concerns about your good health and well-being, and place an "impenetrable steel disk" in your mind to block any desire to smoke.

Hypnosis can be used on an individual basis or in groups. Success rates vary, which may be due to the skill of the hypnotist, or to the suggestibility and motivation of the subject. Hypnosis is not a panacea, but it has been shown to be effective with many people.

Aversive methods In aversive treatment, psychologists or counselors use repugnant or distasteful stimuli to change your desire to smoke. This procedure assumes that (1) if smoking is punished, it will tend to decrease in frequency and (2) if smokers are able to picture a negative experience involving smoking when they have the urge, the desire to smoke will gradually be eliminated. Aversive techniques include rapid smoking, satiation, negative puffing, covert sensitization, electric shock, sensory deprivation, and smoke holding.

Rapid Smoking. This procedure requires you to inhale from one to four cigarettes until the cigarettes are consumed or you become nauseated. The intense dosage of nicotine may cause the body physiologically to resist additional smoke. In addition, rapid and continuous smoking irritates the sensitive mucous membranes of the throat, nasal passages, and lungs, thus further reducing the pleasure of smoking.

Many believe that rapid smoking should be used with great care because of its possibly harmful effects, including increased heart rate and blood pressure, raised carbon monoxide levels in the blood, as well as electrocardiogram abnormalities. Potential subjects should be screened to exclude those who have advanced coronary heart disease or emphysema.

Covert Sensitization. This is a technique designed to make smokers want to avoid smoking. You are asked to imagine yourself smoking a cigarette in various situations. Then you are instructed to picture such disagreeable images as white maggots crawling over the cigarettes, or bitter spit rising in your mouth. You could imag-

ine choking and vomiting sensations, and so forth, accompanying the act of smoking. Next, you imagine yourself not smoking; now you are directed to think pleasant thoughts. Covert sensitization can be used anywhere at any time as it involves no apparatus. When combined with other procedures, covert sensitization yields modest success.

Sensory Deprivation. Sensory deprivation involves putting a smoker on a cot in a dark, quiet room, usually for twenty-four hours. In some conditions, smokers periodically hear messages on smoking's dangers and methods to control the urge for a cigarette. Sensory deprivation has shown a fairly good success rate over a long period of time.

Obviously, however, twenty-four-hour isolation is not appropriate for everyone.

Satiation. This procedure differs from rapid smoking in that you are required to double or triple the number of cigarettes you usually smoke over a given time period, rather than increasing the rate of smoking. No apparatus is needed, but satiation does require subjects to be screened because, like rapid smoking, it produces high doses of nicotine that can damage the cardiopulmonary system. Most results with satiation have been poor.

Negative Puffing. This technique assumes that cigarette smoke itself is repugnant. It is designed to avoid the potentially dangerous effects of rapid smoking and satiation. You puff—but do not inhale—rapidly while holding the cigarette between your lips. Or you hold the cigarette between the last two fingers of your nonsmoking hand and puff on the opposite side of your mouth.

These procedures allow smokers to develop negative associations with cigarettes without absorbing large nicotine dosages. Negative puffing has shown good long-term success rates when combined with other self-control techniques.

Multiple-Treatment Approach. Combining aversive and self-help techniques (also called self-management) can provide a hopeful method to get you to stop smoking. Aversive procedures can effectively produce short-term smoking withdrawal, while at the same time, self-management can make quitting last. In addition, by considering different quitting techniques, you can choose which are most appropriate to your personality, habit, and general health. Such a multiple-treatment approach appears to be highly recommended and, in fact, has shown the highest success rate.

Miscellaneous methods One of the newest techniques to be applied to smoking, *acupuncture*, is really an ancient one. Acupuncture has been used in several countries to help people stop smoking. In one report, four to five sessions were conducted at weekly intervals following electro-acupuncture and the implantation of threads and/or beads in appropriate body points. Although a high success rate is claimed, acupuncture has not yet been thoroughly tested.

Nonsmoking Regulations and Incentives. Recently, some companies have been awarding cash bonuses to employees who refrain from smoking. Others have offered prizes, lottery tickets, and wage differentials. Good results have been reported.

Transcendental Meditation. This Asian meditation technique has gained much popularity in the United States over the past several years. Although transcendental meditation is not usually undertaken specifically to help one quit smoking, reportedly it can reduce smoking as a by-product.

Exercise Programs. Exercise can be very helpful in reducing smoking. Running, swimming, and fitness programs in general demand top conditioning, good breathing, and positive motivation. As smoking impairs the cardiovascular function, it is obviously not compatible with any aerobic exercise—exercise that makes you breathe hard. People who exercise regularly often taper off and many quit altogether.

Cruises and Vacation Programs. A vacation is often a good way to practice nonsmoking under relaxing circumstances. Some programs combine therapy with organized vacations such as cruises. The therapy is attractive and the controlled environment fosters quitting. Help is available from professionals. Breathing therapy, exercises, lectures, and social activities are all used to help the participants stay off cigarettes. However, those who quit usually need help of some kind to keep from starting again once the vacation has ended.

Factors contributing to success

To be successful in quitting smoking you must be committed. It is crucial that you recognize the dangers of smoking and relate them directly to your own health. Those who have a strong personal reason to quit are more likely to succeed than others. For example, studies show that people suffering from heart or respiratory ailments quit much more successfully than others.

Once a smoker has quit, maintenance or follow-up help is vital. It is all too easy to slip back into the habit. A myriad of forces may attack your resolve, including the after-effects of your former habituation (see below). Quitting programs that extend over a relatively long time usually reinforce the commitment to stopping, especially when further extended by maintenance efforts. Programs where follow-up efforts are tailored to your special situation and with leaders who are dedicated to their mission will be more successful than those with no follow-up program.

Maintenance

It has been shown that certain people have a more difficult time staying off cigarettes than do others. Highly anxious persons who have depended on smoking to cope with difficulties often have great problems keeping off cigarettes, as do those with relatively few years of formal schooling. Also, those who have been smoking for many years often find it difficult to stay free of the habit. Environmental factors, too, such as certain social situations and emotional or stressful events may trigger a relapse.

Cessation programs have shown that almost all quitting techniques produce high initial success rates. Unfortunately, however, after a month, three months, six months, or even a year, the initial quit rate declines considerably. Most programs can only claim a 20 to 25 percent quit rate after one year. Relapse usually occurs during the first month after treatment has ended.

To improve this rate, self-management and self-control techniques need to be part of the program itself, rather than introduced after it has been completed. At the same time that smokers are learning to kick the habit, they can also be trained to resist the urge once smoking has stopped. A supportive environment outside the therapeutic setting can also aid former smokers from going back. This may involve using formal buddy systems or enlisting the aid of family members or friends.

Withdrawal symptoms— and how to combat them

Many smokers develop a physical as well as a psychological dependence on cigarettes. This is demonstrated by the various withdrawal symptoms that many smokers experience after quitting. The frequency, intensity, and duration of withdrawal discomfort varies. Happily, most people experience only a few symptoms, and usually for less than a week. These symptoms can include:

Increased appetite Taste buds in the mouth become sensitive when they are no longer dulled by smoke. Thus, food tastes better. In addition, food sometimes serves as an oral substitute for cigarette smoking. Studies have shown that approximately one-third of ex-smokers gain weight (usually five to ten pounds), one-third lose, and one-third stay the same.

When hungry, use sugarless gum or low-calorie snack foods like fresh fruit and vegetables. Increased physical activity will burn off extra calories and prevent weight gain.

Irritability/anxiety Some researchers have found that nicotine serves as a mild tranquilizer for smokers. Eliminating it from the body can cause agitation or nervousness. Others feel that this tension is a reaction to the initial disruption of not smoking rather than an actual withdrawal symptom of nicotine deprivation. In any case, a daily relaxation routine can be helpful

Among ways to relax are meditation, deep muscle relaxation, hypnosis, mental imagery, and deep breathing. A hot shower or bath also helps. (See chapter 7.)

Coughing The cilia (see page 258) that line the bronchial tubes eliminate accumulated mucus. As the mucus is loosened, coughing helps excrete it from the body.

Constipation Nicotine stimulates the adrenal glands that secrete adrenalin. For some smokers, the adrenalin aids intestinal movement. After quitting smoking, you may become constipated. Remedies include eating foods high in fiber like raw fruits and vegetables, bran, and whole grains. A laxative may also help.

Sleepiness Some people find they become drowsy after they quit smoking, again because nicotine is no longer stimulating the flow of adrenalin. This effect can be dealt with by making sure you get your normal sleep each night and taking naps as necessary.

Sleeplessness Others find that the disruption and novelty of not smoking can also precipitate nighttime restlessness. To make sure you are sleeping at night, use up more energy during the day. A glass of warm milk before going to bed may also help.

Dizziness As your bronchial tubes become clear of mucus and are no longer subjected to cigarette smoke, your lungs will absorb more oxygen. Extra oxygen going to the brain initially may cause occasional dizziness.

Depression Smoking may have masked other underlying problems. Quitting may allow them to come to the surface. The depression is generally short-lived, but if it persists, talk with friends or seek professional help.

Sense of Loss Terminating an activity that has been a pervasive part of your life can precipitate a sense of mourning or bereavement. This will pass with time. Keep as busy as possible until then.

The best way to view withdrawal symptoms is in a positive light; indeed, they really are symptoms of recovery.

Additional resources

For more help, the offices listed below are eager to provide anyone with more information on how to quit.

Technical Information Center for Smoking and Health
   Office on Smoking and Health
   Department of Health, Education, and Welfare (now the Department of Health and Human Services)
   Room 1-16, Park Building
   5600 Fishers Lane
   Rockville, MD. 20857
   (301) 443-1690

Office of Cancer Communications
   National Cancer Institute
   Room 10A18, Building 31
   National Institutes of Health
   Bethesda, MD. 20205
   (301) 496-5583

American Cancer Society
   Public Information Department
   777 Third Avenue
   New York, N.Y. 10017
   (212) 371-2900, ext. 254
   (or local chapter)

American Health Foundation
   Health Promotion Services
   320 East 43rd St.
   New York, N.Y. 10017
   (212) 953–1900

American Lung Association
   1740 Broadway
   New York, N.Y. 10019
   (212) 245-8000
   (or local chapter)

American Heart Association
   7320 Greenville Avenue
   Dallas, TX. 75231
   (214) 750-5300
   (or local chapter)

LOW-YIELD CIGARETTES

Some people will continue to smoke in spite of all the accumulated evidence of its harmful effects on the body and educational efforts to persuade them not to. In fact, as of today, we still have some 55 million smokers in the U.S. For these people, we must not only further investigate the effects of smoking, but also attempt to further improve the development of low-tar, low-nicotine cigarettes.

In discussing this subject, several points should be noted. First, as we have seen, tobacco-related diseases are dependent on the quantity smoked and the duration of the habit; obviously, the less exposure to cigarette smoke, the lower the risk. Second, the components in tobacco smoke affect different parts of the body differently. Thus, a "less harmful cigarette" delivers as little smoke and specific tumor-causing substances as possible. It should also be specifically low in substances that contribute to cardiovascular and chronic, obstructive pulmonary diseases. Third, a "safe" cigarette smoked by only 1 percent of smokers would improve overall public health less than a moderately harmful but more appealing cigarette acceptable to 99 percent of smokers. Fourth, it is unlikely that we will ever have a tobacco product that will be as harmless as clean air.

Cigarettes with less toxic substances have been developed during the 1960s and 1970s, primarily in response to reports from the U.S. Surgeon General and the British Royal College of Physicians. The reductions of the harmful agents in tobacco smoke have been brought about in two ways: first, changes in the choice, curing, and growing of tobaccos; and second, the development of filters using cellulose acetate, charcoal, and perforated tips.

Significant progress has been made in the overall reduction of tar and nicotine since 1950. The average yield per cigarette was reduced from 40 to 16 mg. of tar, and from 2.2 to 1 mg. of nicotine. Reduction of several cancer-causing and toxic agents has also taken place. This advance has been reflected by a reduced risk of lung and larynx cancer. For instance, those who smoke filter cigarettes for ten years or more have a 25 percent less risk of getting lung or larynx cancer than those who smoke regular cigarettes (see figure 4.4). The last half of a cigarette has up to 40 percent more tar than the first half. Thus, the fact that filter cigarettes cannot be smoked to the very end may have contributed to the reduced lung and larynx cancer risk.

The benefits of tar reductions in smoke are beginning to be reflected in other statistics as well. For example, the death rate from lung cancer is declining among younger men in England. Part of this decline, which we are also beginning to see in the United States, stems from the fact

that fewer young people are smoking now as compared with the past. However, the reduction of tar in filter cigarettes has played a significant role.

Similar reductions have been reported in the risk of heart attacks and peripheral vascular disease. With both of these diseases, of course, tobacco is not the only causative agent. Much more needs to be known on how elevated blood cholesterol and high blood pressure are modified by, and interact with, smoking. This is vital to understanding whether and how much of the observed risk reduction can be attributed to low-tar, low-nicotine cigarettes. The 14th annual Surgeon General's report on the health consequences of smoking, "The Changing Cigarette," issued early in 1981, restated the health hazards associated with smoking all cigarettes including the low-tar and low-nicotine types.

Studies of chronic respiratory and obstructive pulmonary diseases indicate that smoking filter rather than regular cigarettes has so far not made a difference in preventing these diseases. Chronic obstructive pulmonary diseases involve disease processes that appear to be irreversible, once they have set in.

In this respect we should realize that epidemiological studies are based in general on people who began by smoking the old high-tar cigarettes. As yet, we do not know the risk for tobacco-related diseases for those who have smoked only low-tar cigarettes, and in particular, the low-tar filter cigarettes that became generally available in the 1970s.

Until recently, carbon monoxide has not been reduced as much as tar and nicotine in the smoke of regular as well as of filter cigarettes. In fact, some cigarettes with conventional cellulose acetate filters deliver more carbon monoxide than regular cigarettes. However, newly developed cigarettes with perforated filter tips that dilute the smoke deliver significantly less carbon monoxide than other cigarettes. An estimated one-fourth of all cigarettes sold in the United States in 1979 had such filters.

LUNG CANCER I, MALES

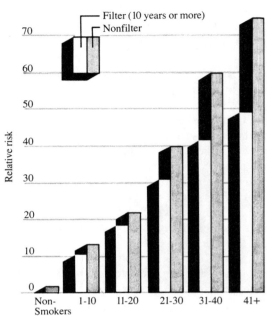

Number of cigarettes smoked per day

LARYNX CANCER, MALES

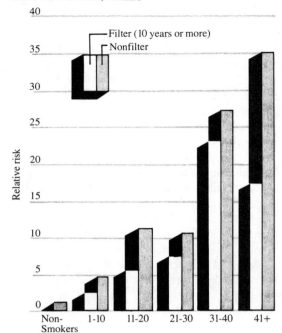

Number of cigarettes smoked per day

LUNG CANCER I, FEMALES

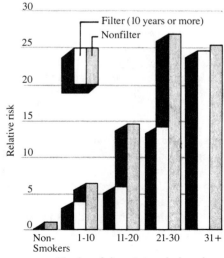

Number of cigarettes smoked per day

LARYNX CANCER, FEMALES

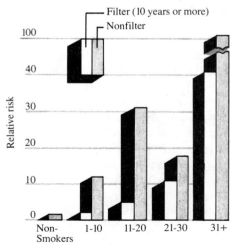

Number of cigarettes smoked per day

Table 4.3

CHANGES IN SMOKE COMPOSITION OF CIGARETTES
MANUFACTURED IN THE UNITED STATES

Smoke constituent	Average delivery per cigarette		
	Before 1960	1978–79	1978/79 (Low tar-cigarette)
Total Particulate Matter (dried tar)	43.0 mg.*	16.0 mg.	8.0 mg.
Nicotine	3.0 mg.	1.1 mg.	0.6 mg.
CO (carbon monoxide)	23.0 mg.	17.0 mg.	8.9 mg.
NO_x (nitrogen oxides)	270.0 μg.†	280.0 μg.	100.0 μg.
HCN (hydrogen cyanide)	410.0 μg.	200.0 μg.	130.0 μg.
Acrolein	130.0 μg.	80.0 μg.	50.0 μg.
Phenol	100.0 μg.	60.0 μg.	20.0 μg.
Benzo(a)pyrene	35.0 ng.‡	18.0 ng.	10.0 ng.

Source: American Health Foundation, 1979

*milligram = 1/1000 of a gram (approximately 1/28th of an ounce)

†microgram = 1/1000 of a milligram

‡nanogram = 1/1000 of a microgram

Cigarettes with charcoal filters allow fewer volatile toxic substances in their smoke than cigarettes with conventional cellulose acetate filters. However, there is as yet no evidence that charcoal filters reduce specific diseases more than conventional filters.

Unfortunately, as the tar and nicotine yield of cigarettes has declined, some smokers, especially those who began with the high-nicotine cigarettes, have compensated by puffing more, inhaling deeper, and retaining smoke in the lungs longer. However, some studies of long-term filter cigarette smokers indicate that some protection results in spite of this compensation, particularly

for risk of lung and larynx cancer. Also, such compensation is less likely to occur in young smokers who began their smoking with low-tar, low-nicotine cigarettes.

Since women tend to smoke cigarettes with low tar and nicotine yields, and since there were considerably fewer women smokers when high-tar and high-nicotine cigarettes were common, the incidence of tobacco-related diseases is expected to be lower for women than men. If flavor additives in the newer, low-tar and nicotine cigarettes are not toxic or carcinogenic, tobacco products are likely to become less harmful as new manufacturing methods are used (see table 4.3).

FIGURE 4.4

Age-adjusted relative risk of lung and larynx cancer for long-term smokers of nonfilter and filter cigarettes by quantity smoked
SOURCE: *American Health Foundation*

It is predicted that by the mid-1980s few U.S. cigarettes will yield more than 15 mg. of tar, about 50 percent will yield 10 mg. or less, and 25 percent will be 5 mg. or less, with corresponding nicotine values ranging from 1.2 to 0.3 mg. We shall be experiencing a relatively greater reduction of tar than of nicotine. These advances are examples of effective "managerial preventive medicine."

Epidemiological studies will have to determine the relative health risk associated with smoking these products. It will be less compared with smoking the old high-tar, high-nicotine brands, although it will be more than the risk for those who have never smoked. But in a real world we need to make realistic decisions, and the development of low-tar, low-nicotine cigarettes is one of these.

In general, upper limits for harmful substances in cigarette smoke can be fixed. It is now technically feasible to provide smokers with acceptable cigarettes having still lower tar and nicotine levels than those on the market today. Even today, if you persist in smoking you can reduce your risk of tobacco-related diseases by smoking the newer low-tar, low-nicotine filter cigarettes.

CHAPTER
5

Physical fitness

Since the early days of recorded history, people have admired the athlete, and many, if not most, ancient societies prized exercise as a virtue. We evolved from a life of physical hardship, but with the industrial revolution, we have become increasingly inactive.

Until the last century, vigorous physical activity was usually an integral part of everyday life. It was necessary for subsistence, transportation, housework, and recreation. Modern technological advances have changed all this. Heavy labor on the job has been largely eliminated by mechanization and automation. Transportation has become motorized. Labor-saving and step-saving devices have reduced physical activity required for housework. Sadly enough, the resulting more abundant leisure time is used by most Americans in passive pursuits, particularly watching television and spectator sports. Thus, most Americans are physically inactive and unfit.

Today we take elevators to ascend a single story; we drive the car to a shopping center half a mile away. Rarely do we exercise to the point where the rate of our heartbeat rises. We have become a nation of spectators preferring to watch a game rather than play it.

Fortunately, although the number of people who jog early in the morning is miniscule compared to the number still snugly tucked into their beds, more and more people are making an organized physical fitness program a part of their daily activities.

But despite periodic surges of interest in exercise and fitness, polls show that fewer than half of all American adults exercise regularly at least once a week. About 70 percent of them feel they should be exercising more. Why don't they? The most common excuses are:

lack of time
lack of willpower
lack of interest
lack of energy
a medical problem

The latest evidence of the benefits of physical fitness indicates that a major advantage of physical fitness is its influence on other lifestyle-related habits. Those who respect their bodies and care for them properly, using them, not abusing them, are those most likely to have the most productive and useful longevity.

283

Glossary

AEROBIC Literally, with oxygen. An aerobic activity is one where a steady supply of oxygen is required for sustained periods of activity such as jogging, rowing, rope skipping, dancing, etc.

ANAEROBIC Literally, without oxygen. A specialized activity in which oxygen is not required for short periods of time—e.g., for short bursts of vigorous activity such as sprinting in which breathing actually stops.

ISOMETRIC A static form of muscular activity in which tension is developed within muscle fibers but little or no movement of joints and bones is involved. Used for increasing muscle bulk.

ISOTONIC Alternate contraction and relaxation of the muscles with rhythmic joint movement.

MAXIMAL OXYGEN UPTAKE The optimal absorption and incorporation of oxygen from the air, delivered to the body's tissue—also called aerobic power.

MITOCHONDRIA Main energy source of the cell.

MYOGLOBIN The protein in muscle tissue that carries oxygen.

The Benefits of Exercise

Is exercise really necessary for good health? Testimonials to exercise are not lacking among the sages of the past.

About 100 B.C., Cicero observed that "exercise and temperance can preserve something of our strength in old age." Aristotle stressed the need for exercise to maintain "a healthy mind in a healthy body."

In the Mishneh Torah, the twelfth century Jewish scholar and physician, Rabbi Moses Maimonides, strongly recommended daily exercise and warned that "anyone who sits around idle and takes no exercise will be subject to physical discomforts and failing strength."

Early in the eighteenth century, the renowned British physician, Thomas Addison, said: "Exercise ferments the humours, casts them into their proper channels, throws off redundancies, and helps nature in these secret distributions without which the body cannot subsist in its vigour nor the soul act with cheerfulness."

In 1799, the Englishman, Thomas Easton, evaluated the lifestyles of 1,712 people over one-hundred years of age in a book on human longevity and concluded: "It is not the rich and the great, nor those who depend on medicine, who become old: but such as use much exercise. For the idler never attains a remarkable great age."

In 1864, an English physiologist, Edward Smith, performed the first systematic studies on the physiologic and metabolic responses to exercise. He reported a higher mortality rate among people in sedentary occupations compared with those who were physically active.

In the United States exercise and fitness were popular with the founding fathers, among them Benjamin Franklin, John Quincy Adams, and Thomas Jefferson. Jefferson was particularly enthusiastic about walking. "Habituate yourself to walk fast without fatigue," he wrote.

SOURCES OF EVIDENCE

All these early but astute observations have been confirmed by modern science. Archeological and anthropological studies on early and primitive humans, current epidemiological studies, clinical and physiological research, and animal laboratory studies all point to the same conclusion: regular exercise improves the quality and, perhaps, even the length of life; conversely, physical inactivity has many deleterious effects on the body.

Our prehistoric ancestors were used to regular levels of endurance exercise as they foraged and hunted for food and ran to escape enemies. Thus, it is not surprising that, *through evolution, our cardiovascular and endocrine systems as well as our metabolism were adapted for rigorous physical activity and still require it for optimal functioning.*

Many anthropologists feel that our early ancestors were probably not unlike the Tarahumara Indians, a cave-dwelling people who live in the remote Sierra Madre Occidental Mountains of northern Mexico. The members of this Uto-Aztec tribe are famous for their extraordinary endurance. The Tarahumara (meaning "foot runner") collect food by outrunning deer and wild turkeys, which finally drop from exhaustion. Their traditional sport (rarhipa) consists of men, women, and children running 50 to 200 miles kicking a wooden ball between villages, non-stop, for twenty-four to seventy-two hours at a time over rugged mountains. This is a vivid example of how, through the evolutionary process, humans have acquired the physical capabilities and endurance of animals.

In the industrialized world coronary heart disease is by far the major adult health problem today. During the past twenty-five years, nearly one hundred epidemiological studies have examined the relationship of regular exercise at work and/or during leisure time to the development of heart attacks. Most of these studies reveal an inverse relationship between physical activity levels and coronary disease. Active people get about half of the heart attacks and reflect only a third of the associated mortality of inactive people. Even milder exercise is associated with lower rates of coronary disease. Walking, stair climbing, cycling, or gardening, if performed several times a week, year-round, appears to be sufficient.

Evaluating the effect of exercise on cardiovascular disease and other illnesses is a complex task, since individuals who strive to be physically fit are also likely to watch their diet and weight, drink in moderation, and are unlikely to be heavy smokers. An accurate epidemiological evaluation of the benefit of physical fitness must consider other lifestyle habits to determine the effect of each of them (see chapters 1. Nutrition, 2. Alcohol, 4. Tobacco). Another consideration is that programs designed to enhance physical fitness cannot be measured as precisely as the number of drinks consumed per day or the number of cigarettes inhaled. These research limitations must be kept in mind as we attempt to evaluate the immediate and long-term health benefits of exercise.

DETRIMENTAL EFFECTS OF INACTIVITY

Frequently, the disabling consequences of physical inactivity have been studied experimentally by putting healthy male volunteers at bed rest. The following are some of the deconditioning effects that may occur as a result of severe inactivity. (Similar disabilities were observed in astronauts returning from space until in-flight exercises were instituted.)

- Rapid deterioration of the ability to do prolonged work and deliver oxygen from the air to the tissues (maximal oxygen uptake or aerobic power)

- Deterioration of cardiovascular function resulting from direct effects on the heart muscle, particularly among the elderly
- Loss of minerals and protein from the tissues leading to musculoskeletal problems
- Wasting of skeletal muscle with loss of tone and strength and decreased joint and ligament flexibility
- Bone thinning or osteoporosis, causing bone fractures, particularly among the elderly
- Chronic low-back pain
- Loss of smooth muscle tone in the veins leading to venous pooling of blood causing difficulty in adjusting to the upright position, varicose veins, and increased risk of venous blood clots (thrombophlebitis)
- Abnormalities of carbohydrate and lipid (fat) metabolism
- Resistance to insulin action leading to an oversecretion of insulin, abnormalities in the handling of sugar, chemical manifestations of diabetes mellitus, and increased risk of heart attack
- Weight gain and increased obesity
- Blood lipid abnormalities that may contribute to coronary risk

Because of the demonstrated detrimental effect of bed rest, early and progressive activity has become the rule following uncomplicated heart attacks. Less illness, fewer deaths, and shorter hospital stays are the results.

FITNESS COMPONENTS

Health, as defined by the World Health Organization, is "physical, mental, and social well-being, and not merely the absence of disease or infirmity." Such a definition implies the positive quality of physical fitness, which means the ability to carry out daily tasks with vigor and alertness, without undue fatigue, and with ample reserve energy to enjoy active leisure pursuits, and the ability to respond to physical and emotional stress without an excessive increase in heart rate and blood pressure.

Table 5.1
DECONDITIONING EFFECTS OF INACTIVITY

1. Reduced cardiovascular function
2. Decreased work capacity (maximal oxygen uptake) or aerobic power
3. Inefficient cardiovascular system (increased heart rate and blood pressure)
4. Skeletal muscle atrophy with loss of tone and strength
5. Decreased muscle and joint flexibility
6. Bone demineralization (osteoporosis)
7. Postural hypotension—low blood pressure felt when one moves suddenly to upright position from a lying position
8. Increased adiposity—excessive body fat
9. Glucose intolerance and insulin resistance (diabetes mellitus)
10. Blood lipid abnormalities

SOURCE: Arthur S. Leon, M.D., Laboratory of Physiological Hygiene, School of Public Health, University of Minnesota.

The basic components of physical fitness are generally agreed to include the following:

1. *Muscular Strength*: the contracting power of skeletal muscles. It is improved by weight lifting and isometric exercises in which static muscle contractions are sustained.
2. *Muscular Endurance*: the ability of skeletal muscles to do prolonged work, either isometric (static) or isotonic (alternately, shorten and lengthen). Weight training and push-ups help here.
3. *Cardiorespiratory Endurance (Aerobic Capacity)*: characterized by prolonged, moderate intensity, rhythmic contractions of large muscle groups during which the circulatory and respiratory systems maintain blood and oxygen delivery to the exercising muscles. This is considered to be the most important aspect of fitness in terms of health and quality of life. It is reached by isotonic exercises such as running, brisk walking, swimming, and bicycling.
4. *Flexibility*: the range of motion in a joint or sequence of joints. It requires stretching exercises that are usually part of the warm-up and cool-down phases of endurance training programs.
5. *Body Composition*: the amount of lean and fat tissue in the body. Strength training increases lean body mass and endurance training usually reduces body fat. Measuring skin fold thickness of various parts of the body is a handy way of estimating relative fatness.

In addition to these five basic components, physical fitness also involves:

Muscular Power: the ability to release maximum muscular force in the shortest time.

Agility: speed in smoothly changing body positions and directions.

Speed: rapidity in performing successive movements of the same type.

Muscle Bulk

Posture

BENEFITS OF ISOTONIC EXERCISE

Most people benefit physically and psychologically from isotonic exercises such as running, brisk walking, swimming, and bicycling. Perhaps all they need to know is that they "feel better." But they are experiencing more than a feeling. Isotonic exercise sets in motion elaborate biological processes involving the skeletal muscles as well as the cardiovascular, respiratory, and endocrine systems.

Skeletal muscle changes

Unlike strength exercise, endurance training such as long-distance running, does not increase skeletal muscle mass or strength. It does, however, increase muscular capacity for aerobic metabolism of carbohydrate and fat. Exercised muscles also extract greater amounts of oxygen from the blood by increasing the number of capillary blood vessels supplying each muscle fiber. This results in improved oxygen delivery throughout the body.

Isotonic exercise also increases oxygen delivery by increasing the amount of myoglobin and mitochondria in the skeletal muscles. Myoglobin helps to deliver oxygen from the cell membrane to the mitochondria—the cell's energy source. Other positive effects of isotonic activity are increased muscle stores of carbohydrate in the form of glycogen and decreased lactic acid production. All of these biochemical adaptations contribute to increased exercise tolerance and increased aerobic capacity.

Table 5.2
BENEFITS OF ENDURANCE EXERCISE

1. **Skeletal muscle changes**
   A. Increased blood supply (capillaries)
   B. Increased oxygen uptake and utilization
   C. Increased metabolic capacity
   D. Increased myoglobin content
   E. Increased energy (glycogen) stores
   F. Decreased lactic acid production
2. **Cardiovascular-respiratory changes**
   A. Increased cardiorespiratory capacity and endurance
   B. Reduced heart rate
   C. Reduced blood pressure
   D. Reduced cardiac work and coronary blood flow requirements
   E. Increased heart muscle (myocardial) blood supply
   F. Increased output per beat (stroke volume)
   G. Decreased cardiac irritability
   H. Increased blood volume and hemoglobin
   I. Reduced blood coagulability
   J. Reduced work of breathing
3. **Metabolic adaptations**
   A. Reduced body fat stores
   B. Appropriate appetite adjustment
   C. Increased tissue sensitivity to insulin and improved glucose tolerance
   D. Improvement in blood lipid profile: Reduced triglycerides and increased high-density lipoproteins

SOURCE: Arthur S. Leon, M.D., Laboratory of Physiological Hygiene, School of Public Health, University of Minnesota.

Cardiovascular changes

A program of exercise training has been shown to increase the capacity of the heart to pump blood (stroke volume), particularly in young people. This mechanism involves several factors: with exercise a direct enlargement of the heart muscle takes place, a more effective return of blood to the heart from the peripheral tissues results, increased blood volume is produced, and a slowing of the heart rate occurs, allowing more time for filling. The resulting increased stroke volume improves one's maximal oxygen uptake and, therefore, increases one's work capacity and endurance.

A reduction in heart rate at rest and during exercise occurs with short-term exercise training. A decrease from 85 beats per minute to 60 or less is not unusual; this is a saving of 1,500 beats per hour or more than a million beats per month. There is usually an associated reduction in systolic blood pressure (the pressure during the contraction part of the heartbeat cycle). Since heart rate and systolic blood pressure are major determinants of cardiac work and oxygen demands, this reduction results in a decrease in coronary blood flow requirements. Further reduction in heart work results from the skeletal muscle changes mentioned above and from decreased work of respiration. The resulting improvement in cardiovascular efficiency may be the most important way in which exercise training reduces the heart attack risk. Exercise training in rehabilitation programs also increases the work capacity of patients with limited coronary reserve due to a heart attack.

Other effects of exercise include a possible reduction in the chance of fatal cardiac rhythm disturbance and of clot formation within arteries.

METABOLIC EFFECTS

Changes in body weight and composition

Physical activity and endurance exercise play an important role in the maintenance of proper body weight, body composition, and appetite. As we know, physical inactivity promotes obesity; physical activity promotes weight reduction.

> The usual fat content of the body as a percentage of body weight of American men is as follows: Age 25 years—14 percent; age 55 years—26 percent, for American women: Age 24 years—25 percent; age 56 years—38 percent. Trained endurance athletes usually have less than 12 percent fat if men, and less than 18 percent, if women. Men are considered to be obese if they have over 25 percent fat and women more than 30 percent.

Simply put, exercise increases caloric expenditure and promotes the breakdown of fat stores. The breakdown of fat is increased during endurance exercise through the associated increased secretion of adrenaline and other hormones and reduced secretion of insulin. These hormonal changes promote the breakdown of fat stores (the fat being released into plasma in the form of free fatty acids) that are subsequently oxidized for energy production. The resulting increase in levels of plasma-free fatty acids provides an important source of fuel during mild to moderate endurance activity. Increased levels of circulating free fatty acids may persist for hours following exercise.

Appetite suppression often occurs with regular endurance exercise and is believed to be related to the elevation of adrenaline levels, related hormones, and fat breakdown.

Change in body composition usually induced by endurance training consists of a decrease in total body fat with no change or a slight increase in lean body tissue.

Changes in carbohydrate metabolism

Endurance exercise has an effect similar to insulin on the absorption of glucose by muscle and fat cells. Thus, the body responds by reducing insulin secretion. Reduced insulin blood levels may persist for days after a single prolonged exercise session. Decreased blood insulin levels serve to break down fat. This metabolic effect also helps prevent and manage adult-onset diabetes where the primary defect appears to be a peripheral tissue resistance to insulin and glucose. (See chapter 1. Nutrition.)

Changes in blood lipid profile

The effect of exercise on total blood cholesterol levels has been studied, but to date the results are contradictory. Most studies fail to demonstrate a cholesterol-lowering effect, although a reduction is more likely if there is an associated weight loss.

Reports that habitually active people have higher levels of high-density lipoprotein (HDL) have recently been confirmed by exercise studies. This is significant because:

- An inverse relationship has been reported between HDL cholesterol levels and risk of coronary heart disease; and
- HDL is associated with a lower risk for atherosclerosis. (See chapter 1, Nutrition.)

PSYCHOSOCIAL BENEFITS

The following benefits are often experienced by people who exercise regularly.

1. A feeling of well-being. For many this provides the primary incentive for regular exercise. The feeling of well-being may be related to a release of morphine-like substances by the brain.
2. Exercise has a tranquilizing and muscle-relaxing effect. One study showed that jogging was as effective as a tranquilizer or a progressive relaxation technique in reducing muscular tension.
3. Exercise appears useful in reducing mental depression. A study found that jogging for as little as a half hour three times a week was at least as effective as psychotherapy in treating depressed patients.
4. Sound sleep.
5. Increased stamina and resistance to fatigue.
6. An improved personal appearance through reducing body fat and improving muscle tone.
7. Improved self-control and self-confidence, and an improved body image. Increased sexual performance may result.
8. Higher motivation in improving health habits, including cessation of smoking and moderation in food and alcohol consumption.
9. Exercise provides a means of fellowship with family and friends.

10. Increased job satisfaction and productivity and lower absenteeism have been reported among workers in exercise programs.
11. Exercise inhibits the decline of many physical capabilities associated with aging. These include loss of strength, vigor, flexibility, and youthful appearance. Ongoing regular activity may possibly postpone the thinning of bones (osteoporosis), which is the cause of much disability in the elderly. Clinical investigations confirm that elderly people who exercise are fitter than young people who don't.

Guidelines for Exercising

The three main approaches to exercising are:

1. A regularly scheduled program. Guidelines for such a program are included in this section.
2. Supplementary active leisure-time activities. Most people, especially those who wish to lose weight, should supplement a regular exercise program with active recreational pursuits such as gardening, home maintenance projects, bowling, and social dancing.
3. Stepped-up daily activities. Take every opportunity to move around more at home and at work. Try consciously to reduce your reliance on the automobile. Walk more. If possible—walk, bike, or jog to work. If you must use transportation, get up earlier and walk to the pick-up point. If you must use a car, park fifteen or twenty minutes walking distance from work. Gradually reduce your reliance on elevators and use stairs.

    At work, when possible, stand instead of sitting. Be active during coffee and lunch breaks. Walk around, go up and down stairs. Find a private place to do flexibility exercises, light calisthenics, run in place, or step up and down on a chair.

While at a desk, you can intermittently perform isometric exercises involving the upper and lower extremities and abdominal muscles, and flexibility exercises such as neck rotation and drawing the knees to the chest. Several books are available about exercises that can be performed in a chair.

These added bits of physical activity can help a previously sedentary person advance from a low to an intermediate level of stamina and improve muscle tone, strength, endurance, and flexibility.

CHOICE OF MODE(S) OF EXERCISE

For a significant effect, a program of rhythmic (isotonic) exercise should be brisk, sustained, and regular.

The exercises must be strenuous enough to produce an increase in heart and respiratory rate that will meet increased demands on the working muscles. They must be sustained at a steady level for a sufficient length of time or, if intermittent, repeated enough during each session to improve cardiorespiratory fitness. They must be done frequently enough on a regular basis to achieve or maintain fitness.

Table 5.3 lists home and recreational activities and sports, their approximate peak of energy expenditures in kilocalories per hour and in multiples of the resting metabolic rate (MET), and the relative value for improving maximal oxygen uptake (cardiorespiratory endurance), body composition, strength, and flexibility. Exercises improving strength also would be expected to improve muscular endurance if enough repetitions are performed. Rhythmic exercises using large muscle groups in which the body is moved continuously against gravity for prolonged periods are the most effective for improving cardiorespi-

ratory endurance, reducing body fat, and achieving other metabolic benefits. These include running, jogging, brisk walking, cross-country skiing, and rope skipping.

Similar benefits can be obtained with activities using large muscle groups in which the body is supported (as in bicycling, swimming, and rowing) if a similar increase in heart rate is obtained and the duration is sufficiently long to make up for not having to move the body against gravity. These are the exercises of choice for people who are grossly obese or have problems with their weight-bearing joints. Intermittent sports activities (e.g. racquet sports, soccer, and basketball) are a great deal of fun, but not always convenient since they require the participation of others. More importantly, because they provide high levels of heart and lung stimulation only in *spurts*, they are thereby insufficient in duration for effectiveness. In addition, they are difficult to measure in terms of prescribing safe levels of exercise, and during the heat of competition, safe limits and warning symptoms may be ignored. Such sports, therefore, are not the best forms of exercise for people with medical problems, such as diabetes or coronary heart disease who need to conform to carefully prescribed limits. Sports requiring long pauses and only occasional brisk efforts are unlikely to be adequate in improving cardiorespiratory fitness. Among these are baseball (except for the pitcher), bowling, golf, and volleyball.

A very efficient way of carrying out a fitness program for improving all the basic parameters of fitness in a relatively small space is by setting up an exercise circuit. This circuit consists of performing a prescribed number of repetitions of different types of exercise in an orderly, progressive manner at different stations within the circuit. Generally, exercises involving the arms and legs are alternated. Exercise stations include isotonic, strength, and flexibility exercises. Isotonic exercises in the circuit are commonly pro-

Table 5.3
APPROXIMATE ENERGY EXPENDITURES AND FITNESS VALUE
OF SPORTS AND RECREATIONAL AND HOUSEHOLD ACTIVITIES

Activity	KCal per hr.*	METs**	Cardioresp. endurance	Fat loss	Potential fitness benefits Strength	Flexibility
Archery	300	4	–	–	–	+
Auto driving	150	2	–	–	–	–
Badminton						
social doubles	300	4	–	+	–	+
social singles	360	5	–	+	–	+
competitive singles	480	7	+	+	–	+
Baseball or softball (except pitcher)	280	4	–	–	–	+ +
Pitcher	450	6	+	+	–	+ +
Basketball	360–660	5–9	+	+	–	+ +
Bicycling						
5 m.p.h. (level)	240	3	–	–	–	+
8 m.p.h.	300	4	+	+	–	+ +
10 m.p.h.	420	6	+	+	–	+ +
11 m.p.h.	480	6	+	+	–	+ +
12 m.p.h.	600	8	+ +	+ +	–	+ +
13 m.p.h.	660	9	+ +	+ +	–	–
Billiards or pool	240	3	–	–	–	–
Boating						
rowing slowly (2 m.p.h.)	240	3	–	–	–	+ +
rowing mod. fast (4 m.p.h.)	500	7	+	+	+	+ +
rowing fast (6 m.p.h.)	900	12	+ +	+ +	+	+ +
sailing	300	4	–	+	–	+
motor	240	3	–	–	–	–
Bowling (while active)	240	3	–	–	–	+

Activity	Calories	**				
Boxing	800	11	++	++	+	+
Brick laying, plastering	240	3	-	-	-	+
Calisthenics						
light	360	5	-	+	-	++
heavy	600	8	+	++	+	++
Canoeing (see boating)						
Card playing	150	2	-	-	-	-
Carpentry, light	360	5	+	+	-	+
Circuit training	300–600	4–8	+	+	+	+
Croquet	240	3	-	-	-	+
Dancing						
slow foxtrot	360	5	+	+	-	-
fast step	560	7	+	+	-	+
square dancing	560	7	+	+	-	+
modern, moderate–vigorous	240–360	3–5	+	+	-	++
Fencing (vigorous)	660	9	+	+	+	+
Field hockey	600	8	+	++	-	+
Fishing						
from pier or boat	240	3	-	-	-	-
standing with waders	300	4	-	+	-	-
walking with waders	420	6	+	+	-	+
Football (while active)	700	9	+	+	+	+

*Caloric consumption is based on a 70 kg. (150 lb.) person. There is a 10 percent increase in caloric consumption for each 7 kg. (15 lb.) over this weight and a 10 percent decrease for each 7 kg. under 70 kg.

**Multiples of resting metabolic rate

(continued)

Table 5.3
APPROXIMATE ENERGY EXPENDITURES AND FITNESS VALUE
OF SPORTS AND RECREATIONAL AND HOUSEHOLD ACTIVITIES *(continued)*

Activity	KCal per hr.*	METs**	Cardioresp. endurance	Potential fitness benefits Fat loss	Strength	Flexibility
Flying	150	2	–	–	–	–
Gardening						
leisurely	360	5	–	+	–	+ +
hoeing	360	5	+	+	–	+
much lifting, stooping, digging	500	7	+	+	+	+
Golfing						
power cart	240	3	–	–	–	–
pulling bag cart	300	4	–	+	–	+ +
carrying clubs	360	5	–	+	–	+
Gymnastics	300	4	+	+	+ +	+ +
Handball						
social	600	8	+	+ +	–	+
competitive	660	9	+	+ +	–	+
Horseback riding						
slow	240	3	–	–	–	–
trotting	360	5	+	+	–	–
Horseshoe pitching	300	4	–	+	–	+
Housework						
Light (vacuuming, mopping)	240–300	3–4	–	+	–	+
Heavy (scrubbing floors)	300–360	3–5	+	+	–	+ +
Hunting	500	7	+	+	–	–

Activity	Calories*	METs**				
Ice hockey	600	8	+	-	+	+
Jogging (see running)						
Karate and judo	700	9	++	++	++	+
Motorcycling	240	3	-	-	-	-
Motor scooting	200	3	-	-	-	-
Mountain climbing	600	8	+	+	++	++
Mowing						
riding	200	3	-	-	-	-
pushing power mower	300	4	++	-	+	-
pushing hand mower	450	6	++	+	+	+
Musical instruments (see also piano)	150-300	2-4	-	-	+	-
Paddleball or Racquetball	600	8	++	-	++	+
Painting	360	5	+	-	+	-
Piano playing						
leisurely	150	2	++	-	-	-
vigorously	225	3	++	-	-	-
Ping-Pong/table tennis	300-420	4-6	+	-	+	-
Pipe organ playing	240	3	+	-	-	-
Raking leaves	360	5	+	-	+	+
Reading	125	2	-	-	-	-
Repairing, auto, radio, TV	240	3	+	-	-	-

*Caloric consumption is based on a 70 kg. (150 lb.) person. There is a 10 percent increase in caloric consumption for each 7 kg. (15 lb.) over this weight and a 10 percent decrease for each 7 kg. under 70 kg.

**Multiples of resting metabolic rate

(continued)

Table 5.3

APPROXIMATE ENERGY EXPENDITURES AND FITNESS VALUE
OF SPORTS AND RECREATIONAL AND HOUSEHOLD ACTIVITIES *(continued)*

Activity	KCal per hr.*	METs**	Cardioresp. endurance	Fat loss	Strength	Flexibility
Rope skipping						
leisurely	300	4	+	+	−	+
vigorously	800	11	+ +	+ +	−	+ +
Rowing machine	840	12	+	+ +	+	+
Running						
5 m.p.h. (jogging)	600	8	+	+ +	−	+ +
6 m.p.h. (jogging)	750	10	+ +	+ +	−	+ +
7 m.p.h. (mod. fast)	870	12	+ +	+ +	−	+ +
8 m.p.h. (mod. fast)	1020	14	+ +	+ +	−	+ +
9 m.p.h. (fast)	1130	15	+ +	+ +	−	+ +
10 m.p.h. (very fast)	1285	17	+ +	+ +	−	+ +
upstairs	1000+	14+	+ +	+ +	−	+
Sawing hardwood	600	8	+ +	+ +	+	+
Sexual intercourse	360–600	5–8	−	−	−	+
Shoveling						
light	420	6	+	+	−	+ +
moderate (10 lb/min)	560	7	+	+ +	+ +	+ + +
heavy (16 lb/min)	660	9	+ +	+ +	+ +	+ + +
snow	560	7	+	+	+	+
Shuffleboard	240	3	−	−	−	+
Singing	150	2	−	−	−	−

Activity						
Skating						
ice or roller, leisurely	420	6	+	+	–	++
ice or roller, rapidly	700	9	++	++	+	++
Skiing						
snow downhill, light	500	7	–	+	–	+++
snow downhill, vigorous	600	8	+	++	+	+++
cross country (2.5 m.p.h.)	560	7	+	++	–	+++
cross country (4 m.p.h.)	600	8	++	++	+	+++
cross country (5 m.p.h.)	700	9	++	++	+	+++
cross country (8 m.p.h.)	1020	14	++	++	+	+++
Skiing, water, or surfing	480	6	–	+	+	+
Skimobiling	200	3	–	–	–	–
Skin diving						
moderate	900	13	+	++	–	++
fast	1200	16	+	++	–	+
Sleeping	70	1	–	–	–	–
Snowshoeing (2.5 m.p.h.)	600	8	++	++	–	+
Soccer	750	10	+	++	–	+
Squash						
social	600	8	+	++	–	++
competitive	660	9	++	++	–	++
Stair climbing (see Walking)						
Standing at ease	125	2	–	–	–	··

*Caloric consumption is based on a 70 kg. (150 lb.) person. There is a 10 percent increase in caloric consumption for each 7 kg. (15 lb.) over this weight and a 10 percent decrease for each 7 kg. under 70 kg.

**Multiples of resting metabolic rate

(continued)

Table 5.3

APPROXIMATE ENERGY EXPENDITURES AND FITNESS VALUE
OF SPORTS AND RECREATIONAL AND HOUSEHOLD ACTIVITIES *(continued)*

Activity	KCal per hr.*	METs**	Cardioresp. endurance	Potential fitness benefits			
				Fat loss	Strength	Flexibility	
Swimming							
leisurely	360–500	5–7	+	+	–	+	+
crawl, 25–50 yds./min.	360–750	5–10	+	+	–	+	+
backstroke, 25–50 yds./min.	360–750	5–10	+	+	–	+	+
breaststroke, 25–50 yds./min.	360–750	5–10	+ +	+	–	+	+
butterfly, 50 yds./min.	840	11	+ +	+	–	+	+
sidestroke, 40 yds./min.	660	9	+ +	+	–	+	+
Tennis							
doubles	360	5	–	+	–	+	+
singles	480	6	+	+	–	+	+
Typing							
	240	3	–	–	–	+	
Volleyball							
noncompetitive (6 or more)	300	4	–	+	–	+	+
competitive	450	6	+	+	–	+	+
Walking							
level road, 1–2 m.p.h. (strolling)	120–150	2	–	–	–	+	+
level road, 3 m.p.h. (leisurely)	300	4	–	–	–	+	+
level road, 3.5 m.p.h. (brisk)	360	5	+	+	–	+	+
level road, 4 m.p.h. (fast)	420	6	+	+	–	+	+
level road, 5 m.p.h. (very fast)	480	6	+ +	+	–	+	+
downstairs	425	6	–	+	–	+	+
upstairs	600–1080	8–14	+ +	+ +	+	+	–
uphill (3.5 m.p.h.)	480–900	6–12	+ +	+ +	+	–	–
downhill (2.5 m.p.h.)	240	3	–	–	–	–	–

Activity						
snow, hard (3.5 m.p.h.)	600	8	++	++	+	+
snow, soft (2.5 m.p.h.)	1200	16	++	++	+	+
hiking, 40 lb. pack (3 m.p.h.)	420	6	++	++	+	+
Watching TV or movies	125	2	-	-	-	-
Weight training	480	6	+	+	+	+
Window cleaning	300	4	+	-	+	-
Wood chopping	560	7	++	+	+	+
Wrestling	900	12	++	+	+	+

SOURCE: Arthur S. Leon, M.D., Laboratory of Physiological Hygiene, School of Public Health, University of Minnesota.

*Caloric consumption is based on a 70 kg. (150 lb.) person. There is a 10 percent increase in caloric consumption for each 7 kg. (15 lb.) over this weight and a 10 percent decrease for each 7 kg. under 70 kg.

**Multiples of resting metabolic rate

vided by motorized treadmills, bicycle ergometers, and rowing machines, but running in place and rope skipping may be substituted. Strength training is usually provided by weight lifting using bar bells or commercial weight-lifting apparatus.

Calisthenics programs are another popular form of exercise. However, most programs fail to improve cardiorespiratory fitness due to the lack of sufficient continuous, vigorous isotonic exercise. The Royal Canadian Air Force has switched from its famous calisthenics program to jogging as the principal conditioning program for its recruits; calisthenics are optional. A set of calisthenics for improving flexibility and strength begins on page 315.

When selecting an exercise program that you will enjoy, persist at, and benefit from, the following points should be taken into consideration:

1. *Initial level of physical fitness, usual physical activity pattern, health status, and age.* If you have not been habitually active, have a relatively low level of cardiorespiratory endurance, and are over thirty-five, strenuous activities such as jogging should be avoided as an initial conditioning exercise. Instead, you should start with lower intensity activities such as walking or recreational swimming or cycling, adding more vigorous activity as your condition improves. A health assessment and exercise stress test given by your doctor will provide information as to which activities are appropriate for your maximal oxygen uptake level. If there are health problems, a safe exercise prescription can be provided by a knowledgeable physician, usually in consultation with an exercise physiologist. If in doubt, stick to a lower intensity program of walking, recreational swimming, or cycling. (see Preventive Measures to Reduce Injuries, page 334).

2. *Previous exercise experience skills are preferred.* Exercise, sports, and recreational activities that you enjoy, are skilled in, or wish to become skilled in are more likely to be continued on a regular basis than a completely new activity.

3. *Benefits expected from exercise.* Exercise should be selected to provide improvement in your own desired fitness objectives. For example, a program designed to prepare an athlete for competition would differ markedly from one for a middle-aged person primarily concerned with losing weight in order to improve health and appearance.

4. *Preference for indoor or outdoor activities.* If you choose outdoor activities that may be affected by the weather, make sure you have alternate activities for times of bad weather.

5. *Preference for individual or group activities.* Companionship is helpful for most people in getting started and remaining in an exercise program.

6. *Availability and cost of facilities and equipment.* Some activities require little or no equipment. Brisk walking, for example, requires only a comfortable pair of shoes. Many communities offer free or inexpensive facilities and physical activity classes. Dress appropriately for your sport to reduce injuries.

7. *Regularity of exercise.* Arrange your exercise program as a regular part of your weekly schedule.

Again, remember to start slowly, and build up gradually.

EXERCISE INTENSITY

Intensity of training is the most crucial factor in successfully increasing cardiovascular endurance. Intensity can be expressed in several ways:

1. As calories burned per unit of time (or as kilocalories, which equal 1,000 calories).
2. As a percentage of the maximal oxygen consumption or aerobic power.
3. In terms of multiples of the resting metabolic rate required to perform the activity (METs).
4. As a particular heart rate or a percentage of the maximum heart rate.

By far the *most practical* means of assessing the strenuousness of an exercise is by measuring the heart rate achieved. During exercise, the heart rate increases at the same rate as the energy output until maximal heart rate is achieved. The points where maximal oxygen uptake and maximal heart rate are achieved are very close.

Studies have shown that, in order for training to improve cardiorespiratory endurance by means of regular, continuous, isotonic activity of twenty to forty minutes' duration, the exercise intensity must be at least 60 percent of the maximal aerobic power. This corresponds to about 70 percent of the maximal heart rate. The greater the intensity and heart rate at which one trains, the shorter the duration of exercise required to improve cardiorespiratory endurance; however, the risk of musculoskeletal injury and cardiac rhythm disturbance are also increased. Conversely, improvement in aerobic power can be achieved with lower intensity exercise if the exercise is extremely prolonged (hours). It is generally recommended that, except for athletes preparing for competition, the upper intensity level for training should not exceed 80 percent of the maximal oxygen uptake, corresponding to 85 percent of the maximal heart rate. Thus, the usually prescribed training heart rate zone is 70 to 86 percent of the maximal rate. This level of exercise is usually associated with some breathlessness and sweating.

Both maximal heart rate and maximal oxygen consumption decrease with age. A rough estimate of maximal heart rate for any age can be obtained by the following equation. (The formula is a rough estimate.)

Estimated max. HR = 220 − Age (in years) (beats per minute)

For example, for a thirty-five-year-old, the maximal heart rate is 220 minus 35, or 185 beats per minute (b.p.m.). The target rate of intensity is from 70 percent to 80 percent of 185, or roughly 137 to 157 b.p.m. Figure 5.1 shows how to find your pulse rate.

The importance of the decrease in heart rate with age is that physiologically an older person may be expending the same degree of intensity of effort as a younger person in spite of a lower heart rate. Table 5.4 shows the average maximal heart rate and recommended target zones for training at different ages. From this table, it is evident that a training effect can be obtained for a twenty-five-year-old by exercising at a heart rate of 140 b.p.m., while a sixty-year-old would require a training heart rate of only 111 b.p.m.

Generally, a training program for a sedentary person should initially aim at an upper limit of 70 percent of maximal heart level, or even lower. Progression to the upper figure in the target zone (85 percent of maximal heart rate) should be carried out over a period of at least three weeks. Since heart rate is reduced by training, as fitness improves, one must work progressively harder to attain the training level. One should not exceed the maximum heart rate, but stay within the target zone levels.

The higher a person's initial level of fitness, the harder he or she must work to increase maximum oxygen uptake. Conversely, a sedentary person with a low initial level of fitness (especially if recently confined to bed rest) would have

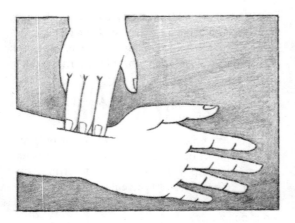

a. Heart rate is found by counting the pulse at the wrist. Press lightly with the first three fingers on the inside of the wrist near the bone that protrudes below the thumb. Count for ten seconds and multiply by six to obtain the heart rate for one minute.

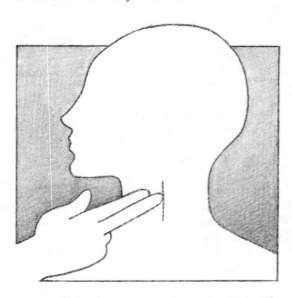

b. The pulse at the carotid artery in the neck is another place to take the pulse rate. This artery can be felt between the windpipe and the large neck muscles.

FIGURE 5.1

Two good ways to obtain the heart (pulse) rate during or immediately after peak exercise. Portable pulse monitoring devices complete with altering systems for too low or too high heart rate, which can be worn during exercise, are available commercially.

a greater improvement with less relative effort than the more fit.

Research has revealed that a variety of different kinds of continuous isotonic exercises yield a similar degree of improvement in maximal oxygen uptake if the same training heart rate zone is employed (e.g., running, jogging, walking, bicycling, or swimming).

Interval exercise training consists of repetitions of alternating moderate to heavy (near maximal) exercise for a specified distance or time with lighter exercise and time for partial recovery. An example of high-intensity interval training is a walk-jog-run program in which a person starts walking, progresses to jogging, and finishes a cycle with an "all-out" run for fifteen to twenty seconds. More physical discomfort or pain is associated with this approach due to the rapid production and accumulation of lactate (a metabolic waste product) and associated marked shortness of breath. This type of training carries a much higher risk of musculoskeletal damage and cardiac complications than more moderate intensity continuous exercise and is, therefore, not recommended for middle-aged or older people. However, interval training in which moderate intensity exercise to achieve the target heart rate is alternated with low-intensity exercise or rest is a good safe way to begin an exercise program. The period of moderate intensity exercise is gradually increased until the activity becomes continuous. Examples of such programs are included in the section on Guidelines for Selected Specific Exercises for Cardiorespiratory Endurance.

Table 5.4
MEAN MAXIMUM HEART RATE IN BEATS PER MINUTE AND
TARGET ZONE FOR EXERCISE TRAINING AT DIFFERENT AGES

Age (years)	Maximum heart rate	Target Zone (bpm) 70%	85%
25	200	140	170
30	194	136	165
35	188	132	160
40	182	128	155
45	176	124	150
50	171	119	145
55	165	115	140
60	159	111	135
65	153	107	130

SOURCE: data adapted from American Heart Association booklet, Lenore R. Zohman, *Beyond Diet: Your Way to Fitness and Health.*

EXERCISE DURATION

An inverse relationship exists between intensity and duration of training exercises required to produce an improvement in maximal oxygen intake. In other words, the harder one works the shorter the time required for improvement. Some studies have shown that training over 90 percent of aerobic capacity or near maximal heart rate may result in improved maximal oxygen uptake with as little as ten minutes of regularly performed isotonic exercise (e.g., rope jumping). However, the risk of injuries is very high at this level of intensity. At the more moderate intensity of exercise recommended above (70 to 85 percent of aerobic capacity), a significant improvement in cardiorespiratory capacity usually results with twenty to thirty minutes of continuous exercise with a much lower injury rate. Some additional improvement will result from forty to sixty minutes of exercise at that intensity.

For those who want or need to lose weight, it should be noted that regular moderate intensity exercise for a minimum of twenty to thirty min-

utes, while increasing aerobic power, may be insufficient to produce a significant loss of body fat and the adaptations in lipid and carbohydrate metabolism that reduce coronary risk factors. For weight loss, exercise sessions should be of sufficient duration to burn at least 300 kilocalories. This corresponds to walking or jogging about three miles. Since a 3,500 kilocalorie deficit is required to lose a pound of fat, 300 kilocalories a day of exercise would result in a loss of a pound of fat every thirty-five days or about ten pounds a year. Improvement in other metabolically related coronary risk factors (glucose tolerance, insulin blood levels, and the blood lipid profile) appears to require a minimum of forty to sixty minutes of moderate intensity exercise. These metabolic adaptations are made easier by an associated weight loss.

Training programs for previously sedentary individuals should be initiated with not more than ten to fifteen minutes of exercise, and gradually increased to the desired duration period of weeks or months. In various studies a high dropout rate because of injuries has been reported for previously sedentary adults whose initial training sessions lasted thirty to forty minutes or more.

FREQUENCY OF EXERCISE

Frequency is another important variable in determining response to exercise training. The majority of experiments indicate that significant improvement in maximal oxygen uptake levels requires at least three training sessions a week for four to six weeks with some further improvement over the next six months. Some additional improvement occurs with five days of training per week. No significant increment in aerobic power results from an increase from five to seven days of training a week, while the possibility of injury increases markedly. Twice a week training sessions will ordinarily maintain the acquired increase in cardiorespiratory endurance.

On the other hand, if exercise is being used primarily for weight control, strong consideration should be given to exercising five or six times a week or even daily. The additional caloric expenditure is considerably greater when compared with training only two or three times per week. A good way to avoid the risk of overdoing is to alternate low and moderate intensity days or to employ a variety of activities emphasizing different muscle groups. For example, jogging could be used three days per week and cycling, playing tennis, or swimming on the other days. Many people like to exercise five or more days a week to relax and help relieve tension or to add to their sense of personal control and self-confidence. If, however, one experiences more than a few hours of transient moderate fatigue following a workout, it may be that the sessions are too frequent and/or too long; cutting down on the frequency and/or the duration of the exercise would be recommended.

Guidelines for Selected Specific Exercises for Cardiorespiratory Endurance

WALKING

Walking is by far the most popular physical activity. More than 60 million American adults walk regularly for recreation. As our natural form of locomotion, it's the easiest, most natural form of exercise. Recreational walking can be carried out safely by most people of all ages, practically anywhere, with no special equipment except comfortable shoes.

Walking is the ideal beginning exercise for sedentary persons who want to become more active. As fitness improves, more vigorous activities such as jogging can be added or substituted. As confirmed in a study by the University of Minnesota's Laboratory of Physiological Hygiene, *brisk walking can provide benefits similar to running* if one follows the general guidelines for exercise training. Obese college students were allowed to maintain their unrestricted diet but were put on a five-day-a-week program of brisk walking, that is, $3+$ miles per hour for one hour a day. In four months there was marked improvement in cardiorespiratory endurance and efficiency. Remarkable metabolic changes also took place, including substantial weight loss, body fat reduction, a marked increase in plasma insulin in response to a glucose challenge, and a significant increase in the anticoronary, cholesterol-clearing factor, HDL.

In order to achieve substantial metabolic benefits from a walking program, it appears that prolonged brisk walking (about one hour) is necessary three to five days per week.

Beginning walkers who are over forty and overweight or inactive can experience muscle strain if they try to push themselves too hard. A progressive walking program for markedly de-

Table 5.5
BASIC PROGRESSIVE WALKING PROGRAM FOR DECONDITIONED SEDENTARY ADULTS

Step no.	Suggested time schedule (weeks)	Distance (miles)	Suggested target duration* (minutes)	Minimum frequency (days/weeks)	Upper % of max. heartrate
1	1	0.25	5	6	60
2	2	0.25	5 X 2	6	60
3	3	0.50	10	6	70
4	5–7	0.75	15	7	75
5	8	1.00	20	5	75
6	9	1.25	25	5	80
7	10	1.50	30	3	80
8	11–12	2.00	40	3	85
9	13–14	3.00	60	3	85
10	15–16	4.00	70	3	85
11	17	4.00	60	3	85

*This is the suggested time for covering the given distance especially for those who do not wish to monitor their pulse rate. The actual walking rate is best determined by the heart rate response. The final target step is potentially possible for most people, but many may find it necessary to accept a lower target step than the final goal in the basic schedule.

SOURCE: data adapted from Bud Getchell, *Physical Fitness: A Way of Life*, 2nd ed., New York: John Wiley, 1979.

conditioned people is shown in table 5.5. Training is gradually increased from a quarter of a mile at an easy gait to a brisk four-mile walk in one hour. Healthy persons enjoying an intermediate level of fitness may start their program at the one-mile level. Initial training heart rate for the deconditioned person should be below the recommended threshold heart rate level as shown in the last column of table 5.5, and only gradually raised to the target heart rate zone. If difficulty is encountered in maintaining a brisk pace, one should periodically slow down for thirty to sixty seconds. A person who has become fit enough to walk three to four miles in an hour is ready for a walk-jog program if there are no health limitations. Wilderness hiking and backpacking are the ultimate walking experience for the fit walker who loves the outdoors.

Another readily accessible high-intensity exercise is climbing stairs (eight–fourteen METs, which is comparable to jogging) for the well-conditioned walker. A steady pace maintained at 100 steps per minute up five or more flights will generally result in breathlessness and perspiration. This exercise should be limited to those in good health, and begun with only one or two flights at a time, with the number of flights and the pace increased gradually. A fitness bonus is that in addition to improving stamina, stair climbing helps develop leg muscles for skiing, bicycling, and modern dancing. Descending aids agility and sense of balance.

JOGGING (OR WALK-JOG)

Running is without question the most effective exercise for rapid improvement in physical fitness with a minimum investment in time. About 40 million Americans are regular joggers including about 20,000 marathon runners. Jogging has become a fashionable symbol of vitality. An entire clothing and shoe industry caters to joggers and people who want to look like joggers. (Figure 5.2 shows the correct jogging posture.)

Although it has some risks and certain precautions are necessary (see below), even markedly deconditioned people can usually progress safely from walking to jogging. In fact, jogging in supervised programs is now widely used for rehabilitation of patients after heart attack or coronary bypass surgery.

Table 5.6 illustrates a basic walk-jog program designed to take the participant from a slow walk through a series of graded steps of at least two weeks each, to the final target of a continuous three-mile jog. The three-mile goal is reasonable for most people of average fitness, although some

may find a lower target more acceptable. Established runners may prefer to continue a progressive training schedule to reach five miles or more per session.

The jogger's level of fitness determines the starting step. Ideally, the person should take an exercise stress test, recommended especially for people over thirty-five and those at risk of heart disease. A deconditioned person should begin with the walking program. The heart rate during training should be 70 to 85 percent of the maximal heart rate. The duration of each training session should be 20 to 60 minutes, not including the warm-up and cool-down phases.

Training sessions should be held at least three days a week. An hour of brisk walking is recommended on alternate days. As conditioning

Table 5.6
BASIC PROGRESSIVE WALK-JOG PROGRAM
FOR DECONDITIONED SEDENTARY ADULTS

Step no.	Distance (miles) alternate between			Target time for 3 miles (minutes)
	walking (@20 min./mile)	and	jogging (@ 10 min./mile)	
1–8	Same as in table 5.5		0	—
9	3		0	60
10	⅛		⅛	40
11	¼		¼	45
12	¼		½	45
13	¼		¾	45
14	½		1	40
15	¼		1½, 1	35
16	⅛		1½, 1¼	30
17	½		2	30
18	¼, ½		2¼	37
19	¼		2½	30
20	⅛		2¾	31
21	0		3	30

SOURCE: see Table 5.5

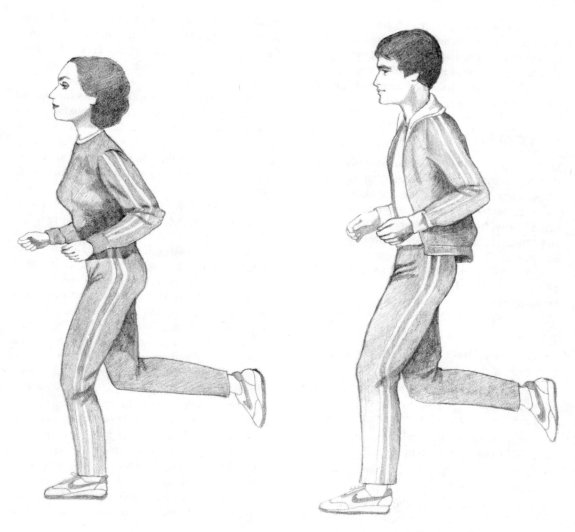

FIGURE 5.2

Correct jogging posture

level improves, the jogger can increase to five days per week, gradually add hills to the terrain covered (which significantly increases energy expenditure and involves new muscles), or progressively increase the speed to a running pace of seven to eight minutes per mile.

BICYCLING

As well as being a useful and economical means of transportation, bicycle riding can be a pleasurable outing with family and friends. Additionally, it can enhance cardiorespiratory capacity as well as provide good conditioning for the legs. Bicycling, however, has a severe limitation: more than one million people are injured in bicycle accidents each year and about 1,000 of them die. (See chapter 10, Traffic Accidents.) Many of these accidents involve faulty equipment or poor riding techniques. Certain rules should therefore be rigidly observed:

- Get a bike from a reputable dealer that meets government safety standards.
- Keep it in good working order by preventive maintenance; periodic checks and adjustments by a qualified mechanic are necessary.
- For training, find a road free of traffic hazards or preferably a bicycle path.
- Obey the vehicular traffic regulations and drive defensively.
- Wear a helmet and cycling gloves to reduce injury. Clips or elastic bands prevent trousers getting caught in the chain sprocket. A chamois crotch pad sewn in biking trousers adds to comfort. Reflectors on the pant legs, or the wheels, and on rear and front of the bike are essential for best visibility after dark.

Once these safety precautions are taken care of, you can plan a bicycle exercise program. An important advantage over walking and jogging,

particularly in the grossly obese or in people with joint problems, is the much lower "G" (gravity) forces operating during cycling. This reduces the likelihood of injury to the feet and ankles, and to the lower back.

To improve your maximum oxygen uptake with a bicycle, you must cycle vigorously, covering ground at least twice as fast as when walking or jogging (eight to ten miles per hour or faster). You need to cycle forty to sixty minutes, at least three times a week, for an adequate training effect.

Intermittent activity similar to the walk-jog technique is a simple, safe approach for progressive conditioning with a bicycle. Table 5.7 shows a gradual progressive interval training program for the bicycle based on either distance or time. Interval training based on distance requires repeat cycling at a vigorous rate for a preselected distance followed by a shorter distance at a slower pace. The suggested intensity or cycling speed during the vigorous phase is adjusted to the initial fitness level of the cyclist and the heart rate response. Cycling speed is increased or decreased to provide a lesser or greater heart rate stimulus. The training heart rate zone after an appropriate adjustment period is 70 to 85 percent of maximal heart rate as with walking or jogging programs.

Interval training based on time consists of repeated vigorous cycling for two- to four-minute periods followed by a recovery period at a reduced pedaling speed. Each step in the training program should be done for at least two weeks.

STATIONARY BICYCLING

A stationary bicycle (bicycle ergometer) with adjustable pedal resistance provides a convenient alternative to bicycling, walking, or jogging for regular isotonic exercise. Working out indoors, you avoid gas fumes, speeding cars, and foul weather. Exercise can be carried out while reading, watching television, or listening to the radio or stereo music. This helps prevent boredom, one

Table 5.7
BICYCLING FOR EXERCISE

Step no.	Suggested speed* (mph)	Vigorous phase Distance or time		Slow (recovery) phase Distance or time		No. of repeat sets	Approx. distance of vigorous cycling (miles)
		(miles)	(min.)	(miles)	(min.)		
1	12	1	5	¼	2	5 to 8	5 to 8
2	15	1	4	¼	2	5 to 10	5 to 10
3	15	1½	6	⅓	3	4 to 10	6 to 15
4	15	2	8	⅓	3	4 to 10	10 to 15
5	12–15	10–20	40–80	Every 5 miles speed may be reduced for 1 mile		—	10 to 20

*The actual cycling speed may have to be adjusted to provide a heart rate stimulus in the target zone of 70 to 85 percent maximal heart rate.

SOURCE: see Table 5.5

of the main reasons home exercise programs are dropped. And for people with orthopedic problems of the lower extremities, it provides a good substitute for brisk walking.

In choosing a stationary bicycle, the following features should be considered: 1) smooth operation without vibration; 2) resistance control adjustment; 3) seat comfort; 4) adjustable seat height (the leg in the down position should be almost straight); 5) adjustable handlebars and

Table 5.8
PROGRESSIVE INTERVAL TRAINING PROGRAM
FOR STATIONARY CYCLING

Step no.	Pedaling* duration (min.)	Rest† duration (sec.)	% Heartrate max.	No. of repeat sets	Total time (min.)
1	2	30	60	5–8	12–20
2	2	30	75	5–8	12–20
3	3	30	75–85	5–8	17–28
4	4	30–60	75–85	4–6	18–28
5	5	30–60	75–85	4–8	20–32
6	10	30–60	75–85	2–4	21–44
7	20	0	75–85	1	20
8	30	0	75–85	1	30
9	40	0	75–85	1	40

*Pedaling speed at 60 rpm's

†Rest can consist of sitting still or pedaling against no resistance, or walking around. Walking also can be used for cool-down.

SOURCE: see Table 5.5

grips; 6) comfortable foot pedals; 7) quiet operation; 8) a rigid frame; 9) a one-way drive; and 10) ease in storage.

Automatic multiaction exercises that provide back-and-forth "swimming" movement of the handlebars in addition to pedaling action are good for improving flexibility, but for the average person these fail to provide sufficient cardiovascular stress.

Principles of interval training similar to walk-jog programs can be used for training on a stationary bicycle. Table 5.8 outlines such a program using repeated cycles of pedaling followed by brief rest periods. The work load, or resistance, is set on the bicycle at a level that increases heart rate to 70 to 85 percent of maximum heart rate after a period of adjustment at a light resistance and lower heart rate. The resistance knob on the bicycle should be set after taking the pulse rate. At least two months should be spent at each stage before progressing to the next higher level of work.

SWIMMING

Swimming is an excellent means of producing high-intensity isotonic activity and cardiorespiratory fitness. *In general, 100 yards of swimming equal 400 yards of jogging in training effects,* or one-half mile of swimming is equivalent to two miles of jogging. An important advantage of swimming over brisk walking and jogging is the reduced pressure on the musculoskeletal system resulting from the buoyancy of the water, which makes it the favorite exercise of obese people and those with orthopedic problems of the lower extremities and back. Swimming has a long history in the treatment, rehabilitation, and conditioning of people with neurological and psychiatric problems. Since the pressure of the water on the body helps promote deeper ventilation of the lungs, its use is being explored for conditioning people with chronic lung disorders.

Complaints common to new joggers, such as muscle soreness and tightening, are unusual in swimmers. In fact, swimming increases the range of movement and flexibility of most muscle groups of the body, especially the shoulders. Muscular strength and endurance are also improved. It is also an excellent way of promoting relaxation and restful sleep.

One drawback to swimming is that lack of skill and total body coordination can bring about rapid exhaustion and discouragement. However, for fitness training, a relatively inept swimmer can have a productive workout by swimming at least one lap. Even a nonswimmer can benefit. For example, a person with joint problems can get some conditioning by walking or jogging in the shallow part of the pool.

Another problem with using swimming for conditioning is the difficulty in judging intensity of effort and caloric consumption. Because individuals vary so greatly in efficiency and speed in swimming a given distance with a given stroke, it is hard to calculate the exact rate of benefit. Even the heart rate during effort may be deceptive because of the occasional reduction in heart rate caused by water contact with the face and chest ("diving reflex").

The simplest training regimen using swimming for a deconditioned person is a swim-walk cycle (table 5.9). This involves swimming a length of the pool, then climbing out and walking back to the other side and repeating the cycle, gradually increasing the number of sets. Later the number of successive swimming lengths can be increased before another walking phase. About two to four weeks should be spent on each stage, starting at the minimum and progressing to the maximum number of recommended repetitions. At the completion of each swim cycle the pulse rate should be checked to determine if the 70 to 85 percent of maximum heart rate target zone is

Table 5.9

PROGRESSIVE SWIMMING-WALKING PROGRAM FOR ADULT CONDITIONING

Step no.	No. of pool lengths* to swim	Walk phase†	No. of repetitions‡	Approximate distance covered (yards)
1	1 (30–40 sec.)	Get out of pool and walk to starting point	10 to 20	200 to 500
2	2 (60–80 sec.)	" " (30 sec.)	8 to 20	400 to 800
3	3 (90–120 sec.)	" " (45 sec.)	6 to 15	400 to 1,200
4	4 (120–160 sec.)	" " (60 sec.)	4 to 16	400 to 1,600

*One length = 25 yds.

†If it is not feasible to leave the pool, rest in the water at the end of the pool the appropriate length of time instead.

‡Start with the lower number of repetitions and add a repetition daily.

SOURCE: see Table 5.5

being achieved. The warm-up and cool-down phase can consist of stretching exercises on the pool deck or in the water or by walking around the pool.

After Step 4 has been achieved, good swimmers may choose to swim continuously for sixteen to thirty-two lengths (400 to 800 yards). Those for whom continuous exercise is not possible can remain at Step 4.

ROPE SKIPPING

Skipping rope substantially raises the heart rate, although not as high as jogging does. Nevertheless, it is a good way to improve or maintain fitness. It can also be a substitute for running or walking during bad weather or while traveling. (See Figure 5.3.)

A certain amount of skill and agility are required, which for most people proves to be no problem. Those with persistent difficulties can go through the motions without a rope. Jumping can impose marked stress on the cardiorespiratory system as well as a sudden severe demand on the hip, ankle, knee joints, feet, and the lower spine. The heart rate can accelerate to near maximal in deconditioned people within a few minutes. Even people who are capable of jogging for thirty minutes often have leg muscle discomfort when they initially jump ten minutes. Therefore, an adequate warm-up session is required, with flexibility and stretching exercises.

Thick-soled tennis or running shoes are recommended to help absorb shock. The rope should be long enough to reach from armpit to armpit while passing under both feet. Handles with weights help prevent the rope from getting tan-

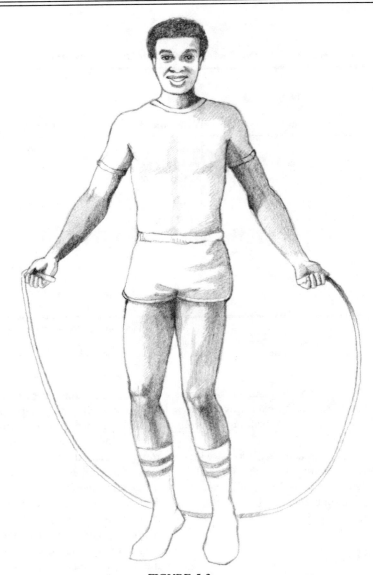

FIGURE 5.3

Rope skipping

Skip rope flat footed with arms extended laterally to permit a comfortable chest position and body mechanics or posture. Use 10−12 foot rope and skip slowly and rhythmically.

SOURCE: *adapted from Bud Getchell,* Physical Fitness: A Way of Life, *2nd ed., John Wiley, New York, 1979.*

gled. Initial training sessions should be brief and intermittent, alternating skipping with rest or walking. The pulse rate should be checked immediately upon stopping to see if the target training zone has been attained.

Table 5.10 shows a progressive rope-skipping regime. One to two or more weeks should be spent on each step. Those who are in reasonably good shape can start at Step 3 or 4. As with other isotonic exercises, three or more sessions per week are required to improve fitness.

RUNNING IN PLACE

Running in place is another alternative to jogging or walking, which can be performed anywhere and can improve cardiorespiratory endurance. Similar precautions as for rope skipping should be observed. The feet should be lifted at least 5 inches off the floor while running. A training schedule similar to rope jumping can be followed.

The heart rate response determines the rate of running. Those at low fitness level should start gradually to build up to the target heart rate zone.

CROSS-COUNTRY SKIING (SKI TOURING OR NORDIC SKIING)

Cross-country skiing among all age groups is a good winter alternative to walking or jogging. It provides vigorous movement of both the upper and lower extremities and has a great potential for increasing physical fitness. Champion cross-country skiers have the highest maximal oxygen uptake values ever recorded.

Cross-country skis and boots are relatively inexpensive compared with downhill equipment. The kind to get depends on the type of skiing one plans to do and the terrain available. A wide variety of attire is possible. Precautions for attire are similar to those described for jogging in the

Table 5.10
PROGRESSIVE ROPE-SKIPPING PROGRAM FOR ADULT CONDITIONING

Step no.	Duration of skipping* (seconds)	Duration of rest (seconds)	No. of repetitions†	Total jumping time (minutes)
1	10	10	12	2
2	20	10	12	4
3	30	10	12	6
4	40	15	12	8
5	50	20	12	10
6	60	30	6 to 12	6 to 12
7	120	30	4 to 8	8 to 16
8	180	30	4 to 8	12 to 24
9	240	30	4 to 8	16 to 32
10	600	120	1 to 3	10 to 30

*Recommended rate is 80 rope turns per minute but should be adjusted to keep the heart rate at 70 to 85 percent maximum heart rate.

†Start with the lower number of repetitions and add one daily until the maximum number is achieved.

SOURCE: see Table 5.5

cold (see below). Water, snacks, and extra clothing should be brought along for extended tours. Injuries are rare.

Little or no instruction is necessary to enjoy the sport because it is as natural as walking. Just a few inches of snow on a golf course, field, or park is adequate cover for cross-country skiing. It is probably most enjoyable in wooded areas.

Both continuous and interval training (similar to walk-jog routines) can be used for training. An example of an interval routine is to ski from fifty to several hundred yards at a pace sufficient to raise the heart rate into the target training zone. This is followed by partial to complete rest for several minutes and five to fifty repetitions depending on one's condition. As one's condition improves, one should be able to perform continuous cross-country skiing for thirty minutes or longer.

OTHER SPORTS

Other popular sports that can contribute to fitness are listed in table 5.3 (pages 292–299). Golf, for instance, provides a great opportunity to walk, climb (occasionally), and enjoy the outdoors. However, unless brisk walking is involved, there is little benefit to the cardiorespiratory system, none at all when electric golf carts are used. Other popular sports listed in table 5.3 such as boating, skating, bowling, and tennis provide varying benefits depending on the intensity and duration of activity. Intense competitive sports like ice hockey, basketball, football, and boxing make great demands on the body and may be dangerous; thus they are not recommended here for the average person.

The "Daily Dozen":
EXERCISES FOR INCREASING FLEXIBILITY AND MUSCULAR STRENGTH AND ENDURANCE

On the following pages are illustrations and instructions for a group of exercises that loosen, stretch, and strengthen major muscle groups of the body. They should be performed at a leisurely tempo. They are ideal for the warm-up and cooldown phases of an isotonic exercise program. They are also good ways to start off a day and to promote relaxation and sleep-inducing fatigue before going to bed.

Potential Risks of Exercise

Exercise does carry some risk, particularly for the previously sedentary adult. The risks include musculoskeletal problems, injuries due to heat, and heart problems. The risk, however, can be minimized by the safety precautions noted below. Happily for most people the risks to health and well-being associated with physical inactivity far exceed the risks associated with sensible amounts of exercise.

MUSCULOSKELETAL INJURIES

Rhythmic isotonic exercise involves the repetitive use of large muscle groups and joints binding them. Therefore, injuries to the muscles and joints are the most common associated risks.

Joggers may develop knee problems, shin splints (pain along the front of the leg), Achilles tendonitis, hip bursitis, sore feet, stress fractures, and many other orthopedic difficulties.

Problems involving the upper extremities such as tennis elbow (olecranon bursitis), tendonitis, painful shoulders due to strain or bursitis, and muscular aches and pain can affect swimmers and tennis players.

EXERCISE 1

Category: Face, neck

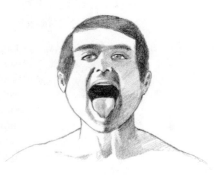

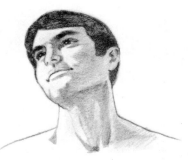

*1. Five seconds.
Do twice.*

*2. Slowly roll your head
around in each direction.
Ten repetitions.*

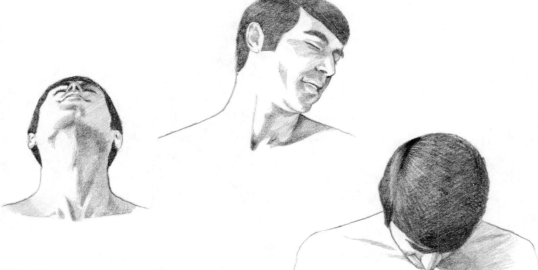

FIGURE 5.4

(Above and on following pages):

Tongue thrust, head circles, and overhead stretch shoulder flex

SOURCE: *adapted from* Stretching © *by Bob and Jean Anderson, $7.95,
Shelter Publications, Bolinas, California. Distributed in bookstores by
Random House. Reprinted by permission.*

EXERCISE 2

Category: Shoulders, arms

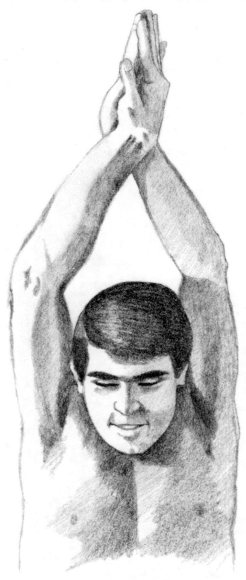

1. Fifteen seconds.

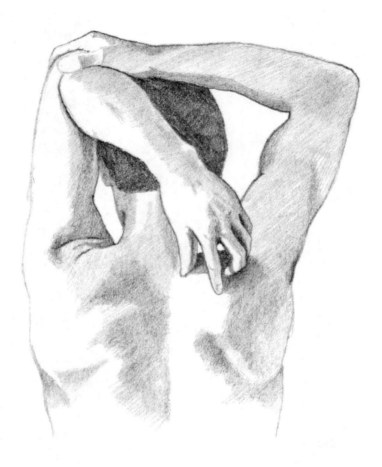

2. *Fifteen seconds for each arm.*

EXERCISE 3

Category: Trunk

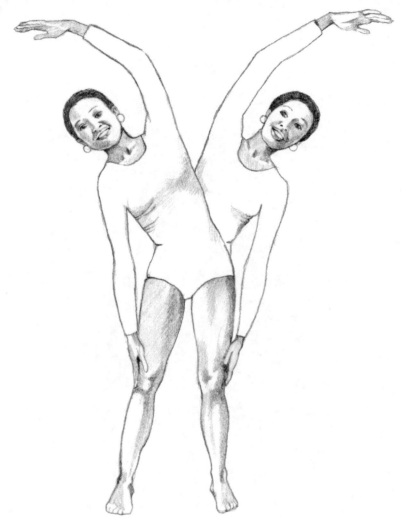

FIGURE 5.5

Side stretcher

Bend your trunk to the side of the lower extended arm. Reach with your lower hand and stretch, sliding the hand down your thigh to the knee. The other arm should be stretched over your head and lean to the side. Return to the starting position and repeat the exercise on the other side. Alternate ten times.

SOURCE: *see figure 5.3*

EXERCISE 4

Category: Trunk, back, shoulders

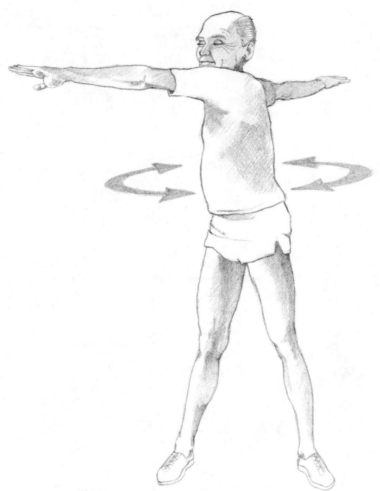

FIGURE 5.6

Trunk rotator

While keeping your heels flat on the floor, twist your trunk to the right slowly as far as you can turn, then return to starting position. Now twist slowly to the left. Repeat the complete movement slowly ten times.

SOURCE: *see Figure 5.3*

EXERCISE 5

Category: Neck, arms, shoulders, back

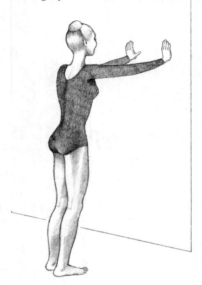 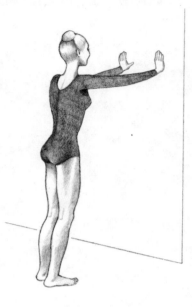

1. *Starting position.*

2. *Count 1.*
   Bend elbows, lowering body
   toward wall until your cheek
   touches wall.

3. *Count 2.*
   Push with hands
   and straighten arms.
   Repeat ten times.

FIGURE 5.7

Wall push-away leg stretches

SOURCE: *see Figure 5.4*

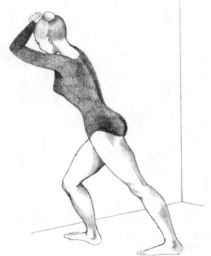 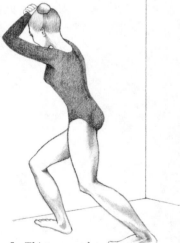

4. *Thirty seconds*
   for each leg.

5. *Thirty seconds*
   for each leg.

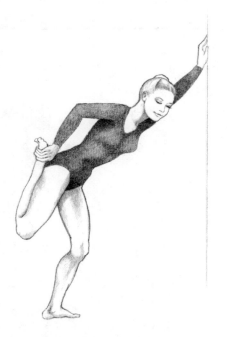

6. *Fifteen seconds.*

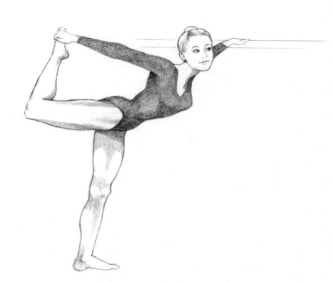

7. *Ten to fifteen seconds.*

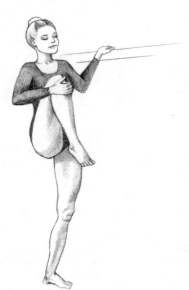

8. *Twenty seconds.*

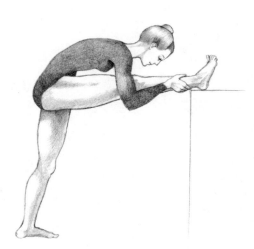

9. *Fifty seconds.*

EXERCISE 6

Category: Hamstring muscles (thighs), back

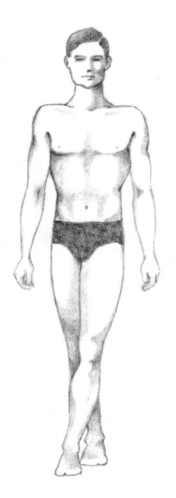 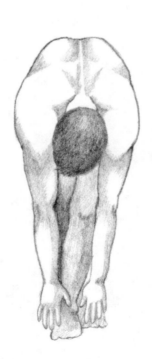 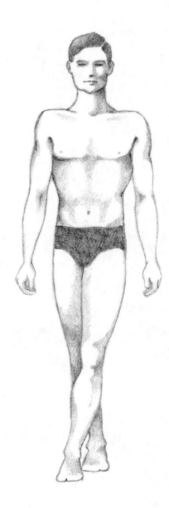

FIGURE 5.8

Cross-leg stretch

Source: *see Figure 5.3*

Bend slowly from the waist and try to touch the floor in front of your toes. Hold the lowest position for a count of five seconds.

Return to the starting position. Relax for a count of three. Switch position of the legs and repeat the exercise ten times.

EXERCISE 7

Category: Thighs, hips, buttocks, lower back

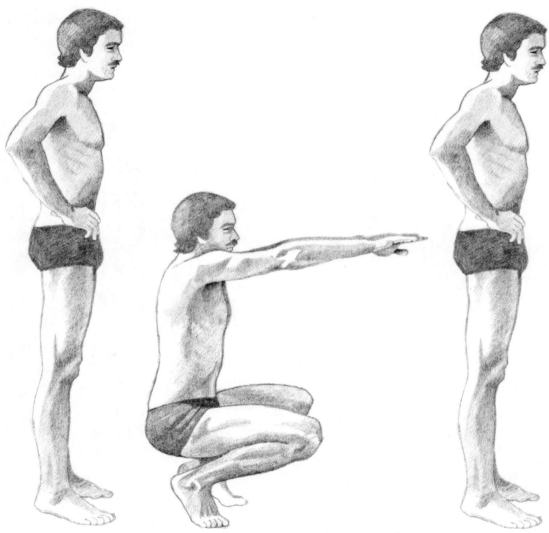

FIGURE 5.9

Half-knee bend

SOURCE: see Figure 5.3

Bend knees to half-squat position while simultaneously swinging arms forward with palms down.

Return to starting position. Repeat ten times.

EXERCISE 8

Category: Abdomen

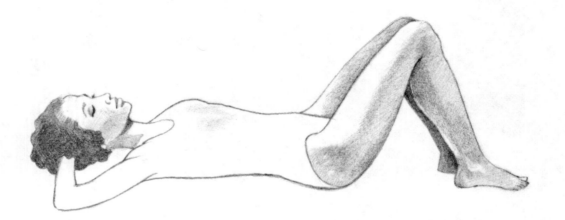

FIGURE 5.10

Bent-knee sit-up

SOURCE: *see Figure 5.3*

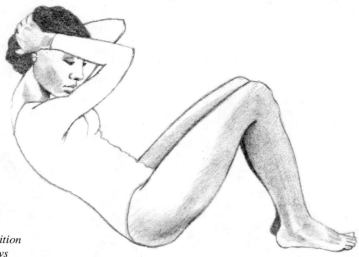

*Tucking chin into chest,
curl forward into a sitting position
until you can touch your elbows
to your knees.*

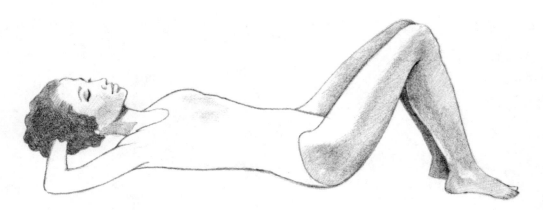

*Return to the starting position.
Start with ten.
Progress to forty repetitions.*

EXERCISE 9

Category: Thighs, hips, buttocks, lower back

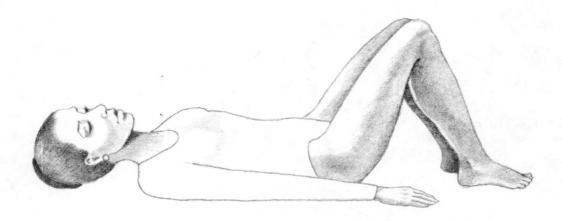

FIGURE 5.11

Hip raise

Source: *see Figure 5.3*

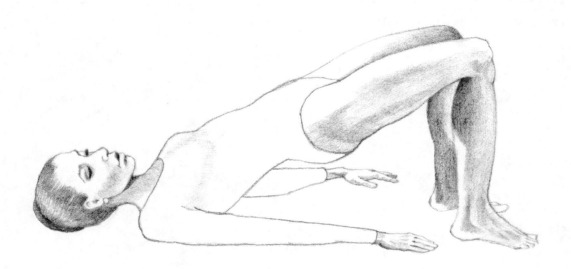

Raise hips off floor as high as possible, but keep shoulders and feet on floor. Tighten buttocks and abdominal muscles, and hold for a count of five seconds. Gradually increase hold count to ten.

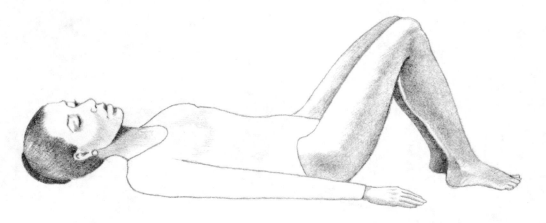

Return to starting position. Repeat five to ten times.

EXERCISE 10

Category: Arms, shoulders, chest

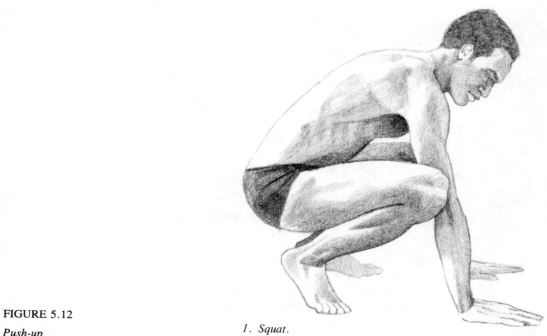

1. *Squat.*

FIGURE 5.12

Push-up

Source: *see Figure 5.3*

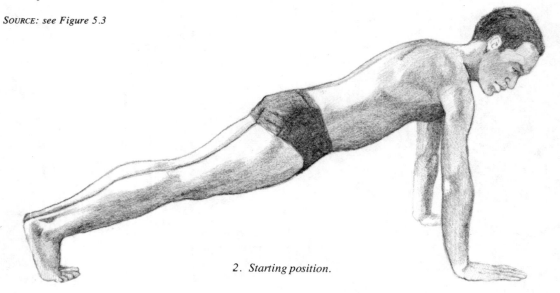

2. *Starting position.*

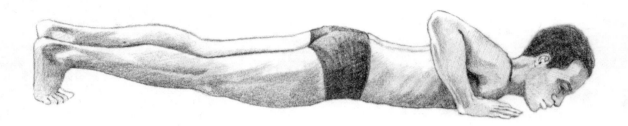

3. Keeping body and legs straight, bend elbows until chest touches floor.

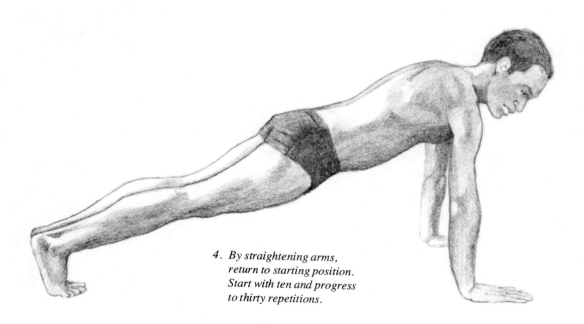

4. By straightening arms, return to starting position. Start with ten and progress to thirty repetitions.

EXERCISE 11

Category: Thighs, back

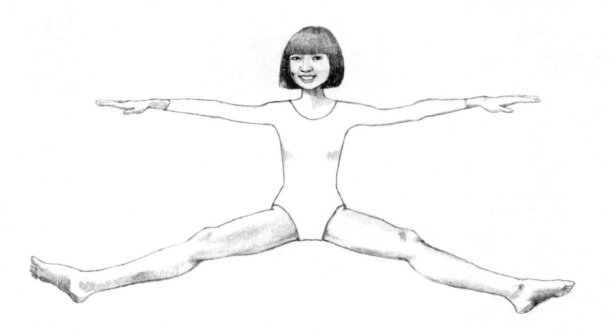

FIGURE 5.13

Alternate toe touching

SOURCE: *see Figure 5.3*

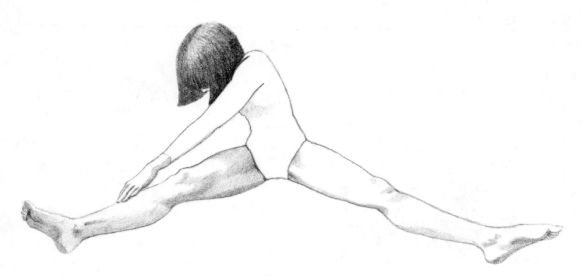

Flex trunk and alternately touch toes with hand on opposite side of body

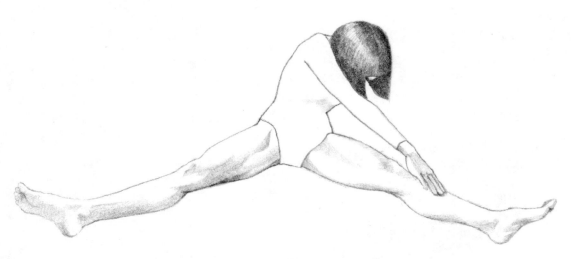

Touch each toe ten times

EXERCISE 12

Category: Hips, lower back

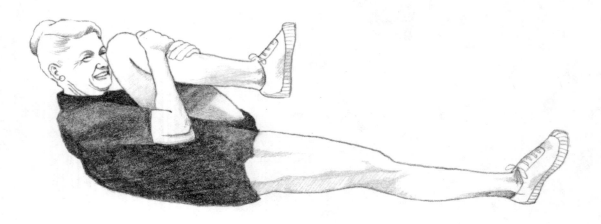

FIGURE 5.14

Hip flexor

SOURCE: *see Figure 5.3*

Grasp the leg just below the knee and pull the knee toward your chest.

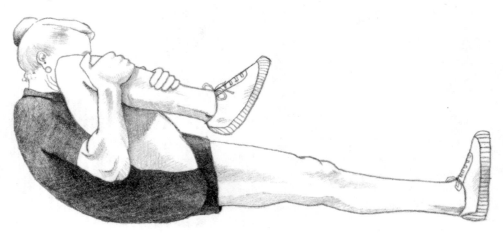

Curl your shoulders and head toward the knee. Hold for 3 to 4 seconds. Return to starting position and repeat exercise with other leg. Alternate. Repeat ten times.

Although some muscle soreness is inevitable for someone beginning an exercise program and accidents are always possible even for the most experienced athlete, most injuries are minor. Serious injuries usually result from exercising relatively too hard or too long. For the jogger, improper running form and hard surfaces can play a role (see figure 5.2, page 307).

It is a common fallacy that regular exercising such as jogging predisposes one to permanent joint damage and degenerative arthritis. Anecdotal reports have raised the fear that joint injury may complicate regular exercise, but this is unproven. It appears that our joints are more likely to "rust out" than give out.

HEAT INJURIES

If precautions are not taken, heavy exercise on warm, humid days may result in dehydration, heat exhaustion, fainting, or even fatal heat stroke. Ordinarily, however, dehydration and heat injuries can be avoided by drinking enough water before and during activities to make up for sweat loss. If the temperature of the environment is approximately the same as the temperature of the blood surfacing to the skin (98.6°F), little body heat can be released to the environment. The body may even absorb heat if the outside temperature exceeds body temperature. Under these conditions exercise should be avoided.

HEART PROBLEMS

Heart attacks and sudden cardiac death during or immediately after exercise have occurred occasionally. Most of the sudden deaths were in persons over forty and were due to cardiac rhythm disturbance (ventricular fibrillation). In a study in Ontario, the frequency of attack was about one episode of ventricular fibrillation for every 100,000 man-hours of exercise. Most of the reported "jogging deaths" were associated with overexertion by persons with known coronary heart disease (often in hot, humid weather). Many were preceded by warning symptoms such as chest pain, irregular heart rhythm, sudden dizziness or faintness, marked fatigue, or extreme shortness of breath. Occasional deaths related to exertion have occurred in young persons with congenital heart defects.

Some heart attacks and sudden deaths that occur after exercise may actually be unrelated to physical exertion. They may occur by chance any time during the day or night; they are actually more common while people are sitting or sleeping. No studies show that physically active people are more likely to have sudden fatal heart attacks than inactive people. In fact, most studies prove the opposite—that there is a reduced risk of sudden or later death following a heart attack for people who are physically active.

PROBLEMS OF WOMEN

Perhaps the first thing that needs to be said is that it is not true that jogging causes sagging breasts, tipped uterus, and associated other problems. A supportive brassiere should be used by women athletes with large breasts to avoid discomfort as well as trauma. Athletic bras are widely available.

As more young women go in for high mileage distance running (sixty or more miles per week), anovulatory amenorrhea (total cessation of menstrual periods) has been observed more frequently. It is unclear whether the cause is the exercise itself, the physical or emotional stress of training, a loss of body fat, or a combination of all these factors. In any case, this condition is not harmful and does not affect future fertility. Periods generally return when the mileage is decreased or with the passage of time. Occasionally, hormonal therapy is used. A warning: exercise-induced amenorrhea is not a reliable means of birth control.

Some pregnant women avoid exercise for fear of inducing miscarriage by jarring the fetus loose. Physiologically, this is nonsense since the fetus is well protected early in pregnancy by the mother's pelvic bones and muscles and later by the cushion of amniotic fluid. A general rule for exercise during pregnancy is "do what you're accustomed to, as long as it feels comfortable."

Runners, ballet dancers, horseback riders, swimmers, and other women athletes who are reluctant to accept a prolonged layoff have been able to keep up their exercising until late in pregnancy without adverse effects. Most obstetricians find that active women have fewer complications during pregnancy, a shorter labor with improved pain tolerance, easier deliveries, and a faster postpartum recovery.

Although there is no evidence that exercise during pregnancy causes birth defects, most physicians, to be on the safe side, advise pregnant women to avoid high-intensity exercise, especially competitive sports and exercising in hot environments. The theoretical reasons for this are to reduce the remote possibility that such activity will cause birth defects by decreasing oxygen supply to the fetus if the mother builds up an oxygen deficit or experiences a fall in uterine blood flow, or if overheating of the mother increases fetal temperature.

Pregnant women should avoid exercise if there is "cervical incompetence"—a dilated or weakened cervix that can lead to a miscarriage. This condition usually requires the cervix to be sutured to prevent premature opening.

Preventive Measures to Reduce Injuries

1. A physician interested and knowledgeable in the effects of exercise should be consulted before embarking on a strenuous exercise program if you are an inactive man over thirty-five, a postmenopausal woman, or a younger person with symptoms of heart disease, or with known coronary risk factors of obesity, high blood pressure, diabetes, cigarette smoking, or elevated blood lipids, or if you have a family history of premature cardiovascular disease.

   The American Heart Association and American College of Sports Medicine recommend that this special evaluation include an exercise test on a treadmill, or a stationary bicycle with electrocardiographic monitoring to assess cardiovascular fitness. (However, many physicians feel that this is being overcautious.) A safe and effective exercise program can then be prescribed adjusted to the person's fitness level and health status. The program should follow basic common-sense principles of exercise elaborated below.

2. Start off slowly. Exercise should not be a "crash program" but part of a gradual lifestyle change. Avoid the tendency to try to undo years of inactivity in a few days or weeks. The body is sure to rebel. No one should attempt to run a mile, swim forty laps, cycle ten miles, or play three sets of tennis the first time out. Activity levels should be gradually built up over a period of weeks. This is especially important for persons forty years of age or older.

3. Warm up and cool down adequately. This precaution is important for avoiding not only serious muscle and joint injuries, but cardiac complications as well. Limbering up gradually by stretching and low-intensity exercise

and walking for five to ten minutes at the start of a session and ten minutes at the end should be the minimum.

4. Choose the best time to exercise. Set aside a regular time and place for exercise sessions and make them part of your regular life pattern. Avoid strenuous exercise for at least two hours after a meal. Food in the stomach requires a significant redistribution of blood for digestion, which can add substantial strain to the heart. If you exercise before meals, allow about twenty minutes to cool down before eating, since blood is diverted to the skin during exercise for heat dissipation.

5. Avoid all-out efforts. The risk of musculoskeletal and cardiac complications is greatly magnified by such displays, especially in middle-aged and older people. Heed the warning symptoms that tend to be ignored during the heat of competition.

6. Listen to your body to avoid injuries to muscles and joints. Don't make the mistake of exercising beyond significant warning pains because more serious injuries may result. Minor muscle and joint injuries respond readily to ice, aspirin, elevation, compression, and rest, or reduction of activities. On the other hand, it is not necessary to discontinue working out for minor muscle soreness, although cutting back on training may be necessary.

Warning signals of possible serious heart problems include pain or pressure during or following exercise in the left or midchest, the neck, left shoulder or arm, dizziness, faintness, irregular heart rhythm, a cold sweat, pallor, nausea, or marked fatigue. If any of these symptoms should occur, stop exercising, and immediately consult a physician.

7. Avoid hot showers, steam baths, and saunas immediately after exercising. Wait until the internal heat generated by exercise has dissipated before exposing yourself to external heat; otherwise the increased burden on the circulatory system can result in a rapid fall in blood pressure with inadequate supply of blood to the brain and heart. This is especially important if you have cardiovascular problems. The cooling-off period with low-intensity exercise of walking is essential before showering, and the water should be neither excessively hot nor cold. If dizziness or faintness develops after exercise, suggesting decreased blood flow to the brain, lying supine with the legs elevated usually helps.

8. Avoid exercise during illness. It can aggravate the illness. An acute infectious disease can adversely affect cardiorespiratory function. Omit exercise until any residual fatigue or weakness associated with the illness subsides.

9. Resume activity gradually after a layoff. A substantial increase of fatigue can result with a few weeks of inactivity, particularly if bed rest was required for illness or injury. To reduce the risk of musculoskeletal and cardiovascular problems upon resuming an exercise program, reduce both the intensity and duration of exercise, and gradually work back to the previous level over a period of time equal to the duration of the layoff.

10. Take appropriate precautions for special weather conditions. During outdoor activities on hot, humid days:

    • Reduce exercise duration and intensity at least until acclimated to the heat.
    • Drink more water. Extra salt is rarely required because of sufficient salt in the typical American diet and because a well-conditioned body conserves salt so that sweat is mostly water.

- Drink about 500 ml. (a pint) of fluid about fifteen minutes before exercising in the heat and frequently during exercise. Water loss during exercise can be estimated by parallel weight loss. Sufficient water intake to replace this loss is necessary to avoid accumulative dehydration, with associated fatigue and cardiovascular deterioration.
- Exercise during the cooler part of the day, in the early morning, late in the afternoon, or after sunset. Competitive racing should be avoided when the temperature exceeds 28°C (82.4°F).
- Wear a minimum of lightweight, light-colored, loose-fitting clothing. A hat and sunglasses help protect against the sun. Avoid rubberized or plastic suits and sweat suits. Such garments are often worn to lose weight rapidly. However, the weight lost by excessive sweating is rapidly replaced by drinking fluids after exercise. In addition to serious dehydration leading to depletion of blood volume, this type of clothing can cause dangerously high body temperatures and can result in fatal heat stroke.

On cold days out-of-doors:

- Wear multiple layers of clothing. An innermost layer of "fishnet" ventilating underwear, both tops and bottoms, combines lightness with warmth while allowing sweat to pass through from the body. The outer layer should be a water-repellent windbreaker that can be un-zipped or removed if overheating occurs.
- Do not overdress since excess sweating can lead to chilling and loss of body heat. A good rule is to wear one layer less of clothing than you would if you were not exercising.

- Wear a hat because substantial heat is lost through the head and neck—up to 40 percent. A wool ski hat also helps protect the ears against frostbite (cold, pain, followed by numbness and pallor).
- Wear mittens to protect hands from frostbite. Mittens are preferable to gloves because the fingers can be kept warm against the palms. For extreme cold, pile-lined leather mittens are best.
- A cold weather mask over the mouth or a ski mask over the face may be worn for comfort and can prevent reflex coronary artery spasm and angina pectoris in people with coronary artery disease. Prophylactic nitroglycerine prior to physical activity in the cold may also be useful in coronary patients.
- Wear leather, wide-soled, flared heel shoes with good lateral stability when jogging on icy surfaces. Wool socks will keep your feet warm even if they get wet.

11. Special tips for joggers:
- Get instructions on proper running form from a reliable instructor or running book.
- Wear good quality running shoes (see figure 5.15). Good training shoes are either leather or lightweight nylon with leather reinforcement, have good arch and heel supports, flexibility, and soles with good impact shock absorption and traction. Above all, they should fit well and be comfortable from the first wearing. Shoes that hurt during the try-on won't improve with repeated wearing.
- Hard or uneven surfaces are more likely to cause injuries. Soft, even surfaces such as a level grass field, a dirt or wood chip-covered path, or a running track are easier on the feet and joints than asphalt.
- Joggers (and walkers) using roadways, particularly during rainy or snowy days

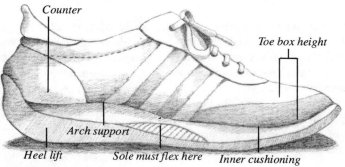

Counter

Toe box height

Arch support

Heel lift

Sole must flex here

Inner cushioning

FIGURE 5.15

Anatomy of a good running shoe

SOURCE: *adapted from "Athlete's Feet: Care and Repair of the Two Most Valuable Tools," Booklet published by* Runners World, *1974, World Publications, Box 366, Mountain View, California.*

of reduced visibility, should face oncoming traffic, watch for cars, never assume that the drivers see them, and wear bright clothing.

- Chafing becomes a problem when running long distances, particularly in the summer. Nylon (or similar synthetic fibers) shirts, shorts (with built-in underwear), and bras appear to be the best nonabrasive materials. Smearing vasoline or vasoline ointment at sites of rubbing such as between the legs, under the arms, over nipples, and between the toes is usually helpful.

- Run with a companion, and carry identification and enough money for a phone call.

Public Health Measures to Increase Physical Activity

In spite of general agreement today on the health benefits directly related to physical activity, public health policy has lagged behind public perception and has been slow in seeking out ways to promote increased leisure-time physical activity. This lack of initiative can be partly attributed to those who have insisted on obtaining "final, experimental proof" of the health improvement and chronic disease prevention that can be effected by increased physical activity in our sedentary society. Such an attitude reflects a misunderstanding of the nature of scientific proof and the type of evidence actually required for public health action. This is unfortunate, especially so because major professional and governmental agencies around the world have agreed in their official recommendations that any strategy for improving health and the prevention of chronic disease in our modern, affluent societies should include the advocacy of increased, regular, leisure-time physical activity.

The reasons for such a position are:

1. There is sufficient available evidence that increased physical activity in high-risk sedentary populations may reduce risk of heart attack, obesity, diabetes, and other maladaptations of sedentary people, and will result in an overall improvement in health, vigor, quality, and perhaps length of life.
2. The benefits of regular exercise appear to outweigh the risks of continued inactivity for most people.
3. The need for regular exercise is universal in sedentary cultures because of the physiological, metabolic, and psychological concomitants of physical inactivity.
4. The goal of more physical activity, including regular exercise, is appropriate and realizable as a public health measure. It is compatible with growing public interest and knowledge about exercise, physical fitness, disease prevention, and quality of life.
5. Promotion of regular exercise imposes little extra burden on health services and can be carried out at relatively low cost to the individual, to industry, to municipalities, and to all levels of government.

Strategies for promoting a general increase in physical activity levels for the American public are discussed below.

START EARLY IN LIFE

Role of the family

Encouragement of a physically active lifestyle should begin during early childhood so that it is more likely to become part of a lifetime behavioral pattern. At this point, parents have the primary responsibility. They can discharge it by setting an example in their own lives and by directly encouraging children to participate in all forms of physical fitness activity. Emphasis should be placed on participation and enjoyment rather than competition. It is not enough to send children off to Little League sports where the pressure is concentrated on winning.

Role of the school

As the children grow, a good physical education program in elementary and secondary schools becomes crucial. According to a recent Canadian study, an ideal school program should include the following elements:

1. *Maximum Participation*. Physical education should be compulsory in both primary and secondary schools. When physical education is made an elective in secondary schools, students who are not good at competitive team sports or who are overweight and self-conscious often choose not to take it, even though they are the ones who need it most.
2. *Daily Instruction*. A weekly total of 150 to 300 minutes of physical education instruction for elementary students. A UNESCO Council recommended one-sixth to one-third of the total elementary school schedule be devoted to physical activity.
3. *Wide Variety*. A good program should offer enough choice of activities to interest all students, both boys and girls.
4. *Lifetime Fitness Activities*. The emphasis should be on sports and activities that can be continued throughout the child's lifetime and that are known to have positive influences on health—such as running, swimming, skiing, and racquet sports, as opposed to team sports.
5. *Qualified Teachers*. A key element is the availability of properly trained teachers with specialties in physical education to lead the program.
6. *Adequate Facilities and Equipment*. Schools in which facilities are inadequate should upgrade them by imaginative use of existing resources in the community, such as community swimming pools, nearby playing fields, and outdoor recreational areas. Conversely, schools with good recreational fa-

cilities should make them available for adult use before and after school and on weekends and holidays. Also, teachers and other school employees should be permitted and encouraged to use the school athletic facilities to promote their own fitness and as a positive example to the students.

7. *Principles of Child Growth and Development.* Activities should be appropriate for the level of physical and emotional development of the child.

8. *Promotion of Positive Attitudes.* The joys of play, physical activities, and fitness should be emphasized throughout the school curricula. The common practice, even among coaches, of using physical activity as punishment, as for example, push-ups and jogging laps, should be emphatically discouraged.

NATIONAL STRATEGY

In 1976, Congress established the Office of Health Information, Health Promotion and Physical Fitness and Sports Medicine within the Office of the Assistant Secretary of Health. Its functions include the establishment of a national information clearing house, fostering research and model projects involving physical fitness, and a national conference exploring education in lifetime sports in the school system.

Though underfunded and understaffed, this office has the potential of playing the prime role in developing a coherent federal health program involving exercise.

STATE STRATEGIES

Only a few states have active Governors' Councils on Physical Fitness and Sports even though federal funds are now available to such councils for physical fitness improvement projects. State health departments should be playing a more active role in the promotion of exercise.

The Massachusetts Department of Public Health actively promotes exercise through the mass media and by developing and disseminating lists of community exercise facilities and other health promoting resources.

Oregon's legislature allocated one percent of highway funds for the construction of adjacent bikeways and footpaths. Thus far, 300 miles of such paths have been constructed. This encouragement to commute to work or school by cycling, walking, or jogging not only promotes fitness, but also cuts down on both fuel consumption and air pollution. Along the same lines, improvement of public transportation systems to make them attractive alternatives to private cars also can indirectly increase physical activity.

State departments of education should promote teaching of lifetime sports and "aerobic" exercises. Legislation is also needed to increase the number of state-mandated physical education programs.

LOCAL COMMUNITY EFFORTS

At the local level, communities should develop more trails for hiking, cycling, cross-country skiing, and nature studies; they should also develop parks, racquet and basketball courts, swimming pools, natural swimming and water sport areas, camping areas, skating rinks, and playing fields.

Since their introduction to the United States from Europe in 1973, fitness trails (parcourses) have been widely initiated. Parcourses are laid out along an approximately two-mile long trail with different types of exercise stations located about every 300 yards.

Increased development of exercise facilities and fitness programs by parks and recreational departments is also needed, particularly in inner cities, to give low-income people a better chance to exercise. The need for this is indicated by a

Gallup Poll showing that exercising is primarily a middle- or upper-income class phenomenon.

Community efforts should also be made to provide special exercise and recreational programs and transportation to and from the activity centers for the disabled and the elderly. Community development of day-care and baby-sitting arrangements would allow women at home with children to participate in physical activity and recreational programs. Support should also be given for activity programs that involve both mother and children. A promising development for these special groups is the inclusion in many new apartment buildings of physical activity and recreational centers. Developers should be encouraged to continue this trend.

PHYSICAL ACTIVITY PROGRAMS AT WORK

Employee physical fitness facilities and programs are becoming increasingly common in private corporations and governmental agencies although only a small percentage of the American work force has access to such programs. Many corporations employ full-time fitness directors. Such programs have been reported to increase productivity, reduce absenteeism, and strengthen morale. Other companies, as an alternative to their own program in the workplace, allow employees time off to participate in outside programs. Some contract with local community facilities such as the YMCA or private athletic clubs to provide exercise training, particularly for executives.

Exercise programs in the workplace should be strongly encouraged because of the accessibility afforded exercisers before and after work and during the lunch hour. Such programs need not be expensive. Suitably located companies can launch walking, jogging, and cycling programs by installing locker and shower facilities in a basement or storeroom. More elaborate facilities including gymnasiums could be incorporated into the design of future workplaces.

In large office towers, an ingenious enticement to physical activity involves making stairways more inviting, dramatic, and safe in order to encourage their use. This approach includes making the stairway locations more obvious and the stairways more pleasing through the use of color, lighting, decoration, and music.

Another suggestion to increase the use of stairways is to require access by stairs to commonly used facilities such as washrooms, eating places, lounges, and meeting rooms. Altering elevator systems so that they stop only at every third or fifth floor (with the exception of one elevator for deliveries and disabled people) could also be helpful. Tax incentives should be provided private industry to encourage the building or renovating of facilities for fitness programs. Walking, jogging, and cycling between home and the workplace can be promoted by staggering work shifts and providing showers, changing rooms, and bicycle storage areas at the workplace.

PHYSICIAN'S ROLE

In a recent survey, it was shown that only about 25 percent of patients ever recall their physicians suggesting that they should exercise. Yet individual physicians can have considerable impact on the exercise habits of their patients. Simply asking about exercise habits during the course of a medical history and physical examination raises exercise consciousness.

Physicians should know the physiological effects of exercise in order to provide patients with proper advice: how to evaluate patients for exercise programs; how to prescribe safe and effective exercise programs for improving fitness in apparently healthy adults as well as those with special medical problems; and how to manage exercise-related injuries. Furthermore, encouragement to exercise can be provided through verbal and printed information and, above all, by personal example.

Rx for physical activity

1. MOVE:
   Climb stairs, ride a bike, lift, carry.
   Dosage: Every day as often as possible.

2. STRETCH & BREATHE DEEPLY:
   Take a fitness break and relax.
   Dosage: Daily upon arising, at bedtime, and as needed when tense.

3. BEND, TWIST, SWING:
   Limber up your body including arms, hips, and back.
   Dosage: At least three times each week.

4. WALK, RUN, SWIM, CYCLE, SKI TOUR, JUMP ROPE:
   Thirty minutes or more of continuous isotonic activity, vigorous enough to increase your heart rate, and make you breathe more deeply and rapidly.
   Dosage: At least three times each week.

5. ENJOY LIFE:
   Spend leisure time at sports, active hobbies, home maintenance, or outdoor activities.
   Dosage: Two-hour period at least once a week.

CHAPTER

6

Family planning and childbearing

Perhaps no decision a young woman makes will be more important than that of having a child. For herself, for the baby, for the father, and for society at large, the importance of a normal pregnancy and normal childbirth cannot be overemphasized. The birth of a child should always be an occasion for celebration—and it usually is. The next generation is assured, the family reaffirmed, a new life begun. Sadly, if an unwanted or abnormal baby is born, there can be unfortunate consequences for many people. The parents may face a lifelong task of raising a physically or mentally deficient child who may ultimately become the charge of society, at great cost, both financial and social. Unwanted children may suffer intensely in their early years and may become ill-adjusted, antisocial individuals in their adult years. Childbirth is a natural event, but the consequences of this natural event can sometimes present individuals or the state with burdens of staggering size.

The care of the prospective mother by herself and by medical professionals is of crucial importance to the birth of a healthy child. The ear-

liest phase of preventive medicine, then, begins before birth. It should continue throughout the pregnancy and be followed thereafter by close monitoring of the baby during its first months of life outside the womb.

In terms of birth control, there are many methods available today to choose from. In the case of a proven defective fetus, several abortion techniques are also available. The risks of birth control methods and of abortion are both being constantly reduced, but they still remain, and every method of birth control must be used judiciously.

The new area of genetic counseling presents the medical and lay worlds with techniques and principles that are exciting, if less well understood.

A society which concerns itself with family planning, prenatal care, infant mortality, and the earliest period in the life of its citizens is inevitably one that gives its citizens the greatest opportunity for a healthy, fulfilling, and productive life.

Glossary

ABORTION Loss of fetus in early pregnancy. It can be spontaneous as in the case of a miscarriage, or deliberate, and, if so, should be carried out by a trained practitioner as early in pregnancy as possible.

AMNIOCENTESIS A diagnostic test during pregnancy used when fetal abnormality is suspected. A sample of amniotic fluid is withdrawn through the mother's abdominal wall and examined.

CHROMOSOMES Structures present in every cell of the body that contain all the hereditary information.

COITUS INTERRUPTUS Withdrawal of the penis from the vagina before ejaculation.

CONDOM A sheath to cover the penis during intercourse to prevent pregnancy.

DIAPHRAGM A flexible metal ring covered with a dome-shaped sheet of elastic material inserted in the vagina to prevent pregnancy.

DOWN'S SYNDROME A chromosomal disorder causing mental retardation and physical abnormalities, caused by presence of an extra number 21 chromosome.

FALLOPIAN TUBES A pair of tubes connecting the ovaries to the uterus. Ovum (egg) travels down one of the tubes. If the ovum becomes fertilized by a sperm that has traveled into the tube, it becomes implanted in the uterus and develops into a fetus.

GENES Units of heredity in the chromosome.

HYSTERECTOMY Surgical removal of the uterus.

INTRAUTERINE DEVICE (IUD) Also known as the "coil." A device placed in the uterus to have a contraceptive effect. IUDs come in different shapes and materials.

LAPAROSCOPY A method of examining the ovaries using an instrument called a laparoscope. Female sterilization can be performed through the laparoscope.

NEONATE Newborn baby.

OVULATION The release of the ovum (egg) from the ovary. This usually occurs during the middle of the menstrual cycle and is followed either by fertilization and pregnancy, or, after fourteen days, by menstruation.

RH FACTOR A substance present in red blood cells of most people, who are known as Rh positive. Those lacking the Rh factor are Rh negative, a genetic characteristic. If a woman with Rh negative blood becomes pregnant and the fetus has inherited Rh positive blood from the father, antibodies against the Rh factor are formed in the mother's blood, causing incompatibility between mother and child, leading to severe complications.

SICKLE-CELL ANEMIA A hereditary blood disorder involving the oxygen-carrying red blood cells, affecting 1 out of every 10 blacks.

SPERMATOZOA (singular: spermatozoon. Both referred to as sperm.) Male sex cells formed within the testes. They are about 1/500 of an inch long and resemble tadpoles. They contain 23 chromosomes which, when combined with the ovum's 23 chromosomes, make up the full complement of 46 in the newly formed embryo.

TAY-SACHS DISEASE A fatal recessive gene disorder caused by an enzyme deficiency, common among Ashkenazic Jews (those of Eastern European origin).

ULTRASOUND Sound waves used to form a diagnostic picture of the fetus in the uterus—now considered safer than X rays.

VASECTOMY A simple operation for male sterilization involving cutting and tying the *vas deferens*, the two ducts passing from the testicles, so that the sperm cannot pass through. It is rarely possible to reverse this procedure to restore fertility.

Family Planning

"All couples and individuals have the basic right to decide freely and responsibly the number and spacing of their children and to have the information, education and means to do so."

In unanimously adopting this declaration in 1974, the United Nations World Population Conference has projected one of the revolutionary predictions of the next century: that it is now medically possible and socially acceptable for men and women to have as many or as few children as they want, when they want them, or to have no children at all.

The aim of this chapter is to provide the reader with the information necessary to make a responsible and informed decision about childbearing from the standpoint of health. Nearly all the options involve some risk (childbearing and childbirth as well as the various birth control methods available). The risks are emphasized not in the way of discouraging any choice or course, but to make the course chosen as risk-free as possible.

BIRTH CONTROL

Birth control is a preventive measure as significant as prudent eating habits and adequate exercise. In general, the health risks inherent in the practice of birth control are fewer than those involved in pregnancy and childbirth, which, in turn, are far fewer than the risks involved in driving a car. For a woman over forty who smokes, however, the potential health risks associated with the use of the contraceptive pill are higher than those in pregnancy complications. (Table 6.1 lists the contraceptive methods available today.)

The risk of problems occurring during pregnancy and childbirth increases with the number of children a woman bears. The stillbirth rate increases sharply after the fifth birth. The risk of infant and early childhood death also increases as the number of children in the family grows.

The best and most successful birth control method is the one that a couple is comfortable with. One contraceptive method may be more appropriate than another at any particular time, and most people use several methods during their reproductive years.

The most effective birth control methods—the pill and the intrauterine device (IUD)—also carry more risk than other methods. (See figure 6.1). Both can cause systemic side effects, both positive and negative, and both are associated with serious complications.

For many couples, the safer barrier methods such as diaphragms and condoms can be just as effective, but they involve much more intercourse-related planning and preparation than the riskier methods. A barrier method of contraception, backed up by early abortion should pregnancy occur, was considered in the early 1980s as the safest reversible birth control method.

Oral contraceptives

About 100 million women throughout the world—10 to 15 million in the United States—use oral contraceptives to prevent conception. The pill's popularity is based on its high effectiveness and convenience when compared with other methods. There are many kinds of pills, but all contain hormonal substances that prevent pregnancy by interfering with the normal reproductive cycle.

The most commonly prescribed type is the "combination" pill, which is up to 99.3 percent effective. The combination consists of two hormonal substances, estrogen and progestin, which inhibit the release of a chemical from the brain that stimulates egg development and ovulation. The action is similar to the inhibition that occurs normally at the end of each menstrual cycle and during pregnancy. Even if ovulation and fertilization occur, the hormones alter the uterine lining so that it is unreceptive to the fertilized egg. In addition, the mucus located at the opening to

Table 6.1
CONTRACEPTIVE METHODS

Type	Effectiveness	Safety and side effects	Convenience
Birth control pills*	combination pills (estrogen and progestin) 99%; mini-pills (progestin only) 97–98%	Greater risk of heart attacks and stroke for users than for nonusers. Possible side effects: nausea, weight gain, depression. Risks increase with age and for smokers.	Reliable. Does not interfere with intercourse. Must be taken daily.
Intrauterine device (IUD)*	94–99%	Infrequent complications: infection, ectopic pregnancy, perforation of uterus or cervix	After inserted, it can be left in place 2 years.
Diaphragm (used with jelly, cream or foam)	80–98% depending on whether used correctly	100% safe. No discomfort or effects on chemical or physical processes of the body.	Takes motivation. Technique to be learned. Must be inserted before each intercourse and remain in place 8 hours. Fit should be checked yearly.
Foam, cream, or jelly alone (including suppositories)	poor, 30–40% failure rate	No serious side effects, except for those with possible allergies to certain brands.	Easily obtained. Must be used 1 hour or less before intercourse.
Condom	64–94% effective depending on whether used correctly	100% safe. No serious side effects. Helps protect against venereal disease.	Easily obtained. Intercourse must be interrupted by putting condom in place before entering vagina.

Method	Effectiveness	Safety	Comments
Condom and diaphragm	100% if used correctly	100% safe	Combines inconvenience of both methods (see above). Requires motivation.
Withdrawal	not effective		
Rhythm		100% safe	Requires motivation, careful record-keeping, and observation of symptoms.
calendar method	53–86%		
temperature	80–99%		
cervical mucus	75–99%		
temp. or mucus only after ovulation	93–99%		
symptothermal**	78–99%		
Sterilization Female	100%	Surgery required. Some risks associated with any surgical procedure.	One-time procedure.
Male	100%	Minor complications possible.	One-time procedure. Can be done in doctor's office. Not effective right away. Other methods must be used for a few months after procedure.

*Requires prescription and/or fitting by professional
**Must observe cervical changes, temperature and mucus

SOURCE: Adapted from U.S. Department of Health, Education and Welfare, Food and Drug Administration. HEW Publication No. (FDA) 80-3069.

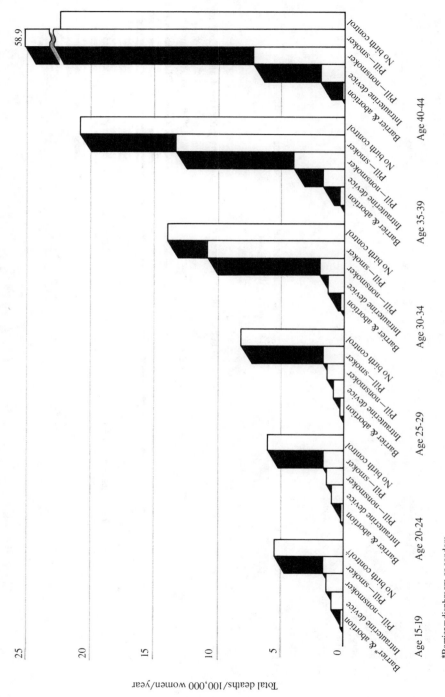

Total deaths/100,000 women/year

*Barrier = diaphragm or condom
†Deaths in women not using birth control = deaths from pregnancy complications

FIGURE 6.1

Birth control and risk of death

SOURCE: *adapted from F.H. Stewart, G.K. Stewart, F.J. Guest, and R.A. Hatcher, My Body, My Health, (New York: John Wiley & Sons, 1979)*

the uterus (the cervix) becomes thick and hostile to the sperm attempting to penetrate the uterus. The combination pill must be taken every day.

Another popular type of pill, the "mini-pill," contains only progestin. Instead of inhibiting ovulation, the mini-pill appears to prevent the fertilized egg from implanting in the uterus and developing. It also may transform the cervical mucus into a physical barrier to sperm. Effectiveness is lower with the mini-pill (97–98 percent) than with the combination pill (99.3 percent). If one of the daily mini-pills is forgotten, the chances of pregnancy are much greater than if a combination pill is missed.

Health effects Side effects of the pill include weight gain, fluid retention, abnormal menstrual bleeding patterns, fatigue, altered libido, vaginal infections, and depression. Serious complications occur most frequently with the combination pill (see table 6.2) and are more likely to occur if certain predisposing factors exist.

Many of the problems associated with the pill have been caused by the hormone estrogen. Over the years it has been found that the amount of estrogen in the pills can be reduced without reducing their effectiveness. Hormonal pills now have been developed that contain no estrogen.

The pill is not recommended for teenaged girls whose full growth has not been attained and whose menstrual cycles are not established. As stated, the risk of complications increases in women over forty and in women who smoke. All women on the pill should have regular and complete physical examinations, including blood pressure checks.

For women with serious medical conditions whose life would be threatened by pregnancy, birth control pills can ensure complete protection. The pill also seems to exert some protective health effects. Pill users may be less likely to develop noncancerous breast tumors and cancer of the ovary than nonusers, although the growth of certain pre-existing cancers may be enhanced by the pill (see table 6.2).

The nutritional changes associated with oral contraceptives are somewhat controversial. A decreased absorption of several B vitamins, vitamin C, zinc, and folic acid have been reported. On the other hand, the pill may reduce the need for some dietary requirements. Because menstrual periods are usually lighter when taking the pill, less iron is lost each month from menstrual bleeding. Some researchers find that oral contraceptives decrease the need for vitamins A and K and the B vitamin niacin, and copper. Estrogen-containing pills seem to increase the body's absorption of calcium.

The pill, while it is being taken, can alter the results of diagnostic medical procedures such as thyroid tests, Pap smears, laboratory blood counts, and biopsies. Health personnel should be told if you are using oral contraceptives so that this can be taken into account when test results are evaluated.

Intrauterine device (IUD)

The intrauterine device, also known as the "coil," is second in effectiveness only to the pill. Used by some four million women in the United States, it is 94–99 percent effective for women who use the method for a year.

The IUD is a small device constructed of inert plastic and is inserted into the uterus by a health professional. The older IUDs were designed to fill the entire uterus. They caused an inflammatory response in the uterus, which, in turn, destroyed sperm or the fertilized egg. The newer devices are smaller and contain contraceptive substances, copper or progesterone, that are slowly released into the uterus. Eventually, the substances are used up and the IUD must be replaced.

Normally, an IUD is inserted during menstruation when the cervix is more open than it is at any other time during the month. It can also

Table 6.2
RISKS OF SERIOUS COMPLICATIONS ASSOCIATED
WITH COMBINATION ORAL CONTRACEPTIVES

Condition	Risk
Cardiovascular disease	
Heart attack	Users have increased risk (2–10 times greater) than nonusers.
	Risk increases for women over 35, for women who had high blood pressure before taking the pill, for those with excessive fat levels in their blood, for women who smoke, and for women with other risk factors.
Blood clots	Risk is 2–10 times greater in users who have no other predisposing factors for blood clots.
	Deaths from blood clot disorders related to pill use—3 per 100,000 users.
	Risk is less with pills containing smaller amounts of hormone, especially estrogen.
	Should not be used by women with a history of blood clots.
High blood pressure	Approximately 1–5% of users develop high blood pressure; hypertension 3 times as likely after 5 years on the pill as it is after 1 year.
	Risk increases for women over 35, for those with a history of elevated blood pressure during pregnancy, a family history of high blood pressure, or a history of excessive weight gain or fluid retention during menstrual cycle.
	Rise in blood pressure may persist after the pill is discontinued and increase the potential for high blood pressure-related medical conditions.
Noncancerous liver tumors	Risk for users several hundred times that for nonusers.
	Risk 1 per 1 million if pill used for less than a year, 1 per 2,000 if pill used for more than 5 years.
	Risk increases for women over 30.
	Complications include rupture of the membranous covering or "capsule" of the liver, extensive bleeding, death.
Gall bladder disease	Risk 2–4 times greater for users to develop disease requiring surgery.
	Risk increases the longer the pill is taken.
Cancer	No confirmed evidence from human studies of an increased risk of cancer; however, oral contraceptives may enhance the growth of certain types of pre-existing breast cancer, uterine cancer, or benign tumors.

WARNINGS OF POSSIBLE COMPLICATIONS: severe abdominal pain, severe chest pain or shortness of breath, severe headaches, visual disturbances (blurred vision, flashing lights, blindness), severe calf or thigh pain.

be inserted following childbirth or an abortion. A Pap smear for cancer and a gonorrhea culture should precede insertion. The IUD should be checked by a health professional three months after insertion and every year thereafter. Its placement should be checked regularly by the woman, with the index finger locating the "tail" of the device, the fine strings that hang down into the vagina.

Health effects Five to 15 percent of all IUD users, particularly those who never had a child, have the device removed because of bleeding and cramps during the first year. Menstrual periods are often heavier (except with the progesterone device), and supplemental iron is recommended when blood loss is substantial. Expulsion occurs in between 3 to 20 percent of women, but is less frequent with the copper and progesterone IUDs.

The IUD is responsible for more serious complications than any other contraceptive method. Three percent of IUD users develop reproductive tract infection. Sometimes the infection is mild and limited to the uterus. Death, however, can occur if the infection is severe and causes abscesses or spreads through the bloodstream. Another complication, perforation of the uterus and retention of the device, is thought to occur once in 1,000 to 2,000 users. Hemorrhage is also a possibility.

The IUD should be removed if pregnancy occurs. If left in, the risk of miscarriage is 50 percent; if removed, the risk is 25 percent. An IUD left in place will not physically harm the developing fetus, however, because the IUD comes in contact only with the tissues protecting the unborn child, and not with the fetus itself. A risk exists with the newer devices containing potentially hazardous chemicals.

Women who become pregnant while using the IUD may have a tubal (ectopic) pregnancy.

In this potentially life-threatening complication, the fertilized egg is implanted outside the uterine cavity.

There are some reports of diminished fertility following removal of the IUD. This is particularly true when infections of the reproductive organs have occurred during the period the IUD was being used.

Early IUD danger signals are: late period or absence of period, abdominal pain, increased temperature, fever and chills, foul vaginal discharge, and abnormal bleeding.

Barrier methods

Diaphragm with spermicide A diaphragm is a dome-shaped rubber device that is inserted into the vaginal canal to cover the cervical opening prior to intercourse. It is used in combination with a spermicidal cream or jelly and acts as a mechanical barrier to the sperm attempting to enter the cervical mucus. The diaphragm must remain in place for eight hours following the last intercourse to ensure that all sperm will be destroyed by the spermicidal agent.

The diaphragm must be fitted by a gynecologist or health professional, and refitting is necessary after childbirth or a significant weight change.

When used correctly, the diaphragm is up to 98 percent effective. Proper use requires a great deal of motivation by the couple. The diaphragm, however, is a highly acceptable form of contraception because it is completely safe and is not associated with any systemic side effects or complications.

Vaginal spermicides Although the effectiveness rate of vaginal spermicides alone ranges between 60 and 95 percent, this birth control method is both simple and safe. Spermicides cause no systemic side effects, they are readily available, and they may provide some degree of protection against venereal disease. They are available in five different forms: creams, jellies, foams in pressurized containers, foaming tablets, and suppositories. They are best used in combination with other methods.

Condom The condom is probably the most widely used form of mechanical contraception. It is a sheath made of lamb membrane or rubber that is fitted over an erect penis to receive the ejaculate. Condoms are relatively inexpensive, easily available, and simple to use. Furthermore, in addition to preventing pregnancy, condoms protect against venereal disease. They are less effective than the pill, IUD, or diaphragm—about 64–94 percent. Failure is generally due to rupture during ejaculation or to incorrect or early removal of the condom. The use of spermicidal agents in conjunction with condoms, and the careful putting on and removal of the condom, can improve reliability.

Coitus interruptus
The earliest method of contraception was coitus interruptus, or withdrawal of the penis from the vagina prior to ejaculation. Although the method's rate of effectiveness is estimated to be only 85 percent, at best, it can be used when no other methods are available.

Periodic abstinence (Rhythm)
This method involves abstaining from intercourse during the fertile time of a woman's menstrual cycle. Today's techniques include a number of newer methods of determining the fertile period. There are no harmful effects from this method, and it is an acceptable form of birth control for many people whose religious convictions disallow other methods.

In the past, a formula based on the menstrual cycle was used to anticipate a forthcoming period of fertility. Today's improved techniques of determining fertility include charting body temperatures, changes in normal vaginal discharge, and other signs and symptoms of ovulation (fertility). Information about this method can be obtained from Planned Parenthood or from a gynecologist.

Postcoital contraception
This method prevents pregnancy after unprotected intercourse or if failure of a protective measure is suspected. It should not be used as a primary method of birth control.

The "morning after pill" contains estrogen and is taken several days after intercourse that might result in conception. Estrogen prevents the survival of a fertilized egg. However, its use for postcoital contraception is controversial. The long-term effects are unknown, and women who are advised not to take estrogen birth control pills should also avoid postcoital estrogens.

Another postcoital method is the insertion of an IUD after intercourse. Although this is still an experimental technique, it has prevented unwanted pregnancies.

Menstrual extraction (also known as menstrual regulation, instant abortion, miniperiod) is a simple postcoital procedure used when a menstrual period is late, but before pregnancy is diagnosed. Tissue is removed from the uterus with a small tube attached to a source of suction—a machine or syringe. Regardless of previous pregnancy status, a menstrual period will follow. The procedure takes ten minutes but should be performed only by a medical professional.

Sterilization
The most effective and an increasingly popular method of contraception is sterilization. It is estimated that one to two million Americans, male and female, choose this method every year. The failure rate is as low or lower than that of the pill.

Sterilization is less risky for men than for women. For this reason, when sterilization is being considered, it is recommended for the male partner. No long-term adverse effects of male sterilization have as yet been noted.

Female Sterilization Of the several procedures available, most involve cutting or cauterizing (burning with electrical current) the fallopian tubes, thereby blocking the passage of the egg from the ovary to the uterus. The egg is then absorbed by the body.

The traditional surgical procedure is tubal ligation, performed in a hospital while the woman receives general or local anesthesia. Surgery is performed through either the vagina or an abdominal incision.

Laparoscopy ("Band-aid surgery") is a simpler and newer method, employing a laparoscope, a long, thin, tubelike instrument with a high-intensity light and magnifying lens. The viewing tube is passed through a small incision made just below the naval and a second incision is made in the lower right part of the abdomen. A portion of the fallopian tubes is cauterized. This results in the growth of fibrous tissue, which blocks the tubes and prevents the passage of eggs. The woman is usually able to go home within eight hours. Because an overnight stay is unnecessary, hospital costs are considerably lower than they are for traditional sterilization procedures. A Band-aid is usually the only dressing applied to the incision, and within ten days the scar disappears.

Complications are infrequent, and the mortality rate is one per 5,000 procedures. Hemorrhage, infection, burns of the bowel wall from the cautery, and deleterious effects from anesthesia are the most common complications encountered. Others include: adhesions (a growing together of tissues that sometimes follows surgical procedures), reconnection of the tubes, swelling of the tubes, perforation of the uterus, and a tubal (ectopic) pregnancy. Sometimes an ovarian cyst forms, possibly because of the disturbed utero-ovarian circulation.

Sterilization usually does not interfere with menstruation. Even though the eggs do not travel through the tubes, the endocrine cycle continues as normal. The procedure does not alter the woman's sex drive, enjoyment, or ability.

It is occasionally possible to reverse the procedure, but until more advanced methods are perfected, sterilization should be thought of as permanent. When surgery is performed to reconnect the tubes, only 15 percent of women are able to have a successful pregnancy.

Hysterectomy, or removal of the uterus, was until recently the most common method of permanent contraception for women. It can be done vaginally or through an abdominal incision, and it is usually done along with other surgery such as a cesarean section. Because of the risks of complications, the cost, and the potential psychological effect of removing the uterus, hysterectomy is recommended over tubal sterilization only when there is some other pathological condition, such as cancer.

Male Sterilization Male sterilization (vasectomy) is simpler to perform, less time-consuming, and less expensive than female sterilization. And there is no risk of death.

Vasectomy is usually an outpatient procedure, performed under local anesthesia, taking about twenty minutes. The sperm duct (vas deferens) in each testicle is cut, making it impossible for sperm to pass from the testicle to the urethra, the passageway through which both urine and sperm pass to the outside of the body.

The hormone-producing area of the testicles is not affected by vasectomy. Male sex characteristics, sex drive, sexual enjoyment, amount of ejaculate, and the quality, duration, and frequency of erection also are not affected.

A cautionary note: pregnancy can occur in the first few months after a vasectomy. Sperm produced before sterilization are stored above the severed duct, and many ejaculations are necessary before the active sperm is cleared out. After the vasectomy, semen samples should be analyzed every month and, until two successive samples are negative, an alternate method of contraception should be used.

Complications such as bleeding, infection, swelling, adhesions, or inflammation can occur. Occasionally, one or both sperm ducts will reconnect. This may happen as often as once per one hundred operations, but when the surgical method used is effective, vasectomy is more reliable than the pill.

As with the eggs in female sterilization, the unejaculated sperm deteriorates and becomes absorbed by the body as part of the general physiological process that constantly removes broken-down tissues. In the first year after vasectomy the body reacts to the increase in sperm cells by producing molecules that destroy sperm. Approximately 50 to 60 percent of men have high levels of these agents in the first year; thereafter, the levels decline.

Vasectomy should be regarded as permanent. Surgery to reconnect the sperm ducts has resulted to date in a fertility rate of less than 15 percent. Corrective surgery may result in sperm being present in the ejaculate, but this does not guarantee pregnancy. It may be that the antisperm agents present in the body destroy live sperm and prevent fertilization from occurring.

Sperm banks, which freeze semen and store it for months or years, will provide a degree of "insurance" for the man who may change his mind about having children. Artifical insemination does not pose any additional risks for the child-to-be, but the length of time that sperm can be safely stored is as yet undetermined. Some experts recommend that sperm not be used after a storage period of three to four years.

Abortion

The earlier an abortion takes place, during a pregnancy the safer it is (see figure 6.2). Of the one million abortions performed annually in the United States, three-quarters take place within the first three months (trimester) of pregnancy. There are approximately 22 complications per 100,000 abortions performed, but the risk of dying from an abortion is less than that of dying from complications of pregnancy.

During the first four months of pregnancy, the abortion procedures used are: suction evacuation (also known as the vacuum aspiration); dilation and evacuation (D&E); or curettage abortion (dilation and curettage—D&C). In the suction method, the products of conception are evacuated from the uterus by means of a small, flexible tube. No anesthesia is required although a local anesthetic often is administered to relax the walls of the cervix.* In the curettage abortion, the products of conception are scraped from the uterine walls. The D&E and D&C procedures must be performed in a hospital or in a clinic under local or general anesthesia. The use of a local anesthetic is safer than a general anesthetic. A ten-day menstrual-like flow is normal following the procedure, and does not indicate hemorrhage.

If pregnancy has progressed beyond four months, other abortion methods must be used. A concentrated salt solution can be injected into the sac that contains the fetus. This is known as a saline abortion. In another technique, prostaglandins—fatlike substances—are introduced into the sac via injection or suppository. Both the saline solution and the prostaglandins stimulate uterine contractions and induce abortion. Both of these methods require hospitalization.

A hysterotomy, removal of the fetal tissues through an abdominal incision, is not recommended as a standard abortion method.

Health effects Complications are uncommon if the abortion facility adheres to prescribed standards of care and employs competent, experienced physicians to perform the abortions. Planned Parenthood groups can provide referrals to approved facilities, throughout the country.

---

*This procedure is normally done during the first few weeks of gestation.

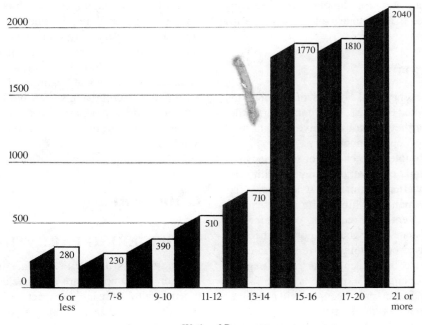

Weeks of Pregnancy

FIGURE 6.2

Major complications per 100,000 abortion procedures
SOURCE: *adapted from F.H. Stewart, G.K. Stewart, F.J. Guest, and R.A. Hatcher,*
My Body, My Health, *(New York; John Wiley & Sons, 1979)*

With the early abortion techniques, there are still some risks—including uterine perforation, cervical laceration, or hemorrhage. Hemorrhage will occur in two to ten women per 1,000 undergoing abortion. It is caused by incomplete evacuation or a flaccid uterus. Infection of the uterus or fallopian tubes following abortion occurs in about 8 percent of the patients, but most infections can be cured with antibiotics.

Complications are more common in abortions performed after the first four months. With the saline abortion, between twenty and twenty-six complications occur per one hundred women aborted. The death rate is four times higher than that in suction or curettage abortions.

If salt is inadvertently injected into a blood vessel at the time of the procedure, sudden death can occur. If salt is injected into the uterine muscle, the uterus may be seriously damaged. Salt injected into the abdominal cavity is another complication that might occur during instillation of the solution. Infection, hemorrhage, and retained products of conception may also occur.

Prostaglandins are thought to produce fewer complications than the saline method. Side effects do occur, however; specifically, women who have prostaglandin abortions may be at a greater risk of fever, uterine infection, retained tissue, and rehospitalization for complications following the procedure than women who have the saline abortion.

INFERTILITY

Some 15 percent of all couples of childbearing age in the United States are involuntarily infertile, which means they cannot conceive after at least one year of adequate opportunity.

For all couples, the chance of pregnancy occurring depends on several factors. Fertility declines rapidly after age thirty for women and after age forty for men; it is highest for both sexes in the middle twenties. Frequency of intercourse affects the chance of pregnancy, not only because of the increased opportunity for fertilization, but also because frequent ejaculations improve sperm mobility. The length of exposure is also a factor; within a year, 80 percent of couples will conceive; within eighteen months, 90 percent. It is thought that psychological factors may also play a role in infertility.

Sixty percent of infertility cases are caused by factors present in the woman, the most frequent underlying cause being a disorder of the fallopian tubes. Other factors include nutritional deficiencies, disorders in the body's hormone-producing system, ovulation failure, and vaginal and cervical conditions.

Women may have trouble becoming pregnant because of a previous method of contraception. Some women fail to ovulate following the discontinuance of birth control pills. Women who have had IUD-related infections may find conception difficult.

Among men, causes of infertility include small ejaculatory volume, a low sperm count, and abnormalities of the penis, testicles, or urethra. Nutritional deficiencies and exposure to hazardous substances such as radiation or heavy metals can cause infertility.

After a thorough medical evaluation, one or both partners may require medical or surgical treatment. Surgery may correct physical abnormalities, and hormonal therapy may stimulate ovulation (see table 6.3 for hormones and associated risks). Hormonal treatment of infertile men has proven unpromising so far, but is sometimes used as a therapy of last resort. Several options for artificial insemination and fertilization are available.

Childbearing

CONSIDERING PARENTHOOD

Among the first things to consider in becoming a father and a mother are the physical and emotional health of each prospective parent. The stresses involved in becoming a parent will demand much from each in the way of flexibility and coping ability as well as in physical stamina. The emotional maturity needed in making a place for a new child is of great importance as well.

The good health of the woman, both physical and psychological, will determine to a great extent the total health of the infant, while the support and affection offered by the father is also necessary to both mother and child.

The woman should discuss the planned pregnancy with her family physician, gynecologist, or other health professional. Any obvious problems can be investigated and treated prior to conception, and tests can be conducted to screen for conditions that could damage the unborn child once pregnancy begins.

Serious chronic disease in the mother creates a major risk due to the medications such women are likely to require. For example, diabetics require insulin, and epileptics require medication to control seizures. These drugs, although necessary to the woman's health, can damage the unborn child.

Table 6.3
DRUGS FOR FEMALE INFERTILITY

Medication	Indications	Risks
Clomid (clomiphene citrate)	An estrogen taken orally to induce ovulation; stimulates production of factors in the pituitary that in turn initiate ovulation; pituitary must be functional and the ovary must be capable of responding. Contraindicated if ovarian cysts are suspected, in malignant disease, and in ovarian failure. Not given to women who have liver disease. For women over 35, lining of the uterus should be tested before medication is prescribed.	Ovarian cysts may develop. Side effects include: hot flashes, drying of vagina, breast discomfort, nausea and vomiting, weight gain, hair loss, visual blurring, menstrual bleeding changes. The risk of a multiple pregnancy occurring increases from 1 in 29 for the general population to 1 in 13. Animal studies have shown medication to have damaging effects on unborn fetus, so basal temperature recording is recommended. After each cycle of medication, the woman is checked to make sure pregnancy has not occurred before another cycle of medication is begun.
Human chorionic gonadotrophin (HGC)	Used in combination with Clomid or another drug, Pergonal®, to stimulate ovulation (should occur 24 hours after HCG injection).	Birth defects have been associated with the drug. Adverse reactions include: overstimulation of the ovaries, ovarian enlargement and rupture, fluid in the lung or abdomen, blood clots. Multiple births may occur.
Pergonal (human menopausal gonadotrophins, menotrophins)	Used to stimulate ovulation when given with HCG or a combination of HCG and Clomid. Not given if there are uterine abnormalities, tubal problems. Thyroid activity must be normal.	Effects from ovarian stimulation may be mild or severe, and include lower abdominal discomfort and ovarian enlargement, weight gain, decreased urination, fluid in the abdominal cavity, increased chance of blood clots, and fluid in the lung. Birth defects have been reported. Treatment must be stopped if effects are severe. There is a 20 percent chance of multiple births.

Habits such as drug addiction and alcohol abuse place the newborn at a risk (see page 370). In addition, the more cigarettes a woman smokes the likelier she is to deliver a defective and/or underweight infant, and low birth weight is closely related to infant death rates. Prospective parents who smoke—particularly mothers—are advised to try smoking cessation programs long before conception. (See chapter 4).

A woman's medical history naturally affects any pregnancy she may have. If a woman has had more than five pregnancies, if these pregnancies have been close together, or if any previous delivery was complicated, the risk for the next pregnancy increases. A previous cesarean section increases the risk, as does a previous infant death or birth defect. Women with previous problems in childbirth, probably because of underlying conditions, seem to be at increasing risk with each pregnancy.

In terms of human physiology, the mid-twenties is the ideal time to have children. Parents who are significantly older or younger are at more risk. High rates of premature births, pregnancy complications, and deaths (of both mother as well as unborn and newborn infants) occur among pregnant teenagers. The social and economic problems of adolescence add to the complexity of the situation, as does the fact that many teenage mothers are unwed.

For women over thirty-five, the risks of complications of pregnancy and delivery, prematurity, and infant death are higher. Down's syndrome and several other genetic conditions occur with a greater frequency among older parents. Between the ages of thirty and sixty, the likelihood that a man will sire a child with a certain type of genetic abnormality increases tenfold. However, the chances of these defects occurring are, in the absolute sense, rare.

When considering having a child, a thorough look at sources of potential problems may help a couple in their decision-making process. If the risk of problems is high, then a couple might forgo parenthood altogether or postpone pregnancy until a time when the risk factors no longer exist or can be reduced. (See table 6.4 for an example of one type of risk-scoring system used during pregnancy).

For all risks to be adequately identified and treated, a risk evaluation should be conducted at various times throughout a woman's pregnancy. The first checkpoint is of course at the initial screening with her gynecologist before pregnancy. After pregnancy occurs, the woman's potential risk factors should be evaluated at her first prenatal visit to her obstetrician, at various times during her pregnancy, at the time labor begins, at delivery, and after birth. The factors at each point may change, and the woman should discuss her condition thoroughly with her physician.

Even after considering the risks involved, a couple might choose to go ahead with the pregnancy, but knowing the risks, make sure to obtain the best prenatal care (care of the woman before birth) and strive to provide the best physical and emotional environment for pregnancy and childbirth.

A woman seriously at risk may be referred to a large medical center for care during her pregnancy. At these regional centers, specialists in high-risk pregnancy and newborns (perinatologists and neonatologists), as well as a team of health professionals specializing in problem pregnancies and the care of the at-risk newborn, are available.

Women who develop serious problems during pregnancy may be transferred to the care of a perinatologist and admitted to a medical center for close monitoring throughout her pregnancy. Women with less serious conditions may continue with their primary clinician but be seen periodically during pregnancy by a perinatal specialist.

Plans can be made before birth of a child to transfer a newborn infant to a medical center should problems occur. Two-thirds of the problems with newborn infants can be detected during pregnancy, and with comprehensive prenatal care

Table 6.4
FACTORS CONTRIBUTING TO HIGH-RISK* PREGNANCY

Contributes a Score of 10 to the total risk

Moderate to severe toxemia† (eclampsia in severe form)
Chronic high blood pressure
Moderate to severe kidney disease
Severe heart disease
Diabetes diagnosed during pregnancy
Uterine malformation
Incompetent cervix (inability of cervix to remain closed)
Abnormal position of fetus in uterus
Excess fluid surrounding fetus
Severe endocrine problem

In previous pregnancies:
    Rh problem in newborn with blood
      transfusion
    Stillbirth
    Pregnancy duration more than 42
      weeks
    Premature infant
    Death of newborn in 1st month of life
Abnormal cervical cells
Multiple pregnancy
Sickle-cell disease

Contributes a Score of 5 to the Total Risk

History of eclampsia
History of kidney disease
Mild heart disease (no symptoms, no limitations on activity)
Mild toxemia
Acute kidney inflammation
Thyroid disease
Potential diabetes
Epilepsy
Small pelvic girdle
Older than 35, younger than 15
Viral disease
Rh factor incompatibility
Vaginal spotting

In previous pregnancies:
    Cesarean section
    Three or more consecutive miscarriages
    Infant weighing more than 10 pounds
    More than 5 children
Blood test positive for syphilis
Severe anemia
Excessive use of drugs
History of tuberculosis or skin test
    positive for tuberculosis
Weight under 100 or more than 200 pounds
Lung disease
Severe flu syndrome

Contributes a Score of 1 to the Total Risk

History of urinary bladder infection
Acute urinary bladder infection
History of toxemia
Family history of diabetes
Alcohol (moderate intake)

Birth defect in previous pregnancy
Mild anemia
Smoke a pack or more of cigarettes per day
Emotional problems

*A total score greater than 10 indicates high risk.
†Toxemia: a condition that begins in late pregnancy and subsides after delivery. It is a serious complication characterized by high blood pressure, swelling, and protein in the urine. In its most severe form, accompanied by convulsions or coma, it is known as eclampsia. Toxemia is associated with high maternal and infant death rates.

SOURCE: adapted from C. Hobel, M. Hyvarinen, D. Okada and W. Oh, "Prenatal and Intrapartum High Risk Screening. I. Prediction of the High Risk Neonate," *American Journal of Obstetrics and Gynecology,* Vol. 117, 1973, pps. 1-9.

many risks that lead to complications can be minimized or eliminated.

For most women, the chances are excellent for a successful pregnancy resulting in the birth of a perfectly healthy baby. Childbearing is, after all, a natural function, and the body is equipped to counter many threats to the pregnant woman and the developing fetus.

GENETIC DISORDERS AND GENETIC COUNSELING

Most human illness has some genetic basis. Until recently, the birth of a child with a genetic defect could not be predicted, but medical technology today can provide prospective parents with much information about the risk of an inherited disease in their unborn child. Many prospective parents do not need genetic counseling. However, if a person or couple has any of the following characteristics, the help of a genetic counselor should be sought before having a child:

1. A history of genetic disease in either parent's family.
2. You have had a child with a genetic disease or a birth defect.
3. Either parent has a genetic disease.
4. Either parent has been exposed to drugs, X rays, or a virus (such as rubella—German measles) prior to or near the time of conception or during the first half of pregnancy.
5. You are a woman thirty-five years or older.
6. You are a man fifty-five years or older.
7. You are a woman who has had several spontaneous abortions.

—adapted from *The Genetic Connection*, David Hendin and Joan Marks, New American Library, 1979.

Genetic counseling, in addition to clarifying any risks present, can provide information on reproductive alternatives, establish an accurate diagnosis, clarify the immediate and long-term consequences of the disorder in question, and provide emotional support to family members during the period of decision-making and adjustment.

Many physicians and other health professionals can provide genetic counseling either on their own or through collaboration with a medical geneticist or genetic counselor. Because of the expertise and sophisticated technology required to provide proper diagnosis and therapy, most genetic counseling services are part of a university-affiliated medical genetics program. Research activity and clinical instruction may be an integral part of the services involved.

Chromosomes, genes, and genetic disorders

Chromosomes are structures present in every cell of the body that contain all the hereditary information of the individual. They are composed of genes, which are the units of heredity arranged in a specific sequence. All normal cells have forty-six chromosomes, with the exception of sperm and egg cells that have twenty-three. There are twenty-two pairs of chromosomes called autosomes and one pair of chromosomes labeled X and Y. Normal men have one X and one Y, while normal women have two X chromosomes.

Each trait of the individual is determined by at least two matching genes, one on each of a pair of chromosomes. Among this vast number of genes, a few in each individual are likely to be abnormal or altered. Some genetically determined defects arise when one or both parents transmit these abnormal genes to their offspring, while others arise from spontaneous mutation occurring in the genes of the unborn.

Genetic disorders are classified into three groups: Chromosome disorders, single gene disorders, and multifactorial disorders.

Chromosome disorders Chromosome disorders are caused by an aberration in the number or structure of the individual's basic genetic material. Such disorders are not usually hereditary and generally affect only one pregnancy. However, about 20 percent are caused by a genetic rearrangement in the genes of the parents and could therefore be inherited. Chromosome abnormalities occur one in every two hundred births. However, all *known* disorders can be detected prenatally.

Down's syndrome, the most common form of chromosomal aberration, is caused by an extra #21 chromosome; a victim of this disorder has 47 rather than 46 chromosomes. The risk of bearing a child with this disorder increases as the mother grows older. The role of the father is not known, although he is believed not to play any role. The risk of Down's syndrome increases from 1 in 2,000 live births among women at twenty years of age to 1 in 300 among women in their late thirties. By the time a woman is forty-five her chances are 1 in 20. The presence of an extra chromosome usually produces mental retardation with additional abnormalities depending upon which extra chromosome is present. For example, an extra #18 chromosome might result in eye and ear defects, an extra #21 chromosome could cause dwarfism, a small head, and facial features of mongolism. However, most Down's syndrome children are educable; they can learn to walk and talk and can become active family members. In addition to Down's syndrome, there are many other chromosome abnormalities that cause severe mental retardation.

Other significant chromosome aberrations affect the *sex chromosomes*, resulting in subtle to profound anomalies. In the *Klinefelter syndrome*, male offspring have two or more X chromosomes and one Y, rather than one X and one Y. This disorder occurs in about 1 in 700 live births. In addition to their mental retardation, the victims are usually tall and have abnormal testicular development. *Turner syndrome* involves female offspring. These children have one X chromosome, rather than two, the incidence being about 1 in 3,000 live female births. They are short, have a wide chest, do not develop breasts, and do not ovulate because their ovaries never develop. Turner syndrome does not appear to affect mental development and IQ; however, some children develop a perceptual problem known as field dependence.

Single gene disorders These are caused by one faulty gene contributed by one or both parents. The risk of this occurring in the children of a couple is the same for each pregnancy. The four types of single gene disorders are: autosomal dominant, autosomal recessive, X-linked dominant, and X-linked recessive (see table 6.5 for typical disorders).

Dominant defects are so-called because the effects of the faulty gene are expressed although the analogous gene is normal. Should one parent be the victim of a dominant disorder, there is a 50 percent chance in each pregnancy that the offspring will have the disorder. Should both parents have the disorder, which is extremely rare, there is a 75 percent chance that children will be affected.

Recessive gene disorders occur when both parents are carriers of the disease. The effect of the normal gene dominates over its counterpart in the parents; therefore, the parents are not diseased. If both parents carry the gene, there is a 25 percent chance that the offspring of any pregnancy will be born with the defect. And if the recessive gene is actually transmitted by each parent, there is a 100 percent chance that the children will express the disorder. If only one parent is a carrier, there is no chance of an infant being born with it. However, there is a 50 percent chance that an offspring of this couple will also be a carrier.

Table 6.5
INHERITED SINGLE-GENE DISORDERS

Types	Typical disorders
Dominant	Huntington's chorea
	Achondroplasia
	Neurofibromatosis
	Adult polycystic kidney disease
	Myotonic dystrophy
Recessive	Cystic fibrosis
	PKU (phenylketonuria)
	Sickle-cell anemia
	Tay-Sachs disease
	Galactosemia
	Werdnig-Hoffmann's spinal muscular atrophy
X-linked recessive	Duchenne muscular dystrophy
	Hemophilia
	Hunter's syndrome
	Fabry disease
	Color blindness
X-linked dominant	Vitamin D resistance
	Rickets

SOURCE: Vincent M. Riccardi, M.D.

Many conditions common to certain ethnic groups fall under the category of recessive gene disorders. *Tay-Sachs disease* is a degenerative disorder caused by an enzyme deficiency. The disease is characterized by a very early onset, paralysis, blindness, and death by age three or four. Tay-Sachs is most common among Ashkenazic Jews—about 1 in 25 is a carrier, and about 1 out of every 3,500 live births among Ashkenazic Jews will result in the disorder. Fortunately, carriers of the disorder can be detected and the disease can also be diagnosed in the fetus.

Cystic fibrosis is the most common fatal childhood illness. Estimates suggest that 1 out of every 25 white people in the U.S. is a carrier, and the incidence is estimated to be 1 in 1,500.

Unfortunately, there is no screening method for carriers yet, nor is there a detection method for the fetus. Carriers are usually identified only after bearing an offspring with cystic fibrosis, although there is a "sweat" test available to determine if one is a carrier. Each subsequent birth from carrier parents has a 25 percent chance of being affected.

One out of every ten black Americans in the U.S. is a carrier of *sickle-cell anemia*. The disease, affecting one out of every 650 black babies, is a hereditary blood disorder affecting the oxygen-carrying red blood cells. Instead of being disc-shaped, the red blood cells of sickle-cell victims are sickle-shaped. The impeded passage of these abnormal cells through blood vessels results in oxygen starvation to areas of the body, causing severe pain. Furthermore, the immune system rids the body of these abnormal red blood cells, resulting eventually in anemia. Blood tests are available to determine genetic carrier status, but diagnostic techniques for the fetus are still in the experimental stage.

Genetic counseling is advised for any person who is suspected of carrying these disorders. The geneticist may be able to allay the fear or clarify the risk.

X-linked disorders are those that are carried on the X chromosome. X-linked recessive disorders most frequently affect men. The X chromosome carries genes that influence factors other than sexual development. Should a woman have a defective gene on one of her two chromosomes, its effect would be eliminated by the normal influence exerted by the analogous gene on the other X chromosome. However, should a woman transmit the aberrant X chromosome to a son, he has only a Y chromosome, not another X, which cannot counteract the negative influence. Should a woman be a carrier and her mate normal, there is a 50 percent chance of a daughter being a carrier.

Hemophilia is the most common sex-linked recessive disorder. The persons affected lack vital factors in their blood that allow normal clotting to occur. Because of this deficiency, the hemophiliac hemorrhages even after minor injuries. Until recently, bleeding episodes could result in death; however, drugs are now available to treat some victims.

X-linked dominant disorders are transmitted in the same manner as recessive disorders; however, the effect is expressed in female carriers as well as in male.

Multifactorial disorders (polygenic). These disorders are caused by the influence of many genes and their interaction with the environment. Examples are disorders such as clubfoot, cleft palate, constriction of the pylorus (the opening of the stomach into the small intestine), and neural tube defects (defects of brain or spinal cord). Any couple has a 1 in 50 chance of bearing a child with any of these defects, but some may now be detected prenatally (for example, neural tube defects). Recurrence rates of these disorders in subsequent births are shown in table 6.6.

Counseling and diagnostic tools

To minimize the risk of bearing a child with a genetic disorder, counseling and diagnostic tests should be undertaken by parents while alternatives remain available. Those who believe they are at risk should seek guidance from a geneticist when planning a pregnancy. Should this preconceptional counseling reveal that they are carriers of a genetic defect, postconceptional counseling will be advised. Diagnoses of genetic defects can be made during the second trimester of pregnancy. If a serious abnormality is detected in the fetus, the pregnancy can be terminated. Prenatal diagnosis can detect many hereditary metabolic disorders, some sex-linked disorders, some anatomic deformities, and all the known chromosome abnormalities.

Many tools are available to determine the health of the unborn fetus where an abnormality is suspected. Ultrasound scanning is a noninvasive technique that utilizes sound waves to detect anatomic defects and is normally accompanied by amniocentesis. In amniocentesis, a small sample of amniotic fluid is withdrawn through the abdominal wall of the mother. The test is generally performed between the sixteenth and seventeenth week of pregnancy when fluid and fetal cells are sufficient to ensure successful analysis of biochemical and genetic abnormalities. Ninety percent of neural defects can be detected by the use of amniocentesis in prenatal diagnosis. The accuracy rate of diagnosis is around 99 percent, and there is little if any increased risk of miscarriage in women undergoing amniocentesis (0.5 percent).

Other techniques are being tested. Amniography involves the injection of a contrast medium into the amniotic fluid allowing a clear picture of the developing fetus to be seen on X ray. This method is being tried during early pregnancy (prior to twenty-four weeks). Direct visualization of the fetus by fetoscopy is available at some institutions. Prenatal diagnostic procedures conducted before the seventeenth week of pregnancy allow the option of terminating a pregnancy. Beyond the twenty-fourth week, genetic counseling can only clarify the risk and define expectations. Abortion at this point is no longer possible because of legal and medical restrictions.

Those undergoing genetic counseling should make sure they understand the diagnosis accurately, the consequences of the prognosis, the likelihood of recurrence, and the choices available to minimize the risk of recurrence. The possibilities for minimizing recurrence risk include foregoing childbearing, prenatal diagnosis with the option of abortion, and artificial insemination if it is the male who is transmitting the aberrant factor.

It is important to emphasize that genetic counselors cannot make decisions for families, but can only help them to make a well-informed choice. The counselor can then assist in carrying

out the decision by arranging for the necessary procedures and interpreting the results.

Emotional and psychological support is critical in genetic counseling, since informed decision-making can be difficult in an emotionally strained setting. The adverse effects of parental anger, guilt, and frustration must be respected and dealt with. Long-term follow-up is often necessary for general support and reinforcement.

Genetic counseling and treatment centers have been established throughout the United States. Check with the pediatrics clinics and with the major medical centers with teaching hospitals in your state.

PREGNANCY

Adjusting to pregnancy

If two people have successfully managed other stages of their life, the prospect of parenthood will probably be handled with a minimum of difficulty. Many influences in each individual's life will prove important during this time, including the relationships of both partners to their own parents. Frequently, one's expectations and behavior at this time reflect how one has gotten along with one's own mother and father.

The need for successful adjustment to pregnancy does not imply that negative feelings about it are unnatural. Ambivalence in both parents is to be expected. Especially at the beginning, there are likely to be gnawing reservations about the whole thing; anxiety about adequacy as a parent, worry about financial stability, doubts about readiness for parenthood, suspicions of rivalry with child, sexual conflicts and fears, fear of loss of independence, concern about changing body shape. Feelings tend to alternate between joy and frustration. The best defense against the qualms of pregnancy is the knowledge that they are not unusual.

Table 6.6
COMMON POLYGENIC DISORDERS

Disorder	Recurrence rate
Neural tube defects (spinal bifida, anencephaly)	5%
Clubfoot	2–8%
Cleft lip	4%
Cleft palate	6.5%
Pyloric stenosis (constriction)	3–5%

SOURCE: adapted from *The Genetic Connection*, David Hendin and Joan Marks, New American Library, 1979.

Health care during pregnancy

Pregnancy provides one of life's best opportunities for preventive care. A woman should take full advantage of it—for herself as well as for her unborn baby. The goal of prenatal care is to maintain the good health of both, to prevent complications, to minimize problems if they occur, and to help make the experience successful and satisfying.

In the beginning, visits to the obstetrician or other health professional should be monthly. Later, when signs of complications are more likely to occur, visits should be more frequent. As the due date nears, visits are scheduled weekly.

The basic examination will include, of course, a complete physical checkup and history, plus matters of special interest during pregnancy. The prospective mother should look for the following when meeting with her doctor:

- A discussion of the normal changes and routines in pregnancy: what to expect, advice about medications, dietary recommendations, vitamin supplements. This is the best time to ask questions about any anticipated problems and to make sure you know what it is all going to cost.

- A complete physical examination (lungs, heart, breasts, rectal examination, etc), including a general checkup of the mouth and teeth.

- A detailed investigation of your medical history—any illnesses, operations, chronic diseases, occupational hazards, family illnesses—to determine whether there are any past or present problems that could increase risk.

- Pelvic examination. A test for gonorrhea and a Pap smear.

- Screening for some genetically carried diseases, if appropriate (see page 362).

- Blood test for anemia, syphilis, abnormal antibodies, blood type, and Rh factor (for possible blood incompatibility problems the baby might develop).

- Urine testing for infection and abnormalities (such as sugar in the urine, which might indicate diabetes).

- Temperature, height, weight, blood pressure (important to monitor during pregnancy to make sure no toxemia of pregnancy is developing), and pulse taken and recorded for later comparisons.

- German measles test to make sure immunity exists (if not, vaccination immediately after delivery).

- Calculation of the estimated delivery date. This is easier if you have kept records of your menstrual periods. If you have a twenty-eight-day cycle and your menstrual periods are regular, calculate the date by adding seven days to the first day of the last menstrual period, subtract three months, and add one year.

Nutrition during pregnancy

If you are well-nourished before and after you become pregnant, the risk of complications during your pregnancy and delivery is much decreased. Most importantly too, you will be providing your unborn child with a solid foundation.

Birth weight is a determinant of a child's survival and future. If you don't eat properly, you are more likely to deliver an underweight baby. The average birth weight in the United States is seven pounds; infants born weighing less than five and one-half pounds are thirty times more likely than normal-weight infants to die during the first month of life. They are also more prone to birth injuries, mental retardation, handicapping conditions, visual and hearing disorders, behavior disorders, and learning problems.

Normally, maintaining a diet that will meet both your and your unborn child's nutritional needs should not be difficult. If you are accustomed to eating a well-balanced diet you need only add calories, protein, vitamins, and minerals (see chapter 1, Nutrition), as discussed with your doctor. However, it will mean altering the pattern of eating by having smaller, more frequent meals, particularly when the enlarging uterus begins to interfere with the normal digestive processes. It may also mean limiting certain items such as those difficult to digest (e.g., fried foods). Excessive alcohol has been associated with birth defects (see chapter 2, Alcohol) and even small amounts of alcohol may affect the fetus; therefore it is suggested that pregnant women do not drink alcohol at all.

For some pregnant women, the nutritional increases normally recommended may not be sufficient. If a woman is significantly underweight when she becomes pregnant, if she has had a previous miscarriage or stillbirth, if she is pregnant within a year of delivering another baby, or if she has a multiple pregnancy (twins or more), her nutritional needs are greater. Emotional stress is also thought to increase nutritional requirements. Women addicted to drugs and alcohol often have nutritional deficiencies that need to be remedied when they become pregnant.

Recommendations about weight gain and salt restriction have changed over the past few years. Previously, women were told to limit their weight gain—sometimes to no more than fifteen pounds—and to eliminate all salt in the diet. These precautions were thought to prevent toxemia, a serious complication of pregnancy. Recently, it has been found that these restrictions can actually cause toxemia or lead to the development of other complications.

Today it is recommended that women gain twenty to twenty-five pounds (see chapter 1, page 144). A weight gain of more than thirty pounds, however, can begin to create problems for both mother and infant. The additional weight puts the body under added physiological stress and thus adds to risk. Also, the fetus may gain extra weight, making labor difficult and placing the fetus at risk. After delivery, the mother's excessive weight will be difficult to lose.

You can tell if your diet is adequate by recording what you eat for a week or two and comparing it with the recommended daily amounts (see table 1.3, Recommended Dietary Allowances, page 102). To evaluate weight gain as pregnancy progresses, weigh yourself weekly (see table 1.13, Overall Weight Gain During Pregnancy, page 145). If you are eating a nutritious diet and gaining steadily, you are probably in good shape. A sudden drop or increase in weight (two pounds per week or more) should be investigated. Normally, the pattern of weight gain is two to six pounds during the first three months and about one pound per week after that.

Exercise

The standard recommendation has long been that mild exercise would do no harm. It may be possible to go further. There is now evidence that pregnant athletes have fewer complications during pregnancy and delivery than women who are not in top shape. Physical fitness not only improves a woman's physical and emotional health but also seems to help her during labor. Therefore, pregnant women accustomed to a schedule of regular and vigorous exercise should continue this regimen. However, an exercise program should not be started during pregnancy (see chapter 5, Physical Fitness).

Sexual intercourse

Physical and psychological changes occur during pregnancy that may increase or decrease sexual desire. The great changes that take place in the woman's body can affect both partners negatively or positively. Emotional reactions to the pregnancy itself on the part of both parents can in turn affect sexual relations.

It is generally thought that sexual intercourse and orgasm will not harm the fetus or cause a miscarriage. However, some studies indicate that intercourse early in pregnancy can increase the chances of a miscarriage while intercourse in the last month of pregnancy may increase the risk of developing an interuterine infection that can harm the fetus.

Bleeding after intercourse, if it occurs, is likely to be the result of pressure against the cervix. However, any such bleeding could indicate a serious complication and should be evaluated by a professional.

Sexual intercourse should not take place if there is a possibility of a miscarriage, if the membranes surrounding the fetus have broken (usually right as labor begins), if there is uterine bleeding, or severe abdominal pain, or vaginal pain.

Before delivery, the couple should decide on a form of contraception to use after the baby is born. Although ovulation may not occur immediately after childbirth, some form of contraception should be used once sexual relations resume. The risks of pregnancy in a breast-feeding mother are 25 percent at twelve weeks after delivery and 65 percent after twenty-four weeks.

Relief for common discomforts of pregnancy

The following are simple remedies for certain universal complaints that occur during pregnancy. They should be tried first. *Only as a last resort and only under professional supervision should medications be taken.*

Heartburn Eat small, frequent meals. Avoid gas-producing, fatty, highly seasoned foods. Alternate dry and liquid meals. Drink milk, hot water, or peppermint tea between meals.

Nausea (morning sickness) Eat dry crackers or toast before arising. Lie quietly for thirty minutes before getting out of bed. Drink hot tea or milk before breakfast. Eat frequent, small light meals containing low-fat foods. Dress slowly and avoid tight-fitting clothes. Rest after meals.

Constipation Get adequate exercise. Eat foods containing roughage (wholegrain cereals, fresh fruit and vegetables). Eat laxative foods (prunes, dates, figs).

Minor aches and pains Moderate exercise will improve muscle tone, and frequent rest periods will help in avoiding fatigue. A small pillow beneath the back when in bed can relieve backache. Good posture will alleviate problems. Pelvic rocking exercises, a snug maternity girdle, or local heat and massage may help. Sleep with a firm mattress and a bed board. Avoid standing in one position too long.

For leg cramps, which may be caused by a calcium-phosphorus imbalance, extend the leg, bend the foot, and point toes toward the knee. A hot water bottle may also help.

Insomnia If insomnia is due to breathing difficulties (from the pressure of the upward growing uterus on the lungs), sleeping with the head elevated by several pillows, or in a side-lying position, will help.

Vaginal discharge An increase in vaginal discharge is normal during pregnancy because of material secreted by the cervix. Normal discharge appears watery or whitish in color. If it becomes bubbly and yellowish, white and chunky, or if there is burning and itching, an infection may be present. If the condition persists, let your physician know.

If no pathological organism is found upon examination, yet symptoms persist, douching may be recommended. If the area begins to itch, apply petroleum jelly to the skin in the genital area to prevent irritation. Wear cotton underwear.

Hemorrhoids Gently replace protruding hemorrhoids into rectum with lubricants. Keep hips and legs elevated as much as possible. Hot baths or cold compresses of witch hazel may relieve pain. Prevent and treat constipation. These measures should eliminate the need for medications. If the hemorrhoids do not subside, the doctor can recommend the use of stool softeners.

Varicose veins Avoid standing for long periods. Clothing should not restrict any part of the body. Support hose will help. Frequently elevate legs and hips above the heart. Rest frequently.

Swelling Elevate legs frequently. Increase water intake to promote removal of fluid from tissues. While in bed, lie in a side position, promoting fluid flow through the kidneys by removing pressure from the uterus.

Hazards during pregnancy

Although the unborn child is well-protected within the mother's body, it is extremely vulnerable to almost everything the pregnant woman inhales or ingests. Medications, food, viruses, noxious fumes, cigarette smoke—all these substances are passed on to the fetus. Early in pregnancy, these agents can cause organ malformation; later exposure can mean functional failure in organs or systems within the body. Fortunately, many of these hazards can easily be reduced or eliminated.

Alcohol Since alcohol interferes with the absorption of nutrients, pregnant women should not drink (see page 119, chapter 1, and chapter 2). Women who drink heavily during pregnancy (more than two drinks per day) risk having infants with birth defects, collectively called Fetal Alcohol Syndrome.

Tobacco A pregnant woman who smokes is at higher than normal risk of miscarrying and of having a child with birth defects or low weight. The chance of delivering a low-birth-weight baby decreases if the mother stops smoking by the fourth month. If she smokes, she is also at risk of heavy bleeding late in pregnancy, which may cause complications endangering the fetus.

Nonmedicinal drugs Although nonmedicinal drugs, such as marijuana have not been established as dangerous to the fetus, there is the possibility of unknown long-term effects. (See chapter 3, Drugs.) Prolonged use of barbiturates during pregnancy can cause symptoms of nervousness and irritability in the newborn baby, usually at about seven to ten days old. The fetus of a woman addicted to heroin, morphine, or methadone is likely to be drug-dependent and to develop withdrawal symptoms within the first few days after birth. In addition, the addicted mother is likely to be undernourished.

Medications In a recent study of 50,000 women, it was found that 900 different drugs were being taken during their pregnancies. In general, the average woman takes between four and nine different medications during the course of her pregnancy. This rather heavy use of drugs occurs in spite of the fact that no drug—either over the counter or prescribed—has actually been proven safe for the unborn child. (See Table 3.1, Chapter 3, Drugs, for commonly prescribed medications that should *not* be taken during pregnancy.)

Very little is known about how drugs affect fetal development. When a defect occurs, it is almost impossible to say exactly what caused it or how. The effect of a particular medication depends on many factors, including the genetic susceptibility of the fetus, the stage of development when the drug is taken, and the amount and duration of use.

Naturally, taking *no* medication during pregnancy is the safest solution to this dilemma. Sometimes, however, drugs are necessary whether to relieve the discomforts of pregnancy, or to treat a medical condition. Some complications of pregnancy must be treated with medication to prevent serious harm to the fetus.

Several medications, however, have proven to be counterproductive. Diuretics ("fluid pills"), which were given to pregnant women in the past, are no longer recommended. They can cause clotting, chemical imbalance, and respiratory distress in the unborn child, and they may upset the woman's chemical balance.

For any medication that is being considered, the benefit-to-risk ratio should be carefully assessed. If the value of the drug to the woman outweighs the risk to the fetus and to the woman, then one might want to take the medication.

Occupational hazards With more women working outside the home than ever before, hazardous conditions on the job are a growing problem for the pregnant working woman and her unborn child. If a woman develops a serious complication of pregnancy, such as threatened miscarriage, anemia, bleeding, infection, or debilitating nausea, she should stop working. If the environment poses risks that cannot be minimized or eliminated, a transfer to a less hazardous environment is advised.

Potential hazards include toxic gases, fumes and vapors, solvents—particularly benzene—X rays, metals, and pesticides. Work that requires constant standing or sitting for long periods, extremely strenuous activity, rotation of shifts, and unreasonable lifting and carrying are all particularly risky for a pregnant woman. (See chapter 16, Occupational Health, or Reproductive Health, page 610.)

Household hazards Hazardous substances used around the house should be avoided or used with utmost caution. Aerosol spray products propelled by fluorocarbons are chemically related to an anesthetic gas that has been implicated in birth defects among children of female anesthesiologists and nurse anesthetists. The effect of other chemicals released in aerosol mist is unknown.

Insecticides and herbicides, paint fumes, turpentine, and furniture stripper absorbed through skin or lungs, can also harm the unborn child. Painting should be avoided, especially if an oil-based paint is used.

Rubber gloves should be worn when using household cleansers and polishers.

All products emitting fumes, such as ammonia and all the substances mentioned above, should be used in well-ventilated areas—if they must be used.

Because the ingredients in cosmetics are not known, the effects on the fetus of using cosmetics are uncertain. Any known to contain mercury, arsenic, or lead should clearly be avoided during pregnancy.

All the safety precautions listed in chapter 9, Home Accidents, apply especially to pregnant women.

Infections during pregnancy

Infections in the pregnant mother may account for more than 20 percent of infant deaths within a month after birth. There are several routes of infection. Table 6.7 shows a list of the most common infections, the effects upon the fetus, and suggestions for prevention and treatment.

Diagnostic tests for problem pregnancies

In some pregnancies, an abnormal development noted by the prospective parents or discovered during a prenatal visit may warrant special investigation. The sooner the tests are made, the sooner the physician can diagnose the problem and the better the chances are for a favorable outcome.

Table 6.7
COMMON INFECTIONS

Infection	Effect on fetus	Prevention
Chicken Pox	May cause shingles, an acute skin inflammation.	Avoid contact with infected persons.
Common Cold	Unknown	Avoid contact with infected persons.
Gonorrhea	Causes ocular gonorrhea at birth from passage through infected birth canal.	Drops of silver nitrate or other medication are placed in newborn's eyes immediately after birth.
Herpes Simplex Virus II (in vaginal area)	Miscarriage if infection occurs during 1st or 2nd trimesters. If contracted within a month of giving birth, infant should be delivered by cesarean section.	Abstain from intercourse if there are lesions.
Hepatitis B	Can cause jaundice, liver and spleen enlargement, and liver damage.	Pregnant women with a history of liver disease, hepatitis, or drug abuse, or who have been exposed to hepatitis, should have blood tested to determine presence of disease.

Although these tests involve some degree of risk, the benefits generally outweigh the possible risk to the woman and the unborn child. However, because a number of these tests have only recently been developed, their long-term effects are not known. Most women will not require any of them.

Some of the commonly used tests are:

X rays Unless vital to the health of the woman or the fetus, X rays should not be used during pregnancy. X rays of the abdomen or lower back, in which the fetus is placed in the direct beam of radiation, are particularly hazardous. Early in pregnancy, X rays would effect serious risk of miscarriage, brain damage, and birth defects. (See chapter 13, Radiation.)

X ray measurement of the dimensions of the pelvic bones is used only under special circumstances. Prenatally, it is usually performed if there

Table 6.7
COMMON INFECTIONS *(continued)*

Infection	Effect on fetus	Prevention
Influenza	Can cause premature labor, miscarriage, or birth defects.	Vaccination of mother with immune serum.
Mumps	Can cause premature labor, miscarriage, or birth defects.	A mumps skin test should be performed before pregnancy. If the prospective mother is not immune, mumps immunization should be given.
Rubella (German Measles)	Can cause severe birth defects if contracted by mother during first trimester.	Women of childbearing age who have never had the disease should be vaccinated. However, the vaccine should *not* be given to anyone who is pregnant or trying to become pregnant.
Toxoplasmosis*	Can cause miscarriage or stillbirth. Infant may be born with abnormally sized brain, enlarged spleen, and blindness.	Cats are carriers. Pregnant women should avoid outdoor cats and if cats are in household, should avoid changing cat litter. Pregnant women should also avoid eating raw or undercooked meat as cattle, sheep, and chickens are also carriers.

*In toxoplasmosis, the infected mother can develop a rash, swollen glands, painful joints. For the effects of other infections on adults, see chapter 15.

were difficulties during previous pregnancies or if the fetus is in an abnormal position. During labor, it is used if the labor fails to progress.

In suspected abnormalities of the placenta or fetus, a special contrast material is used to aid X ray visualization. In one test, sodium iodine is introduced into the woman's bladder to help determine the exact position of the placenta.

In a procedure known as amniography, contrast material is inserted into the sac that surrounds the fetus. This material mixes with the fluid in the sac and outlines the fetal head, trunk, and limbs. Contrast material can also reveal the internal digestive tract of the fetus and make possible the diagnosis of gastrointestinal obstruction, serious fetal distress, or death.

Various radioisotopes are used to diagnose problems. Radioactive substance injected into a woman's vein can determine the location of the placenta.

Thermography using nonionizing infrared radiation is useful in diagnosing certain complications of pregnancy, especially breast conditions and circulatory problems in the legs. (See chapter 13, Radiation.)

Ultrasound Also known as sonography, ultrasound uses sound waves above human hearing range to form a "picture" of the fetus in the uterus. The exact location of the fetus and placenta, the size of the head, and the extent of fetal growth and development can be determined. In addition, fetal heart tones can be heard early in pregnancy with this equipment. It can be used to record uterine contractions and the fetal heart rate before or during labor.

The long-term effects of sound wave testing are not known, but the availability of ultrasound makes it possible to obtain information about many problems that formerly could have been diagnosed only with X rays, which are clearly hazardous. For most purposes, ultrasound is superior to X rays for visualizing and measuring both bony and soft tissues.

Oxytocin challenge test (OCT) Also known as the oxytocin stress test or the contraction stress test, this diagnostic procedure is performed to determine the ability of the fetus to tolerate labor and the continuation of pregnancy. It determines the respiratory reserve of the uteroplacental unit.

Oxytocin, a uterine stimulant, is given to the woman while external recording devices monitor the fetal heart rate and uterine contractions. This test may be recommended for women with high blood pressure, chronic kidney disease, or diabetes. One potential complication is the precipitation of labor. The OCT is contraindicated if the woman has had a previous cesarean section, if her cervix is known to be faulty, or if certain placental abnormalities are present.

Nonstress test (NST) Also known as the fetal activity-acceleration determination, this test measures the fetal heart rate during spontaneous contractions.

Amniocentesis This procedure is usually done to determine if the fetus has a genetic defect. Some conditions that can be diagnosed are Down's syndrome, metabolic abnormalities, neurological defects, a form of muscular dystrophy, and hemophilia. During the latter part of pregnancy, anmiocentesis may be done to determine the maturity of the unborn baby or to obtain fluid for examination in Rh incompatibility.

Some risks are involved—infection, hemorrhage, or miscarriage. But the complication rate is reported to be less than one percent. Ultrasound, which is done to locate the placenta, usually precedes amniocentesis and lessens the risk of complications. (See Genetic Counseling, page 362).

Biochemical tests The amounts of various substances in the pregnant woman's blood or urine or in the amniotic fluid can indicate fetal distress or growth retardation. For example, one particular substance, a hormone called *estriol* found in the mother's urine, increases as the fetus grows and decreases when growth stops providing a useful tool for measuring the fetus' rate of growth. Another test, on amniotic fluid, measures the maturity of the fetal lung tissue. Testing of other substances can identify such conditions as placental damage, cancer, or an ectopic pregnancy.

The availability of biochemical testing during the prenatal period makes it possible to anticipate problems that can occur during delivery. In some cases, medical intervention in the pregnancy may be necessary.

CHILDBIRTH

For most pregnant American women—more than 85 percent of them—childbirth will be normal. That is, they will have normal (vaginal) deliveries of normal, healthy babies. For these low-risk women, many childbirth options are available as to the method of delivery and the physical and human surroundings in which it takes place.

Managed vs. natural childbirth

There are two basic approaches to childbirth: managed and natural.

In managed childbirth, most decisions will be made by the obstetrician, birth is treated as a potentially hazardous event, medications are routinely used, and delivery is always in the hospital.

Natural childbirth developed as a reaction against what was felt to be a cold, clinical, drugged experience in managed birth. Natural childbirth allows the mother more responsibility and options in planning how and where to deliver. It also involves advance preparation on the part of the parents.

Answering the following questions may help you in deciding which would suit you more—managed or natural childbirth.

1. What would be your ideal childbirth experience? Would you want to be asleep or awake during delivery? Why? At home or in the hospital? Why? Who would be there?
2. Are you afraid of drug-free childbirth? Why? Of drugs and anesthesia? Why? What would help you overcome these fears?
3. Do hospitals frighten you or reassure you? Describe the best possible hospital experience for you. Would you prefer a small, private hospital, or a large training hospital with every facility? Do you want to be in the room alone or with other women? Do you want the baby in the room with you? Do you want your husband there frequently? Do you want many visitors? Who may come?

4. How important is it to you as a couple to share the birth experience? This is an important question. Some husbands do not want to be present, or are halfhearted about it. Some wives would rather not have their husbands there, even though it is unfashionable to admit this. You must both be honest in your answers. If you aren't sure how you feel, discuss it and explore it by seeing films and attending classes together.
5. How much time and effort are you willing to invest in motherhood? Full time? For how long? Do you want to continue a social life? Work? (Your decision about breast-feeding, is at issue here. For most women, breast-feeding means full-time motherhood in the first one to six months.)

–adapted from Dr. Silvia Feldman, *Choices in Childbirth*, Grosset and Dunlap, 1978.

After answering these questions and then exploring all the possibilities of both methods, you will be in a better position to choose which is best for you.

Although hospital births are still by far the most common (over 90 percent), natural childbirth methods are gaining in popularity.

Most natural methods involve breathing techniques, exercises, and active support from the husband. The methods are often known by the names of their originators—Lamaze, Dick-Read, Kitzinger, and Bradley, for example.

Choices can be investigated by discussing the alternatives with your doctor, or with childbirth educators in local hospitals, and by contacting local chapters of such organizations as the International Childbirth Education Association (ICEA) and the American Society for Psycho-Prophylaxis in Obstetrics (ASPO).

There are also decisions to be made as to *where* to have the baby, in addition to *how*. Choices in family-centered hospitals, for instance, include partner involvement in the birth, active support of breast-feeding, rooming in, early discharge, and liberal visiting privileges. Midwifery care and delivery are available in some hospitals and out-of-hospital centers. Birthing rooms (homelike rooms in which the couple stays during labor and delivery) and Leboyer delivery are two of the newer alternatives. In some communities, home birth and childbearing centers provide additional alternatives.

It is important for couples choosing natural childbirth to be aware that unforeseen complications can occur and that they should not feel guilty or inadequate if medications, and even induced or cesarean deliveries, become necessary to ensure a safe birth.

Although the great majority of women deliver without a problem, there are a number of risks involved in taking pain relievers and other medications commonly used during delivery. All types of anesthesia involve some risk—usually to the unborn baby. Because of the potential hazards of such medications, prospective parents should consider taking classes to prepare for a childbirth that will require the minimal amount of medication and anesthesia. *The childbirth setting that is chosen should be appropriate, medically safe, and acceptable.*

If you expect to have problems, you will probably prefer to have your baby in a setting that offers the most advanced clinical and technological assistance for labor and delivery. Instead of delivering at a local community hospital, you may prefer to give birth in a facility which has had a good deal of experience with complicated deliveries, usually at a large medical center.

In some labors requiring continuous medical supervision, electronic monitoring may also be necessary. Monitoring would probably be recommended for women with toxemia, diabetes, infections, or in premature labor, or with serious cardiac disease. Complications during labor such as fetal distress could also necessitate its use. In such cases, the uterine contractions and the fetal heart rate are monitored to assess the condition of the fetus.

Two methods of monitoring are used. External monitoring involves strapping devices to the woman's abdomen. In internal monitoring, the measuring devices are attached directly to the fetus and placed next to it within the uterus. Blood samples may be taken from the fetus via an internal tube. Both external and internal monitoring may be used during the same labor.

Monitoring has some risks and should be carefully considered before using. Various complications can occur such as infection, perforation, and fetal damage.

Other methods of delivery

If normal delivery is impossible, two alternative methods of delivery are commonly used: cesarean section and induced labor.

Cesarean section　A cesarean section (C-section) is the surgical removal of the infant through incisions made in the abdominal and uterine walls. In the 1970s, the C-section rate increased dramatically in the United States, inspiring much controversy about the necessity for this increase.

One controversy centers on the formerly standard practice of requiring a woman who has delivered once by cesarean section to have a cesarean delivery for all subsequent pregnancies. It is now known that many women who have delivered via cesarean section can deliver normally (vaginally) for future pregnancies. However, there is risk that the uterus might rupture.

Another unresolved issue is the method of delivering a woman whose baby is positioned upside down (breech) in the uterus. Because of the risks involved in delivering a breech baby, many physicians prefer to deliver by cesarean section.

For many other abnormal conditions of pregnancy, a C-section is the safest delivery method. This might be the case if there are placental abnormalities, a disproportion between the mother's pelvis and the unborn baby, or if the woman has a serious medical illness. The normal risks attached to surgery and anesthesia are involved, but a C-section is one of the safest of all operations.

Many organizations are available to help couples prepare for the C-section experience and share the birth together. (Consult local childbirth groups.) Films are available, discussion groups meet regularly, and some hospitals can arrange for the prepared father to be present at the birth.

Induced labor Labor can be initiated artificially, either by giving the woman a drug that stimulates the uterus to contract or by rupturing the membranes that surround the fetus. Sometimes both methods are used.

Certain conditions of either the mother or the fetus call for induction. For women with high blood pressure, other cardiovascular conditions, or diabetes, induction may prevent complications that could occur during normal labor. In fetal immaturity or postmaturity, if growth is delayed, or if defects are present, induction may be recommended. During induction, close monitoring is necessary.

There are risks, both to the fetus and to the woman, in inducing labor. The uterus may contract too much or too little. The woman may develop an infection. The fetus may be premature or be unable to withstand the stress of childbirth. Respiratory distress or metabolic complications may result. In some women, induction is not recommended.

An encouraging word

For most people, childbirth is a natural, healthy process and presents few risks. A healthful lifestyle, as described here and in the other chapters of this book, is the best preparation for parenthood.

There are many aspects of child-bearing not covered in this chapter. These have been covered amply in other publications and in material published by the following sources.

RESOURCES

Family Planning

Planned Parenthood Federation of America, Inc.
810 Seventh Avenue
New York, N.Y. 10019
(212) 541-7800

National Family Planning and Reproductive Health Association, Inc.
Suite 350
425 Thirteenth Street, N.W.
Washington, D.C. 20004
(202) 783-1560

American College of Obstetricians and Gynecologists
Resource Center
Suite 2700
1 East Wacker Drive
Chicago, Ill. 60601
(312) 222-1600

National Clearinghouse for Family Planning Information
6110 Executive Blvd., Suite 250
Rockville, Md. 29852
(301) 881-9400

Pregnancy and Infant Care

Office of Maternal and Child Health
Program Services Branch
Bureau of Community Health Services
Health Services Administration
Room 7A20, Parklawn
5600 Fishers Lane
Rockville, Md. 20857
(301) 443-4273

National Foundation—March of Dimes
Public Health Education Department
1275 Mamaroneck Avenue
White Plains, N.Y. 10605
(914) 428-7100

American College of Obstetricians and Gynecologists
Resource Center
Suite 2700
1 East Wacker Drive
Chicago, Ill. 60601
(312) 222-1600

American Academy of Pediatrics
1801 Hinman Avenue
Evanston, Ill. 60204
(312) 869-4255

ICEA
(International Childbirth Education Association, Inc.)
P.O. Box 20852
Milwaukee, Wis. 53220

For membership that includes subscription to *ICEA News*, and discounts on publications and meetings:

ICEA, Membership Clerk
195 Waterford Drive
Dayton, Ohio 45459

For catalogs of ICEA publications:

ICEA Publications Distribution Center
Box 9306 Midtown Plaza
Rochester, N.Y. 14604

P.E.P.
(Preparing Expectant Parents, Inc.)
Box 838
Pomona, Calif. 91769

Local Red Cross Chapters

NAPSAC
(National Association of Parents and Professional for Safe Alternatives in Childbirth)
Marble Hill, Mo. 63764

ASPO
(American Society for Psycho-Prophylaxis in Obstetrics)
(Lamaze method)
1523 L Street, N.W.
Washington, D.C. 20005

Institute for Childbirth and Family Research
2522 Dana Street
Berkeley, Calif. 94704

La Leche League International
(self-help information)
9616 Minneapolis Avenue
Franklin Park, Ill. 60131

American College of Obstetrics and Gynecology
(ACOG)
1 East Wacker Drive
Chicago, Ill. 60601

Cesarean Birth Association
125 North 12th Street
New Hyde Park, N.Y. 11040

C-Sec International
(for more information on cesareans)
15 Maynard Road
Dedham, Mass. 02026

Bradley Method
P.O. Box 5224
Sherman Oaks, Calif. 91413

American College of Nurse Midwives
1012 14th Street, N.W.
Washington, D.C. 20005

The National Midwives' Association
P.O. Box 163
Princeton, N.J. 08540

Home Birth Information:

Home-Oriented Maternity Experience
(HOME)
511 York Avenue
Takoma Park
Washington, D.C. 20012

The Association for Childbirth at Home, Inc.
(ACHI)
Box 1219
Cerritos, Calif. 90701

The American College of Home Obstetrics
664 North Michigan, Suite 600
Chicago, Ill. 60611

CHAPTER
7

Stress

To paraphrase Mark Twain, stress is what everybody talks about but nobody does much about. Medical science has difficulty even defining which stresses are "normal" and which are not. There's no question that too much stress, whether emotional or physical, weakens the body's defenses against disease. On the other hand, it is also apparent that in evolutionary terms stress has contributed to our development as human beings. Thus it is probably not a good idea to eliminate stress totally from our lives, even assuming that this were possible.

It should be possible, however, to create environments at home, at work, and in the community where stress is minimized. We should aim at this goal even though human beings are unlikely to achieve it in the foreseeable future. Since the reality of living necessarily involves stress, we should learn how to cope with it. Self-confidence and self-respect are both potent defenses against stress. Close links to family and friends, coworkers, and religious and community groups also provide essential support systems that help us cope with unavoidable crises in our lives.

Additional means of coping with the stress of modern living are also available. New techniques of meditation and biofeedback-monitored relaxation can be employed when we are alone with our stress. Indeed, stress can be managed with resources within ourselves and which we must learn to call upon.

Glossary

ADRENALINE An excitatory chemical produced by the adrenal glands, which plays a major role in the arousal of the human system.

DISTRESS "Bad stress" which taxes us beyond our coping limits and can contribute to our being ill.

EUSTRESS "Good stress" resulting from any change in the environment that causes us to adapt; it makes us forge ahead against obstacles.

FIGHT-OR-FLIGHT REACTION Also known as the emergency response or alarm reaction, this primitive bodily response provides the system with the extra energy and preparedness necessary to fight a situation or to flee from it. Some of the characteristics of the fight-or-flight reaction include muscular tension, increased blood pressure and heart rate, a sharpening of the senses, and the production of extra adrenaline.

GENERAL ADAPTATION SYNDROME A generalized arousal effect on the body produced by hormones. It is intended to stimulate bodily defense mechanisms against disease and thereby to increase the chances for survival through appropriate adaptation. It is characterized by an initial alarm reaction (the fight-or-flight reaction), a stage of resistance to disease, and, if unrelieved, a stage of exhaustion.

STRESS The nonspecific response of the body to any demand made upon it, i.e., the generalized arousal of the psychological and physical systems aimed at adapting to or coping with internal and external change.

STRESSOR The triggering event making demands upon the human system for psychological and physical adaptation.

STRESS-RELATED DISORDERS Also known as the "diseases of adaptation or of "coping," these are the functional disorders that result directly or indirectly from the chronic excitation of the stress response.

History and Definitions

Late in the nineteenth century, Charles Darwin's theory of natural selection and Edmund Spencer's concept of "survival of the fittest" focused attention on the idea that human survival involves adaptation to the "natural" demands of living. Physicians soon began to view illness as the result, in part, of man's perpetual struggle with social as well as natural forces.

Early in the twentieth century, the means by which humans and animals adapt to stress came under scientific study. In the United States, Walter Cannon studied the "fight-or-flight" phenomenon, an arousal reaction called forth in time of danger. This primitive response helps animals and humans to stand and fight or to flee the enemy and is therefore called an adaptive survival mechanism. Cannon observed animals under laboratory conditions that required them to adapt to such demands as cold, lack of sleep, and low oxygen. He noted that reactions to these conditions could be measured by the amount of certain hormones the animals produced.

Later in this century, Dr. Hans Selye, a stress physiologist, further documented Cannon's findings and coined the term *stress* for the nonspecific response of the body to any demand for adaptation made upon it. He defined stress as a General Adaptation Syndrome: "general" because it is produced by hormones that have an arousal effect on the entire body, "adaptive" because it stimulates body defense mechanisms and thus increases the chances of survival, "syndrome" because its individual manifestations are coordinated and interdependent. Stress involves an initial alarm reaction similar to Cannon's fight-or-flight reaction. This is followed by a stage of resistance to disease or recovery. Finally, if the organism is unable to adapt, there is a stage of exhaustion leading to death.

It is now agreed that the ability of a person to function physically, psychologically, and socially plays a role in both health and disease. Stress is a dynamic process of interaction between an individual and the physical, psychological, and social demands of living; it is not a single phenomenon but a continuing process. Stress is a response that occurs when there is a perception of threat (real or imagined): an expectation of future discomfort that arouses, alerts, or otherwise activates the human organism.

THE STRESS MECHANISM

The following will illustrate both the psychological and physical aspects of the stress response. Let us assume a mother's child gets caught under a heavy log on a camping trip. The mother perceives a threat that makes demands on her for an adaptive response. The most adaptive response is to remove the log (figure 7.1). She is able to do this with great alertness because messages from her brain, acting through the hypothalamus, stimulate the sympathetic (or excitatory) nerves and the pituitary gland. The pituitary gland triggers an outflow of adrenaline from the adrenal glands. In turn, this reaction stimulates the heart

and blood pressure and the muscles and the lungs, thereby improving blood flow, oxygen consumption, and strength. Simultaneously, this reaction activates the liver, spleen, and other organs, and inactivates others such as the digestive system. What the mother experiences is sharpened senses, muscular tension, heavy breathing, an increased heart rate, cold hands and feet (as the blood flow is redirected from the extremities to the deep muscles for greater strength and to the brain). Thus aroused, she is able to move the heavy log and rescue her infant.

In this example the stress response was adaptive and appropriate to the situation. In today's world the stressors are more often emotional ones rather than physical ones. Yet our body systems respond in the same way as the mother's did. If this intense response occurs constantly in our lives, our systems are subjected to undue wear-and-tear.

How much stress is good for us? Is it always better to have less stress? The demands of living, in fact, are all stressors. Stressors include everyday activities as well as unusual events or crises in our lives. Rushing to catch a train, entertaining guests, or shopping for Christmas are ordinary events that require us to readjust our lives for a short while and, thus, are stressors. Within this continually demanding environment we must rely upon our coping and adaptive skills in order to maintain an equilibrium between the status quo and change or growth. *Stress is an inherent quality of life, neither good nor bad in itself.*

MEASURING STRESS

What is important about stress is how we react to it. Whether you experience stress as good or bad depends on many factors among which are the nature of the demand, how you perceive it, the social context in which it is made, and the quality of support received from others. How you perceive the nature of the demand is, in turn, a

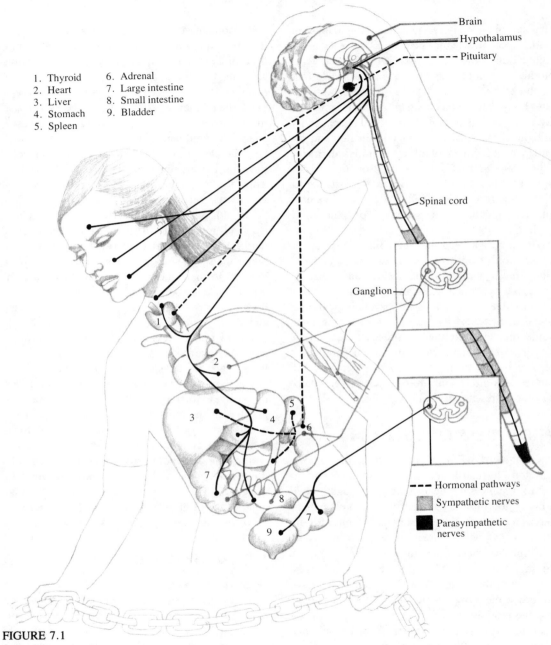

1. Thyroid
2. Heart
3. Liver
4. Stomach
5. Spleen
6. Adrenal
7. Large intestine
8. Small intestine
9. Bladder

Brain
Hypothalamus
Pituitary
Spinal cord
Ganglion

- - - Hormonal pathways
Sympathetic nerves
Parasympathetic nerves

FIGURE 7.1

The stress mechanism
SOURCE: *adapted from W. McNerney, et al,* Stress, *"Blue Print for Health," Vol. 25, No. 1, 1974, Blue Cross Association*

product of your genetic inheritance, your psychological and physical development, as well as your prior experiences. For any given set of stressors, each person will have a different interpretation and a different response.

When the response is appropriate, or adaptive, you experience eustress (good stress) and a sense of mastery, psychological well-being, and increased self-esteem. This positive feeling will, in turn, influence your attitude toward the next stressor and stimulate personal growth.

On the other hand, when your response is nonadaptive, it is experienced as distress (bad stress). If unrelieved by social support, relaxation techniques, or rest and recuperation, distress can become a chronic state. The emotional consequences of chronic distress are broad, including anxiety, tension, anger, helplessness, hopelessness, and depression. Nonadaptive physical changes caused by chronic distress include heightened blood pressure, increased muscle tension, and a raised heart rate and oxygen supply, all of which have no appropriate outlet.

These psychological and physiological responses interact to produce a self-perpetuating cycle of chronic distress. Locked into your distress, your ability to receive feedback and support from others is reduced and the chronic distress may become a prolonged distress syndrome, giving rise to various diseases of adaptation, or stress-related disorders.

In Table 7.1, a Social Readjustment Rating Scale charts the amount of stress involved in various events of living. Too many life changes (such as marriage, job changes, holidays, moving, etc.) within a short period often are followed by some form of physical illness in the ensuing year. We can adapt to only so much in a short period. The mediator seems to be stress.

Table 7.1, the Social Readjustment Rating Scale, provides a means of estimating your risk of undergoing a health change as a result of changes in your life. Each life event has been given a corresponding mean value, which is based on responses of thousands of persons who were asked to rate how much readjustment was required by various events in their lives. Death of a spouse requires the greatest amount of readjustment and, hence, has a mean value of 100. Getting married also requires significant readjustment, but the degree, duration, and severity of the readjustment is only half that demanded when a spouse dies; hence, marriage has a mean value of 50. To estimate your risk of a health change in the next 24 months or so, list the events in your life during the last year. There may be some that do not appear on this list—if so, assign them a value. Add up the mean values of each life event that occurred. The higher your score, the more likely you are to have a health change. If you score below 150 points, you have a one-in-three chance of serious health change in the next two years—fairly safe ground, considering today's complex world. Between 150 and 300 points, your chances rise to about 50–50. If you score more than 300 points, your chances are almost 90 percent.

What this rating system teaches is that we should try to space out those life events we can anticipate and control. Four job changes and remarriage following the death of a parent within two years may be too much to adapt to. Pace the timing of inevitable changes and regulate the occurrence of voluntary changes. Try to keep your yearly life-change score out of the danger zone.

Not all stressors of course are major life events. Any day-to-day activity that excites the emotions can also serve as a stressor. Table 7.2 lists the main categories of everyday stressors as reported by a group of people suffering chronic headache or anxiety. As you review this table, consider what your typical day is like. When you experience one of these stressors, try using one of the stress management techniques outlined in this chapter (see page 406). You cannot, nor should you wish to, avoid daily stressors. However, you can learn new ways of adapting to them.

Table 7.1
THE SOCIAL READJUSTMENT RATING SCALE

Life event	Mean value
1. Death of spouse	100
2. Divorce	73
3. Marital separation	65
4. Jail term	63
5. Death of close family member	63
6. Personal injury or illness	53
7. Marriage	50
8. Fired from job	47
9. Marital reconciliation	45
10. Retirement	45
11. Change in health of family member	44
12. Pregnancy	40
13. Sex difficulties	39
14. Gain of new family member	39
15. Business readjustment	39
16. Change in financial state	38
17. Death of close friend	37
18. Change to different line of work	36
19. Change in number of arguments with spouse	35
20. Mortgage over $10,000	31
21. Foreclosure of mortgage or loan	30
22. Change in responsibilities at work	29
23. Son or daughter leaving home	29
24. Trouble with in-laws	29
25. Outstanding personal achievement	28
26. Wife begins or stops work	26
27. Begin or end school	26
28. Change in living conditions	25
29. Revision of personal habits	24
30. Trouble with boss	23
31. Change in work hours or conditions	20
32. Change in residence	20
33. Change in schools	20
34. Change in recreation	19
35. Change in church activities	19
36. Change in social activities	18
37. Mortgage or loan less than $10,000	17
38. Change in sleeping habits	16
39. Change in number of family get-togethers	15
40. Change in eating habits	15
41. Vacation	13
42. Christmas	12
43. Minor violations of the law	11

SOURCE: adapted from Holmes, T. H. and Rahe, R. H. "The Social Readjustment Rating Scale" *Journal of Psychosomatic Research* 11:213–218 (1967).

Table 7.2
DAILY STRESSORS

Work related (47% of all daily stressors)

1. Monotonous, repetitive tasks such as assembly line work, clerical, or typing jobs
2. Work-related meetings
3. Daily deadline pressure
4. A discussion with the boss
5. Taking and making work-related phone calls

Friendships (accounts for 14% of all daily stressors)

1. Argument with opposite sex (boyfriend or girlfriend)
2. Waiting for a friend who is late
3. Anger over an interpersonal event
4. Arguments with friends
5. Socializing with a group of friends

Home responsibilities (accounts for 10% of all daily stressors)

1. Doing housework (cooking, cleaning, etc.) after a full day's work
2. Shopping (especially when crowded)
3. Machinery (heater, auto, etc.) not working
4. Short-run financial concerns

Traveling (accounts for 9% of all daily stressors)

1. Riding the bus, train, or subway
2. Transportation delay on either side of a commute
3. Driving a car
4. Rushing to be somewhere on time
5. Being stuck in a traffic jam

Educational (accounts for 7% of daily stressors)

1. Being in class
2. Studying, reading, etc. (homework)
3. Taking a test
4. Asking questions in class
5. Teaching others in a class

Family (accounts for 5% of daily stressors)

1. Visiting relatives
2. Worrying about an offspring
3. Playing with and/or caring for an offspring after a day's work
4. Argument with your spouse
5. Scolding an offspring

Miscellaneous (accounts for 8% of daily stressors)

1. Insomnia for 30 minutes or less due to your thinking about the day's activities
2. Going to the doctor or dentist
3. Being alone and feeling lonely

SOURCE: adapted from J. Manuso, "Executive Stress Management," *The Personnel Administrator*, pp. 23–26, November, 1979.

RESPONSE PATTERNS

The fight-or-flight response is an automatic survival response, stirring both new and primitive areas of the brain. As we have seen, in this response increases in heart rate take place, the respiratory rate rises, and blood pressure increases, while the shunting of blood flow to muscles and away from other organs occurs. The result is the improvement of the entire musculoskeletal system and enhancement of the ability to fight or to run away from the enemy. In animals this acute response usually lasts about one hour after the threat has passed; the animal then returns to normal and replenishes the energy expanded. This is a highly adaptive system where acute, brief responses are required, as in true emergencies, such as jumping out of the way of an oncoming car.

In modern man and woman, however, the "enemy" or the threat is not always so easily discernible, and the mere memory of the danger can call forth a prolonged response persisting long after the perceived danger has abated. Such chronic "emergency" response patterns may bring on the development of low back pain (prolonged muscle tension), or insomnia (prolonged arousal), to mention two possibilities. The body's immune system, which helps avoid and combat disease, is also affected by the fight-or-flight response. Because the body's resources are continually strained in responding to stress, it cannot always fight disease effectively.

Chronic stress cannot be dispelled by the normal processes of rest and recuperation. Scientists are aware that anxiety, stress, and fatigue can work hand-in-hand to prevent recuperation. A very high work load is stressful and fatiguing, but the feeling of fatigue is delayed because there is no time to be tired during working hours. The anxiety component in this syndrome would most likely interfere with rest and recuperation after the actual event, leading to further fatigue and distress.

In short, the human distress response is generalized and involves the entire system of psychological and biological emergency mechanisms. Chronic distress makes an abnormal demand on the energy resources of the system. The degree of chronic distress depends primarily on the duration of the stress response, not necessarily on the duration of the stressful event. How we react and not what we react to is the important factor. Distress, a demand response, strains the physical and psychological coping capacity of the individual producing disturbances not only in functioning, but in the normally recuperative processes of sleep and rest as well.

Health Effects

It is well recognized today that stress is an important contributor to disease. Physicians in general practice estimate that one-half to three-fourths of all their patients come seeking relief from stress-related symptoms. In fact, the President's Commission on Mental Health found that one out of every four Americans is suffering "severe emotional stress" although no diagnosable physical illness is present.

Health effects that may be stress-induced are difficult to diagnose because one cannot always determine whether the stress preceded or followed the health effects. If you have a specific disease, you are likely to recall past stressful events differently than someone without such an illness. Also, stress often leads to increased consumption of alcohol, drugs, and smoking which themselves contribute to disease. We need to keep these aspects in mind while reviewing the following common disorders that may or may not be stress-related.

HEADACHE

Half the people who go to a doctor for medical advice report having headaches as one of their symptoms. Headache has many types and many causes. One factor that seems to be present in many of them, however, is stress.

Tension headaches

The most common type of chronic headache is the tension headache, also known as the muscle contraction or "psychogenic" headache. Whatever it's called, it feels the same: a persistent, dull, squeezing ache in the head, neck, or shoulders, beginning and ending gradually. Occasionally, there are sudden jabs of pain. Tension headaches may last for hours, or even weeks, or months, but are not usually accompanied by any physical symptoms other than stiffness in the neck or clenching of the jaw.

Stress is responsible for most tension headaches. A person under stress reacts physically with the fight-or-flight response that involves, among other things, tensing of muscles. Although the body is well-suited to coping with this reaction on a short-term basis, when the stress persists and the muscle contraction is relentless, the nerve nets in the head begin to register pain.

The best approaches to the prevention of muscle contraction headaches are: (1) remove the apparent environmental causes or remove oneself from them; (2) learn to cope better with the causes through stress-reduction techniques and/or psychotherapy. Neck and shoulder exercises, consisting of alternate tightening and relaxing of muscles, can relieve some of the pain, although the headache usually has to run its course.

Migraine

Unlike tension headaches, chronic migraine headaches throb and pulse, and tend to be associated with nausea, blurry vision, vomiting, and loss of appetite. Usually the pain is on one side. Most patients seen by physicians for migraine are women, and there is some evidence linking it to hormone levels. It is thought that the condition may worsen at menopause, with the use of oral contraceptives, or around the time of menstruation. It often disappears during pregnancy.

Migraine headaches often involve a hereditary predisposition. In persons with this predisposition, stress can cause constriction of the brain's arteries (the pre-headache phase). This is followed by a sudden dilation or opening up of portions of these arteries (the headache phase). The dilation stretches the nerve endings that encircle the arteries, causing the pain.

CHRONIC NECK AND BACK PAIN

Neck and back pain often may be a symptom of physical illness, but it is sometimes caused by a chronic stress response. Recall that one of the major features of the stress response is bracing or muscle tension in anticipation of fighting or fleeing. In modern society we no longer fight or flee in the face of daily events, but we nevertheless experience the muscle tension of the stress response. How often have you heard the expression, "Brace yourself!" Chronically bracing in response to daily stressor events builds up lactic acid in the muscles and causes reflex spasms. This is experienced as pain.

Sometimes we have a painful illness and, by bracing, we increase the pain. Lower back pain is often referred to as a "headache that slipped down the back." Many people have neck and shoulder pain, which is also related to bracing efforts. Relaxation techniques can be useful in helping people alleviate chronic pain related to incorrect bracing efforts.

GASTROINTESTINAL DISORDERS

Peptic ulcer

One of the public's most widely held beliefs is that stress can give you ulcers. While this notion lacks solid proof, there is some evidence that suggests it might be true.

Some research suggests that people with certain personality characteristics may be prone to developing ulcers. In one study psychoanalysts were able to pick which male patients had an ulcer, as opposed to some other disease, simply on the basis of a psychiatric interview. But this type of study cannot determine whether the psychological characteristics that were noticed had truly caused the ulcers, or whether the ulcers were a result of some other cultural (see chapter 4, Tobacco), environmental, or dietary factor, or whether the psychological differences were simply the result of a reaction to having the ulcer.

No stress reduction technique has been shown to be useful in either the treatment or the prevention of peptic ulcers.

Ulcerative colitis

Ulcerative colitis is a disease of the large intestine that typically is associated with symptoms of diarrhea and rectal bleeding. Its cause remains a mystery, despite intensive study. The belief that stress contributes to ulcerative colitis has waxed and waned over the years.

During the first half of this century ulcerative colitis achieved a reputation as a classic psychosomatic disease. It is still so regarded by many psychiatrists, although their supporting evidence does not meet modern standards of scientific proof. The early theory held that victims of ulcerative colitis have personalities susceptible to stress. In the late sixties and early seventies new studies found that those with ulcerative colitis were no more anxious or psychologically abnormal than others. Stress is not now considered to be a significant cause of ulcerative colitis.

Irritable bowel syndrome

Irritable bowel syndrome rivals the common cold as a leading cause of absenteeism from work. Symptoms include abdominal pain, constipation, or diarrhea, which almost always occurs during the day, rarely at night. Unlike ulcerative colitis, irritable bowel syndrome is never life-threatening, and people with this disorder have normal intestines. The syndrome usually begins its irregular course in adolescence or early adulthood.

There are two overall patterns the irritable bowel syndrome usually follows. The first, spastic colon (also known as spastic colitis) is characterized by lower abdominal pain often accompanied by constipation and small stools. People who react to emotional arousal with hostility, tension, and defensiveness may be more prone to spastic colon than others. The second pattern is painless diarrhea, also known as nervous diarrhea or mucous colitis. People who react to emotional arousal by expressing hopelessness, helplessness, and defeat may be more likely to experience painless diarrhea. Obviously, not all victims fit neatly into one or the other of these patterns.

For some people stressful emotions are an important cause of this syndrome. Attacks often occur after major stressors in their lives. Compared with others, people with irritable bowel syndrome are more likely to be anxious, depressed, and to have experienced stressful events. However, all the studies that established this association leave open the possibility that these psychological symptoms are a result rather than a cause of the disorder. Some experiments have shown that changes in the activity of the intestine may be as much a part of emotional reactions as crying.

Why only some people react to stress with colonic symptoms is a question that remains unanswered. For example, some people with the syndrome have colons that are particularly sensitive to various drugs and painful stimuli. The role of this sensitivity is unknown as are its causes, although emotional makeup may indeed be a factor.

There is no known medical therapy that is effective with irritable bowel syndrome; stress reduction techniques may have the potential to help. So, too, may regular exercise.

CANCER

Different cancers have different causes, many of which relate to environmental factors. Among the risk factors associated with cancer are cigarette smoking, alcohol abuse, radiation exposure, diet and exposure to certain chemicals (see chapters 2, Alcohol, 4, Tobacco, 13, Radiation, and 16, Occupational Health).

Stress certainly can increase the risk of getting cancer if it causes you to smoke more cigarettes, or if it prevents you from kicking the habit, or if it causes you to increase your exposure to any other factor thought to cause cancer. Scientific studies so far undertaken have not been able to link stress directly with cancer.

Some researchers feel, however, that there are two stress factors that increase the chances of cancerous growth. One is brain activity that depresses the immune system, thereby decreasing the body's innate ability to fight cancer. The other is brain activity that creates hormonal imbalances. More work still needs to be done in this area before any definitive claims can be made that stress is a primary causative factor in the development of any cancer.

CORONARY HEART DISEASE

Sir William Osler, a noted physician, commented as long as seventy years ago that in addition to the hereditary factor and a rich diet, the typical patient with coronary disease was a "keen and ambitious man, the indicator of whose engines is always set at 'full speed ahead.'" Most doctors can recite instances of a patient who, at an exciting ball game or upon receiving stressful news, has suddenly suffered severe chest pain and a heart attack. Surprisingly, such evidence rarely has been formally evaluated in a controlled scientific study.

Debate continues to focus on whether stress per se directly increases the risk of heart attack or whether stress affects traditional risk factors such as lipids, blood pressure, and smoking, all of which in turn promote the development of cardiovascular disease (see chapter 1, Nutrition, and chapter 4, Tobacco). Studies of medical students during examinations and of accountants at tax time have shown that blood cholesterol rises during such times of stress.

Stress-prone personalities

In a famous study, Drs. Ray H. Rosenman and Meyer Friedman developed a classification system dividing people into "Type A" and "Type B" personalities. They pointed out that the highly stressed Type A people have higher cholesterol levels than Type Bs.

Type A behavior is characterized by an excessive sense of time urgency, a well-developed competitive drive, a propensity to meet deadlines, and a high degree of impatience. These people always take their work home with them. They try to do two things at once and are superachievers needing to reassure themselves of their value. In contrast, Type B people chronically arrive late, never meet a deadline, and are not generally tense; they sit and talk with relaxed hands and no twitches. It is also possible that the stressed, Type A person is self-indulgent and overeats, which in the fat-rich American environment leads to increased lipid levels in the blood. Most Type A people tend to smoke more than Type Bs. The rate of blood clotting is accelerated in Type As, and the stimulation of their autonomic nervous system also appears to be accelerated. However, they do not appear to have significantly increased blood pressure.

(While it is true that stress can temporarily raise blood pressure in the fight-or-flight reaction, this is an acute response and does not lead to a chronic elevation of blood pressure. In other words, there is no tension in hypertension. Most people probably feel that having hypertension means they are tense. However, hypertension simply means "high blood pressure.")

Does stress actually play a role in health beyond its impact on the standard risk factors? Several recent studies indicate that the highly stressed, Type A person has about a two to three times greater risk of a heart attack than the Type B individual. In most of these studies the increased risk could not be completely explained by the higher cholesterol level and increased smoking behavior found in the Type A person. Some other element in this personality type appeared to increase risk.

The cardiovascular impact of stress is not uniform for everybody. Blue collar workers appear to be affected more than white collar workers. Among women, the risk of heart attack remains the same, whether she works or stays at home, or whether she is a Type A or a Type B. However, the woman who is married to a blue collar worker and works as a clerk or secretary for an insensitive boss has an increased risk of heart attack.

In addition to the stress imposed by competition, job dissatisfaction, and excessive time urgency, there is some evidence that increased social and geographical mobility, loss of a sense of social cohesiveness, low job status, and overloads that exceed coping capacity also exert increased tension on individuals.

Whether it is possible to reduce stress by converting the Type A to a Type B is largely unknown. The few studies attempting to make these transformations are still too preliminary to suggest that great success can be achieved. In view of this, the main advantage of identifying highly stressed persons lies in urging them to make other efforts to reduce the risk of heart attack. Everyone who has anything to do with improving the health of such persons should insist that they pay even greater attention to controlling traditional risk factors such as high blood cholesterol, high blood pressure, cigarette smoking, overweight, and lack of physical activity. In many instances the Type A will do especially well in controlling these risk factors because it is in the nature of the Type A to work diligently to achieve success. They may tend to overdo in this area as well. Type As could benefit from learning how to pace themselves—how to manage their time in such a way as to allow for more frequent respites.

GYNECOLOGICAL DISORDERS

The menstrual cycle

Although the relationship between menstruation and stress has long been accepted, the progression from superstition and anecdotes to case studies and clinical research has been slow. Nevertheless, stress is thought to be linked with gynecological problems. For one thing, the menstrual cycle itself causes stress. Since there are sex differences in the hormonal response to stress, it is reasonable to suppose that the menstrual cycle, with its accompanying hormonal changes, should also be susceptible to the effects of stress. Many women have had the experience of a late or skipped menstrual period immediately after a stressful change in life, but there is very little information on the effects of stress on menstrual disorders. This may be due to the difficulties of evaluating cause-and-effect relationships.

The symptoms of premenstrual depression include psychological ones such as tension, anxiety, depression, irritability, and insomnia, as well as headaches, dizziness, nausea and vomiting, increased frequency of asthmatic attacks, and extreme water retention and edema. Dysmenorrhea (painful menstruation) and premenstrual depression are separate disorders, although they may occur together. Research shows that stress is one of the multiple causes of dysmenorrhea. Premenstrual depression, on the other hand, is an example of a physical change causing a psychological reaction. In fact, emotional disturbances are often exacerbated during a woman's premenstrual time.

It is difficult to determine the severity of menstrual depression, elation, or irritability before deciding whether the use of drugs can be justified. All that can be stated with certainty is that many menstrual cycle hormonal changes cause many behavioral changes. What treatment, if any, to employ is a matter of trial and error.

Amenorrhea, or the cessation of menstruation for reasons other than normal menopause, has been related to severe environmental stress. For example, women imprisoned in concentration camps showed a high incidence of amenorrhea, which could only be partially accounted for by poor nutrition. However, it also occurs in dancers or athletes who are extremely physically active (see chapter 5, Physical Activity).

Miscarriage

Repeated miscarriages have in some cases been correlated with a low tolerance for frustration and conflict, sex identification problems, and emotional instability. Psychotherapy has increased normal births in this group.

Pregnancy

In labor itself, pain is an obvious stressor. The attitude and performance of nurses and physicians have been found to exert a profound influence on the degree of stress reported in labor.

One researcher found that women who experienced many life changes both before and during pregnancy were twice as likely to have complications such as premature births, prolonged labor, breech births, and miscarriages.

Infertility

Infertility, or the inability to conceive within one year (as opposed to sterility or the total inability to conceive), long has been related to psychological conflict such as uncertainty over the desirability of pregnancy or a lack of sexual satisfaction. However, age is a more common cause of infertility than anxiety, with women over thirty-five often experiencing difficulty in conceiving. There appears to be only circumstantial evidence linking infertility to stress.

EPILEPSY

More than one million Americans have repeated seizures and are considered "epileptics." These seizures may consist of convulsions or they may be disturbances in sensory awareness, unconsciousness, or some combination of these. Despite the magnitude of this problem, the cause or causes of the seizures are yet to be identified. The role of stress in exacerbating seizures is still uncertain. Emotions may sometimes play a role but estimates of how much vary widely.

Biofeedback has been used successfully as a treatment technique for certain types of epilepsy. By using biofeedback equipment that tells patients what their brain wave patterns look like from moment to moment, the patients learn to normalize their brain wave patterns to some extent and to control the frequency of seizures.

ASTHMA

Asthma is a common and potentially serious disease. The characteristics of an asthmatic attack are wheezing and difficult breathing, caused primarily by a spasm of the lungs' passageways. While asthma is most common in early childhood, it can start in middle age as well. The disease frequently disappears spontaneously; about three-fourths of all asthmatic children outgrow it by age thirteen. However, it may recur after many symptom-free years. In the United States, 2 to 5 percent of school children below the ages of twelve or fifteen have asthma.

The causes of asthma are largely unknown. Allergic reactions, drugs, tobacco smoke, physical exercise, and emotionally upsetting events can precipitate an attack. But no one factor can account for the course of asthma. One theory of asthma is that people who hold in their anger under stress do not increase their adrenaline flow even though their bodies continue to reflect the stress. Their air passageways then contract, causing them to wheeze.

If this theory is true, then some asthmatic attacks would appear to be under partial voluntary control. Indeed, it has been reported that people can "think themselves into asthma." One study investigated this phenomenon by spraying asthmatics with a substance to which, they were told, they were allergic; but which, in fact, was inert. Half of them showed a narrowing of the airways in their lungs and more than a quarter of them had asthmatic attacks. This demonstrates the importance of one's perception of events in triggering symptoms.

There are several possibilities for prevention of asthma by stress reduction. Obviously, one is to stay away from stressful situations. However, this often is not practical or desirable. Other methods for which success has been claimed include hypnosis by a professional, self-hypnosis, behavior therapy, biofeedback, group therapy, family therapy, and individual psychotherapy. None of these methods has been subjected to rigorous experimentation for efficacy, but group and family therapy have produced the most dramatic results. All these preventive tools should be used in conjunction with whatever medical treatment is indicated. Asthma is not purely a psychosomatic disease. Most cases have an allergic component.

DIABETES MELLITUS

Scientific evidence suggests that stress is intimately linked with both the onset and the course of diabetes mellitus. It is a disorder of carbohydrate metabolism, and is the result of poor insulin function or utilization. In adults it often results from overnutrition (see chapter 1, page 135). The insufficient amount of insulin or the ineffectiveness of the insulin produced may be due to the interference of hormones produced by the pituitary, adrenal, or thyroid glands, which are active in the stress response (see figure 7.1).

The primary result of diabetes is hyperglycemia, or too much glucose in the blood. Research on nondiabetic patients indicates that stress such as that experienced in starvation, infection, or emotional trauma leads to a delay in the disposal of carbohydrates in the body. This delay results in an undue elevation of blood glucose level. However, the nondiabetic's glucose levels generally return to normal following the removal of the stressor. This may not happen in the diabetic. Thus, stress often is treated as a factor precipitating symptoms of an already dormant condition rather than a direct causal factor. Attempts to define the diabetic personality have been inconclusive.

Appropriate treatment for diabetes requires medical supervision and appropriate insulin dosages. More research is needed before definitive statements can be made regarding the onset and course of this illness as it relates to stress.

MENTAL ILLNESS

The primary question in mental illness is why some persons remain healthy and why others get sick when exposed to the same stressors. The answer seems to be in the interaction of a variety of factors: the nature of the stressor, an individual's susceptibility based on his or her genetic predisposition or early environmental influences, behavioral practices, available social supports, and the health care system.

Depression

The many determinants of mental dysfunction are best observed in depressive illness. Common situations such as bereavement can produce temporary disturbances indistinguishable from depression. Depression often is characterized by a variety of physical symptoms such as poor appetite and weight loss or increased appetite and weight gain, sleeping too little or too much, fatigue, and immoderate tearfulness or crying.

Patients with depressive disorders often report the loss of a loved one as an important factor, whereas patients with anxiety disorders are more likely to report problems with test or job performance. This is an important distinction because many depressed patients also suffer a great deal of anxiety. Psychological symptoms of depression include restlessness, irritability, guilt, poor concentration and short-term memory, social withdrawal, pessimism, loss of interest in pleasurable activities such as sex, feelings of hopelessness, worthlessness, and suicidal thoughts. The predominant role of agitation in depression has to be distinguished from anxiety, which requires different treatment.

Manic-depressive illness, where people experience mania (excitation), depression, or an alternating combination of these moods in the extreme has a strong genetic component, and usually is not the result of stress. However, psychological stressors can serve as triggers.

Stress can have delayed effects, as in the case of a young child losing a parent. Such children often experience frequent and severe depression and psychological stress when they reach adulthood.

Schizophrenia

Schizophrenia, a thought disorder that distorts perception of reality and is characterized by disjointed thoughts and feelings, appears to be strongly influenced by genetic predisposition but not by stress factors. Studies show that children of schizophrenic parents who are adopted and raised by normal families experience the same frequency of the disorder as children raised by their schizophrenic parents. Here again psychological stressors may serve as triggers, though they are not necessary.

Anxiety disorders

Once referred to as "neuroses," anxiety disorders include phobias, hypochondria, nonpsychotic depression, and generalized anxiety. They are often developed and maintained by a poorly managed stress response.

Fear of flying is an example. First, people with this phobia perceive a danger. Whenever they think about flying, the fight-or-flight stress response is aroused. Because this is nonadaptive, they begin to avoid thinking about or being anywhere near flying in order to avoid the discomfort of the nonadaptive stress response. The more they avoid flying, the greater becomes the fear. If not addressed, phobias can exert strong influences over behavior. Such irrational fears often can be successfully treated through behavior modification.

The anxiety disorders include many reactions. Some, such as the obsessive-compulsive and generalized anxiety disorders, are thought to be influenced by genetic predisposition. However, the likelihood of their occurring most often depends on the stressors exerting demands for adaptation. As was mentioned earlier, distress occurs when there are demands on you which tax or exceed your adjustive resources. Which response is brought forth, whether phobia or depression, depends on your experience and genetic predisposition.

SUICIDE

Suicide, the tenth most common cause of death in the United States, occurs throughout the life cycle, the rate progressively rising with increasing age. Approximately 25,000 to 50,000 deaths per year are attributed to suicide, although the number of attempted suicides may run as high as 250,000 per year.

Since the 1960s, the incidence of suicide has increased to epidemic proportions. The suicide rate for teenagers (ages fourteen to nineteen), doubled between 1960 and 1970, as did the rate for men in their twenties. Among women in their twenties, the rates quadrupled during those years.

The dramatic changes in physiology, personal responsibility, and social role which take place during adolescence have always made adolescence a period of high stress in modern societies. The breakdown of the traditionally supportive family and church, and the encouragement of immediate gratification through "fly now, pay later" values, along with our permissive attitudes toward alcohol and drug abuse have dovetailed at this critical stage of life to produce the epidemic of suicide in adolescents.

To stem the epidemic will require a massive educational effort to assist young people to prepare for the rigorous demands and responsibilities of adult life, of marriage, and parenthood. Improvement of their communication and conflict resolution skills is necessary in order that they may survive the emotional turbulence of adolescence.

The risk of successful suicide is three times greater for men than for women, presumably because women attempt suicide by means of less lethal methods (pills and wrist slashing versus guns and hanging). Marriage seems to protect against suicide while divorce and widowhood seem to increase the risk.

Additional factors include a previous suicide attempt, a family history of suicide, a recent major loss (loved one, relationship, job, limb), alcohol and drug abuse, unsympathetic and conflict-ridden relationships, and a failure to recognize the need for professional help in the presence of persisting and disabling psychiatric symptoms. Social and psychological stresses may precipitate, complicate, and perpetuate suicidal risk by contributing to the nonrecognition of psychiatric illnesses, including alcoholism.

Depressive illness is the most frequent psychiatric diagnosis associated with suicide (50 percent). Character disorders (30 percent) follow with schizophrenic illnesses (20 percent) also of significant impact. Symptoms of depression occur in almost all suicidal patients and include:

- disturbances of appetite, sleep, energy, sexual drive, concentration
- feelings of hopelessness and helplessness
- morbid thoughts, anxiety, fears, pessimism, guilt, and sad or depressed moods
- increase of alcohol or other drug consumption
- uncontrollable crying fits or lack of ability to cry
- misperceptions of the intentions of others
- withdrawal

Failure to control symptoms through self-medication or willpower may create a sense of guilt and despair; these feelings can be heightened when others criticize the depressed person's nonfunctioning or attempt to minimize his or her distress. Advice to work, socialize, or "feel happy," well meant as it may be, will only deepen the sense of helplessness and guilt and heighten the need to escape, which may evolve into a brief and self-limited tension state lasting several days, during which the potential suicide may seem to be improving.

As far as treatment goes, potential suicides may be usefully divided into three categories:

- those with acute depressive illness who make the most serious suicide attempts, and require treatment with antidepressant medication, electroshock therapy, and possibly hospitalization
- those without serious psychiatric illness but with long-standing interpersonal conflicts who can benefit from psychotherapy and efforts to reduce these conflicts and discrepant attitudes between themselves and others about their difficulties
- a socially isolated group including chronic schizophrenics, alcoholics, and the elderly who must be brought into the mainstream of medical care through outreach and follow-up programs

No matter what program is followed, it is important that suicidal people and their families recognize the person's needs for treatment and reduction of responsibilities. It must be understood that improvement generally follows a zigzag course, and that the recurrence of symptoms does not usually mean a relapse has occurred. Families and potential suicides should know that proper medication can relieve much of the suicide drive rapidly, economically, and in a relatively simple way, but must be taken in adequate doses for a reasonable period of time, and that individual psychotherapy, family therapy, or cognitive skills training (Life Strategy Workshops) can reduce conflicts at home by helping to change the division of responsibilities among the members more in line with their particular skills, needs, and temperaments.

Handling a suicidal crisis on the telephone or in person

Dr. Ari Kiev suggests the following in dealing with a potentially suicidal person:

Don't panic. Talk calmly and reasonably.

Keep the lines of communication open. The person wanted someone to talk to and needs to know that you understand how he or she feels.

Focus on the problem. Don't get sidetracked. Find out what precipitated the crisis. Try to get the person to externalize the problem by putting it into a realistic perspective.

Identify the loss. Was the precipitating event the loss of a spouse, friend, job, position, status, or what? Empathize, but try to put the loss into realistic perspective.

Latch on to the will to live. Remember, a potential suicide is ambivalent; *part of the individual doesn't want to die.* Something the person says will most likely give you the opportunity to point out that "part of you wants to live."

Don't get into a debate. Don't argue the merits of life versus suicide. In particular, don't get trapped into answering a question like, "Give me one good reason why I should go on living." Any answer you can give to such a question will be shot down. Avoid platitudes like, "Life is so wonderful" or "You have everything to live for." These comments, although well-meant, will only convince the person that you don't really understand how he or she feels.

Be supportive. Look for the person's positive, attractive qualities and previous successes, however small, in order to evoke his or her awareness of alternatives.

Suggest feasible options. Suggest some objective that can be easily accomplished to break the cycle of defeat and provide an avenue for achievement and a sense of mastery over the situation.

Don't give direct advice. Encourage the person to make his or her own choices.

For information about suicide prevention programs that can be helpful in assisting people cope with the early stages of suicidal crisis, check your local telephone book, the nearest medical school, or the county medical society. You may also write to the Social Psychiatry Research Institute, 150 East 69th Street, New York, New York 10021, for more detailed information and for a free booklet, *Guidelines for Friends and Relatives of Psychiatric Patients*.

Stress Management and Prevention

PERSPECTIVE ON STRESS

The following overview on dealing with stress is by Herbert Spiegel, M.D. Modern medicine puts such extreme emphasis on high technology and the use of drugs that it often overlooks the oldest and, at times, the most effective therapeutic instrument that people possess—the mind.

Stress by itself has a potential for self-sabotage on the one hand, or growth and expansion on the other. When the executive style of a person is faulty or inept in a given situation, the resulting misdirection of the stress leads to frustration, self-impairment or counterproductive activity expressing itself in tension which has been associated with a wide variety of psychosomatic diseases.

However, when the person's executive judgment is competent and able more or less to synchronize inner expectations with the outer context of stimuli, experiencing events as a series of challenges, stress can serve to stimulate the imagination. Stress may offer an opportunity to apply experiences of the past to new situations and occasionally may help one see new connections in an inventive or creative way. In this sense, stress can be a desirable asset leading to growth, exhilaration, and a sense of well-being.

A prevalent error that many people commit in coping with stress is to assume that the only way to negotiate with stress is to fight it. Fighting stress, however, only aggravates the tension and is self-defeating. A more effective approach to resolving the tension and its symptoms is a deceptively simple one. Accentuate the positive. That is, restructure your perspective by focusing upon what you are for rather than what you are against. By consciously and deliberately planning your daily life emphasizing respect for your body, observing proper eating habits, using alcohol moderately or not at all, not smoking, and taking appropriate physical exercise, you can generate a continuous affirmation of yourself and life, which not only avoids tension but simultaneously transforms the daily stresses of everyday life into expressive and, at times, creative living.

Centuries ago, Aristotle proposed a plan for a healthy and satisfied life. Aristotle proposed a balance among work (to earn food and shelter), sleep (to reconstitute one's energy), play (the pursuit of an activity for the simple joy and relaxation of it without deep meaning or significance), and leisure. By leisure Aristotle envisaged an interest that stimulates one's curiosity, imagination, and inventiveness, possibly, but not necessarily, leading to an innovative or creative experience. These elements—work, sleep, play, and leisure—balanced together can, with a little luck, be the ideal way to convert anxiety into that productive stress which yields a sense of living well.

If and when this effort fails, then adopting the more formal techniques and exercises elaborated in this chapter is the choice of last resort. A variety of techniques are available to help you respond to stressors more effectively. Many of them involve learning to recognize your own response patterns and then learning new ones. The main point is that you can learn to affect your own health in a positive manner. Self-regulation of stress response is not easily learned. It requires considerable time and effort. Try working with one method at a time and don't expect miracles the first week. Living is synonymous with stress as we adapt, change, and interact with the demands of life from moment to moment. *It is the inability to cope with stress—adequately and over time—that produces distress.*

The techniques described below for preventing distress share two goals: diminishing the stress response and the time required to reestablish a balanced state and increasing the ability to perceive real danger, thereby adjusting the intensity and type of response required for survival. Both techniques embrace social changes that can alter the intensity and quality of stressors, and both techniques emphasize improvement of individual attitudes and coping skills.

PRESCRIPTIONS FOR STRESS MANAGEMENT

It should be clear by now that stress management involves complex attitudes, social and psychological practices, as well as specific behaviors. There are no single, simple answers. You must find out what works best for you. For example, if you experience mainly psychological stress, some of the mental techniques reviewed here may be most appropriate for you. If, on the other hand, your stress response is primarily physical, some of the deep relaxation techniques may be preferable. Think about how your stress management techniques fit into the situations outlined below. Which ones work best for you? How can you refine them?

The individual

Most people are not aware of their own behavior. They know very little about how they operate, or what their defenses are. As a result, they do not fully recognize their own stress responses, and are not aware when a stress overload begins. Once you have learned how you behave, you can choose the stress load that is appropriate for you. It is also imperative to learn a method of self-regulation of the stress response to help you in achieving and maintaining low levels of arousal. These methods can break the sequence of the stress response and avoid the cumulative effects of stress.

Try to regulate the frequencey and intensity of your emotional responses. If you tend to hold things inside, try to talk them out. If you find this difficult to do, start with friends and other people you trust, and work your way up with others. If you are easily excitable, try to think before you act. Give yourself five seconds to think over a response before you begin to react.

Try to reconsider those situations that you usually perceive as stressful. When you are faced with a situation that you expect will be stressful, rehearse your reaction to the point where you feel comfortable with the situation. Such role-playing may facilitate your responses in many situations.

As the likelihood of experiencing a stress response is closely tied to general health, avoid excesses and observe the tenets of good health: avoid cigarettes, get proper rest, avoid excessive alcohol, get proper exercise, and limit caffeine intake. Make sure that poor health habits do not induce your stress response.

Try to become as adaptable as you can to situations that are out of your control. Although most people seem to seek control of their lives, there is only a very limited area that we can in fact control. Recognize what this area is, and accept as random chance the outcomes in other areas over which you have no control. When you find yourself stuck in a traffic jam, take a deep breath, relax your muscles, and say, "What is, is."

Social support systems in the family, community, and on the job can provide you with realistic appraisals of your expectations, perceptions, and adaptation. Groups with a common purpose, in your neighborhood or at work, can prevent much distress produced by isolation, and fulfill the need for social acceptance. In addition, participation in a group providing a service to others can be self-rewarding and diminish your distress. Those who provide the service and those who receive it often share common goals, and both can gain social skills and a sense of self-mastery.

Preparation for dealing with stress must begin early. Schools should teach how to recognize and cope with it. In our highly mobile society, extended families are important. Furthermore, in a world where most stressors are psychosocial and involve others, the importance of human interaction and social networks in distress prevention cannot be overestimated.

Develop a philosophy for living a purposeful life. It will make you feel more secure and less responsive to everyday stressors. If you find yourself constantly seeking the approval of others, think of yourself as your own "higher authority." Research has demonstrated that ego strength is one of the major methods for avoiding stress-related disorders. You can build up your ego strength and self-confidence by gradually setting yourself more demanding tasks. As you succeed on a lower level, your confidence will be bolstered and you can move on to more difficult tasks.

Treat others with whom you have regular contact in such a way as to minimize their stress response. Develop the trait of equanimity. If you are responsible for developing stress carriers around you, they will ultimately become sources of stress for you.

Organize your life so as to provide periodic respites from your responsibilities through vacations, hobbies, and diversions. Remember, trying too hard to do any task tends to have exactly the opposite effect of what is desired. This is perhaps most commonly observed in sports, where trying too hard leads to focusing more on performance than on enjoyment of the sport itself.

Because anxiety and other stress-related symptoms are subjectively uncomfortable, sufferers sometimes try to medicate themselves. Alcohol, marijuana, and minor tranquilizers often are abused in an attempt to allay stress (see chapters 3 and 4). Tranquilizers are intended, even mandated, as short-term medications. Don't treat stress with inappropriate palliatives. In the long run they are ineffective and may cause you to become dependent on them.

The family

The most common sources of stress in the family are money, sex, child-rearing, and lack of communication. If not addressed, these problems can give rise to family dysfunction. Since social support, primarily from the family, is the best method known today of coping with stress, any stressor that interferes with the social support function of the family must be managed as quickly as possible.

Lack of communication probably is the most significant problem in families. Most people seem to feel, like the ostrich, that if they avoid seeing a problem it doesn't exist.

Whenever issues are not properly dealt with, however, they can result in suppressed feelings which set the family up for a breakdown. All family members should take the time to listen to each other and to share feelings of fear, anger, frustration, and worry. Feelings must be accepted, acknowledged. Once acknowledged, these feelings can be dealt with. Sharing more responsibilities may be an answer, or giving a family member greater freedom, more regular periods of discussion. The importance of self-help, of course, should never be underestimated, but family members should learn to help each other.

Learning the skills of assertiveness is important as is abandoning the striving for perfection in family life. Pieces of problems can be handled, regardless of the continuation of the larger problem.

Sibling rivalry, or feelings of resentment and jealousy toward brothers and sisters, is normal. Expressing these feelings, though difficult in the short run, is most adaptive and enhancing of family life in the long run. Families should provide for sharing time to get negative feelings out in the open.

Put aside one hour per week when the whole family is together, and designate it as the sharing hour. Encourage each other to talk about issues of individual and family importance. Be supportive, even if you have a different point of view. Make sure that at least one meal per week is spent with the whole family together.

It is important also to recognize the fluctuating joys and frustrations of the life cycle. At different stages of family life different problems naturally occur. At birth, children are dependent and are relatively easy to manage. When they enter adolescence, however, there is usually a period where children reject parental values. Later, conflicts between the generations may be further complicated. For example, you may be dissatisfied with your child's mate and the way your grandchildren are brought up. On the other hand, they may resent any interference on your part.

Money problems can be eased by careful planning and budgeting. Whatever your family's priorities, these must be examined in relation to the necessities and needs of different family members. There will be costs and benefits to virtually any budget you develop. To encourage financial

management abilities in children, those over age three should be given a small allowance to spend as they see fit, with no questions asked.

A cohesive, loving, intimate, and supportive family cannot be bought. Spouses who spend all their time in achieving wealth discover later in life that this has not purchased what they may have wanted most—a family.

Sex is perhaps the most intimate interpersonal relationship possible, and if the other facets of a marital relationship are suffering, they will quickly be reflected in a couple's sex life. Sexual fulfillment, which is capable of significantly reducing the other sources of stress in a marriage, is more likely to unfold within a committed, loving, supportive, and communicative relationship.

Another source of possible difficulty in family life today has to do with the changing roles of both men and women. Today, more than 50 percent of the wives in this country are wage earners, bringing new perspective to the issues of who carries out what role in the family or how family responsibilities should be shared. The age of sexual stereotypes is disappearing, and we must discover creative ways of lessening the stressful impact of the transition.

Child-rearing brings with it a unique set of stressors. Although parents often feel totally responsible for the development of their children, childrens' lives are also products of the larger society as well as the family. Now, more than ever, the school system, the neighborhood, television, and other societal influences may determine the socialization of the child, often more than do parents. Parents cannot hope to shield the child from such influences, although their values and priorities should be the starting point of a child's socialization. The imperfections of normal family life are adaptive in that they serve to prepare the child for living in the real world. An overprotected child who has never faced any of the real problems of living will be less adaptive in later life. Accept the challenge, the diversity, and the enjoyment of imperfection and variation over which you have no control. Try to view raising your children as a creative experience rather than as a strenuous series of responsibilities and sacrifices (which it also is!).

Finally, don't forget your own needs, regardless of your role as spouse, parent, or child. If you ignore your own needs, suppressed anger and frustration may build up only to surface at a later time to jeopardize the security of the family. Don't ask the impossible of your children or yourself. Accept reality.

The workplace

The employee If you find that you are working too hard at your job, examine those tasks that can be easily delayed, shared, or delegated. Consider sharing tasks with co-workers who are not presently overloaded. Learn how to manage your time.

On the other hand, you may be underutilized in your job, leading to a sense of dissatisfaction. Make sure that your supervisors are aware of your availability for additional tasks. Assert yourself in your discussions with the boss and make yourself available to others in the company.

If your management's perception of your job role is ambiguous or rigid, clarify with your management exactly what your responsibilities are. It is of the utmost importance to keep the lines of communication open with your boss and with others to whom you report, lest misunderstandings and grudges develop and ultimately induce a stress-related reaction.

Role conflict is a stressful element in many jobs. For example, being an employee, a parent, and an active member of a community means playing several conflicting roles. If your job causes you to feel conflict between your role at work and at home, or if you feel unchallenged by responsibilities and lack of opportunity to experience and grow, you should examine your goals and the roles you choose to play. Perhaps you are limiting the roles you could assume.

When your job demands that you cope with either a great amount of daily variability, or with deadening stability, discussion aimed at reaching a solution is vitally important. If you can trade off responsibilities with others, this may serve as a reliable respite. Alternating tasks during such periods also may be of help. Whenever daily variability is high, it is important to get away from your workplace for a short while each day, even if only for a five-minute walk, preferably in the middle of the day.

Whenever your job brings you into a lot of contact with people who are tense and burdened with stress, realize that you are not responsible for their personalities. Reaffirm your belief in yourself, taking responsibility only for what you can control. Employ stress-reduction techniques whenever you can. Develop additional social contacts when you find that your job is isolating. Also, ask yourself if you are seeking the approval of a person who is important to you but who is a stress carrier. If you are, try to let go of this approval seeking, for it is often impossible to achieve the approval of a stress carrier.

The assertive style, combining directness, honesty, and respect for others' feelings is usually the most adaptive way of expressing your anger when you are in a job situation. Most job situations discourage any emotional reactions, particularly the open expression of anger. Get some perspective, and remember that you are not your job.

When you find that there is an incompatibility between your career opportunity and your boss's style, begin by assessing and reevaluating your own career. A career plan forces you to realize what your desires are. When you do a certain job, carry it out to the best of your ability. It will strengthen your self-confidence. You will gain the respect of your fellow employees and of management. The satisfaction of a job well done will help immunize you against the common stressors of any work environment.

The employer Increasingly, corporate executives are recognizing their institution's role as a stressor to their employees, and have begun to provide policies and programs to help their employees deal with it. The costs of ignoring this stress at work are considerable, resulting in higher medical costs and lower productivity.

Many large companies are beginning to provide direct services to employees through their own medical departments. Such departments typically offer health screening examinations and some limited treatment. Some medical departments offer extensive alcoholism and drug abuse services to employees. Some employers offer employee counseling programs, handled internally or by outside practitioners. The program offers employees short-term counseling and psychotherapy aimed at assisting them in adjusting to problems in living, and teaching them methods of coping with stress.

Some corporations employ external consultants who offer stress management training programs. These programs typically last one to two days and involve the employees in a training sequence that assists them in managing their stress response. Employees learn to recognize and to modify their stress response in a variety of situations. They generally learn a method of deep relaxation, some thinking strategies for coping with stress, and some form of time management, managerial styles, and other coping techniques.

Other ways of helping employees are career development programs, time management workshops, managerial style workshops, preretirement workshops, and conflict management workshops. Because the work environment provides significant stresses in an individual's life, there is a great need for companies to teach employees how to best manage the stress that develops in the workplace.

Since women and minorities are subject to unique sets of stressors, in addition to the stressors common to all groups, they require special attention. Through workshops, Equal Employment Opportunity and Affirmative Action programs, women and minorities may be offered a support network and a series of strategies for coping with occupational stress.

A positive work experience requires the opportunity to communicate freely with management and an established method for the adjustment of employee grievances. In large companies this is most frequently handled through employee representation by unions or other groups.

Society

In many industrial societies, people seem to "wear out" faster, partly because of the demanding expectations made on them. They have low boredom and very high achievement thresholds, feeling vaguely guilty when not working. Also, the greater social mobility in our society tends to foster greater social instability, making for an increased burden of adaptation. Yet our society tolerates only a limited set of stress-reduction techniques such as tears, the expression of anger, or even laughter. Even these outlets seem to be traditionally limited along sex lines.

The physical environment we live in all too often produces stress, with noise, dirt, poor public transportation, lack of adequate space, and other minor environmental irritants. Our urban designers and architects should be encouraged to design for social needs, and town planning boards should include experts in stress management and social engineering. (Refer to chapter 11, Air Pollution, chapter 12, Water Pollution, and chapter 16, Occupational Health.)

Noise in particular is becoming intolerable in many of our cities; we should be aware of the toll noise pollution takes and work for stricter enforcement of anti-noise ordinances and provisions. As we can all testify, traffic congestion has also become seemingly unmanageable in many towns and cities. Nonresidents of cities should be taxed if they drive their cars in the cities; the resulting revenues could be used to upgrade public transportation. Better parking facilities, bicycle paths, and other means could go a long way to improving the environment for us all. A general unawareness of how our environment affects us, adding to our burden of stress, must be combated early in the educational process. Our high schools, colleges, and professional schools should express a commitment to educating us for wellness. Normally, health professionals are trained to deal in sickness, not in wellness, a situation which need not be perpetuated.

Leisure

Unfortunately, Western society has neglected to pace itself and has continuously attempted to squeeze higher and higher levels of production out of its work forces. In some areas in this country, even Sunday, formerly a day of rest, has now become just another "business as usual" day. We need to provide ourselves with leisure time and we need to know how to best use that leisure. Too often, people become anxious, bored, or otherwise dissatisfied with their leisure time, spending it in unhealthy ways (smoking, drinking, overeating). With the advent of the technological revolution in information processing, leisure time may become increasingly important. Preretirement counseling programs offered by corporations focus on the need to develop strategies for the productive use of leisure time. When people have been defined and have defined themselves solely as workers, and are then cast into a "nonfunctional" role in retirement, there are significant needs for adaptation. Training in the appropriate uses of leisure time should begin in grade school, and this ability should be cultivated throughout life so that vacations and retirement do not serve more as stressors than they otherwise would.

Technology and Communications

It appears that the decades of the 1980s and 1990s will usher in a true technological revolution. Its introduction will be increasingly evident in our service and manufacturing institutions, with a resulting displacement of many workers. Most workers subsequently may be reemployed in other work, but in the meantime, most of us retain a fear of automation, which naturally serves as a stressor.

The great blessings of our world of instant communications sometimes seem lost in the additional burden of stress that it can frequently confer upon us. Many of the television and radio news programs seem to focus inordinately on violent crimes, natural and man-made disasters, intruding sometimes even upon the victims' expression of grief and sorrow. "Entertainment" offered by the weekly variety shows often never rises above the level of the sordid, the violent, the abnormal, the murderous, or the perverse. The coverage of the war in Vietnam may have been responsible for the national reluctance to continue it, but on the other hand, it may have desensitized many people to the atrocities and processes of war. One does not have to ask for censorship of bad news, but other countries have found different means of providing television news and entertainment, and our own media would do well to consider some of these different ways.

STRESS REDUCTION TECHNIQUES

The following stress reduction techniques are means to decrease the fight-flight response and increase the relaxation response. Many of them can speed up a return to equilibrium once the acute stress is dealt with. They also increase perceptual skills and allow one to be realistic about expectations.

Although these techniques require some discipline and daily practice, they involve "letting go" and "letting it happen" rather than making it happen. They also encourage suspension of expectation to allow awareness of the immediate experience. Many persons who have tried these techniques report an increased sense of well-being, a receptive attitude, an increased sense of mastery, and enhanced self-esteem. The ability to master one's response pattern diminishes the fear of being controlled and the need to react by attempting to control others.

Often, the effects of stress reduction techniques do not include the immediate relief of particular physical symptoms such as headache. What first becomes apparent is a more easygoing attitude; in other words, the first gains often are psychological, and are only later followed by relief of symptoms. The problem for many people is that they give up when their symptoms are not alleviated immediately. We are not accustomed to taking responsibility for our own health and we are not always willing to exert the required self-discipline. When using one of the following techniques, both motivation and patience are necessary, but the mental and physiological effects often are well worth it.

Books by the score have been written to describe some of the following techniques; this is a brief overview. If you are interested in pursuing any one approach, look at the popular literature on the specific technique that interests you, and seek guidance, at least in the early stages.

Meditation

Most types of meditation were developed by Asian cultures where meditation is part of an integrated world view, a spiritual expression, and a lifetime commitment. Some of these techniques have been adapted to Western culture, where they are not necessarily used for the evolution of the inner self into cosmic awareness, but to diminish stress and induce a relaxed state that is both inherently pleasant and useful.

All forms of meditation share the goal of "mastery over attention," that is, focusing one's attention either inward or on an external object or idea. For example, in transcendental meditation (TM) attention is focused on the mantra, a short word or sound chosen for the individual by a teacher. The mantra is repeated over and over again for ten to fifteen minutes at a time. Often, in other methods the focus of attention is your own rhythm of breathing.

At first, focusing so intently seems totally beyond control and extraneous thoughts intrude. It can be frustrating, especially to those who need it most. A teacher can be helpful in the early stages. Later, you can practice on your own. The importance of patient practice cannot be overemphasized in meditation.

If you have physical symptoms, meditation alone may not be sufficient, but it is certainly valuable in setting up the proper framework for more specific approaches. Combining meditation with biofeedback (see below), for example, may be effective in the treatment of high blood pressure.

Some researchers consider meditation to be a unique physiological state, different from both sleep and wakefulness, yet with attributes of each. The important factor is that this physiological state is almost diametrically opposite the stress state. The state of meditation rapidly produces physiological changes during the time it is practiced, and thus it can disrupt the cycle of chronic distress even if it only reestablishes physiologic balance for twenty minutes at a time.

Both stress and activity involve an increased body metabolism with associated increases in oxygen and carbon dioxide exchange, in respiration and heart rates, and in levels of lactic acid and stress hormone. The regular practice of transcendental meditation produces opposite effects during its twenty-minute practice periods. Body metabolism decreases 20 percent as does oxygen and carbon dioxide exchange, and so forth. These changes, brought on minutes after beginning transcendental meditation, would take hours of sleep to produce.

Drs. Herbert Benson and R. K. Wallace, in studies of transcendental meditators, presented evidence that the ability to induce the physiological changes observed during meditation are innate. Meditation "lets it happen," uncovering abilities usually hidden by stress responses. Their key concept of "letting it happen" and "passive focus" are shared by some other stress reduction approaches, for example the Jacobson technique described below.

Autogenic training

In the 1920s Dr. J. H. Schultz, a psychiatrist, developed a self-generated technique combining Western methods of self-suggestion with ancient yoga. Joined by Dr. Wolfgang Luthe, he taught patients to use repetitious phrases and imagery to induce bodily sensations first of heaviness and then of warmth. Patients felt more relaxed and less stressed. Their technique received wide acclaim.

Autogenic training is done best in a relaxed setting in a quiet room with reduced lighting. It can be practiced in a sitting or reclining position, the crucial criterion being lack of strain or muscular tension. Many people prefer sitting in order to avoid confusing relaxation with sleep. The next important element of preparation is to develop an attitude of passive receptivity. An actively striving, goal-oriented attitude will not work in this or in other stress-reduction approaches.

Once you are comfortably positioned, you begin passive concentration on a repetitive phrase or image focused on your body. You can repeat to yourself, "My right arm is heavy" for about one minute. If you are left handed, begin with the left side. Then open your eyes and flex your muscles. This step is necessary to learn to attain relaxed feelings while in an alert, active state.

The progression should be repeated four times before doing the same with the nondominant arm. Then the same series of exercises is repeated with the legs: first the dominant leg, eyes closed, then flexing it with eyes open. Repeat four times. Then do the same with the other leg.

When feelings of heaviness have been experienced for one or two weeks of practice, you begin doing the same thing for the sensation of warmth, in addition to the exercises for heaviness. This stage may take four to eight weeks of practice, before moving on to such areas of focus as a slow, even heartbeat, rhythmic respiratory pattern, relaxed abdomen and forehead. Each new stage is added on to the repertoire. Eventually you should be able to go through the entire series in a few minutes. After several months, you are ready to begin the next stage of autogenic meditation, which involves visualization and incorporates the techniques of meditation.

Progressive relaxation

In the 1930s Dr. Edmund Jacobson, a psychophysiologist, developed the technique of progressive relaxation. He noted that tension and stress often were accompanied by a generalized increase in muscle tension of which the patient was unaware. He developed a technique in which patients are asked to actively tense, then actively relax muscle groups in an attempt to increase awareness of both states. One could learn to identify stress in its early stages and the preferred relaxed state could be induced. Dr. Jacobson's training period of fifty-six one-hour sessions was subsequently abbreviated to six twenty-minute sessions. This latter schedule is commonly used and is known as the modified Jacobson technique. One version is given here. Have someone read it to you slowly or read it into a tape recorder and play it back for the best results.

Active relaxation exercise (Relaxation tape—approximately twenty minutes).

Sit in a comfortable chair in a quiet, semi-darkened room, and loosen all tight clothing.

Concentrate on both your lower legs, then the upper legs, the buttocks, abdominal wall, chest wall, lower arms, upper arms, shoulders, back of neck, forehead, and face.

Now, close your eyes and keep them closed if you can do this comfortably. Focus your mind on both lower legs and check for any differences between the left and right. Continue to do the same with your upper legs, buttocks, abdominal wall, chest, arms—compare left to right, and right to left. Continue on with upper arms, back of neck, forehead, and face muscles.

While you are concentrating on your face, allow yourself to focus on your right nostril and picture the air flowing in and out, easily, on its own, as if it's occurring in someone else. Allow your focus to shift gradually to your left nostril and do the same there—just passively picture the air flowing in and out on its own. Then repeat with both nostrils together for about forty-five seconds. Note the natural, easy breathing pattern in and out, while maintaining your focus on both nostrils.

Now let your focus to shift to your right lower arm; tense those muscles. Hold the tension with your fist clenched for several seconds so that you really feel the tension, and then let go. Relax all the muscles in your lower arm, wrist, and hand, and note the difference between the now relaxed state and the previously tense one.

Shift your focus to your right upper arm. Dig your elbow into your side and tense it. Hold the tension and feel it, then let go, relaxing all the muscles in your upper arm. Maintain your focus there, and again note the difference between the relaxed state and the previously tense one, enjoying the relaxed state.

Repeat the same thing with your left lower arm first, and then your left upper arm.

Let your focus shift to your forehead and wrinkle your brow. Hold it and feel the tension there for several seconds, across your forehead and into your temples and scalp. Relax all the muscles in your forehead, search for any ideas of residual tension, and loosen any knotted areas. Enjoy the state of muscle relaxation.

Allow the focus to shift now to your facial muscles. Spread your lips back in a grimace, showing your teeth, and hold it. Really feel the muscles tensing throughout your face, and then relax each and every one. Check your jaw for any residual tension, and relax it.

While concentrating on your face, repeat your focus on breathing in and out of your right nostril first, then your left nostril, and finally both. Enjoy the easy rhythmic flow of your own breathing. Take a minute or so to do this.

When you're ready, allow your focus to gently move to the back of your neck; tense it by allowing your chin to drop forward and touch your chest. Hold this position for a few seconds and feel the tension. Then relax and enjoy the difference.

Now focus on your chest and expand it by leaning forward in your chair and arching your back, taking care not to hurt your back. Feel the muscles between each rib as you hold the position briefly and then relax by sinking back into your chair. Allow yourself to enjoy this relaxed position. Note the air flowing in and out of your chest cavity, massaging the inside of your chest wall, relaxing your chest muscles even further.

Now shift your focus to your abdominal wall and tense it by bearing down *briefly*. Then relax fully and completely, and note the new state of relaxation. With each breath, feel the inside of your abdominal wall being massaged and enjoy the further relaxation this brings.

Allow your focus to shift to your right upper leg and right buttock and tense that area now.

Hold it for a few seconds, and then relax all the muscles there. While focusing, continue to relax any areas of residual tension. Enjoy the state of relaxation.

Drop your focus to your right lower leg and tense the muscles there by raising your toes so that you plant your heel on the ground. Feel the tension in the back of your calf, hold it, and then relax all the muscles in your lower leg, noting and enjoying the difference.

Repeat the same way with your left upper leg, followed by your left lower leg.

With your eyes closed allow your focus to take in both lower legs, relaxing them even further. Then the upper legs, buttocks, abdominal wall, chest wall, both lower arms, upper arms, shoulders, back of neck, forehead, and finally allow your focus to come upon your face muscles, relaxing them even further. Search your body for residual areas of tension and spend some time relaxing them.

Allow your focus to return to your breathing and repeat the focus on your right nostril, then your left nostril, and then both at the same time. Allow some time for this part of the exercise. Feel the fresh air as you inhale, and feel all the tension leaving your body as you exhale.

Still keeping your eyes closed, allow your focus to return to your surroundings, and allow everyday thoughts to come back to mind. When you feel ready, gently open your eyes and slowly begin to take in the room, while still noting your breathing. You may note a difference in your perception of your surroundings—enjoy them and sit quietly for a few more moments. You have now finished the relaxation exercise. Used twice a day, it will help you to be more relaxed throughout the day.

The relaxation response

Some people have felt that the mystical experience and "giving of mantra" in TM made it unappealing for Western clinical practice. Dr. Herbert Benson, therefore, decided to explore whether other approaches such as prayer, breathing exercises, or the repetition of a word could produce the same effects. He found that they could. As the Maharishi Mahesh Yogi, the TM guru, has not permitted research on his methods, there is still debate as to whether TM can offer benefits beyond those of the Benson Relaxation Technique.

Dr. Benson's approach also requires a quiet environment, a mental device, and a passive, "letting it happen" attitude. The relaxation response typically involves repeating the word "one" over and over, while in a quiet, relaxed state for fifteen to twenty minutes.

The quieting response

Dr. Charles Stroebel, a psychologist and psychiatrist, decided that the meditation techniques requiring fifteen to twenty minutes daily were unsuitable for the time-urgent Type A personality who needs techniques to combat his or her stress response in very brief periods of time. Stroebel also felt that meditation turned some people into "walking zombies." As a result he developed a technique called the Quieting Response.

The Quieting Response takes only six seconds and is intended to counteract the initial phases of the fight-or-flight response, which also appears to last six seconds. Thus, instead of practicing a system of deep relaxation for twenty minutes once or twice a day, this approach requires that you employ the Quieting Response fifty to one hundred times daily, as the need arises. Dr. Stroebel found that, after about six months of regular practice, the Quieting Response becomes a quieting reflex—what was originally a deliberate effort becomes virtually automatic.

The Quieting Response pays special attention to what might be considered "gearshift" mechanisms in the stress response. For example, the facial muscles, which are capable of 250,000 individual expressions, are important gearshifts for expressing emotion. Likewise, the diaphragm, which regulates breathing, is a gearshift in terms of regulating the basic rhythm of life. Thus, the Quieting Response relates particularly to the facial muscles and to our breathing pattern.

If you are prone to Type A behavior, and cannot sit for long periods of time, perhaps the Quieting Response is appropriate for you. Here is a brief description of the Quieting Response and how to make it work for you. Remember, it takes about six months of regular practice for this technique to become automatic.

The six-second quieting response

1. Begin by recognizing the cue of your fight-flight reaction. Notice whether or not you are tense, annoyed, anxious, or otherwise upset. This is your cue for mobilizing the Quieting Response. Typical events that trigger the fight-flight response are: missing a train, losing a coin in the coffee machine, or a brief disagreement with a friend.
2. Immediately after recognizing the cue, make yourself smile and allow your eyes to sparkle. This is to avoid the tensing of the facial musculature, which signals negative emotions to the brain. In the event that you are in a situation where you cannot smile overtly, smile inwardly to yourself and make sure that your facial muscles do not make a grimace.
3. Now say to yourself, "Alert, amused mind—calm body." Because most stress responses carry with them self-suggestions of tension, anxiety, and impatience, these negative messages must be counteracted with a positive message.
4. Let yourself enjoy your ability to "shift" to the right "gear." Say to yourself, "I am on top of this situation. I can handle this."

5. Take two easy, deep breaths. Imagine that you are breathing through holes in the bottom of your feet. Fill up the lower lobes of your lungs first, and then fill up the middle and upper sections of your lungs. Breathe deliberately and deeply, counting slowly to four as you do. If you find that you get dizzy, this is because more oxygen is reaching your brain. You will adapt to this over time.
6. While exhaling, pay attention to your jaw, your tongue, and your shoulders. These body parts are highly responsive to stress. Make sure that your jaw is loose and relaxed, that your tongue is resting on the lower part of your jaw, and that your shoulders are limp and relaxed.
7. Feel a wave of heaviness and warmth flowing from your head to your toes. This counteracts the otherwise automatic tension response, which is part of the stress process.
8. While exhaling the second deep breath, say to yourself, "I am not going to let my body get involved in this. I can allow myself to relax and to handle this situation better." Again, you are giving yourself positive suggestions, which are consistent with coping.
9. Resume normal activity. Now that you have counteracted the fight-flight reaction, do not dwell on the reaction or augment it, but return to what you were doing previously.

Biofeedback

Biological feedback, or biofeedback for short, is the measurement of biological or physiological phenomena and the simultaneous visual and auditory feeding back or display of this information. It requires instruments to measure and record the biological information so that the patient can see it or hear it. Learning by trial and error, the patient is aided in establishing voluntary control over aspects of his or her physiology that previously were not controlled. The instrument is, in effect, a temporary bridge between a person's awareness and his or her physiological functioning, providing information otherwise unavailable.

Various physiological phenomena such as muscle tension, brain waves, and hand temperature, previously thought to be involuntary, have been demonstrated to be voluntary, once the appropriate information is provided. When information concerning the stress response, such as muscle tension or increased heart rate, is provided, the patient can learn to control them, lessen them, and experience relaxation. With continual feedback provided, the individual learns under conditions which are closer to real life situations than are the eyes-closed meditation techniques.

Clinically effective biological feedback must include both general relaxation training and specific biologic feedback via instruments. Proof that patients have learned generalized relaxation includes diminished respiratory oxygen-carbon dioxide exchange, blood pressure, pulse rate, and lactic acid levels. Until this is accomplished, and generalized to situations outside the laboratory, additional training will not be clinically effective.

If it is to be clinically useful this new learning must be both generalized and reinforcing. Many factors, including the learning climate, play a role in this situation. The type of learning involved is not unlike the learning that children of two, three, or four undergo as they increase the ability to control motor and automatic functions. The environmental setting, therefore, should include continuous reinforcement, love, and steady support. This allows an adult as well as a child to learn, by trial and error, control over previously uncontrolled body functions. The attitude and therapeutic skill of the trainer are crucial.

In the biofeedback setting, patients are asked to perform tasks that normally stimulate the fight-or-flight response, but in which success can be achieved only by producing an opposite response. For example, people often "try hard" to relax, as they do in competitive situations, whereas only

by "letting go" or "letting it happen" will relaxation occur. The instructions must be given in a relaxed setting in which stress is minimized. In essence, patients learn to follow the signal of the biofeedback instrument rather than lead it and compete with it. They become aware that the signal is produced by themselves and that the machine is producing nonjudgmental, therefore nonstressful, information. How the actual learning occurs, however, remains uncertain.

Thus, biofeedback training has three main goals. First, to increase awareness of what you are doing with your body arousal. Second, once you are aware, to permit you to learn to control or to modulate this bodily arousal in the laboratory. And lastly, if you can control your arousal in the lab, to teach you how to transfer this control to everyday life, where it counts.

Self-hypnosis

Hypnosis is a goal-oriented, active technique that can produce an antistress response when the patient is ordered to enter a meditative state. The trance state induced with hypnosis has some similarity to the meditative trance state.

In addition to the hypnotic trance's general effects of relaxation and sensation of well-being, self-hypnosis can be used to focus on specific problems that often are stress related. These sometimes involve the reduction of a stress response when confronted with stressors such as visits to a dentist.

Other uses of self-hypnosis focus on specific stress-response patterns. For example, it is a valuable tool in breaking such habits as smoking, alcohol abuse, drug use, and overeating.

Exercise

Exercise is a stressor, and therefore can be either helpful or harmful depending on whether it is appropriate to your physical condition and to the situation. This point often gets overlooked in the enthusiasm for physical activity.

The response of a nonconditioned person to exercise is similar physiologically to a distress response—increased heart rate, increased arousal of the sympathetic nervous system, and increased muscle tension.

The athletic conditioning of such a person is similar to relaxation training in that a similar activity or stressor, when repeated over a period of time, no longer evokes as dramatic an arousal response. Stronger muscles, of course, help one deal with physical stressors. For example, lower back pain experts find that in many cases it is weak muscles rather than any bone or nervous system damage that are at fault.

What types of exercises will be relaxing rather than distressing?

Stretching is helpful in conditioning and relaxing. In using stretching exercises to increase flexibility, gradual stretching is better than a rapid bouncing motion, because the latter causes a reflex contraction of the muscle leading to tension rather than relaxation, and may possibly cause muscle damage.

In general, regular exercise leads to greater cardiovascular fitness and increased muscle strength. The former is particularly helpful in preventing physiological distress responses to any stressor. For instance, increased pulse rates and blood pressures often are found in otherwise normal patients who react to the stress of a physical exam; this is not found in patients who exercise regularly.

Aerobic exercises such as running, dancing, bicycling, tennis, and volleyball are relaxing as long as you build up your endurance gradually and sensibly.

Your attitude toward exercise also is crucial. Exercising for enjoyment is relaxing, but exercising to win is not. Professional athletes are not particularly relaxed. Being more relaxed does not mean achieving less, and this is worth remembering not only in exercise, but in other aspects of living. When you respond in a more relaxed manner, more energy is left to deal effectively with other stressors.

Don't be demoralized if you don't like structured exercise. Twenty minutes of brisk walking once a day provides your body with the minimum of exercise necessary. However, do get this twenty minutes of walking exercise each day. Don't give up on your body! (See chapter 5, Physical Fitness).

PSYCHOTHERAPY

Psychotherapy is a treatment designed to produce a response primarily by psychological, psychophysiological, emotional, or behavioral means rather than by physical means. There is a wide variety of schools and practitioners. Psychotherapy has evolved from helping the client achieve relief from psychologically induced discomfort and social ineffectuality to helping the client achieve positive mental health and growth. Psychotherapy has been used successfully for both physical and psychological disorders.

Credentials for practicing psychotherapy have been broadened, but the main practitioners today are psychologists, psychiatrists, and psychiatric social workers. There are three major schools of psychotherapy, one of which appears to be particularly well-suited for the treatment of the stress-related disorders.

The oldest school of psychotherapy is derived from Freudian psychoanalysis and is called the analytic or psychodynamic approach. This form of psychotherapy tries to relieve the patient by unraveling internal problems and by bringing unconscious historical conflicts into the patient's present consciousness. The target of treatment is not the patient's symptoms, but rather the psychodynamics that are believed to generate these symptoms. The therapy clarifies, confronts and interprets, but is generally more passive, and examines the relationship between the patient and the therapist as a mirror of the patient's unresolved childhood conflicts. This school of psychotherapy has not enjoyed much success when examined scientifically and experimentally. It is typically a long-term approach and may be quite expensive.

The second major school of psychotherapy is called behavior therapy or behavior modification. Most behavior therapy derives from laboratory studies of learning processes. The therapist treats only the observable symptoms and does not postulate an unconscious. The aim of this treatment is to change the frequency, intensity, and appropriateness of certain behaviors. The behavior therapist believes that the patient has learned maladaptive responses and must be taught new ones. Behavior therapy typically is short-term, and has enjoyed the greatest success in alleviating the stress-related disorders. Some of the techniques used by behavior therapists include relaxation techniques discussed in this chapter.

The third major school of psychotherapy is called humanistic therapy. Humanists believe that a person has a need for self-actualization, and a higher level of experience involving goodness, truth, beauty, justice, and the like. Humanists believe that the failure to express and to realize the potential of higher human needs, motives, and capacities is the cause of emotional distress. The goals of humanistic therapy are self-actualization and the enrichment and fuller enjoyment of life, not the cure of "disease" or "disorders." The humanistic goal is to develop increasing sensitivity to one's own and to others' feelings. Such awareness will help establish warm relationships and improve ability to perceive, intuit, sense, create, fantasize, and imagine. Some of the techniques humanists use include sensitivity training, encounter groups, and sensory awareness train-

ing. Because humanists do not believe in treating disease, there has been little research showing the impact of this school of psychotherapy on the stress-related disorders.

In order to choose the most appropriate practitioner and type of psychotherapy for you, contact the local psychological or psychiatric association, or the local social work organization. Ask for two or three referrals and consult with each before you choose. Also consult your physician for a referral.

Each case of distress is different but the answers to some general questions may be helpful.

1. Have you identified the problem area(s)?
2. Have you considered that your own unfounded expectations or misperceptions may be contributing to your problems?
3. Have you discussed your concerns with friends or colleagues who will be honest yet supportive?
4. Have you placed yourself in the other person's shoes to gain understanding?
5. Have you tried to communicate or just present your point of view?
6. Have you tried to listen, to learn, and to become more empathetic toward the views of others?
7. Do you try to do too much too quickly so that you are always racing the clock?
8. Do you interrupt others?
9. Have you identified which parts of your body signal that you are acutely distressed?
10. Have you tried to relax, using one of the relaxing techniques?
11. Have you tried to remember how your body feels immediately afterward and tried to reproduce these feelings?
12. How much time and energy do you invest in your welfare, your family, your friends, and other people upon whom you depend?
13. Do you think you need professional help?

Stress reduction techniques dovetail with the mental attitudes necessary for coping. The ability to listen with suspended judgment, the desire to understand rather than to explain, and the wisdom of empathy are all aided whenever you relax your physiological systems. Physical and mental tension produces tension in others, who then help to create a vicious cycle by serving as a stressor to you!

The need for family and social groups cannot be overestimated. An intact family or group of friends helps develop skills as well as provide support when we need it most. With social support during our time of distress we may grow, and at our height of joy we may share and increase our happiness. In order to deal with our mundane irritations a haven—quiet, nourishing, and therapeutic—can shift our focus to more joyful aspects of our lives.

CHAPTER

8

Dental hygiene

While almost nobody dies from dental disorders, the cost of not keeping teeth in good condition is considerable and increases with age. The prevention of tooth decay and gum disorders has a significant impact on the total health care cost of society as well as on the well-being of all of us. And dental and gum diseases belong to the group of disorders that are most responsive to simple preventive measures.

Such protective procedures include careful cleaning of teeth coupled with vigorous gum massage, reduction of intake of refined sugars, and the application of fluorides either in drinking water or in toothpaste.

Like so many programs in preventive medicine, the earlier in life preventive activities are started, the more likely it is that they will be most effective. The early years at home and at school need to be used for preventive dental education so that we can develop a generation relatively free of dental disease. No new knowledge or techniques are needed, only the determined application of principles with which we are already familiar.

Glossary

CALCULUS: Tartar, or hard, calcified deposits formed on the teeth near the edge of the gums

CARIES: Tooth decay or cavities, caused by organic acids

GINGIVITIS: Inflammation of the gums caused by plaque

PERIODONTAL DISEASE: Chronic inflammatory disease of the bone and gums

PLAQUE: A sticky mass of bacteria that accumulates on and around the teeth

PYORRHEA: An inflammatory periodontal disease, resulting in loosened teeth and receding gums

TRENCH MOUTH: Acute gum infection causing excessive bleeding

Prevalence of Dental Diseases

Dental diseases are a particularly frustrating paradox.

They are and possibly always have been the most prevalent chronic diseases in the United States; yet they are probably the most easily prevented of all chronic diseases. Dental caries, commonly known as tooth decay or cavities, are almost completely preventable and most periodontal disease (*pyorrhea*—disease of the bone and gums that support the teeth) can also be prevented. Obviously, the proven and easily applied methods of preventing these diseases are widely ignored.

Dental diseases are among the oldest recorded human afflictions. Both dental caries and periodontal disease have been observed in the preserved skulls of ancient people, and descriptions of tooth decay can be found in the writings of Aristotle. All evidence indicates, however, that dental diseases were a minor health problem for our ancestors compared with their epidemic presence in modern societies. Tooth decay, in particular, can be characterized as a disease of contemporary civilization because its prevalence has increased steadily as foods and eating habits evolved toward our present-day diet, which is rich in carbohydrates and refined or processed foods.

Tooth decay now affects more than 95 percent of Americans. The onset of the disease occurs in children shortly after the eruption of their first primary teeth, and decay continues to attack most people's permanent teeth, into late adolescence or early adulthood. It is slightly more prevalent among females than males of the same age, and is higher in the Northwestern U.S. than in other parts of the country, for reasons not fully understood. *It is estimated that, by age 17, two-thirds of our population have five or more decayed, filled, or extracted permanent teeth.* Tooth decay is the major cause of extracted permanent teeth until about age thirty-five, after which most tooth loss is the result of destructive periodontal disease.

In addition to the pain, infection, and disfigurement that result from dental diseases, they constitute a major economic burden. In 1978, the American public is estimated to have spent more than $10 billion on dental care. Even so, more than half the population receives no dental care at all during any year. Nor could they get adequate treatment if they sought it. To provide such treatment for the existing amount of tooth decay and periodontal disease is far beyond the total capacity of our present or projected dental human manpower. Clearly, this pervasive problem can only be controlled by preventive measures, individually undertaken. Prevention begins with an understanding of causes. *In spite of the fact that many people believe that loss of teeth is an inevitable part of the aging process, with proper care it is possible for them to keep all of their natural teeth—for a lifetime.*

Causes of Tooth Decay

Dental caries may be defined as localized, progressive destruction of the tooth, beginning with the outer enamel layer, as a result of attack by organic acids.

Because tooth decay is so widespread, many have come to regard it as practically inevitable. It is common to hear, "Bad teeth run in my family," or "I inherited soft teeth." In fact, tooth decay is not inherited and is certainly not inevitable.

Decay is caused by the interaction of three factors:

- the growth of specific bacteria on the tooth surface
- the presence in the mouth of fermentable carbohydrates—especially sugars
- a tooth surface with less than ideal resistance to acid

Should any one factor be eliminated or suitably modified, tooth decay will not occur.

BACTERIA

In searching for the bacteria essential to causing decay, several types have been implicated. Certain streptococci, called *Streptococcus mutans*, are especially suspect. These microorganisms,

which are normal inhabitants of the mouth, readily metabolize sugars to form acids. In addition, they have the peculiar ability to produce—from sugar—sticky, insoluble polysaccharide molecules called glucans. It is believed that these glucans enable the organisms to adhere to the tooth surface where they rapidly multiply into an almost invisible bacterial mass called dental plaque, which coats the tooth surface. Because plaque is very adherent, it can be removed by only the most thorough and regular use of the toothbrush and dental floss; and it reforms rapidly—probably within twenty-four hours.

SUGARS IN THE DIET

When sugars in the diet are introduced into dental plaque, the plaque bacteria rapidly convert the sugars to acids. Concentrations of acid in plaque may remain at levels high enough to endanger the tooth for thirty minutes or longer after sugars are eaten.

TOOTH ENAMEL

Whether these acids will damage the tooth depends in part on the resistance of the tooth enamel, the third factor in the causation of tooth decay. Enamel that lacks sufficient amounts of the fluoride ion particles in its outer layers is much more likely to be damaged.

At first the damage is slight. The acid dissolves a small amount of mineral from the enamel, producing a defect far too small to be visible to the naked eye. This early defect is reparable by the natural processes in the mouth. If no further acid attacks occur, minerals in the saliva will gradually replace those lost, and the enamel will be restored to normal. The process will be greatly enhanced if fluoride is also available at the enamel surface. More commonly, however, additional acid attacks *do* occur because of frequent ingestion of sugars—by eating sweet snacks several times a day, for example—and the cumulative destruction of enamel finally overcomes the natural repair mechanisms of saliva.

The result is an actual loss of tooth structure: a cavity has formed. From this point on the lesion can only be repaired by a dental filling. If left untreated, the cavity will continue to enlarge and will eventually destroy the entire crown of the tooth.

Because three factors are involved—bacteria, eating habits, and tooth resistance—we cannot tell how long it takes an irreversible cavity to develop or how many acid attacks are required or at what intervals. These factors differ for different individuals and perhaps for different teeth in the same mouth. But we do know that at least two of the causative factors, eating habits and tooth resistance, are within the control of each individual and that, if controlled, tooth decay can be prevented.

Causes of Periodontal Disease

Periodontal disease is chronic inflammatory destruction of the soft tissues (gingivae or "gums") and the bone that surround and support the roots of the teeth. This problem affects more than three-fourths of the adults in the U.S. and is the leading cause of loss of teeth in persons over thirty-five.

PLAQUE

The major causative factor of periodontal disease is the accumulation of bacterial plaque on a tooth at or beneath the point where the gingival tissues contact the tooth crown. The bacteria responsible for this plaque formation are thought to be different from those involved in tooth decay. When plaque remains in contact with the soft tissues, inflammation results, characterized by redness, swelling, and bleeding—a condition called *gingivitis*. At this stage, the process can be reversed by prompt institution of careful oral hygiene procedures to keep the teeth free of plaque. Localized gingivitis may also be associated with decayed teeth or rough dental fillings, in which case it can be eliminated by corrective dental treatment.

If left untreated, however, inflammation progresses and the gums become detached from the root of the tooth, resulting in the formation of periodontal pockets between the roots and gum. Pocket formation signals a serious, though not yet critical, phase of periodontal disease. The pockets provide an ideal environment for further bacterial growth and are very difficult to keep free of plaque and food debris. As the pockets become deeper, the inflammation process eventually involves the adjacent supporting bone, which is gradually destroyed, resulting in loosening, drifting, and ultimate loss of the tooth. At advanced stages of the disease, abcesses and associated pain frequently occur.

Population surveys consistently show that periodontal disease is related to the presence of plaque and to increasing age, the latter probably reflecting the longer exposure to chronic bacterial irritation. It has not been established that either nutrition or heredity plays a direct role in the causation of periodontal disease. However, it is clear that a person's defense mechanisms, possibly the immune system, are important factors in regulating how well the tissues resist the irritants produced by bacterial plaque.

TARTAR

In many persons hard calcified deposits called calculus, or tartar, form at or beneath the edge of the gums. These deposits, primarily dead bacteria, probably do not directly contribute to periodontal disease, but they do encourage the accumulation of bacterial plaque on their rough surfaces.

Prevention of Tooth Decay

A way has not yet been found to avert the formation of bacterial plaque on teeth; but the tooth decay encouraged by plaque can nevertheless be almost totally prevented. This can be done by enhancing tooth resistance and altering the harmful aspects of diet. *For maximum effectiveness, the preventive process should begin in childhood—ideally, before the first teeth appear—and should continue at least into the early adult years.*

FLUORIDE

The essential first step is to increase the resistance of the teeth to acid attack by exposing them to adequate amounts of fluoride (see chapter 1, Nutrition). The best way to accomplish this is to adjust the fluoride content of public water supplies to approximately one part fluoride per million parts of water (ppm). In twenty-one American cities tooth decay decreased steadily as the water fluoride concentrations approached 1 ppm (figure 8.1, p. 424). Other studies throughout the world have proved conclusively that if children are exposed to optimally fluoridated water from birth, they will experience 50 to 70 percent fewer cavities than otherwise expected, and that these preventive benefits will persist throughout life.

Community water fluoridation is very inexpensive and totally safe. No adverse health effects of fluoridation have been demonstrated, except for some mottling and discoloration of teeth among persons exposed to water containing naturally occurring fluoride at concentrations two and a half or more times higher than recommended. In the United States about half the population, 115 million people, now have the protective benefits of water fluoridation.

For those who do not, several alternative sources of fluoride are also effective in preventing decay. These include fluoride solutions, gels, and pastes, which are applied directly to the teeth by a dentist or dental assistant. Self-applied fluoride mouth rinses and tablets also are available. Especially effective are fluoride rinse and tablet programs conducted in schools, supervised by classroom teachers or adult volunteers. These programs cost as little as 50 cents per child per school year, and more than 10 million schoolchildren are currently participating in them. All these alternative methods of fluoride application will prevent from 30 to 50 percent of new cavities.

Fluoride-containing toothpastes should be used by every one, in combination with other methods of fluoride application. They provide somewhat less preventive benefit, presumably because they contain low concentrations of fluoride and are not thoroughly applied by most people.

For maximum benefits, exposure to fluoride should begin at birth and continue without interruption at least through the teenage years. A dentist or physician can prescribe the most appropriate method of supplying fluoride for each person.

SEALANTS

Recent research has demonstrated that adhesive sealants, a thin film of plastic that looks much like nail polish, can be applied to the biting surfaces of the teeth and will provide 100 percent protection against cavities on those surfaces so long as the sealant remains in place. Sealants can be applied by the dentist, dental hygienist, or dental assistant in the dental office or in school-based programs. They must be checked at regular intervals and reapplied as necessary. *Sealants are a highly recommended method to increase tooth resistance and should be used with fluorides.*

DIET

While fluorides and sealants are effective, the entire job of preventing tooth decay must include correcting the dietary practices that are its major causes.

Most people have heard the advice, "To prevent tooth decay, stop eating sweets." Although this advice is scientifically well-founded, few people are likely to make such a drastic change in their eating habits. In any case, eliminating sugars is not necessary for caries prevention. What is essential is to reduce the *frequency* with which sugar-containing foods are eaten; in particular, to avoid sugar-containing snacks between regular meals. Most children readily accept such snacks as raw vegetables, nuts, fresh fruits, and cheese when these are offered from early child-

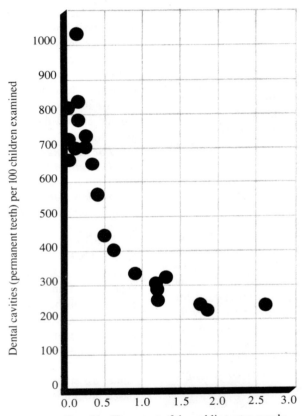

Fluoride (F) content of the public water supply in PPM (parts per million)

FIGURE 8.1

Effect of fluoride on dental caries.
This test observed 7,257 white schoolchildren,
12–14 years old, in twenty-one cities of four states.
SOURCE: adapted from H.T. Dean, F.A. Arnold, Jr., and E.
Elvove, Public Health Reports *57: 1155 (1942)*

hood instead of sweet snacks. *The practice of giving infants a nursing bottle with sweetened formula or other sugared liquids to suck on overnight—or even for a short time—is particularly dangerous to the teeth and should be completely avoided.* The liquid constantly bathing the infant's teeth makes a prime breeding ground for bacteria, leading to a condition known as "milk bottle cavities."

Improved methods to prevent tooth decay are being actively researched. It is likely that antibacterial chemicals to remove dental plaque or prevent its formation, and even a vaccine against tooth decay, will some day be available. But it is not necessary to wait. With fluorides, adhesive sealants, and carefully controlled dietary practices, almost all tooth decay is preventable.

Prevention of Periodontal Disease

BRUSHING AND FLOSSING

Most periodontal disease can be prevented by regular, thorough personal oral hygiene—toothbrushing and flossing—to keep the teeth as free of bacterial plaque as possible. Ask your dentist to demonstrate the correct way to brush and floss your teeth, and what sort of toothbrush is best for you. It is critically important that the correct methods of tooth cleaning be learned and begun early in life and that they be routinely continued at least daily. Although severe periodontal disease is most often seen in adults, the early stages of pocket formation are sometimes present in adolescents. Prompt action can reverse the early stages of gingivitis. But neglect means long drawn-out treatment, frequently involving surgery, with no guarantee against the ultimate loss of teeth.

CHAPTER
9

Home accidents

The saying, "A man's home is his castle," refers not only to our constitutional rights to privacy but to the fact that we feel most secure in our own homes. It may come as a shock to learn that so many accidents—easily as many as occur in the workplace—happen at home.

The responsibility for this situation is all our own. There are no annual drives, and no inspections dedicated to reducing catastrophes that occur regularly in the apartments and houses where we spend most of our time.

At a minimum, we can look closely at the features of our own dwellings which, when cor-

rected, can reduce the chances of accidents. Most of them can be prevented by simple, inexpensive measures that take only a few minutes to implement. If special attention is paid to electrical and heating devices, the location of equipment and furniture, stairs, bathroom, and kitchen, our homes can really be as secure as we like to imagine them. As we share our homes with older people or children, we must share the safety, too.

The Most Commonly Overlooked Source of Accidents

In theory, and assuming a reasonable use of caution and common sense, every accident in and around the home is preventable. *We know far more about accident prevention than we know about how to avoid the major diseases. Yet, in a single year in the U.S., 240,000 people are accidentally killed in their own homes.* The annual figures for nonfatal accidents in and around the home are just as alarming: Accidents requiring confinement to bed total more than $5\frac{1}{2}$ million; those imposing activity restriction, 8 million; those causing no restriction of activity but still requiring medical attention, about 10 million. The total is $23\frac{1}{2}$ million nonfatal home accidents a year, one for every ten Americans.

Luckily, in the area of home accidents, every man and woman can be a practitioner of preventive medicine. No academic degree is required, no arcane technical training is necessary; it is simply a matter of knowing the rules and following them. Do you, for example, insist on the Underwriters Laboratory (UL) seal on all electrical equipment, showing that the manufacturer meets prevailing standards of reliability and safety? Do you read and save manufacturers' instructions, especially those dealing with safety hazards and how to avoid them?

The most common and dangerous types of hazards are outlined in this chapter. Also included are reference points for checking home equipment and tips on how you use it or may possibly abuse it. Less frequent yet important ways in which accidents occur are indicated as are general principles alerting you to home accident potential. There is information about what to do when all safety precautions have failed and someone's life is threatened.

Because this chapter presents warnings about household equipment, supplies, and practices, the "Don'ts" must be stressed. Family safety rules, however, involve positive, not just negative, considerations. The approach should be: "We have this object. It is useful. We like it. It also has dangers. Let's figure out how to use it safely and avoid those dangers." If a family discussion cannot agree on how to avoid real danger, then serious consideration should be given to doing without the item. Don't let exaggerated safety precautions stultify your enjoyment of life but, at the same time, don't let it be ruined by carelessness, thoughtlessness, or ignorance.

Each of us takes calculated risks almost every day. We cannot isolate ourselves from all risk. A life without such minor gambles would be monotonous and unproductive. People will always be killed or injured in the course of reasonable, healthy adventure or because of "freak accidents." What we are dealing with here, however, is the predictable, preventable accident.

The principal causes of deaths from home accidents

Age group	Cause
Under 1 year	Suffocation and ingested objects
1–14 years	Fires and burns
14–44 years	Poisoning by liquids or solids
45–64 years	Fires and burns
65 and over	Falls

Falls

FALLS AMONG OLDER PEOPLE

Among all fatal falls, about three-fourths occur in people sixty-five and older; nearly half of these falls take place in the home. *In fact, falls lead all other causes of death in home accidents.*

Falling hazards remain about the same for adults of all ages, but the hazards are exaggerated for the older group by physiological and health changes due to aging.

The shuffling gait, deteriorating muscle coordination, and loss of sense of balance characteristic of many older people are all conducive to tripping. As these conditions advance, they make recovery from a fall less and less likely. A harmless tumble in younger years might be a crippling fall later in life.

With age, vision becomes impaired. A wearer of bifocal or trifocal lenses should use extra caution in walking, particularly going down steps, because the person must move his or her head to look through the distant vision of the bifocal lenses. As we grow older, our accommodation to changes in lighting is also greatly slowed, and much more light is required to see well. Dimly lighted stairways are hazardous at any age, but far more so in old age, especially when coming into a house from bright sunlight.

Elderly people are sometimes confused after awakening from a sound sleep. They may start out for a room that existed in a previous home, even embarking on a walk outside to get to it. Falls are all too common during these distressing situations.

The circulatory problems of old age can also induce accidents. It is particularly dangerous to ascend a stepladder and then look up to reach some object. In doing so, the vertebral arteries may be compressed and reduce an already impaired circulation to the brain. The person may become faint or actually lose consciousness momentarily and fall. There is also the so-called drop-attack in which the person suddenly and unpredictably falls to the ground without loss of consciousness, possibly from loss of posture and gait control, due, in turn, to nerve degeneration.

A common and serious injury to older people is the fractured femur or thigh bone, the longest bone in the body and a weight-bearer. One doesn't have to fall to sustain this injury. Older people's bones are often so brittle that even a slight wrench, as from a trip on a rug, can fracture the femur. The resulting fall often produces further injury.

WINDOWS AND HEIGHTS

Small children, especially under five years old, are the principal victims of fatal falls from windows. This is a particularly serious hazard in high-rise buildings, though a fall from even the second floor of a house can easily kill a small child.

The ingenuity of a child should never be underestimated; a bed placed near a window is an obvious invitation to disaster, but it is easy to build an access to a window ledge out of chairs, books, and boxes. Children not only fall out of bedroom windows, but also living room and kitchen windows; they fall off roofs and fire escapes. These falls occur most often when children are left alone or are indulging in horseplay. Parents should be especially alert from July through September when most falls occur. Leaning against faulty screens is a major cause of falls.

There is an easy, inexpensive, and effective way of preventing many of these accidents. New York City enacted a law requiring owners of multiple-occupancy buildings to install window guards in all apartments where children aged ten years and younger reside. The result: falls were virtually elimated from windows with guards. However, a guard should be used only for the lower part of the window; this is to avoid trapping people in a room in case of fire or making entrance by firemen difficult.

Adults also fall out of windows. The leading causes appear to be: alcohol abuse, lack of caution in repairing or washing windows, hanging screens, hanging clothes, shaking out rugs, opening or closing windows when not fully awake, and sleepwalking. These are chiefly behavioral rather than environmental causes, although some of them might be avoided if window sills were higher.

FALLS ON STAIRS

Stairs are the most dangerous area in the home and the site of about 350,000 serious accidents yearly. As already noted, stairs pose a particular hazard at the extremes of age.

General precautions

1. *Adequate lighting*, especially in halls and stairways.
2. *Stair risers*. These should be of uniform height in each stairway, preferably 7½ inches.
3. *Marking of stairs*. The bottom step and the top step should be marked with a signal—a white or colored strip or something distinctive. Many falls are caused by mistaking the next-to-last step for the last one on the way up or down.
4. *Gates for children*. Small children, exploring on their own, are likely to try the stairs, thus inviting falls. At this age, they must be watched closely and constantly, but this safeguard may fail. Therefore, installation of a gate at each stairway is absolutely essential.
5. *Carrying packages on stairs*. Be extra careful when carrying large or heavy packages, and never carry anything in such a way that your vision is at all obscured by it.

6. *Circular stairways*. These steps usually narrow toward the center of the stairway, and a fall can result if a foot is placed on a narrowed step. Use the outer side of the circle where the steps are of normal width.
7. *Footwear*. Beware of walking up or down stairs in stockinged feet—at least wear good slippers. Beware of high heels as well as long dresses on stairs.
8. *Handrails*. These are essential for all stairways. Each handrail should be stout and, where attached to the wall, it should stand out sufficiently to allow a hand grip around the rail. If practical, each stairway should have handrails on both sides. The rails themselves should be at least 2 inches in diameter, and be installed at a height 30–33 inches above each step. For baluster-supported rails the balusters should be spaced not more than 4 inches apart to keep a child's head from slipping through.
9. *Stair surfaces*. Stairs should be nonskid. Stair mats help, but proper carpeting is still better. Providing a firmer grip for one's feet, carpeting also provides more cushioning in the event of a fall. However, carpeting carries its own hazards: it must be firmly secured in place so that it cannot slip or shift; carpeting with long, deep piling, such as shag, should not be used on stairs because heels may catch in it.
10. *Articles on steps*. A serious tripping hazard can be created by leaving articles of clothing, toys, books, or any other items on stairs or, for that matter, anywhere on walking areas of the home.
11. *Outdoor steps*. Handrails are most needed here. The distance to fall may be shorter than in an inside stairway, but the steps are likely to be made of concrete or some other un-

yielding material. An extra hazard is created by snow, sleet, or ice on outside steps, especially as one emerges from a comfortable interior onto an unexpectedly slippery surface. Sand or rock salt can be spread on these surfaces to provide a safer foothold.

REACHING FOR ARTICLES

Avoid the temptation to stand on chairs, boxes, books, open drawers, and other makeshifts as a convenient way of getting something from a high shelf or putting a ceiling light on. You can topple too easily, as well as damage whatever you're standing on.

There are suitable alternatives. A sturdy, light stepladder belongs in every household. It should have a strong spreader that locks securely when the ladder is set up; its steps should not be less than 3½ inches deep, and it must be properly set up, regardless of its height.

Ladders also present hazards. Reaching too far to one side can result in tipping the ladder or, more likely, losing one's balance and falling off. Do not climb higher than the second step from the top, and never stand on the platform. Another useful article is the "kikstep," which provides two steps. It is unlikely to slide on any surface once stepped on because of a special stopping mechanism. It can be readily stored out of the way.

Remember that this kind of equipment should be avoided by older people who are quite likely to lose their balance. Store things so that the elderly can reach them without having to do any climbing.

Outdoor ladders
The outdoor ladder involves a hazard because it allows the user to climb much higher and, therefore, to fall farther. Each year, falls from ladders kill 300 to 400 people, mainly those doing home tasks, such as washing windows, painting, or cleaning gutters. Ladder accidents probably cause as many as 40,000 disabling injuries annually in

falls from the ladder itself or from a work area to which it gave access. In the latter case, sloping roofs, especially when wet, are a particularly dangerous area.

Ladders should be of good quality, unpainted wood (so that defects are readily seen). Buy the best—your life will be suspended on it. Look for the label of the American Ladder Institute. Store it carefully, and check it each time before you use it. Metal ladders should be used with great care near electric wires. In setting up the ladder, make sure the bottom is far enough away from the house to provide solid support. For each 4 feet of height from the ground to the resting point of the ladder, place the bottom of the ladder one foot out from the vertical. You can measure the height with the ladder, allowing one foot per rung. Be certain that the footing for the ladder is solid and not slippery. If possible, have another person steady the ladder while you are using it. If it must be placed in front of a door, lock the door first. Do not rest the top of the ladder against any surface that can crumple. For access to a roof the ladder top should extend at least 3 feet above the point of support at the roof line.

TRIPPING HAZARDS

Tripping hazards are a common form of easily prevented accidents. A loose rug is always a hazard. It may slip on the polished floor underneath; or the edge of it may easily be kicked up to form a tripping hazard. If the room is not carpeted, rugs should be firmly fastened to the floor—and periodically inspected to make sure that the anchoring remains secure.

Waxed floors
Waxing is almost certain to produce a slippery surface, especially on linoleum or tile floors. Use care.

Electric wiring

An extension cord that provides the slightest opportunity of being accidentally kicked up constitutes a tripping hazard and should be moved. If such a cord cannot be relocated or covered with heavy furniture, the possibility of installing a new electrical outlet should be considered. Where an extension cord is laid over a floor for only a short period—for example, to provide electricity for an hour or so to a slide projector—the cord should be moved to a safe area if possible, and if this cannot be done, its presence should be advertised by covering it with a brightly covered article. A recent innovation is a brightly colored, spring-retractable extension cord. If UL-approved, its use might be considered.

Spilled liquids on floors

Water or melting ice cubes on a linoleum or tile floor (or on a cement patio) can create a slipping hazard. Spilled grease is even more apt to cause slipping accidents and injuries. Always wipe up such spills promptly.

Fires and Burns

More than 600,000 fires, responsible for 5,000 deaths occur every year in American homes. Fires are the second leading cause of death in home accidents after falls, taking their greatest toll in the age groups 1–15 and 45–64.

With our dependence on oil, gas and electricity for heating, cooking and powering appliances, we live constantly exposed to potential hazards of fire and electrocution. We are not likely to reduce this dependence; therefore, we must deal with the hazards involved.

WHO STARTS FIRES?

Anybody can accidentally start a fire. However, it is most likely to be done by elderly adults and children.

Elderly adults often forget to turn off appliances. Their senses, particularly vision and smell, are diminished, and discovery of a fire is likely to be delayed. Their reaction in an emergency is slowed and their sense of touch may be so diminished that burns fail to register immediately and thus produce more extensive tissue damage.

Children and matches

For children, the process of lighting a match is fascinating to watch and to imitate. Some of the danger of playing with matches has been reduced with the development of the "safety match," but even this type is not "fail-safe," particularly in the hands of children with some ingenuity—that is, most children. Pocket and table lighters are obviously just as dangerous.

The basic preventive action here depends on constant supervision. One study showed that of all children under fifteen who died in home fires, one-third had been left unattended. It is not enough to teach a child not to play with fire. Even the most conscientious parents forget the suddenness with which a fatal event can occur. It takes only a few seconds to strike a match, drop it on clothing, and start a fast, fatal fire.

WHAT STARTS FIRES?

Food and grease are heavily involved in appliance fires. The leading ignition sources are, in descending order: electric stoves, electric wiring, cigarettes, gas stoves, matches, and television sets.

Ignition of clothing

This is the most lethal of all fire hazards. It victimizes 150,000 Americans annually, 2,000 of whom die. If a person's clothing catches fire about six times as much skin is deeply burned, and the death rate is four times greater than when clothing is not involved. Some types of clothing are less flammable than others, but nothing one would wish to wear is absolutely fireproof. The vulnerability of fabrics to fire varies. Wool, for example, is more fire resistant than lightweight cotton. Some of the synthetic fabrics are greatly flammable. Loose-weave fabrics burn fastest because they allow more circulation of air to encourage flames. The same thing is true of loose clothing. The risks have been lessened somewhat by the introduction of flame-retardant clothing ("flame resistant" is the official designation on the labels). The federal government requires that all children's sleepwear be made of such material. With the possible exception of cotton products, most flame-resistant clothing looks as good as any other, although it is a little more expensive. It should be noted that after many washings, the flame retardant chemical washes out and its protection is lost. The manufacturer's instructions for washing should be strictly observed. *Remember, the material is "flame-resistant," not "flameproof."* Also, some flame-retarding treatments of clothing are suspected to have a carcinogenic (cancer-producing) effect. However, until this controversy is settled, the calculated risk involved is heavily weighed on the side of burn prevention.

Seldom do persons escape serious injury when their clothes are ignited. One can flee from some types of fires, but clothing cannot be re-moved rapidly enough, nor the fire put out fast enough to prevent much injury. A blanket or similar wrap should be used to envelop the victim to try to smother the fire as water in sufficient quantity is rarely at hand. If the burned person tries to run, this only fans the flames and increases the probability of breathing in flames and smoke. The fact is that extinguishing fire in clothing will not often be successful enough to prevent serious and painful burns.

Cigarettes, cigars, and pipes

The careless use of such materials is estimated to cause one-third of all deaths from fires. It is estimated that smoking materials started 138,000 fires in 1975.

Smoking in bed Smoking cigarettes in bed after a few drinks at night is potentially suicidal. Alcohol and drugs not only heighten the possibility of the smoker dropping off to sleep, but also delay awakening by smoke or flames. Mattresses, instead of bursting quickly into flames, are likely to smolder, giving off poisonous carbon monoxide and other gases that can kill victims or render them unconscious.

Upholstery fires The dangers here are similar to those arising from smoking in bed, with the same causes. The chief difference is that upholstery material often includes plastic which, on burning, adds to the assortment of toxic gases.

Guests who smoke For the host or hostess: never go to bed after a party without carefully checking for live cigarette or cigar butts, especially in upholstery and other furnishings. Smoldering upholstery fires are not always put out merely by dousing with water. Sometimes they start again, even hours later. If in doubt, call your fire department.

Electrical equipment

About 15 percent of home fires are caused by improper use of electrical equipment. Often, the first sign of trouble is a blown fuse. If a fuse blows, the cause should be ascertained. Don't just substitute a new fuse, or switch to a higher amperage fuse. Never use a coin as a temporary measure.

Before replacing the fuse, check all electrical equipment that was plugged in when the fuse was blown. Electrical circuits should never be overloaded. If you cannot discover the cause, don't take a chance—call an electrician. You face a triple disaster if you do not heed the warning: fire, electrocution, and ruining an expensive piece of equipment.

Extension cords Avoid multiple extension cords plugged into one receptacle—the so-called spider. Promptly replace frayed cords and broken plugs; do not run cords over metal fasteners, such as hooks. Be cautious about running extension cords under carpeting.

Hot spots in walls If you discover unaccountable heat when placing your hand on a wall, and there is no heating or plumbing line running in that location, suspect an electrical fault and immediately get an electrician to investigate.

Accessory heaters Radiant heaters and space heaters are heavy users of electrical power and are possible fire hazards. Be sure that the equipment bears a UL seal on both the heater and its cord. An extension cord must also be heavy duty, just as the original plug-in cord is.

Do not use such a heater where inflammable material, such as clothing or draperies, might somehow come into contact with it. Floor models should be firmly seated to assure that they will not topple. Preferably, you should purchase a heater that shuts off automatically if knocked over.

Fireplaces, wood-burning stoves, and kerosene stoves

Fireplaces must be carefully screened to prevent embers and sparks from being shot into the room. Keep all flammable materials away from the hearth area. Learn how to operate the damper to obtain maximum effectiveness from your fireplace, and also how to prevent filling the room with smoke and carbon monoxide. Have the chimney checked yearly before using the fireplace. Do not build a roaring fire just before going to bed.

Kerosene heaters are unsafe and their use has been widely outlawed. They present both fire and carbon monoxide hazards.

Outdoor grills

Never use an explosively flammable fluid such as gasoline to start a charcoal fire. Use long forks or tongs and heat-proof gloves and an apron, to prevent burns.

Kitchen fires

Kitchen range and oven This equipment should bear the seal of the American Gas Association or, for electric ranges, the UL seal. With *gas burners*, most accidents not caused directly by the burner arise from defective flues, leaking pipes, faulty pilot lights, and improper usage, such as allowing a pot to boil over and extinguish the flame, or allowing children to play with the controls or brush against them.

Escaping gas produces serious hazards of fire, explosion, and carbon monoxide poisoning. Fuel gas is odorized, naturally or artificially, and you can smell it. Never disregard this warning. If the odor is strong, do not take chances. First, open the windows both top and bottom. (Natural gas rises to the ceiling; liquified petroleum gases and bottled gas accumulate near the floor.) Then get out of the house and call the gas company—

from a neighbor's telephone. En route do not turn on any electric switches, and do not pull out any electric plugs—the small spark thus created is enough to explode the gas. Do not light a match. Too often, someone returns home, smells gas on opening the door, either turns on the nearest light switch or lights a match to investigate, and is killed in the immediate explosion or the fierce fire that ensues.

Always keep the gas burners clean and free from sticky substances from spilled food. Have the burners adjusted by an expert if the flame is yellow and flickering, instead of blue and upright.

Many of these problems, excluding those of escaping gas, can also arise in the use of electric stoves (see page 450).

Food that bursts into flame during cooking Cooking oil is the usual cause. This scary emergency can usually be brought under control quickly. Often, merely dropping a pot lid on the cooking utensil will smother the fire immediately. Baking soda or salt dropped onto the fire can also extinguish it. Never use water on burning grease or oil; it will probably spread the fire. If your countermeasures fail and the fire spreads, do not waste time; get out and call the fire department.

Gasoline

Never store gasoline anywhere inside your home. Do not store it outdoors, either, if a safer fluid is available. If gasoline is essential as a fuel for a power mower, for example, store it in a well-ventilated area, in a closed, safety can. Do not buy more than your immediate use requires. Pour it into the gasoline tank of your equipment when you are outside, and never smoke in the vicinity.

Scalds

Most scald victims are children. Scalds occur most commonly in the kitchen, but bathtub scalds tend to be more serious because they cover a larger surface of the body.

In the kitchen, do not leave pans with their handles protruding from the stove. A small child can pull over a utensil full of boiling water or, even worse, hot grease, or can pull on the cord of an electric frying pan with the same results. Unwary adults also become victims in such accidents.

In the bathroom, never leave a small child alone in a bathtub where he can turn on the hot water tap, even for a few seconds. Be careful about leaving elderly or otherwise infirm household members unattended in a bathtub.

FIRE PREVENTION AND CONTROL

What to do in case of a home fire

If it is a general conflagration, get out as fast as you can, making sure that everybody else in the house gets out, too. Don't stop to collect personal belongings. If your exit is more than a few steps away, crawl, don't walk or run. Telephone the fire department from a neighbor's phone.

In smaller, localized fires, you may try to deal with it yourself with water or a fire extinguisher, but do not persist after a few seconds of failure. *It is only a matter of seconds between life and death.* If your home is filling with smoke, do not stop to ascertain the source: get out. Bear in mind that flames are only part of the menace—carbon monoxide and poisonous smoke are just as dangerous.

Above all, do not box yourself in; be sure you have a clear escape route. After it's all over, check for suspicious smoldering, in upholstery, for example. If there is the least doubt in your mind that the fire has been totally and finally extinguished, call the fire department.

Fire and smoke detectors

One or more such devices should be installed in every home depending on its size, without exception. In some areas of the nation, installation is required by law in all new construction. They are easily installed in existing homes.

There are two main types: the photoelectric detector, which is especially sensitive to smoke, and the ionization detector, which is especially sensitive to flames. Both are effective. Both are available as either battery-powered or house-current powered units. The battery type seems preferable because it works during a power failure, is easier to install, and cannot become a fire hazard itself.

Most detectors emit a continuous-tone warning, some a warbling sound, and some can be connected to a remote warning device. At least one brand combines an emergency light with the audible alarm. Look for the UL seal. The gravest danger from home fires occurs during the night when residents are asleep. The detector warning is designed to awaken anyone who is not deaf.

Proper placement of the detector improves its efficiency. It should be ceiling mounted because most smoke rises to the ceiling. It should be strategically placed: in a hall, within about 10 feet of bedroom entrances; at the top of basement stairs, and so forth. If possible, avoid installation in the kitchen where smoke from food preparation could set off the alarm unnecessarily.

Test the equipment after installation, and at periodic intervals. A convenient method is to blow smoke into it. This may require standing on some type of step. Be careful, because the sudden blast of the alarm may startle you enough to make you fall off the step.

A prearranged plan of action in a fire or smoke emergency

Such a plan should include at least the following:

1. *A method of escape* for each member of the household from every area of the house, each with an alternative plan in the event that the primary escape route cannot be used. Second and third floor bedrooms should be equipped with emergency chain or rope ladders. Consider installation of a bar to hang onto beside selected windows to decrease the danger of falling out when yelling for help. In case of fire, teach all household members to crawl on the floor, not walk upright, because nearly all poisonous gases of a fire rise to the ceiling; they are lowest in concentration nearest the floor.

2. *Have a prearranged plan for all household members to meet at a designated place outside the house or apartment.* This is a life-saving measure. Many deaths occur when a family member rushes back into a burning house to rescue another member, who has already escaped but could not be found. Do not select a spot that predictably would be occupied by firemen or their equipment. This could easily deny the preselected spot to sole possession by household members and thus upset your precautionary plan.

3. *Make each member of the household practice the plan.* Speed is critical to effective action in a fire. The ability to act quickly is likely to be impaired in a person suddenly awakened and who already may have inhaled enough poisonous gas products to increase confusion. The plan's actions should be rehearsed enough so as to make them automatic in a real emergency.

Fire extinguishers

Each home should be equipped with one per floor. Their use should be based on good judgment. A rule should be agreed on that if there is any doubt at all, forget the extinguishers, get out of the house, and call the fire department. If you are confident that you can control the fire quickly with an extinguisher, use it promptly and properly. Stand away from the flames, aim at the source of the fire, not at the flames, and move the spray from side to side.

Select a fire extinguisher with a UL or FM (Factory Mutual) label. Do not use a liquid content extinguisher or water on a grease fire or on an electrical fire. A 2A:10BC extinguisher will handle a small fire of almost any source or type. Be certain that you understand the manufacturer's specifications and directions. Check the dial on the equipment periodically to be certain that it still has sufficient pressure to be useful in an emergency.

Fires in high-rise apartment houses

The problems here are different from those in one or two-family residences. Modern multistory apartment buildings usually are constructed of fire-resistant materials that make them considerably less susceptible to a conflagration than are private homes. However, old apartment buildings with much wood construction and in poor repair are hazardous.

Your actions during fires generally will have to be a compromise between the measures recommended for private homes and for modern apartment buildings. You should ascertain what past experience and future probabilities are concerning fires in your building. Then decide on a plan for yourself and your family.

The plan should be based on two contingencies: fire in the building and fire in your own apartment. The general rule in properly constructed high-rise buildings is not to leave the building and, in fact, not to leave your apartment unless it is the site of the fire.

Fire in the building

Call the fire department immediately. Don't assume someone else has already done so. If small amounts of smoke are seeping into your apartment under the doors, quickly stuff wet towels about the doorway and *partially* open a window—full opening may create too much of a draft. Then stay in your apartment at the opened window, preferably close to the floor, and await the arrival of firemen to tell you what to do next.

If you feel that you must leave, press your hand against the door first. If it is abnormally warm to the touch, do not open it—there is probably a dangerous fire in the corridor. If it is not warm, open it cautiously. If there is not much smoke in the corridor and you feel certain the corridor can be used, alert other occupants of your floor quickly and go to the stairwell.

Do not use an elevator. Close the stairwell door behind you to prevent an increased draft for the fire. If you encounter increasing smoke during your descent, either try the corridor of another floor or, probably best, return to your own apartment.

Naturally, you could use an outside fire escape if the building is so equipped, but be careful not to fall or to descend to what proves to be the floor where the fire is. If you have a balcony, this might be a good refuge, depending upon its location in relation to the fire. Either take your keys with you or be certain that the door to the balcony will not lock you out and trap you there.

Fire in your own apartment

Your apartment building may be almost totally fireproof, but the contents of your apartment are flammable. Actions during a fire in your own apartment are quite similar to those described for private homes, including selection of a prearranged meeting place for household members. Except for very minor fires—and remember that minor fires can become major ones in seconds— leave your apartment *immediately*. Alert your neighbors. Then proceed as for fires in the building.

Don't use the elevators. Elevators may stick between floors in a fire and thus trap the occupants, and heat-controlled elevator operating panels may automatically send the elevator to the very floor on which the fire is located.

First-aid measures for burns

Improper immediate treatment can adversely affect subsequent medical care.

Minor burns   Any burn is painful. Minor ones should be treated immediately by soaking in cold water. This relieves the pain, prevents extension of the burn deeper into the tissue, and may prevent or at least reduce blister formation.

Extensive and deep burns   Insist on treatment by a physician. Do not smear ointments onto burned areas. Cover them with sterile bandages or clean linen and immediately get the patient to a hospital, preferably by ambulance.

Carbon Monoxide and Smoke Poisoning

Carbon monoxide poisoning is produced whenever incomplete combustion of carbon or carbon compounds occurs. It is an insidious threat to life in practically all fires. Its chemical formula is CO, which can also mean "colorless and odorless."

HOW IT WORKS

The affinity of CO for the hemoglobin of human blood is about three hundred times that of oxygen. Thus life-sustaining *oxy*hemoglobin can quickly be converted into poisonous *carbox*yhemoglobin, and unless the process is stopped quickly, death by asphyxiation is inevitable. When the brain is deprived of normal oxygen supply, consciousness is dulled and then lost. In some cases an equally disastrous state of euphoria occurs that can lull one into giving up trying to escape, even when the escape route may be clear.

FIRES AND CARBON MONOXIDE

Most fires start with some kind of material smoldering before bursting into flame. In this process, smoke is given off. Smoke consists of any of a large variety of toxic chemicals, and is accompanied by CO. In fires where the victims are found in their beds or on the floor near the bed, generally they died from asphyxiation by carbon monoxide and smoke, not from flames. Even when the bodies are badly charred, it is obvious that the victims must have been unconscious, usually from CO poisoning, when the flames reached them.

Only in movies can the hero enter a fiercely burning building, search endlessly for the heroine, and emerge with her unscathed. The likelihood of the victim already being dead of carbon monoxide and other toxic gas inhalation is so great as to be almost a certainty, and the chances are overwhelming that the foolhardy rescuer would also become a victim, if not during his search, then certainly while struggling, upright, to carry the victim out.

The other ingredients of smoke are also asphyxiants, and in today's home, the assortment is almost limitless. Most of the plastics widely used in home furnishings are more flammable than wood and many give off highly toxic fumes when they burn. There is no practical possibility of eliminating plastic material from the home. The hope is that manufacturers will build into these products the maximum possible fire resistance. Meantime, be alert to this additional hazard and, as a precautionary measure, have smoke detectors installed.

OTHER SOURCES OF CARBON MONOXIDE

In addition to fires, there are further sources of carbon monoxide and other poisonous gases in the home. These include the gasoline engine or motor. Many people die of CO asphyxiation each year because their cars are left running in a garage, with suicidal intent or otherwise. If the garage is attached to the house, CO can seep in and endanger other members of the household. Never allow an automobile motor to run in your garage for any period of time, whether the garage door is open or closed.

LENGTHY EXPOSURE TO SMALL CONCENTRATIONS OF CO

This is perhaps the most treacherous of all types of CO poisoning. It involves a series of hard-to-detect nonlethal poisonings. Its victims experience symptoms only after being in the home for hours and are free from them after leaving the home. Headache probably is the most common symptom, along with nausea, loss of appetite, vomiting for no apparent reason, and many other nonspecific complaints. Often the real cause of such symptoms goes unsuspected for some time, while the victim remains exposed to the possibility of unconsciousness and death. A physician who suspects the real cause will insist on a detailed check of the home for CO sources. Removal of the offending source usually leads to a quick and dramatic cure.

Home heating and hot water units

Look for an AGA (American Gas Association) or UL seal on all heating equipment. A heater must be properly vented and the vent must remain unclogged. Before starting it in the fall, have it checked by an expert. A previously safe vent may have become clogged with bird or squirrel nests, soot, or other debris. A defective flue damper is also dangerous.

Kitchen stoves

Modern gas ovens usually do not require venting. If they are working properly they give off only minute quantities of CO. But they were not designed to heat a home. When an oven door is left open with a full fire inside, grave danger of CO poisoning is introduced. A gas kitchen stove (or any gas heating unit) can become a hazard when the flame is not properly adjusted (it should be blue, not yellow), or when the pilot light malfunctions. Never disregard the odor of gas no matter how slight.

Charcoal burners and hibachis

Never use charcoal burners or hibachis inside the house. They give off dangerous amounts of CO when used where venting is inadequate. When used outdoors, there is no CO hazard.

TREATMENT OF ACUTE CO POISONING

Open the windows. Get the victim outside as quickly as possible. Administer mouth-to-mouth resuscitation if the victim has stopped breathing or is barely breathing. Get the patient to a hospital, even if recovery seems to be occurring. A careful medical checkup is necessary for all victims because of possible delayed effects of the poisoning.

Carbon monoxide has one compensating characteristic: it tends to rise from the floor to the ceiling. Thus it is important for anyone in a fire to crawl on the floor, rather than try to walk or run upright.

Poisons

After falls and fires, poisoning by solids and liquids is the most frequent cause of death from home accidents, with a toll of about 3,400 deaths yearly in the United States. About two-thirds of these deaths are caused by chemicals, drugs, and other medicines. Food poisoning is usually a bacterial disease, not classed as an accident (see chapter 13, Infectious Diseases).

Twice as many males die of such poisonings as females. In the age groups 15–24 and 25–44 poisoning from solids and liquids is the most common cause of accidental death in the home. The full extent of the problem, which is a major one at all ages, is difficult to estimate because statistics are usually limited to deaths. Nonfatal poisonings, no matter how serious, are grossly underreported by comparison.

The list of substances that may be poisonous when ingested by humans is infinite and preventive measures vary accordingly. (See page 447 for what to do in case of poisoning.)

POISONING BY DRUGS AND MEDICATIONS

The most ubiquitous drugs found in homes across the nation tend to cause the most deaths. Thus, aspirin and aspirin-related drugs lead the list, causing nearly one-third of fatal drug poisonings. Similarly, and because improperly used they are much more deadly, the second most frequent cause of death is the group of sedatives, hypnotics, barbiturates, and related preparations. Drugs for treatment of diseases of the heart and cardiovascular system rank next. The prevalence of these drugs around the house also accounts for the serious nonfatal poisonings, especially in the case of aspirin drugs. (See chapter 3, Drugs.)

Precautions

Follow the directions Get complete instructions from the pharmacist, including a list of the medication's limitations. Do not assume that if one tablet produced some relief of symptoms, five tablets will accomplish five times as much improvement.

Never remove medicines from their original containers and transfer them to unlabeled or mislabeled receptacles. This invites confusion. Ask your pharmacist to divide the prescription into smaller labeled containers if you do not wish to carry a large one.

Before taking any drug, inspect the label or directions before removing it from the shelf, again before uncapping the bottle, again before taking the dose—and perhaps once more before returning it to the shelf. This may seem an elaborate ritual, but it is the type of system usually taught—for good reasons—to all physicians, pharmacists, and nurses.

Discard remaining, unused medicine when the illness ends for which it was prescribed. Do not keep it for the next attack, unless the illness recurs frequently. Old drugs may lose their potency; they may be confused with some other preparation and be taken accidentally. Discard all drugs no longer in use.

Keep all drugs away from small children Discipline is not enough. Children are curious and ingenious. High shelves are better places for drugs than low shelves, but there should also be a safety catch or, better yet, a lock on the cabinet door. Handbags containing drugs should be kept out of the way of prying hands. Avoid taking drugs in front of children; they like to emulate adults.

Don't let your frustrations with opening "childproof" caps keep you from insisting on them.

After the law requiring safety caps went into effect in 1972, the reports of harmful aspirin ingestions in children under five years was cut nearly in half. If older or handicapped adults in the household cannot use these safety caps, other packaging can be provided by the pharmacist, but do not disregard your consequent extra responsibility for protecting children from drugs.

Don't buy substances of questionable or limited value and, above all, do not keep them around after current usage is ended. For example, although boric acid has uses as an insect killer, it is poisonous if swallowed and there are nontoxic substitutes. Infants have died as a result of the accidental mixing of boric acid into the milk formula. Camphorated oil, sometimes accidentally substituted for cod liver oil, is highly poisonous; it has no function that cannot be carried out as well or better by less poisonous substances. As many as five hundred camphor poisonings have been reported in a single year.

HOUSEHOLD CHEMICALS

Of the enormous number of such preparations used in the modern home, some of the most frequent are:

Drain and toilet bowl cleaners These usually are, or can produce, powerful acids or alkalis that eat through fats and other material in clogged drain pipes. They have a similar effect inside the human body.

Furniture polishes Most contain mineral seal oil, which is a petroleum distillate, as are naphtha, kerosene, gasoline, and related products. All are poisonous to the stomach when swallowed and also to the respiratory system when vomited. In the respiratory system they cause chemical pneumonia, which is not responsive to antibiotics. Most such products carry the warning: "If swallowed, do not induce vomiting."

Wood panel cleaners These preparations often contain solvents and additives, and a pine oil, that can also produce chemical pneumonia.

Soaps and detergents Because mild soap is relatively harmless, many people assume that detergents are equally benign. They are, in fact, alkaline and extremely toxic. When children rub their eyes with hands that have been in detergent, eye burns can result.

Ammonia Frequently used in household cleaning, it is poisonous when swallowed.

Aerosols There are at least five types of hazards:

1. Explosion of the can, if it is overheated or punctured. Never throw it into a furnace, and don't try to crush or puncture it.
2. Children, and even adults, may release the aerosol contents in such a way as to strike their eyes.
3. The contents of the can, if inhaled, may be toxic.
4. Both the contents and the propellant may be inflammable. Never use an aerosol can near a flame. The path of the aerosol may ignite, leap back toward the can, and explode it in a mass of flames.
5. Under some circumstances, the propellant may be dangerous in a confined space.

Gasoline Aside from the enormous fire hazard it presents, gasoline is extremely toxic. Don't try to siphon gasoline by mouth—the risk of swallowing it is too great. In general, gasoline is dangerous to handle anywhere on the home premises.

Carbon tetrachloride "Carbon tet" is used as a cleaning agent. Because its fumes are highly dangerous and the effects are unpredictable, it has been banned from interstate shipment. Some people are more susceptible than others; alcoholics are at particular risk. Inhalation of the fumes can cause acute, fatal liver failure.

Paint removers Some types are highly flammable, irritating to the skin, and dangerous to inhale in closed areas. Nonflammable paint removers also contain toxic ingredients, which, when inhaled or splashed on the skin, can damage the central nervous system as well as bone marrow and blood cells.

Household paints Most are safe when appropriately used, but can be poisonous when swallowed. Paint solvents or thinners may contain petroleum distillates, with the inherent dangers mentioned under Furniture Polishes above.

Plastic epoxy resins Used for many mending purposes, they can produce severe dermatitis to exposed skin and are highly toxic if taken internally. Respect the manufacturer's cautionary label.

Combining chemicals Never mix a bleaching or cleaning agent with an acid-type toilet bowl cleaner, ammonia, lye, rust remover, vinegar, or oven cleaner. The mixture can liberate chlorine gas, which is so lethal that it was used as a weapon during World War I. This can—and does—happen in the seemingly harmless act of dumping a cleaning agent into a toilet bowl for disposal, when the bowl already contains an acid cleaner. Don't try to memorize the various chemicals involved. Simply follow the rule of never mixing household chemicals, cleaners, and related substances in any kind of container. The same precautions apply to chemicals used to clean a home swimming pool or to treat the water in it.

Rodenticides It should be obvious that any poison strong enough to kill a large rat might also kill, or at least induce, violent illness, in a human being, especially a child. There are at least one thousand cases of such childhood accidents each year. When using rat poison in the home, it should be inaccessible to either humans or animal pets. There is practically no area of any house that is inaccessible to a determined rat.

Insecticides Follow the manufacturer's instructions, but do not place absolute confidence in a statement that the preparation is nontoxic to humans. What may be safe in normal usage by an adult may become dangerous if ingested in substantial quantities by a child. Keep these preparations in a locked cupboard away from children. Aerosol insecticides may be toxic to humans, but even if they are not, they are producers of the hazards described above for aerosols.

Other pesticides For children and adults there are hazards related to the use of all pesticides in both the home and garden. DDT was banned in January 1973. Safety problems have now arisen from the chemicals developed as DDT replacements. Their names alone should inspire caution: organophosphates, such as demeton, dimethoate, disulfoton, phorate, mevinphos, parathion, and azinphosmethyl; or carbamates, such as aidicarb, arprocarb, carbofuran, methomyl, amino carb, and carberyl; chlorinated hydrocarbons, such as BHC, lindate, methoxychlor, chlordane, aldrin, dieldrin, heptachlor, and endrin. These preparations may be introduced into the human body in several ways: accidental contamination of food; drinking them from an unlabeled container or a container contaminated by a pesticide; siphoning by mouth; ingestion of the chemical from contaminated hands; absorption through the skin, particularly when not protected by clothing; splashing or spraying the substance into the eyes or onto the skin; inhalation of dust, mists, or fumes, or from smoking or contamination of cigarettes.

Such substances should be bought only in quantities required immediately and should not be stored for future use.

Utmost care must be taken to prevent contamination of food. Protective clothing must be worn and goggles and masks may be necessary, depending on the type of chemical and its usage.

Obviously, the greatest exposure will be on farms, where wider areas and greater varieties of pesticides are used. But the home garden or fruit trees can also produce serious hazards from such operations, and to a lesser extent such dangers are introduced into the home, even in cities.

Moth balls should be singled out because some look invitingly like candy balls. They contain naphtha and are poisonous. A child who puts one in its mouth and is shocked by its bad taste may gasp, aspirate the ball, and be strangled by it. Call your poison control center (see page 447) for information or treatment, or take the child to an emergency room at the hospital.

General precautions

Most of the categories listed include materials that are so helpful to running a household that to eliminate them would be unthinkable. Nevertheless, some general precautions can be taken to minimize their dangers.

1. *Store the substances securely.* The area under the kitchen sink is convenient, but it can be easily reached by a child. Store the chemicals in a relatively inaccessible place such as on a high shelf, though not so high that it requires standing on something to reach it, thus substituting an adult falling hazard for a child's poisoning hazard. A lock on the door of the storage cupboard is inconvenient but

highly desirable. Also, try to keep all toxic products in one place. The more storage areas used, the more difficult it is to make them secure or to remember to take the necessary routine precautions for each.

2. *Avoid toxic products with unusual containers and pleasant odors added that appeal to children.* This precaution is not always possible but is worth remembering.

3. *Never rebottle or repackage these products.* Don't store cleaning solutions in soft drink or wine bottles, or some other unsuitable container. It is not enough to put your own label on a bottle to which you are transferring such substances. Your label may not be sufficiently legible, it may not display a prominent poison warning, and it will not include the ingredients that should be known in the event of a poisoning.

4. *Never store toxic products near foods.* Cake made accidentally with cleaning powder instead of cake flour will, at best, be inedible and, at worst, lethal. Unlikely as it may seem, this frequently happens.

5. *Avoid over-buying of preparations only occasionally used.* Buy only what is needed; discard the rest.

6. *After using a toxic material, put it away immediately.* If this is delayed because of other tasks, a child may be the next person to use the substance.

7. *Do not relax precautions because no children live in your home.* Other people's children may visit and grandchildren often visit for days or weeks. Such exposure is fraught with special danger because people who have long had no need to child-proof their homes are unprepared for the invasion of small children. Joyous family get-togethers may end in tragedy because, in the excitement of reunion, the absence of one small child exploring on his own goes unnoticed.

PLANTS AND BERRIES

These are natural products, bought for enjoyment. In general, they are not thought of as having poisonous possibilities, but in fact some of them do.

The sprig of mistletoe, hung overhead at Christmas, is decorative, but its berries, which can drop to the floor and be eaten by a small child, are poisonous.

One leaf of the poinsettia, another popular Christmas plant, contains enough poisonous juice to kill a child who chews it.

Castor beans are planted to produce lush green plants and are often strung into necklaces. Well-chewed by a child, however, one bean can produce death. Rosary pea beads, also used to make necklaces, have the same lethal potential.

There are other hazardous plants that can be brought into the home or raised in home gardens:

Jack-in-the-pulpit and elephant ears may burn your mouth and throat with crystals of calcium oxalate. Cherry twigs and leaves, as well as peach tree leaves, release cyanide when chewed. Petals of rhododendron, laurel, azalea, lily-of-the-valley, and many other plants can cause violent illness, even death, when chewed. Poison hemlock looks like a wild carrot and contains a deadly poison. This is not to be confused with the evergreen tree with the same name. Moonseed, which looks like wild purple grapes, can be lethal if eaten. Thorn apples can cause delirium and coma, even death, if eaten. Deadly nightshade berries are aptly named.

The leaves and vines of tomato and potato plants should not be eaten. Pie made of rhubarb stalks is safe, but rhubarb leaves should not be eaten; they may damage your kidneys with oxalic acid.

The safest rule is never to eat any plant not known to be an established foodstuff. Keep all plants, berries, and so forth away from small children, and vice versa. Teach these principles to older children who may encounter unsuspected poisonous plants in their own backyard or be tempted by them on hiking excursions.

FIRST AID FOR POISONING

In spite of the urgent need for immediate action in poisoning cases, expert advice should be obtained before doing anything, in order to avoid doing precisely the wrong thing. Telephoning the family physician is desirable, but many families have no family physician and those who do have one can rarely reach him or her *immediately*.

The alternative is to phone one of the six hundred poison control centers scattered around the nation, located mainly in hospitals and health departments. Most of them provide twenty-four hour answering service. All of them have extensive files on computer tape of most known types of poisons or, if the poisonous substance is rare, each center can make immediate contact with the comprehensive files of the National Clearing House for Poison Control Centers. The inside cover of most telephone books contains a printed list of emergency numbers for their areas. One of them is usually listed for "Poison Control Center." Don't wait for an emergency to occur. Look for the number in your telephone directory *now*. If you cannot find it immediately, make appropriate inquiries as to the number to call and record it where you can find it quickly.

If an emergency does occur, don't waste precious time by trying to look up things to do—in this or any other book. Call the Poison Center before starting any other measures, with the exception of artificial respiration where it is necessary.

The following progression of steps is recommended:

1. If the victim has stopped breathing, give artificial respiration, preferably by the mouth-to-mouth method. Otherwise, no additional steps could possibly accomplish anything.
2. If no other person is present, and you must concentrate on artificial respiration, try to summon help by yelling or screaming.
3. In most cases, it is unlikely that artificial respiration will be required immediately. If it is not, quickly find what caused the poisoning, take the container to the telephone, and call the poison center. Be sure you have a piece of paper and a pen or pencil to write down the instructions you receive.
4. Describe the source of the poison and the age and physical condition of the victim.
5. If you are told to administer milk, water, or other liquid, be certain to inquire about the amount (usually 1 to 2 cupfuls to small children, a quart to older children and adults). If you are advised to administer some fluid which you know or suspect is not available, ask about a substitute.
6. *Vomiting induction.* If you are told to induce vomiting, follow these directions. *In every household, especially if there are children, there should be a bottle of syrup of ipecac in the medicine cabinet.* It can be bought in a pharmacy without prescription in a one-ounce bottle. Be sure it is properly labeled—something like "Syrup of Ipecac. Poison antidote," or "To induce vomiting." If instructed to induce vomiting, give one-half the contents of the 1 oz. bottle by teaspoon, using a cup or more of water to wash it down. Don't mix the syrup of ipecac in the water, because if the patient is not able to drink the whole cup of water, some of the drug will be lost. The dose will almost certainly induce vomiting. If it does not, give the other half of the bottle within twenty minutes, but then no more.

If you have neglected to keep syrup of ipecac on hand, induce vomiting by making the victim gag: tickle the back of the throat with your finger. During vomiting the patient should be placed face down, with head lower than body, in order to prevent inhalation of vomitus. Do *not* give salt water, soapy water, or mustard water to induce vomiting; you will only add another danger to an already critical situation.

Remember: *Do not induce vomiting until you have been instructed to do so by the poison center or by a physician.*

7. Last, depending on the nature of the poisoning, and the advice from the poison center or physician, you are ready to await further assistance, or get the victim to the nearest hospital. Take the poison bottle or package with you.

8. Once again, don't try to be an expert on poisoning treatment, and don't take the advice of any other amateur. Get expert advice quickly and act on it. You may thus save a life or prevent great suffering.

Home Appliances, Tools, and Equipment

Accidents arising from the use and misuse of home appliances include mechanical mishaps, fires, or electric shocks. Appliances may be unsafe when purchased, or may become so with long use and the wearing out of parts and wiring; they may be improperly maintained or used. Appliance-caused accidents can occur anywhere in or around the home. One of the more useful sources of information on such appliance hazards is *Consumer Reports*, published by the Consumers Union, which includes a consideration of relevant safety factors in all its ratings of home appliances.

THE BATHROOM

Because lots of water is used in bathrooms, they are potentially hazardous sites of electrical accidents when appliances are used there. *Blow-dryers* are probably the most dangerous. A blow-dryer with the current on can easily be dropped into a basin full of water. Without thinking, the user may grab the appliance out of the water, causing a severe, even lethal electric shock. Instead of following that natural but lethal reaction, you should unplug the appliance immediately. Only then can the dryer be removed from the water without risking electrocution. Make it a rule always to disconnect the appliance when not in use, even for a brief time. This rule also applies to *electric hair curlers* and *curling irons*, *electric toothbrushes*, *electric razors*, and *water-picks*. Whenever possible, use these items in the bedroom.

Never set a portable *plug-in radio* on the edge of the bathroom tub or on a shelf above the tub and turn it on. It could accidentally fall into the bath water and electrocute the bather. Also, a person immersed in bath water who decides to turn the radio dials can be electrocuted because of defective wiring.

Portable electric heaters should not be used anywhere in the house without proper precautions, but especially in the bathrooms. Never touch one when you are grounded; for example, when you are wet or in contact with a wet surface, or a water pipe, radiator, water faucet, steel sink, or other conductor of electrical current. A heavy-duty extension with a rating high enough to carry the required load should be used, not an ordinary lamp extension cord.

THE KITCHEN

The kitchen, showplace of electrical equipment, is also a minefield of potential hazards. The *electric toaster*, in addition to sharing the dangers common to all electrical appliances, has a unique one of its own. Sometimes, the pop-up mechanism may not work, or the object being toasted gets stuck. If, through ignorance or carelessness, you try to dig out the toasted article with a metal instrument such as a fork or knife, electrocution can occur instantaneously. The toaster should always be unplugged before such a maneuver is attempted, or before the risky method of turning the toaster upside down is tried. Children should not be allowed to use the toaster until they are old enough to be instructed in how to use it and to remember its electrical dangers.

The kitchen sink counter shelf Be cautious about using even the most shock-proof appliances on such a shelf, particularly if it is metal. The danger can be lessened by using a nonconducting base—a wooden cutting board, for example—between shelf and appliance. Do not allow the electrical cord to come into contact with water or with any part of the appliance that may become hot and melt the insulation on the cord.

Garbage disposer If the disposer is a continuous feed type, its off-and-on switch should be installed where an adult could not accidentally turn it on by brushing against it; it should be high enough to prevent children from reaching it. To unclog and restart it, if you need a tool other than the one provided with the machine, use a dry broomstick.

Food processors, blenders, and mixers are almost standard equipment in today's home kitchens. Most of this equipment is electrically safe with proper usage. The precautions regarding electrical shock apply. Some special ones: Before changing blades or other attachments, any machine must be unplugged. Merely turning off the switch is not enough. What a food processor does to a piece of meat in a second, it can do to your fingers. Don't attempt to stir the contents of a blender or processor without first shutting off the motor. The least that can happen is that your rubber or plastic spatula will be mixed with your food, or if a metal implement, ruin the blades of your appliance. Never leave any of the blades and slicers where children can pick them up.

Electric carving knives Be certain that they are UL approved. Never remove or insert the blades of the plug-in types without first unplugging it.

Dishwasher/washing machine/dryer Most of this equipment is foolproof against opening while in operation, but read the manufacturer's instructions carefully. The chief danger arises from the possibility of electric shock, since both clothes washers and dishwashers come in contact with plumbing. Three-wire plug-ins and receptacles should be installed for all such equipment. There can be serious hazard for *small children* who may try to climb inside a drier or turn on the switch, or both.

Stoves The particular hazard in electric stoves is that the burners can be "on," but because they are not always red, they may seem to be "off." This must be explained to children. In all types of stoves, there is always the danger of loose clothing catching on fire. Window curtains should not be hung near the stove.

Pot handles should be turned away from the front of the kitchen range to avoid scalds.

Cupboard doors and drawers should not be left open. High ones may produce a scalp laceration when you straighten up; low ones are a tripping hazard.

Knives and other implements Store knives carefully, preferably in individual slots in a wooden knife holder. This will make it harder to grab a knife by its cutting blade, and also will protect the edge. Remember that a *sharp knife* is safer than a dull one. More effort is required to cut or chop with a dull knife; therefore, more possibilities of accidental cuts arise from dull knives. Do not walk around carrying a sharp knife; do not leave sharp kitchen implements lying on a kitchen counter where curious children can pick them up and play with them.

Bottles and containers A study of thirty-seven instances of *exploding pop bottles* revealed that in ten cases the bottle exploded without any apparent cause; fourteen occurred during normal handling, and thirteen after an impact—being dropped, tipped over, or merely jarred against another bottle. In thirty incidents medical treatment was required, largely for hand lacerations or eye injuries (one victim lost an eye).

Another type of explosion accident is the *sudden ejection of a bottle cork or cap*. The larger the bottle, the greater is the explosive force. One such bottle exploded within a refrigerator, and its fragments penetrated the refrigerator walls.

Do not store bottles of carbonated beverage in a hot closet; avoid knocking them down or jarring them against other objects; store them on lower shelves to reduce the impact if they are accidentally dropped; do not shake the bottle; and, above all, direct the cap or cork away from yourself or anyone else when opening the bottle.

When opening a champagne bottle, wrap the bottle neck and cork with a napkin and ease the cork out, without pointing the bottle at anyone.

Cans of food explode if they are heated to a high enough degree without being opened.

Plastic cooking bags present hazards when they are tightly sealed with food inside and placed in the oven. An explosion can occur and spattered grease from the contents of the bag may start an oven fire. The bag should be ventilated with holes that are large enough so that cooking juices will not seal them during baking or roasting. Another safety measure is to add flour to the contents of the bag.

Steam pressure can power a railroad locomotive that pulls a hundred freight cars. In the same way, steam pressure can build up within a sealed metal container such as a *pressure cooker*. Such cookers can blow up, causing severe or fatal injuries from shrapnel-like pieces of metal; in other cases, escaping steam can scald the cook. Do not use a pressure cooker until you have made yourself thoroughly aware of all its dangers.

OTHER APPLIANCES AND EQUIPMENT

Television sets

The *only* part of a television set the viewer should deal with is the control panel on the front of the set. The inside wiring and all other arrangements are for professional experts. The amateur repairperson will rarely succeed in remedying a malfunction and is highly vulnerable to electrocution; he or she can also set fire to the set and to the house.

Allow enough room about the set to permit adequate ventilation of the considerable amount of heat that a TV set generates. Prohibit horseplay in the vicinity of the set; knocking into the front of the set may cause the TV tube to implode and hurl bits of jagged glass across the room. Unplug your set if you are going away for any extended period of time. Consult your repairman concerning lightning hazards.

Use care in cleaning the viewing area. Turn off the set first, and do not use a liquid cleaner because it might seep into the electrical circuits and cause shock or a fire as well as damage the plastic tube cover.

Electric fans

In these air-conditioned times, many people are not familiar with the potential dangers of electric fans. Children and adults have received severe finger lacerations or amputations from curious poking into an electric fan that was turned on. An object introduced into fan blades may become a propelled missile. Fans with a mesh guard to prevent introduction of an object into the blades are not popular because they seem to decrease the flow of air. Whenever practical, installation of an electric fan should be on a wall bracket, solidly anchored, above the reach of prying hands.

Vacuum cleaners

Be aware of frayed electrical cords. Turn off the motor before attempting to dislodge any item stuck in the intake. Indoor vacuum cleaners should not be used on a patio, around a swimming pool, or elsewhere outdoors because of the increased possibility of electrical shock.

Power tools

Because of the wide variety of injuries that power tools are capable of causing, these general precautions should be taken:

1. The tools should be grounded (three-pronged plug) or be labeled as double insulated (two-pronged plug) and should be used only in dry areas. The electrical shock potential is all the more serious because such equipment is usually used in the basement where the possibility of electric shock is greatest. Use three-pronged extensions and sockets for grounded tools.
2. Insist on equipment having a UL-approved seal.
3. Do not keep combustible materials in the vicinity of any such tools.
4. Read carefully the accompanying manual and keep the guards supplied with the equipment in place, as instructed. If adequate guards are not available, do not use the equipment.
5. Don't forget to use safety goggles.
6. Always disconnect the electrical power before adjusting for a changed task.

Your chance of serious injury from home power tools is greater than that arising from similar equipment in industry. Most industries have strict safety rules. Workers who neglect to use guards and other safety precautions do so at the risk of losing their jobs. Supervise yourself and members of your family just as strictly.

Lawn mowers

Many hazards have been reduced by manufacturers' improvements, but they still exist. You should be well aware of them and make sure they are known by anyone using your mower.

Foot injuries Amputation or mangling of toes can result from a foot sliding into the rotary blades under the mower. Although this can take place on level ground, it is more likely to happen on an incline. Wear heavy shoes, preferably with a hard toe, but realize that even these will not provide complete protection against the blades. Never pull a mower toward you.

Hand injuries The usual cause of hand injuries is a foolhardy attempt to dislodge something from jammed rotary blades without first shutting off the motor.

Propelled objects A piece of wood, stone, glass, or metal on a surface being mowed can be propelled by rotary blades at so great a velocity that the object becomes, potentially, a lethal missile. Before mowing, rake the lawn to remove such objects. The danger to the operator of the mower is chiefly to his or her lower extremities; a bystander is in greater peril because as the object travels from the mower blades it is likely to rise.

Some additional precautions Mow during daylight hours, when you can see what you are doing. Do not mow wet grass; you are more likely to slip into the blades, and if you are using an electrical mower, the danger of electrical shock is increased. Keep all guards on the equipment. Always shut off the motor before refueling, and allow it to cool. Stand clear of the appliance when starting it. Do not stand in front of the mower when the motor is idling. Disconnect the spark plug before attempting any adjustment or repair.

If you are using a gasoline-powered motor, store the gasoline in a well-ventilated area in a safety container. Follow the manufacturer's instructions concerning upkeep. Always allow the mower's motor to cool before refilling the gasoline tank. Gasoline spilled onto a hot motor—and such spills occur often—can produce a fire or explosion.

Keep children away from the area of operation of a power mower.

These warnings apply to all rotary power mowers, although some brands are relatively safer than others.

Garden tools

All garden tools are somewhat dangerous, but hedge clippers are particularly so. Use a brightly colored extension cord to avoid accidentally cutting the cord and receiving a shock.

Snow throwers

Snow throwers, gas-powered or electric, present hazards similar to those of lawn mowers. They may be more hazardous, in fact, since they are operated on wet and slippery surfaces and they have more exposed moving parts.

Some desirable features are: a safety or "dead-man" control, usually a clutch that stops the wheels when it is not squeezed by the operator's hand; a safety control on the reverse lever to prevent it from backing into the operator; an easily operated throttle to allow instant shutting down of the motor; guards over the open ends of the chute; and an efficient, adequately guarded deflector that regulates the height to which the snow is thrown.

Consumer Reports recommends that the operator wear ear plugs if the equipment is to be operated continuously for several hours to protect the user from hearing damage (see chapter 14, Noise).

The precautions that apply to freeing a power mower from obstructions apply also to the snow blower. One additional warning that may also apply to some power mowers is that shutting off the blower motor before cleaning it may not afford sufficient protection. There may be enough tension remaining from the suddenly halted motor to force a few turns—all it takes to produce severe hand injuries—after the blocking object is removed. Use an implement, not your fingers, to remove an object, even with the motor shut off.

As with power mowers, do not allow children in the vicinity of operation of a snow thrower. Unless you enforce this rule it is likely to be broken because children probably will find a snow thrower even more fascinating than a mower.

Paint sprayers

In addition to poisoning from paint, paint removers and paint thinners, the sprayer itself introduces hazards of its own. If the spray is accidentally triggered while the opening is pointed at your hand or other parts of your body, the paint can be injected through your skin into the deep tissues with damaging results.

In using a paint sprayer indoors, wear a mask, ventilate the room as much as possible, and extinguish all flames within a wide distance of your spraying—flames, pilot lights, cigarettes, and the like, including electric heaters. The same precautions should be observed for spraying in a comparatively confined space outdoors.

Power saws

Use full protective equipment, goggles, hearing protectors, gloves, and snug-fitting clothes with nothing left dangling or flapping to be caught in the saw. Do not operate such equipment in the rain, because of the increased electrical hazard. These precautions apply to other power saws, both inside and outside your home. Always use the guards available for each type of power saw. Always shut off the power and wait for the saw to stop running before changing the saw to a different location.

Antennas

Antennas have become the leading cause of electrocution in the United States. With millions of CB radios in use, many people are installing tall antennas to produce better reception. Although any kind of antenna can be an electrocution hazard, those for CB radios are especially hazardous because of their greater height. Electrocution occurs most frequently when the antenna, usually 20 to 60 feet high, is being erected or taken down. An overhead power line may go unnoticed, or may be concealed by foliage; or the tall antenna may easily get out of control and lean over onto a power line. In these situations, people holding on to the antenna are almost always electrocuted.

The most effective preventive measure against this accident is to have the antenna installed by an expert. One other precaution: the antenna and its tower should be grounded to reduce the chance of damage from lightning strikes.

If electrocution does occur, act fast but carefully. Assuming that the victim still will be in contact with the current, your first problem is to break this contact. Do not use your hands, or you also will become a victim. Use a dry wood pole or plank or other nonconductor of electricity to make the separation. Be sure the separation is far and secure and will stay that way.

Only then, administer cardiopulmonary resuscitation to the victim until an expert arrives. Courses in cardiopulmonary resuscitation (CPR) are offered in most communities.

Glass doors and windows

An estimated 40,000 people each year try to walk through glass doors and windows that they don't realize are there, and 6,000 of them require hospitalization. Children often run or stumble into glass doors and windows and, if the glass breaks, they can suffer severe injury. A storm door may be caught by a gust of wind as it is being opened and a glass pane may slam into someone's outstretched arm. Often a person intent on an errand walks into what appears to be an open doorway but actually is a sliding glass panel. This sort of thing causes as many injuries to adults as to children.

Large, distinctive decals should be applied to solid glass doors at several eye levels to give adequate warning to any person approaching that the door is made of glass and that it is a closed door.

Decals will minimize the danger but do not provide a guarantee that such an accident will not occur anyway. Therefore, tempered glass is recommended; it has about five times the strength of ordinary glass. Even if it does break, it almost undoubtedly will crumble into granules instead of shattering into shards and slivers.

Other safety glazing materials are: laminated glass, the middle layer being a plastic sheet; wire glass, which is seldom acceptable to home owners; and rigid plastic sheets. Some form of such safety glazing should be installed instead of ordinary glass in all totally or partially glass doors, including storm doors, throughout the house. In some areas, storm doors are legally required to be installed with plastic rather than glass panels.

Outdoor play equipment

It is estimated that more than one hundred thousand people require hospital emergency room treatment for playground injuries each year. These injuries are about equally divided between those occurring at public playgrounds and those occurring on the home premises.

In home surroundings more than two-thirds of the injuries occur on swings. Slides also are responsible for many accidental injuries. Swimming pool slides now must conform to Consumer Product Safety Commission standards, which specify materials, strength, and related matters, and also minimum water depths under such slides. (See page 461 for further information on swimming pool hazards.)

Be certain that playground equipment on your property is sturdy, well maintained, clean, and in good repair. Children, especially visitors, should be taught the proper use of this equipment and should be supervised in their play.

Cluttered areas

The garage often becomes the repository of a variety of dangerous equipment and materials, and more keeps on being piled on it. This creates the perfect setting for injury to a child, usually an older one. He or she can explore tools, electrical equipment, paints, solvents, and other materials, in relative seclusion.

There is not much point in placing poisonous materials in locked cupboards inside the house to keep them away from children, and then leaving equally dangerous materials in the open in a garage. Don't tempt your children. Clean out the garage. Dispose of everything that serves no immediate specific need; throw away old solutions, even new ones, that cannot be reused. Throw away gasoline, benzene, and other highly flammable materials and rebottled fluids, using great care in the disposal process. Provide wall shelves, racks, or other anchoring and storage devices for as many implements as possible. Then keep the garage door locked.

Go through a similar process with your basement and attic. This will be rewarding in several ways: you will be able to find and use things more readily without searching for them (you may even find a valuable tool that had been missing); and you certainly will find satisfaction in the number of family safety hazards you have eliminated from all three areas.

Suffocation

INGESTION OR INHALATION OF OBJECTS OR FOOD

Suffocation from ingestion or inhalation of objects or food with obstruction of the breathing passages ranks sixth in causes of fatal accidents in the U.S., with nearly 3,000 deaths each year, more than one-half of them in the home. These deaths occur at all ages, but people aged seventy and over are more than twice as likely to die from this cause as are those in any other age group. Luckily, death usually is preventable if a simple first aid measure is used promptly.

That uncomfortable feeling from food or liquid going down "the wrong way" is due to its partial entry into the opening of the respiratory tract. Coughing to expel the offending material starts automatically, is usually promptly successful, and the victim quickly recovers.

Strangulation on food is an extension of this process: the substance enters the respiratory passage far enough to act as a plug blocking inhalation and exhalation of air. In adults, the most common offending substance is meat. The victim cannot breathe in or out, cannot speak, cannot cough to expel the food because one must inspire air and then expel it to produce a cough. *Death from asphyxiation is only a minute or two away.*

Because this condition bears some resemblance to a heart attack and often occurs in public eating places, it came to be known as the "café coronary." The victim arises abruptly from the table, staggers toward the toilet, collapses, and dies.

Infants and small children can choke from any kind of food, especially peanuts, but also soft, mushy preparations, especially when the child stuffs too much into its mouth. Most of these cases are taken care of by dangling the child head down and slapping its back. If this fails, as it sometimes does, the maneuver described below for use in choking adults should be used promptly on the child.

It is not always possible to prevent such episodes, but some precautions can be useful.

For children under one year old, food asphyxiation is the leading cause of accidental deaths in the home. Avoid hurried feeding, which is likely to lead to cramming more food into the mouth before the previous mouthful has been swallowed. When the child can feed itself, supervision is essential, both to prevent choking and to treat it if it does occur.

During childhood, choking comes from the incredible variety of objects that find their way into the mouths of toddlers. Once in the respiratory tract, they can either produce strangulation or be aspirated into smaller breathing passages in the lungs, from where they must be removed with specialized instruments.

In adults, most cases are caused by eating too fast, particularly by gulping down large pieces of meat. Imbibing alcohol before eating is an important predisposing factor: it increases appetite or hunger while lessening inhibitions against wolfing down food. But alcohol does not have to be present. For example, someone makes a remark that produces instant laughter. The quick inspiration of air that accompanies the laughter may suck food or liquid into the air passage. Usually, the resulting episode of choking is brief, but strangulation can occur. It is important to remember this cause-and-effect relationship when someone eating at the table suddenly shows signs of strangulation during hearty laughter.

A heart attack is an emergency that demands fast action in summoning expert help. But choking demands *instantaneous* help that must be administered by someone on the scene. Later is far too late. The heart attack victims, unless they have experienced sudden cardiac arrest, are still breathing and probably can talk. The choking victims can neither breathe nor talk, even though at first they are fully conscious. The choking victim soon "turns blue." The heart attack victim is likely to be pale at first, but also may become blue.

If the event occurs suddenly during a meal, it is better to assume that the cause is choking and treat it as such. If it turns out to be a heart attack, the chances of having done real harm are not great. Professional help should be called for in either event, by someone other than the would-be rescuer. The calculated risk of treating a heart attack victim mistakenly thought to be a choking victim is, in general, one that should be unhesitatingly taken.

Hopefully, a choking victim knows the widely accepted signal for choking, and will grasp his neck between his thumb and finger, telling you in sign language, "I am choking on food." The diagnosis is made for you. You must know what to do.

HEIMLICH MANEUVER

The old method of hard slaps on the back has been largely replaced by the *Heimlich Maneuver*, named after Dr. Henry J. Heimlich, the physician who devised it. Its principle is to exert pressure on the abdomen in such a way as to force residual air out of the lungs and thus expel the foreign object by air pressure. It produces an effect similar to that of squeezing the sides of a flexible, lightly corked, plastic bottle: the cork pops out. In choking victims on whom this maneuver is used, the offending material often pops out with enough force to propel it across the room.

Following is a description of the maneuver in Dr. Heimlich's words:

If the victim is standing, (1) stand behind the victim and wrap your arms around his waist. (2) place your fist (thumb side against the victim's abdomen) slightly above the navel and below the rib cage. (3) Grasp your fist with your other hand and press into the victim's abdomen with a quick, upward thrust. Repeat several times if necessary.

If the victim is supine (lying on the floor, face up):

1. *Place the victim face up and kneel astride his hips.*
2. *With one hand on top of the other, place the heel of the bottom hand on the abdomen slightly above the navel and below the rib cage.*
3. *Press into the victim's abdomen with a quick upward thrust. Repeat several times if necessary.*

(Figure 9.1 illustrates the Heimlich Maneuver.)

The method is simple and effective in most cases. Practice it gently a few times so that you will remember it. Remember, too, that your action must be immediate: *the victim has at most about four minutes to live*, and by the time others realize what is happening, some of that precious time already will have elapsed. If the victim already has lost consciousness, he probably has only seconds left.

What to do if choking on food when alone

If alone it is possible to perform a modified maneuver on yourself, based on the same principle, provided you do it immediately, before beginning to lose consciousness. Instantly pick a table, shelf, sink, or similar object that will catch your abdomen at about the level described for the fist or hand of a rescuer in the regular maneuver. Fall on the edge of it, hard enough to produce the necessary abdominal sudden compression. Repeat if necessary, as many times as you are able to. It offers a good chance of being successful.

A by-product of this method is the discovery that it sometimes works when conventional methods have failed to resuscitate a person who has drowned. It may provide just the necessary expulsion of water, and perhaps debris, from the respiratory passages.

The maneuver is not completely safe. A few injuries, such as fractured ribs, even rupture of a stomach, have occurred. These are survivable injuries. Asphyxiation is not.

MECHANICAL SUFFOCATION

Although this type of suffocation causes fewer deaths than ingestion or inhalation of food or other objects, it nevertheless is one of the major categories of fatal home accidents, causing about seven hundred deaths each year. It includes smothering by bed clothes, thin plastic materials, and like substances; suffocation by cave-ins or confinement in closed spaces; and mechanical strangulation.

The suffocation of children who put *thin plastic bags* over their heads became for a while a national tragedy and is a striking illustration of how a useful product could become a dangerous thing. All such bags now carry a warning against this specific misuse, and the number of deaths has been greatly reduced. Proper precautions must still be observed. Plastic bags and containers should never be carelessly left where small children can get to them; the hazard should be recognized in supervising children's play.

The possibility of suffocation in *cave-ins* similarly requires disciplining of children, to prevent them from playing in areas where cave-ins might occur. There should also be discipline among adults, who must foresee situations in which these accidents can happen and take the necessary preventive measures.

A good example of the danger of suffocation in enclosed spaces is presented by the *discarded refrigerator*. This hazard has become well known and in many places the law requires that the doors must be removed from any discarded refrigerator. Unfortunately, there are still violations of this rule; and children are ingenious in discovering such hideaways and climbing into them.

Accidental mechanical strangulation also chiefly affects children. Do not let children play with *rope lassos*. Unintentional misuse can produce strangulation; it seems that periodically a group of children attempt to simulate a hanging and succeed all too well.

Wires and cables stretched across drives to prevent children from entering on bikes can go unnoticed by the child running into the barrier at full speed. The results can be serious.

A long, *trailing scarf* used while riding in a wheeled vehicle or on a snowmobile, even in a home driveway, is an invitation to either a broken neck or strangulation if the scarf gets caught in the wheels or other moving parts of the vehicle or some object that the vehicle is passing.

FIGURE 9.1

Choking on an obstruction—the Heimlich Maneuver

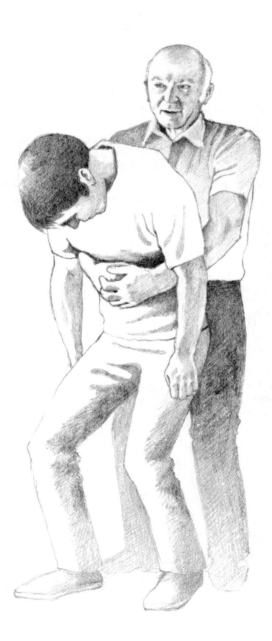

The Heimlich Maneuver to remove an obstruction from the throat has two variations. The first is when the victim is standing: Grasp him around the waist (as at left) *and quickly press your fist upward into his abdomen* (see above right).

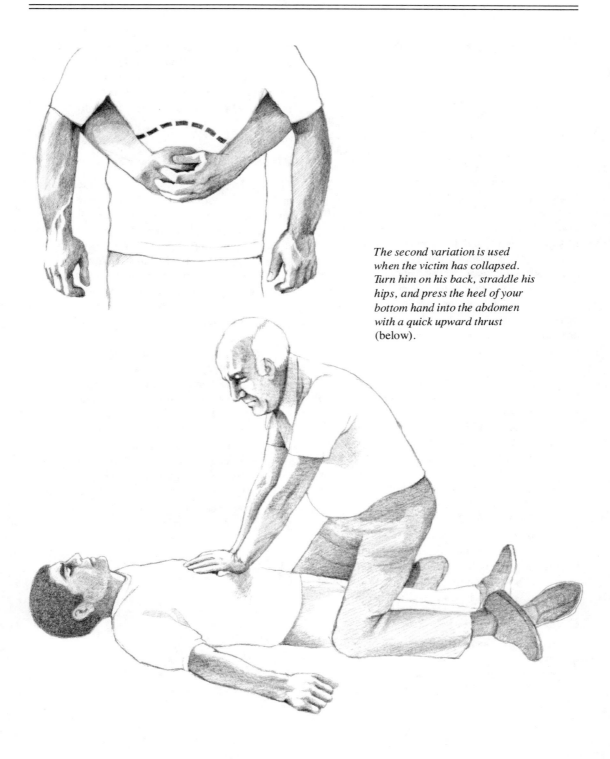

The second variation is used when the victim has collapsed. Turn him on his back, straddle his hips, and press the heel of your bottom hand into the abdomen with a quick upward thrust (below).

Firearms and Explosives

FIREARMS

Of all the dangerous objects in the home, firearms would seem to be the most obvious and, therefore, easiest to deal with. Yet, fatal accidents from such weapons and explosives rank as high as fifth in the causes of death from home accidents, with a toll each year of about 1,200 people. Practically all of these result from carelessness.

American children under fifteen are victims of more than 30 percent of home firearms deaths. Most children involved in gun accidents—shooters and victims—are unfamiliar with either guns or the safety rules for their use. They are exposed from a very early age to stories of our fabled "Wild West," where the use of guns appeared extremely casual. Furthermore, the child who used to go to the movies to live out these fantasies now has them brought into his or her own home, via television.

"Toy" pistols should be prohibited in the home. Frequently, they are the start of a deadly succession which moves from pistols, to cap pistols, "BB guns" and finally to the real pistol, rifle or shotgun discovered in the child's own home. If the gun is loaded, tragedy may be seconds away. The danger is by no means confined to youngsters. Adults, who should know better, can do the same thing, with equally tragic results.

No firearm should ever be left around the house, either loaded or unloaded. This includes leaving a gun in a belt or shoulder holster, or throwing a coat with a gun in its pocket over a chair. If, for some compelling reason, a gun must be loaded, it should be kept in a locked drawer or cabinet with the key kept on the person of its owner.

If you are handed a gun, never be satisfied with the assurance, "It isn't loaded." Make sure for yourself, being sure to check the firing chamber for a bullet, and having done so, never point it at anyone or pull the trigger. That these fundamental precautions are widely neglected is apparent in the number of people who, each year, shoot themselves or others in the process of cleaning, or even just examining, a weapon.

FIREWORKS

The yearly toll in blown-off or mutilated fingers and hands, permanently blinded eyes, severe burns, and a variety of other accidental injuries, as well as deaths, is highest during the fireworks season—the Fourth of July and the weeks preceding and following it. Sale of fireworks is illegal in many urban areas; sometimes the use of them by unauthorized persons is not allowed. However, the accidents that occur each year provide ample evidence that these laws are widely disregarded.

With recognition that the admonition will be frequently disregarded, it is urged that fireworks be left to professional fireworks experts (they, too, sometimes are injured or killed in their work).

Even "sparklers," which are not generally used except by children because they seem too tame, can be injurious. It is not generally realized that the sparks can ignite clothing, produce eye and other burns, and—more frequently—can produce severe burns of fingers and hands when picked up while still hot.

Swimming Pools and Bathtubs

POOLS

The pleasures and health benefits that pools offer all family members need never be interrupted if a few simple precautions are heeded.

The most obvious precaution is to minimize the danger of *drowning*. A significant difference between a private and public pool is that the home pool is far more likely to be used by one person, with nobody at poolside or even in the house. Here, the "buddy system" is recommended. It provides the swimmer with the relative security of having someone constantly present to come to the rescue if he or she gets into trouble.

Every home pool should have some kind of *rescue device* at poolside—a ring buoy or a long pole, for example. Inflated life rafts are not foolproof, and small children tend to become overly venturesome in their use. Children in a home pool should be constantly supervised by a responsible older person.

Whether the bathing locale is a home swimming pool or a bathtub of some kind, no small child should ever be left alone in it even for seconds. *An infant can drown in a few inches of water*. If the telephone or the doorbell rings, either remove the child from the water and from the vicinity of it, or ignore the bell.

Every home swimming pool should be enclosed with an effective *fence*, with a gate that can be locked to prevent anyone, but particularly a child, from getting to the pool. If the pool is filled with water, drowning is the danger; if it is empty, a fractured skull is a possibility. Many towns have adopted ordinances requiring pool fences.

Slipping on a concrete or similar surface around a swimming pool is another hazard that should be anticipated. Wet feet on a normally nonslippery surface that is also wet can be a hazardous combination. Forbid horseplay around the pool.

If you wish to use the pool at night, install *adequate lighting*. The switch for the lights should be in the house, not near the pool. Radios and other electrical appliances should never be used near the pool.

Diving boards present their own peculiar hazards. Be sure that it is firmly anchored and is stout enough to support a heavy diver safely. In many places there are regulations governing the minimum depth of water in a pool under various heights of diving boards. Follow the regulations. Many accidents are caused by dives into shallow water.

For adults, the greatest danger from home swimming pools probably comes from using the pool after *imbibing alcoholic beverages*. A safety expert once proposed the slogan: "Drinking like a fish doesn't make you one."

BATHTUBS

Although swimming pools are the most obvious sites for drownings at home, the bathtub is also hazardous. About two hundred people drown in them each year. A warning has already been recorded about leaving infants unattended in a tub, either regular or infant size, even for a few seconds. But adults can also be victims. A tub is a special menace to people with convulsive seizures, heart disease, and similar conditions. It can also be the site of a fall that produces unconsciousness, while bathing or showering. Old people are in special danger from this type of accident (see falls, page 431).

Children's Toys, Vehicles, and Clothing

The variety of toys available for children is so enormous and so subject to change that only some broad principles can be recorded concerning their relative accident potentials. Many youngsters are injured by toys every year, and the situation is complicated by the fact that play things are not thought of as being injurious or deadly. Since the types of toys sold vary according to age, toy safety principles are presented for six age groups, with some overlap:

0-2 years

(Period for exercising new-found senses.) Be certain that toys do not have parts, including inner fillings, that could become loose and be put into the child's mouth, to be swallowed or aspirated. Examples are materials used inside rattles, eyes on teddy bears or dolls, and squeaking mechanisms inside dolls and toy animals. Balls, and all other toys, should be too large to insert into the mouth. Beware of sharp edges on toys that might break and present sharp edges.

2-3 years

(Period of exploration.) Wheeled vehicles for children should be tip-proof and pinch-proof. Avoid toys that are run by electricity or have removable parts or sharp edges.

3-4 years

(Period of fantasy.) Doll clothing and children's play clothing should be made of nonflammable material. Avoid pins; use fasteners that will not separate from the material to which they are attached. Avoid cutting edges. Keep in mind that even after discipline through reasoning has become possible, small objects left in the play area by children of these and older ages may be picked up by younger siblings.

4-6 years

(Creative period.) Limit construction sets to simple ones. Avoid clay, paints, and related materials that you have any reason to suspect may be made of toxic materials. Avoid toys that shoot things. The use of small sports equipment or of electrically operated toys should be prohibited or carefully supervised.

6-8 years

(Period of developing mechanical interests.) Use of all previously mentioned toys, with some additions such as carpenter tools, should be supervised. Look for the UL seal on all electrical toys and supervise their use. Avoid sharp-edged toys and those that are excessively complicated to use. For all wheeled vehicles, buy sturdy equipment that will not tip easily. Insist on toys being put away when not in use, to prevent younger children from using them, and also to prevent cluttering the floor with tripping objects for adults.

8 and over

(Period of specialization of interests and skills.) From here on, the problems become more complex. Insist on the UL seal on all electrical equipment, avoid shoddy sports equipment, supervise at least the beginning stages of use of chemistry sets, tools, skis, water equipment, and the like. First be aware of the hazards yourself, and then teach the youngster how to work with toys constructively and safely. Children of this age can be reasoned with; but allow them to participate in decisions. Again, guard against inadvertant use by younger brothers and sisters.

Elevators

Elevators are, in general, remarkably safe, considering their almost constant vertical travel throughout each day. Local laws usually require periodic inspection by an elevator expert who, after each inspection, issues a certificate posted in the elevator.

Elevator doors can be hazardous to children. Getting caught when the door closes will be painful to children and perhaps cause serious injury, although this is probably not enough to injure an adult more than slightly. Do not allow children to fool around in an elevator.

To be caught in the door of a moving elevator almost certainly will mean death. This could result from an ill-advised attempt to pry open the door of a stalled elevator. If you are in a stalled elevator, press the emergency button and stay in it until it again operates normally or until an expert rescuer tells you what to do.

Older children sometimes try to open the top of the elevator car and climb on top of it, or pry open the closed door to the elevator shaft. Although these episodes are not common, their fatality rate is very high.

Be especially careful about allowing visiting children to ride in an elevator without adult supervision. For children who do not live in apartments, an elevator is a novelty and they may not realize that it is not a toy.

Hazards from Hobbies and Workshops

It is estimated that more than 75 million Americans participate in one or more crafts, and the number increases steadily each year. Photographic darkroom work, painting, sculpture, ceramics, decoupage, stained glass making, and a great many other hobbies give pleasure at home to people of all ages. Unfortunately, few people realize that hobbies often present health hazards. Toxic or explosive fluids, fumes, and dust may be encountered in all of the above hobbies. Even stamp collecting can be risky—many of the commercial fluids sold to make the stamps' watermarks more visible are as flammable and explosive as gasoline. Fortunately for the hobbyist, most of these materials must be used frequently and over a long period to do real damage, but their hazards should be understood.

One very common material is glue. Used not only for hobbies but also for ordinary household repairs, it has several hazards. Be especially careful when using any type of "superglue" advertised as able to bond anything. This claim can be dangerously correct; in a very short period it can *glue fingers* together or to other objects. It has been known to glue eyelids shut after they were touched by fingers with glue on them. Washing skin with water to remove the glue will only make the glue set faster.

Use glue with great care and do not let young children use it at all. Provide them with a safer paste. An additional hazard of glue not often seen in the past is *glue sniffing* by children, which can cause sudden death.

To make sure you are working safely with your hobby materials, the following *general precautions* should be heeded:

- Use a room with adequate ventilation, forced by a fan, if necessary.
- Do not use kitchen utensils, and be extremely careful if the kitchen is your workshop.

- Keep all materials out of the way of children.
- Carefully read all manufacturers' directions and warnings.
- It is unlikely that you will attempt any craft without some instruction, usually in the form of manuals, books, or other materials. Read all the precautions as carefully as you read the "how to" material. If in doubt, consult your library or an expert.
- If you are planning to start a new hobby, or are not sure what hazards may be present in the materials you are already using, check carefully as to the possible short-and long-term effects they may have, especially if you are pregnant or nursing.
- If you have severe allergies, be doubly careful in selecting your hobby.
- Store all materials safely in labeled, unbreakable containers rather than glass. Cover them when not in use—even for a few minutes.
- Keep your hands clean and, if advised, wear rubber or other protective gloves and an apron. Wear a mask where dusts and other air contaminants may be produced.
- Do not allow food or beverages in your work area. They may become contaminated with toxic materials. Similarly, do not allow cigarettes or other smoking materials in the area, not only because of fire hazard, but also because of the danger of contaminating them.
- Do not use flammable materials anywhere near flame, and if they are explosively flammable, do not use them near an electric switch. Have a fire extinguisher handy.
- In general, substitute less hazardous materials and methods wherever possible.

Enjoy your hobby, but do it safely. If you are not willing to make concessions to safety needs, discontinue your hobby and choose one with fewer safety hazards.

Alcohol Abuse

Although alcohol abuse is not an accident, it is discussed briefly here to record a warning that all efforts to prevent home accidents may fail when a member of the household drinks alcoholic beverages to excess. Chronic alcoholism presents the most difficult problem, but even occasional imbibing can impair muscular coordination, reaction time, and good judgment with the result that the drinker can cause or abet most types of home accidents.

The association of alcohol with falls and fires is well proved. But we need more research on the problem. How many injuries are initiated by a tipsy cook? How often do power tool injuries come from attempts to use such equipment after having had too much to drink? How many children have been injured at home when an intoxicated parent relaxed supervision?

It is suggested that those involved in a home accident question themselves about the careless action that produced it. If the accident took place after more than a small consumption of alcohol, they should honestly evaluate the role of drinking in the incident. This might lead to more caution about overindulging in alcohol, particularly when household chores must be done.

If someone in the house is afflicted with chronic alcoholism, the problem is much more complex. (See chapter 2, Alcohol.) The first step toward prevention of home accidents caused by an alcoholic is to get him or her into an alcoholism rehabilitation facility or program. It has been amply demonstrated that chronic alcoholics, who want to be rehabilitated, can be. But until the alcoholism is under control permanently, safety violations by that person in the home and elsewhere will be a constant threat.

Farm Home Accidents

More than half a million disabling injuries strike American farmers each year. The accident death rate is about half again as great as that from all accidents to American people. About one-half of these deaths are caused by motor vehicle accidents. However, these figures include occupational accidents. Farm home accident rates are only a little higher than those of all other home accidents, although the death rate from them is clearly higher. There is no reason to suppose, however, that the problems of farm home accidents are greatly different from those that occur in non-farm homes.

One difference may be worth mentioning, as a warning. Farm homes are likely to be more removed from emergency medical service, including ambulance transportation, than are those in cities. The first aid procedures for common accidents therefore should be thoroughly learned by all farm residents.

Keeping Current

The material in this chapter emphasizes the dangers to which everyone is exposed in the home, but home as the safe haven of tradition is an attainable goal if its residents exert constant efforts to make it so. It is not enough to be aware of existing hazards in the home and how to prevent them. By the time you read this chapter, new products will have been evolved and new hazards will have been introduced into American homes.

Newspapers, magazines, and television can help you keep abreast. Two publications are especially valuable: "Family Safety," published quarterly by the National Safety Council, which some companies make available to their employees, is obtainable by individual subscription; and "Consumer Reports," published monthly by Consumers Union. Materials from these two publications were extensively used in the preparation of this chapter. Both of them are published by non-profit organizations and their findings can be counted on to be thoroughly researched and objectively presented.

Also, learn to use governmental agencies and civic organizations as sources of information about product safety. Examples are local, state, and federal consumer protection agencies; the local or state health department, or the U.S. Public Health Service; the local or national safety council, the nearest Poison Control Center, the Better Business Bureau. Most of these, and others, are listed in your local telephone book. Do not hesitate to request information from any of them.

No book can cover everything. To the extent that you exclaim, "But I know a home accident hazard that wasn't mentioned at all," this chapter has been doubly useful because it has produced greater awareness, on your part, of the vast extent of the home accident problem, and has set you to thinking constructively about the subject.

CHAPTER
10

Traffic accidents

The issue of traffic fatalities is a serious one today because so many children and innocent adults are involved, suffering injury or death as a consequence of driver irresponsibility. While we can always make further progress in the development of safer cars and safer highways, we need to concern ourselves more effectively with the driver. A driver's irresponsibility affects himself or herself and many innocent others.

Driver education is crucial. This education should probably be a mandatory aspect of the school curriculum. We can penalize a driver for irresponsible driving, adopting penalties similar to those of many other countries, particularly of those in Europe where serious measures have produced results. Americans, however, view any legislation that affects their "freedom" on the highway as interfering with their basic rights as Americans. Yet, as this chapter shows, drunken driving, excessive speeding, or not wearing seat belts, cause the disability and the deaths of thousands of drivers and innocent citizens every year. Many countries have strong and forceful laws against drunken drivers and practice a far greater usage of seat belts than our own. Why can we not duplicate such achievements? Murder and suicide on the highways by means of an automobile are not the kind of "rights" we should tolerate.

We expect that all readers would agree with this concept. If so, why do we not act accordingly, as a society and as individuals?

Glossary

BLOOD ALCOHOL LEVELS   For drivers: Illegal level in most states is 0.1 grams of alcohol per liter (g/L). In Michigan it is 0.07 g/L, and in New York, Ohio, and South Carolina it is 0.05 g/L.

PASSIVE RESTRAINTS   Automatic crash protection for car occupants in the form of automatic seat belts released as the door opens, or air bags consisting of inflatable cushions.

The Price of Mobility

It is characteristic of our society that the primary reason for reducing the national speed limit to 55 miles per hour was to save gasoline, and only secondarily to save lives. The money Americans spend at the gas pumps seems to arouse more concern than does the financial cost to the nation of the carnage that takes place on the highways— $50 billion in 1979 for law enforcement, medical costs, and productivity losses, plus the incalculable cost of pain and disfigurement. Only about 11 percent of American drivers fasten their seat belts despite evidence that doing so can reduce highway collision deaths by 9,000 to 12,000 yearly (or up to 25 percent) if used universally. Our laws against drunken driving and speeding remain lax and lightly enforced despite the fact that alcohol and inappropriate speed are the major causes of all car accidents.

Unlike the many mysteries surrounding diseases, such as cancer and stroke, there are few mysteries about the causes of car accidents, yet auto fatality is the sixth leading cause of all U.S. deaths—50,331 in 1978—and the leading cause of accidental death.

Moreover, for every highway fatality, there are nearly one hundred injuries, ranging from scratches, bumps, cuts, and bruises to concussions, sprains, dislocations, ruptures, fractures, brain damage, and paralyses. It is estimated that each year traffic accidents create 1,800 paraplegics and quadriplegics.

Highway death strikes especially at the young. Auto accidents are the leading cause of all deaths for persons fifteen to twenty-four and are the second leading cause of death for those one to fourteen. More than half of all highway deaths occur between the ages of fifteen and forty-three (see figures 10.1–10.5, and table 10.1). Some 1,000 children under the age of five die annually in road accidents and an estimated 100,000 are seriously injured. One out of every fifty infants born in the U.S. will eventually die in a motor vehicle accident. The special vulnerability of young people to highway death is dramatically demonstrated in these figures. Crippling highway injuries follow the same pattern. Such brutal statistics raise the question of whether present parental supervision and public laws are adequate.

The statistics on the distribution of death on the highways also show that more men than women are killed. This may be at least in part because women drive less than men and less often at rush hour or in bad weather. Drivers account for almost half the total deaths, passengers for one-fourth, pedestrians for 16 percent, motorcyclists for 9 percent, and bicyclists for 2 percent. The death *rate*, however, is highest for motorcyclists (see figure 10.4 and tables 10.2 and 10.3).

Table 10.1
HIGHWAY FATALITIES BY AGE GROUPS (1978)

Ages	Fatalities
All Ages	50,331
0–5	1,511
6–9	1,112
10–14	1,586
15–24	18,532
25–34	9,452
35–44	4,752
45–54	4,032
55–64	3,634
65 and over	5,426
Age unknown	294

SOURCE: National Highway Traffic Safety Administration.

While deaths from most other causes are not always preventable, the vast majority of highway fatalities are. They are preventable in several ways; by using caution, by obeying traffic laws, and by incorporating technological devices such as seat belts more rigorously. Above all, our traffic laws need strict enforcement while violations call for strong preventive measures. *Prevention begins with a clear understanding of the causes.*

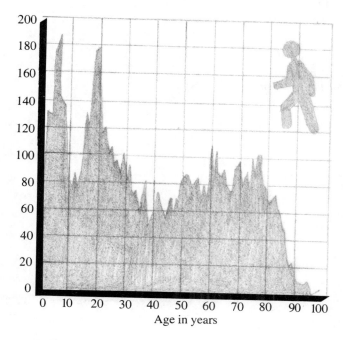

FIGURE 10.1

Number of pedestrians killed
SOURCE: *National Highway Traffic Safety Administration (NHTSA), Fatal Accident Reporting System (FARS), 1978*

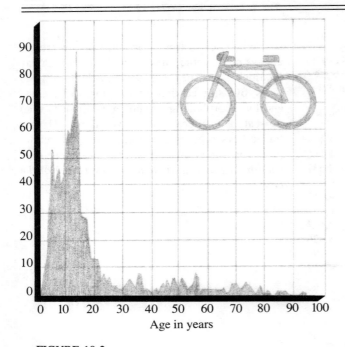

Age in years

FIGURE 10.2

Number of pedalcyclists killed
SOURCE: *National Highway Traffic Safety Administration*
(NHTSA), Fatal Accident Reporting System (FARS), 1978

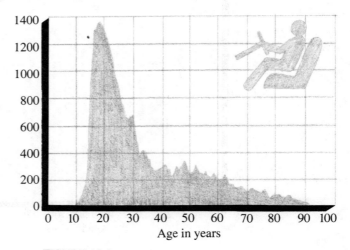

Age in years

FIGURE 10.3

Number of drivers killed
SOURCE: *National Highway Traffic Safety Administration*
(NHTSA), Fatal Accident Reporting System (FARS), 1978

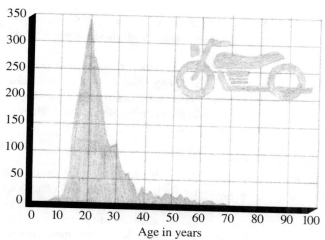

FIGURE 10.4

Number of motorcyclists killed
SOURCE: *National Highway Traffic Safety Administration
(NHTSA), Fatal Accident Reporting System (FARS), 1978*

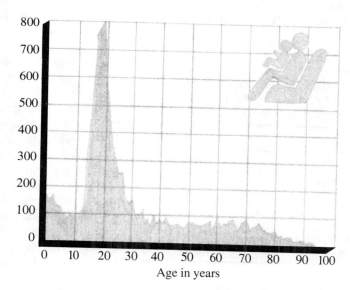

FIGURE 10.5

Number of passengers killed
SOURCE: *National Highway Traffic Safety Administration
(NHTSA), Fatal Accident Reporting System (FARS), 1978*

FACTORS AFFECTING TRAFFIC ACCIDENTS

Alcohol

Drinking drivers are involved in about half of all fatal auto accidents. A classic 1963 study conducted in Grand Rapids, Michigan showed that drivers with blood alcohol levels in the range commonly considered illegal are fifteen to twenty-five times more likely to be involved in crashes than are nondrinkers on the road at the same time and place. Even moderate amounts of alcohol measurably raise the probability of an accident. More recent surveys confirm that the drinking-driving patterns in the U.S. have not changed much since the 1963 report.

Weekends and nights are the deadliest times on American roads. On Friday and Saturday nights around midnight, one out of three drivers on the road has drunk some alcohol during the evening, and about one in ten is legally drunk.

Table 10.2

FATALITY RATES AMONG
OCCUPANTS OF VARIOUS VEHICLE TYPES
(PER 100 MILLION VEHICLE MILES) 1978*

Vehicle	Rate
Total	3.3
Passenger Cars	2.4
Motorcycles	19.8
Buses	0.7
Trucks	2.3
Single Unit Trucks	2.5
Combination Trucks	1.4†

*Final

†The fatality rates for combination trucks do not include fatalities in other vehicles involved in collisions with them.

SOURCE: National Highway Traffic Safety Administration.

Studies consistently show that drinking is involved in about three-quarters of all nighttime fatal accidents.

In addition, alcohol is thought to be involved in a significant proportion of pedestrian deaths. (For physical effects of alcohol intake, see chapter 2. For the effects of combining alcohol with other drugs, see chapter 3.)

Speed

Speed in itself is not necessarily dangerous if it is not excessive for the prevailing road conditions and for the driver's ability and experience. For example, accident statistics show that interstate highways with 55 mph speed limits have approximately half the death rate of roads posted at lower speeds, probably because the interstate highways are frequently better designed and less traveled. What raises the likelihood of an accident is speed combined with poor road conditions. Sudden changes in speed and a wide range of speed and vehicles on a road can also lead to accidents.

A car moving too slowly on a 55 mph highway can be as much a hazard as the car traveling too fast. Yet, in one ranking of factors that contribute to highway accidents (table 10.4), driving over the speed limit was 11th after such other factors as driving while intoxicated (#1), driving within the speed limit but too fast for conditions (#2), driver distracted by passengers (#8), and improper turns (#9).

However, the higher the rate of speed at which a crash occurs, the greater is the likelihood of a fatal injury. Analysis of crashes shows that the percentage of occupants killed as a result of cars hitting a brick wall at 20 mph is virtually zero. As speed increases, the percentage shoots up and at a speed of 50 mph an average of 46 percent of car occupants are killed (figure 10.6). Another way of comparing the impact of crashes at various speeds is shown in figure 10.7 where the effect of crashing at 30 mph is similar to dropping a car out of a fourth story window.

Table 10.3

FATAL TRAFFIC ACCIDENT VICTIMS IN THE U.S. (1976 THROUGH 1978)

| Year of accident | Total occupants | Non-Occupants | | | | Total |
		Motorcyclists	Pedalcyclists	Pedestrians	Others	
1976	32,780	3,312	914	7,427	1,090	45,532
1977	34,215	4,104	922	7,732	903	47,878
1978	36,956	4,577	892	7,795	111	50,331*

*1978 Fatalities (final)

Non-Occupants:	13,375	Light Trucks	6,636
Motorcyclists:	4,577	Heavy Trucks	1,008
Pedestrians:	7,795	Unknown—Trucks	496
Pedalcyclists:	892	Buses	41
Others:	111	Other Vehicles	370
Breakdown of Total Occupants	36,956	Unknown Vehicles	252
Passenger Cars	28,153		

SOURCE: National Highway Traffic Safety Administration, (NHTSA), Fatal Accident Reporting System, (FARS), 1978.

Table 10.4

ORDER OF PRIMARY COLLISION FACTORS IN FATAL VEHICULAR ACCIDENTS (CALIFORNIA, 1976)

Order	Primary Collision Factor	Number	Percent*
1	Driving while intoxicated	1,126	28
2	Driving within speed limits, but too fast for conditions	584	15
3	Pedestrian stepped into road	375	9
4	Driving on wrong side	237	6
5	Failed to yield at intersection	237	6
6	Disobeyed stop signal	190	5
7	Improper driving maneuver	141	4
8	Driver distracted by passenger	140	4
9	Improper turns	103	3
10	Pedestrian failed to yield	98	3
11	Driving over speed limit	90	2
12	Improper passing	53	1
13	Improper lane change	48	1
14	Under the influence of drugs	18	.4
15	Improper parking	17	.4
16	Brakes failed	14	.3
17	Following too close	11	.2
18	Other equipment failure	9	.2
19	Improper backing up	7	.1
20	Headlights failed	2	.05
21	Undetermined	438	11
Total		3,980	

*Percentages rounded off

SOURCE: California Highway Patrol Analysis Section.

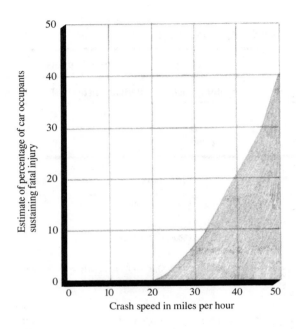

Crash speed in miles per hour

FIGURE 10.6

Likelihood of an occupant fatality at different crash speeds
SOURCE: *National Highway Traffic Safety Administration (NHTSA), 1979*

Age of driver

As shown in figures 10.1–10.5, young people are involved in fatal accidents more than are any other group, probably because of their inexperience and because of their greater willingness to take risks than more mature drivers.

Type of vehicle

The fatality rates per 100 million miles are given by vehicle type in table 10.2. The highest rates by far are for motorcycles. The rates for passenger cars are somewhat higher than for all trucks as a group while the lowest rates are for bus occupants.

Prevention

Over the past ten years, there *has* been a significant overall reduction in the vehicle fatality rate in the U.S. (table 10.5). Most of the decrease must be attributed not to better driving behavior and habits, however, but to "outside" factors over which the individual behind the wheel has little control. Among these are: highway safety design that helps the driver to avoid a serious mistake or a bad move; improved federal auto safety standards; better local programs for licensing, testing, policing, and controlling traffic; and built-in improvements by automakers that make cars less susceptible to crash damage and accidents.

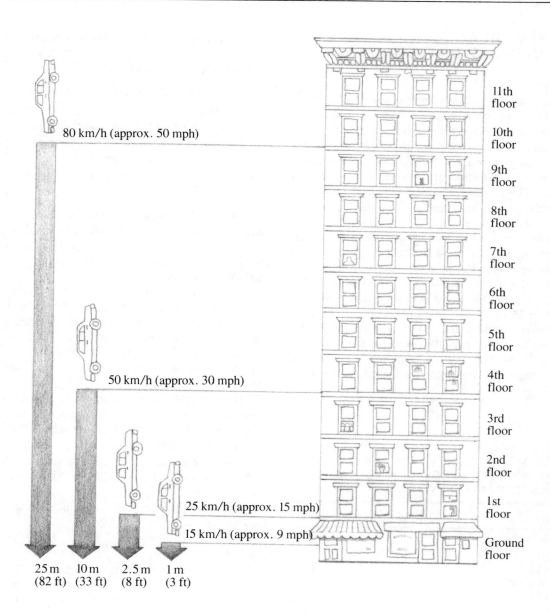

FIGURE 10.7

Comparison of impact of crashes at various speeds
SOURCE: *adapted from data from Mercedes Benz*

INDIVIDUAL PREVENTIVE MEASURES

Drivers

Be fully alert. Don't drink if you plan to drive. By the same token, avoid drugs or medications (barbiturates, antihistimines, amphetamines, tranquilizers, marijuana, and so forth) that can impair your reflexes or make you drowsy. Don't drive when overtired; if you become drowsy at the wheel, stop for a break—a cup of coffee, a little exercise and fresh air, or a nap.

Fasten your seat belt and be sure everyone else in the car has done the same before you start the engine. Half of all fatalities and injuries could be prevented if every rider wore seat belts.

Don't use the excuse that you're only going for a short trip: most accidents take place less than 25 miles from the driver's home. And get special restraints for children too young to wear seat belts (See page 482 on Child Restraints).

A fundamental aspect of road safety is the constant exercise of good judgment and common

Table 10.5
U.S. MOTOR VEHICLE DEATH RATE
(MOTOR VEHICLE DEATHS PER
HUNDRED MILLION VEHICLE MILES)

Year	Rate
1971	4.68
1972	4.53
1973	4.27
1974	3.61
1975	3.45
1976	3.31
1977	3.38
1978	3.39

SOURCE: National Safety Council, *Accident Facts*, various years.

sense. *Be a defensive driver*. Try to anticipate all possible contingencies, especially sudden ones. For example, be prepared—

- for the driver ahead of you to stop suddenly;
- for drivers on either side of you to cut in front of your path when changing lanes;
- for the driver who enters an intersection on your right without stopping;
- for a pedestrian or child darting into the street.

Don't weave in and out of traffic; keep your speed constant; keep a safe distance behind the car in front of you (at least one car length for every 10 mph of speed and an even greater distance when the road is wet).

Don't create situations that cause problems for others. Know your territory, and your own limitations. Everyone has different reaction times and vision capabilities. Drive with yours in mind.

Don't start up at a green light until you are certain the car approaching the cross street will stop.

If you are following an erratic driver (perhaps someone you sense is unfamiliar with the area), hang back so that you do not hit the vehicle if he or she stops suddenly.

If you are a pedestrian, don't step into a street without having eye contact with the driver of an oncoming car.

Check for obstacles and small children when backing up.

Bicyclists

Bicyclists should observe all the "rules of the road" that apply to drivers, such as riding in the same direction as traffic, signaling when turning, and obeying traffic signs. Such actions will permit car drivers to anticipate a cyclist's moves.

For bicyclists, one important way of minimizing the risk of being hit by a motor vehicle is to be clearly visible under all conditions. During daytime, the cyclist should wear a bright jacket, preferably yellow and reflective. For nighttime, rear and side reflectors and a front light should be permanent equipment on the bicycle; and strips of reflecting tape on the cyclist's clothing.

Motorcyclists

Motorcycle accidents killed 4,300 people in 1978 and, although fewer than one hundred people were killed in moped accidents in 1978, it is estimated that by 1984 fatalities will have risen to 1,200 per year due to the growing popularity of mopeds.

Head injuries are the leading cause of death in motorcycle and moped crashes, and the regular use of a proper helmet is the most effective means of reducing their incidence and severity. *Riders who do not wear safety helmets triple their risk of dying in a motorcycle accident.* A tragic experiment supports this statement: since 1976, twenty-seven states have repealed or weakened helmet laws, lowering usage as much as 50 to 60 percent. During this period motorcycle fatalities increased by half. *In fact, per mile of travel, the motorcyclist has a seven times higher fatality rate than that of the occupant of an automobile.* Three-quarters of all motorcycle collisions are the result of a car or truck making a left turn in front of the oncoming motorcycle, hitting the cycle from the front.

The Department of Transportation has established standards for helmet construction and design. These should be followed when choosing a helmet. The helmet should have a full-face shield, but one providing good ventilation to prevent steam-up. A helmet without a shield mandates shatterproof goggles for protection of the eyes. The goggles must be clean and free of scratches to be most visually effective and provide full safety.

The visibility of riders and vehicle is a critical factor in reducing accidents. Reflective clothing and equipment and rider strategy can maximize this visibility for day and night riding. Motorists should learn to look for motorcyclists. Driver education can assist in this process.

In addition to wearing a proper safety helmet, motorcyclists should wear clothing that will offer maximum protection. Inadequately clothed motorcyclists involved in accidents often receive deep abrasions and lacerations that can require skin grafting or amputation. Sturdy clothing—leather pants, leather jacket, boots—offer the best protection. We can't emphasize too strongly: wear a helmet when riding any kind of cycle, including mopeds.

All states should pass and enforce strong laws requiring riders of motorcycles, mopeds, and other cycles to wear helmets.

What you can do about your car

Car maintenance Keep your car in good working order. Although most states require regular inspections, you should also periodically check certain parts of your car and correct problems as soon as they arise. Following is a list of the major items to be checked and what you should look for.

Brakes. Your brakes should work smoothly and rapidly. If your car tends to pull to one side when you brake, the brakes may be wet. If so, they can be dried by riding *lightly* on the brake pedal. If wetness is not the problem, have the brakes checked immediately to find the reason for their malfunction.

Most state laws require foot brakes to stop a car within 30 feet at 20 mph, and a parking brake that stops the car within 75 feet at 20 mph or holds it in place on a 25 degree incline.

Brake lights. These are absolutely essential in warning drivers behind you that you are slowing down or stopping. They are easily checked. Do so frequently.

Directional signals. Also essential to enable you to communicate with other drivers. If the usual clicking sound is not audible when the signals are turned on, they are not working properly. A change in the dashboard light indicator also indicates a mechanical problem. If your electrical directional signals fail, you are required by law to use hand signals until they are fixed.

Taillights. Taillights and side marker lights warn other drivers of your presence. Make sure they work.

Horn. Use the horn to warn pedestrians and other drivers of your approach. Use it when passing another vehicle, when driving out of a blind driveway or alleyway, or before entering a blind curve.

Steering. On a straight, level stretch of road the car should hold its course with little or no correcting of the wheel. If there is a pull to one side or excessive vibration or if the steering wheel has too much "play," take the car to a mechanic.

Tires. Tire condition affects steering ability as well as traction. If tires are unevenly inflated, the car can pull to one side. Maintain the recommended pressures at all times. When traveling with a heavy load or at high speeds for a long distance, inflate tires as recommended in the instruction manual for such conditions, generally four pounds extra pressure. Tire pressure must be measured only when the tires are cool and before driving any great distance. Proper pressure also helps to prevent blowouts. Finally, tires should be checked periodically for cuts, knots, and bulges, and of course for wear—they should have at least 1/16 of an inch tread.

MECHANICAL AND PASSIVE PREVENTIVE MEASURES

Roadways

Until recently, roads were laid out to fit the land. Sharp turns were frequent, and bridge-builders sought out the narrowest points to minimize construction costs. Today, highways cleave to the countryside in geometric patterns to make driving easier and safer. Their curves are gentle, and banked so that a car can easily be driven around them. Bridges are built with straight approaches to minimize risks. Interstate roads nearly eliminate the possibility of head-on collisions, and lower the probability of many other accidents. Even though these are high-speed roads, the number of fatalities per hundred million miles traveled on interstate roads is 1.6, about half the national fatality rate.

Today's interstate highways have guard rails designed not simply to stop a wandering car from going off the road, but to redirect it back onto the travel lane with minimal damage. They also have new "breakaway" poles that are designed, like the new guard rails, to reduce the damage to cars striking concrete abutments, utility poles, or trees. Abutments are often protected by energy-absorbing barriers that bring cars to a relatively safe and gentle stop before they hit immovable objects.

With construction of the interstate highway system virtually completed, the major needs now are maintenance, repair, and improvement. All states, and many smaller jurisdictions, have data systems that identify the sites of frequent accidents and determine whether highway factors cause them. The Federal Highway Administration, working through state highway departments, helps to finance the spot safety improvements needed. Responsible drivers, as citizens, can help see to it that such improvements are made.

Car design

Statistics show that roughly 85 percent of fatal accidents are related to the driver or the road, whereas 15 percent are due to the vehicle. Most vehicle deficiencies are due to faulty maintenance, such as bald tires, lack of brake fluid, and so forth. Only 1.5 percent or fewer of all fatal accidents are directly caused by faulty car construction, although continued improvements in occupant protection can significantly reduce the number of motor vehicle fatalities, should an accident occur. The federal agency responsible for highway and vehicle safety programs is the National Highway Traffic Safety Administration, a unit of the Department of Transportation. This agency has established three groups of standards that must be met by all vehicles sold in the U.S.

The first group, called the "crash-avoidance" standards, is intended to reduce the likelihood of an accident. They include minimum performance requirements for windshield washers and wipers, defrosters, brakes, tires, lights, mirrors, and various vehicle control systems. Shift lever sequences for automatic transmissions, for example, are now standardized so that a driver is not confused in changing from one car to another.

The second group, called the "crash-worthiness" standards, is concerned with occupant protection in the event of a crash. These include performance requirements for seat belts, an energy-absorbing collapsible steering column, windshield retention to keep occupants from being ejected through a windshield opening in a crash, locks that prevent a door from springing open during a roll-over, and padding on the dash.

The final group, the "post-crash" standards, is concerned with after-crash injury. This group has requirements such as a fuel system that withstands crashes without leaking flammable fuel and interior fabrics with a slow burn rate.

These safety standards have been gradually upgraded and extended to cover light trucks and vans, as well as passenger cars. At the same time, procedures have been evolved for safety testing of new cars both by the manufacturers and the government to ensure that the standards are complied with. As a result, newer cars are demonstrably safer than older ones. A 1976 study by the General Accounting Office showed that the occupant of a 1974 model year car was about 25 percent more likely to survive a crash than the occupant of a 1966 car—the difference being the government's "crash-worthiness" standards. To date, these standards have saved over 64,000 lives.

Protective equipment

In an auto crash there are usually two collisions: first, the collision between the car and another object, and second, the collision between the car's occupants and the interior of the car. Injury prevention measures must involve both. Seat belts and padded interior appointments are examples of innovations already in use.

Seat belts The most common type is a three-point restraint, consisting of a lap belt and shoulder belt coupled together. Such a combination prevents sliding forward of the hips, minimizing tilts with the upper body, and the chance that the legs will strike the instrument panel, and prevents contact with the steering column, the windshield, and the dashboard.

The seat belt is the most effective form of protective equipment in automobile crashes. Yet, according to the Department of Transportation, only about 11 percent of drivers put them on. Among drivers involved in crashes, even a smaller percentage (8.4 percent) were wearing seat belts.

The majority of Americans appear to strongly oppose laws that require seat belt use. Two to one, they favor automatic crash protection over manual belts. Why? The reasons are legion. Some claim seat belts are uncomfortable to wear, difficult to keep straight, difficult to adjust, and inconvenient to store neatly. Others fear being trapped if the car catches fire in a crash or is submerged under water. Some think they will be safer if they are thrown clear of the car. And many people simply resent being told to do anything, under the delusion that society is not affected if they are injured.

In fact, rather than trapping people inside the car, seat belts protect passengers from severe injuries and allow them to escape more quickly. As for being "thrown clear," the odds of getting killed are considerably higher if one is ejected than if one remains inside the car.

AUTOMATIC PROTECTION SYSTEMS

An automatic (or passive) restraint is one that does not require any special act on the part of the occupant, such as fastening a buckle. The two most widely used devices are automatic seat belts and air bags. Studies have shown that a lap belt used in conjunction with an air bag is comparable in effectiveness to a full automatic seat belt system. If used universally, it is estimated these two systems can reduce highway fatalities by 9,000 yearly and serious injuries by about 65,000 yearly.

Passive Seat Belts. As one opens the door, the automatic belt swings away, allowing easy entry. As the door is closed, the belt automatically moves into position across the shoulder (and waist, in some models). The belt remains in place at all times when the vehicle is in operation.

Air Bags. Air bags, or air cushion restraint systems, consist of inflatable cushions which, in a front-end collision, automatically fill the space between front seat occupants and the steering wheel, dashboard, and windshield, preventing occupants from being thrown against the interior of the car. In some models, lap belts or knee restraints are needed to prevent the occupant from sliding over or under the air bag.

Most experts believe that the air bags will provide at least as good protection, and probably better, to front seat occupants in front-end collisions as will a lap-and-shoulder belt, because they move evenly, distributing the crash forces, and they do this without requiring the occupant to take any action. The air bag, however, offers only limited protection in side impacts, rear-end collisions, and roll-overs, and the use of a lap belt is still highly recommended.

CHILD RESTRAINTS

Properly designed restraints for small children are even more important than for adults because in a collision a small child is more likely to be thrown against the car interior. Contrary to what many parents think, a child is *never* protected by being held in an adult's lap; not infrequently a child is crushed between the adult and the surface of the car.

It has been estimated that three-quarters of the injuries in car accidents suffered by children under five can be prevented by the proper use of approved commercial car seats. It is important for all who drive with children in their cars to remember and act on this statistic.

In order to protect children, a well-designed child seat must be properly secured. Infants should be placed in infant car seats in a semi-reclining position facing the rear of the car. The seat should have adequate padding and a harness system and should be held in place by the car seat belt.

After infancy and up to age four, children should ride in an approved child seat. The best of these are made of hard molded plastic with energy-absorbing padding and harness straps for the shoulders, lap, and crotch. Like the infant seat, it is secured with the car seat belt. Some child seats have tethers—straps that are attached to the top of the plastic seat and can be attached to the metal frame of the car—that are designed to hold the top of the seat in place in a crash. The tether that comes with some models must be used for the carseat to be fully effective.

Children become accustomed quickly to the idea of riding restrained. Parents report less distraction when they chauffeur restrained children, and the biggest plus, outside of lives saved, is that habits learned at an early age are more likely to be continued in later years.

LEGISLATIVE PREVENTIVE MEASURES

Alcohol
Even very small quantities of alcohol in the blood (0.02 or 0.03 grams per liter) can impair driving ability and increase the risk of a traffic accident. But rarely in the U.S. do legal definitions of "drunkenness" behind the wheel reflect that fact.

Following federal guidelines, all states have enacted some form of "implied consent" law, which requires anyone accepting a driver's license to agree to testing for blood alcohol content by law enforcement officials.

In most states, a blood alcohol level of 0.1 grams of alcohol per liter (g/L) of blood is presumptive evidence of being "under the influence," a level quickly attained by drinking three martinis, five beers, or five glasses of wine in a short period of time.

A few states, such as Michigan, define a blood alcohol level of less than 0.07 g/L (approximately two drinks) as adequate proof one is not legally under the influence of alcohol. In New York, Ohio, and South Carolina, a blood alcohol level of 0.05 g/L is the limit.

Several other states distinguish between a person "under the influence of alcohol" and "in-toxication," primarily for the purpose of determining penalties. But in virtually every area, measurement of alcohol in the body is done with a test based on alcohol concentration in the breath—the so-called breath test. (A few states also use blood, urine, and saliva tests.)

Unfortunately, the implied consent law has not been notably effective in deterring drunken driving. Violators involved in fatal accidents are often successfully prosecuted, but rarely jailed. Most are released with suspended sentences and a brief revocation of driving privileges. Penalties for drunken drivers, and for drivers who refuse to take breath tests, vary from state to state, but only where driving laws are seriously applied do they do any good.

Scandinavian countries are a case in point. In Sweden, for example, the penalty for driving with a blood alcohol content of 0.15 g/L or greater is usually imprisonment for one to two months and license suspension for at least one year—which the police regularly enforce—even if the driver was not involved in an accident but was merely stopped for a routine check. If the blood alcohol level is less than 0.15 but greater than 0.05 g/L, the offender must pay a fine and suffer license suspension for at least one month. These legal measures have dramatically reduced fatal accidents involving drunken drivers.

In 1974, several Canadian provinces enacted stiffer penalties for drunk driving, which in Canada is defined as driving with a blood alcohol content of at least 0.08 g/L. They also passed a mandatory seat belt law and mandatory reduced speed limits. Probably as a consequence of these measures, the fatality rate was reduced by 31 percent in the first three years of the program, in spite of a yearly increase in the number of vehicles and the amount of travel.

Speed

After the preliminary imposition of 55 mph national speed limits in the fall of 1973, fatalities per vehicle mile traveled dropped suddenly and significantly (see table 10.5). Lowering the speed limit on highways has been credited with about one-half of the reduction—about 9,000 lives. The trends of motorist compliance with the 55 mph speed limit have shed additional light on relationships between speed and fatalities. A disproportionate share of fatalities occurred in the western and southwestern states where resistance to (and violations of) the 55 mph speed limits is most widespread.

It is generally accepted that deaths and injuries could be reduced even further if speed limits were further lowered. But such efforts face strong resistance in a nation that believes in the inalienable rights of personal mobility and fast travel. Thus, the 55 mph speed limit for highways seems to many the best available compromise between saving time and increasing safety.

Protective equipment

Seat Belts. All cars sold in the U.S. must be equipped with fabric belts that can be fastened around the occupant to limit motion in case of sudden impact. Even airbag cars must have a lap belt to provide protection in side and roll-over crashes. But the use of these belts is not enforced

in the U.S. In countries that do enforce belt use, the wear rates are much higher than in the U.S. The state of Victoria, Australia, for example, mandated seat belt usage in 1971. The result was that about 90 percent of all drivers "buckled up," and highway fatality rates went down.

Should society legislate the use of seat belts as is done in certain parts of Canada and Australia? Should such legislation apply to passengers as well by making the drivers responsible? In view of the resistance people have toward using seat belts, even in spite of their demonstrated advantages, we believe some legislation is indicated. It could be enforced by the police in the same way they deal with drivers who speed or make wrong turns. No doubt, it would initially demand a great effort by the police and the traffic courts. But at times it is necessary to motivate people legislatively to modify injurious habits, particularly if they harm others as well. Another inducement could come from insurance carriers if they were to refuse to pay when injuries are caused by the nonwearing of seat belts. The Federal Republic of Germany is trying this approach. The benefits derived from all of these efforts are clearly worth the effort.

Automatic Restraints

Because seat belts are not used by many, the U.S. Department of Transportation in June 1977 issued a regulation requiring "passive," or automatic, restraint systems in all passenger cars sold in the United States by model year 1984. However, these regulations may have to be changed to allow for the fact that U.S. auto manufacturers currently could not designate cars as six-passenger vehicles if passive restraints were required. No such restraints have been developed for the middle passenger on a bench-type front seat, other than airbags.

PART

II

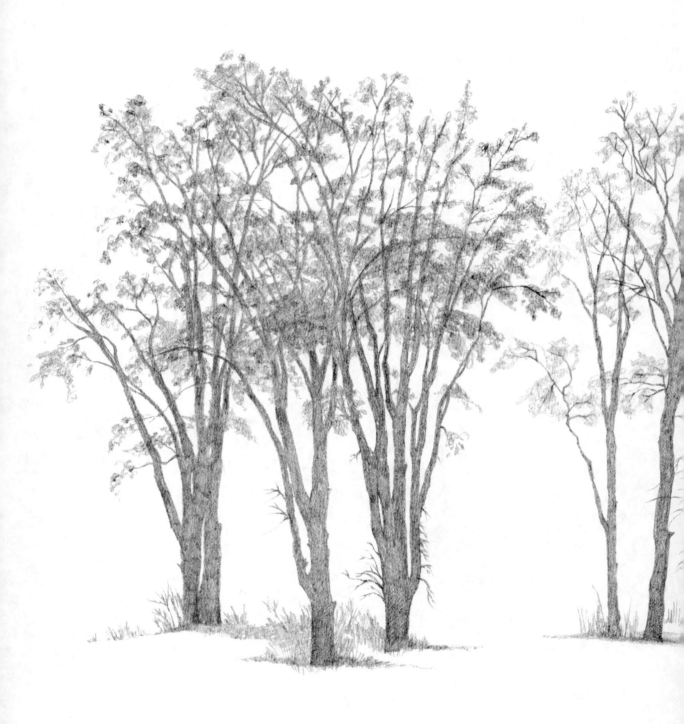

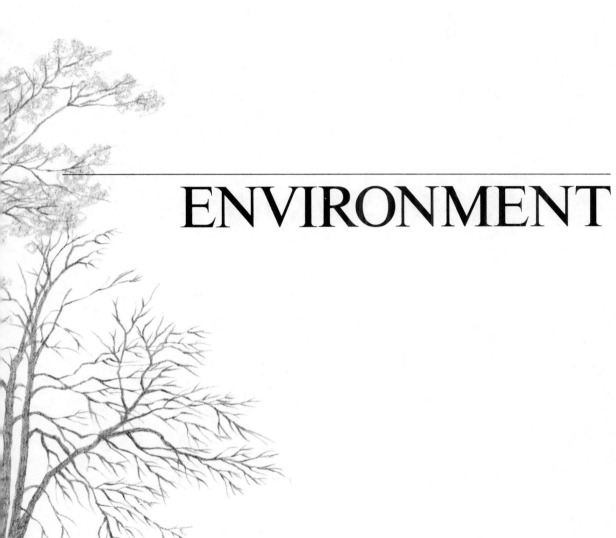

ENVIRONMENT

CHAPTER
11

Air pollution

Surely one of our most important freedoms is the right to breathe air free of harmful gases and particles. Clean air is essential to life. Yet, we have allowed many elements in our modern lifestyle to contribute to pollution of our planet's precious air. Among the most important sources of air pollution are industrial wastes vented into the air, motor vehicle exhaust, and garbage incineration.

In the past decade, thanks to a phalanx of new laws, we have made important strides toward control of all three of these sources of dirty air. As a result, the air in our cities and near our highways and factories is less polluted than it was fifteen years ago. But there are still areas of the nation where, because of geographical factors affecting the movement of air and because of rapid industrial growth, air pollution persists as a health problem.

Although it is very difficult to pinpoint such air pollutants as direct causes of disease, we do know that they impose an extra burden on those who are elderly or who already have respiratory problems. The battle for cleaner air is a continuing one in which all of us can participate, both by monitoring our own environment and by supporting legislative efforts to force the polluters to clean up.

Glossary

ACID RAIN   Chemicals from industry, automobiles, and home heating rise into the atmosphere and are spread over the earth by air currents, then come back to earth in the form of acidic rainfall.

FOG   Condensation of natural water vapor in the air.

GREENHOUSE EFFECT   Theory that carbon dioxide in the air absorbs heat energy and reflects it back to earth while permitting ultraviolet energy from the sun to pass through, thus raising air temperature on earth.

INVERSION   Layer of cool air trapped under warm air.

PARTICULATE   Particle of dust or soot in the air.

PPM   Concentration of a chemical in parts per million.

SMOG   Photochemical reaction of hydrocarbons from automobile exhaust, together with nitrogen oxides and sunlight, creating a mixture of irritating chemical compounds.

TPM   Total particulate matter.

History and Definitions

A PRIMEVAL PROBLEM

With the discovery of fire by our cave-dwelling ancestors came indoor air pollution, in the form of smoke-contaminated caves. In fact, it is likely that those smoky caves contained more concentrated air pollution than that encountered today in many communities.

Until Elizabethan times, Europeans heated their homes by building fires in pits located in the center of the room. Outlets for smoke were minimal, causing serious indoor pollution. With the introduction of chimneys, indoor pollution abated but outdoor pollution increased. Chimneys made possible the use of coal for domestic purposes and, by the seventeenth century, there were as many as 360,000 chimneys in London belching forth gritty smoke. This chimney smoke, along with emissions from factories, combined with sea fog to produce a noxious gaseous mixture. For the next three hundred years the industrial centers of England, Wales, and other countries were mantled in this fog, sometimes resulting in dramatic effects on human health (see table 11.1).

The most deadly episode on record occurred in Greater London in December 1952. Five days of stagnant air and intense fog greatly increased the concentrations of smoke from coal-burning homes, power plants, and factories. There were 4,000 excess deaths—those exceeding the number normally expected for that time of year—the majority among persons already suffering from heart or lung disease. Ten years later, another episode in London caused 700 excess deaths.

Air pollution episodes had long-term as well as immediate effects. Nine years after the October 1948 pollution episode in Donora, Pennsylvania, a follow-up study found that persons who had become ill during that event suffered a greater prevalence of disease and higher death rates than those who had not become ill during it.

Many cities have achieved dramatic improvement in air quality since these incidents took place. Inhabitants of cities such as London and Pittsburgh are particularly aware of the progress that has been made in reducing urban air pollution. Coal has been largely replaced by oil, electricity, and natural gas for home and industrial heating. The government has required air pollution controls in power plants, major industries, and motor vehicles. As a result of reducing pollution at its source, the lethal episodes of the past are not likely to be repeated. Nonetheless, air pollution continues to cause human health problems, toxic effects on plants and animals, and damage to buildings and works of art. It causes concern among scientists that the world's climate will be altered by carbon dioxide accumulations in the atmosphere, due in part to people's destruction of forests.

MEASURING AIR QUALITY

One measure of air quality is the concentration of total suspended particulate (commonly referred to as "dust" or "soot").

To measure air quality and provide uniform advice to the public, the Environmental Protection Agency (EPA) and the Council on Environmental Quality have devised the Pollutant Standards Index (PSI). The PSI reports levels of five major air pollutants: carbon monoxide, photochemical oxidants (approximately 90 percent of which is ozone), nitrogen dioxide, sulfur dioxide, and particulate matter. These measures are converted to a scale graded from 0 (good) to 500 (significant harm), representing the potential adverse health effects associated with concentration of pollutants (see table 11.2). All state and local agencies responsible for monitoring urban areas of more than half a million people have adopted the PSI. Its nationwide acceptance is expected by 1983.

The EPA has also established three levels of air pollution episodes—alert, warning, and emergency—roughly corresponding to scale values of 200, 300, and 400. Each level of warning is accompanied by recommended actions such as reducing traffic, limiting fuel use, restricting incineration, and reducing manufacturing activities. Air pollution actions are not based on pollution concentration and predicted weather/wind conditions alone. Other factors considered are total area, total population, population density, pollution duration, and the number of people exposed to high levels. Therefore, the healthfulness of different cities is difficult to compare based on the PSI alone.

Table 11.1
SELECTED AIR POLLUTION EPISODES

Date	Place	Excess Deaths
December 1930	Meuse Valley, Belgium	63
October 1948	Donora, Pennsylvania	20
December 1952	London, England	4,000
November 1953	New York, New York	200
December 1962	London, England	700

Table 11.2
POLLUTANT STANDARDS INDEX (PSI)
(SET BY U.S. ENVIRONMENTAL PROTECTION AGENCY, 1978)

Index value	PSI descriptor	General health effects	Cautionary statements
500	Significant harm level*	Premature death of ill and elderly. Healthy people will experience adverse symptoms that affect their normal activity.	All persons should remain indoors, keeping windows and doors closed. All persons should minimize physical exertion and avoid traffic.
400	Hazardous (Emergency)	Premature onset of certain diseases in addition to significant aggravation of symptoms and decreased exercise tolerance in healthy persons.	Elderly and persons with existing diseases should stay indoors and avoid physical exertion. General population should avoid outdoor activity.
300	(Warning)		
200	Very unhealthful (Alert)	Significant aggravation of symptoms and decreased exercise tolerance in persons with heart or lung disease, with widespread symptoms in the healthy population.	Elderly and persons with existing heart or lung disease should stay indoors and reduce physical activity.
100	Unhealthful	Mild aggravation of symptoms in susceptible persons, with irritation symptoms in the healthy population.	Persons with existing heart or respiratory ailments should reduce physical exertion and outdoor activity.
50	Moderate		
0	Good		

*State and local agencies are required to take emergency action to prevent air pollution from reaching this level, such as restricting auto traffic and manufacturing activities.

Air

Only 21 percent of the air we breathe is oxygen; most of it, 78 percent, is nitrogen. The rest is carbon dioxide (0.3 percent) and argon (0.07 percent), with trace amounts of a few other gases and differing amounts of water vapor. Most—95 percent—of what we call air is found in the troposphere, an approximately six-mile layer between the surface of the earth and the stratosphere. The troposphere receives thousands of tons of manufactured wastes daily. The earth's natural rotation creates winds and air currents that help disperse them, but if the air becomes stagnant, acute air pollution follows.

A wide variety of natural and artificial substances are found in the air in the form of suspended particulate matter, mist, and gas. Artificial sources contributing to this pollution include grinders, sanders, welders, sprayers, and drillers; industrial processes in which heat and pressure are used to produce vapor; and combustion in the production of energy by furnaces and engines.

Sources of Pollution

Industrial processes—those emitting toxic metals such as lead, arsenic, mercury, or toxic organic compounds—and motor vehicles are the major sources of air pollution. Two-thirds of the sulfur oxide in the air is thought to be emitted from coal and oil burned in power plants, while the primary source of carbon monoxide is the automobile's combustion engine. The recent increased use of wood-burning stoves as a substitute home-heating source will only add to the air pollution problem.

Oil burners used in apartment houses or commercial buildings for space heating are another major source of particulate pollution. While home burners use grades of oil from which most of the mineral matter has been removed, commercial oil burners use poorer grades that produce more particulate matter. Control of particulate pollution from oil burners requires that combustion equipment be well maintained and operated, although even the best equipment will emit black smoke when the equipment first starts up. Once proper combustion is established, however, a well-designed and well-operated unit should not produce visible pollution.

Sulfur dioxides, an important class of pollutants, are produced when the sulfur in fossil fuels is oxidized during combustion. The oxidation process often continues when the sulfur dioxide enters the atmosphere and sulfuric acid and other sulfates are produced. Control of sulfur dioxide and sulfates can be achieved by limiting the sulfur content of fuel or eliminating sulfur dioxide from fuel gases. Petroleum from some areas of the world is naturally low in sulfur, but generally the fuel must be desulfurized to meet the standards established by the regulatory agencies. A valuable and reusable by-product of such a process is sulfur or sulfuric acid, thus demonstrating that pollution control can have indirect benefits as well.

INDUSTRIAL POLLUTION

Prior to the 1970 Clean Air Act, industrial emissions and combustion of bituminous coal were considered the most serious sources of air pollution. Technological advances in pollution control devices and the increasing public demand for cleaner air have helped to reduce dust fall and gaseous pollution substantially, although most urban areas have not yet met all the established standard levels.

Polynuclear aromatic hydrocarbons (PAH), nitrosamines, pesticides, mineral dusts like asbestos, and metals like lead, cadmium, beryllium,

Table 11.3
PARTICULATE AIR POLLUTION

Source	Particulates* $(mg./1,000m^3)$
Cigarette smoke	95,000,000
Cigarette smoke, sidestream	3,700,000
Incinerator, garbage	820,000
Power plant stack	620,000
Stack, home heating, coal	470,000
Diesel engine exhaust (undiluted)	170,000
Outdoor burning of grass and leaves	140,000

*Mg. particulates per 1,000 cubic meters

SOURCE: Division of Environmental Carcinogenesis, Naylor Dana Institute, American Health Foundation, Valhalla, New York.

arsenic, chromium, and manganese have been identified as particulate contaminants with potential adverse health effects (see chapter 16, Occupational Health). Maximum limits have been set for several of these contaminants. The determination of their total particulate matter (TPM) is still being studied. The EPA is investigating the possibility of instituting a standard based on particulate size. Table 11.3 summarizes the sources of particulate air pollution and their relative concentrations per cubic meter.

AUTOMOBILE POLLUTION

Automobiles account for about 60 percent of the total weight of the pollutants discharged into the atmosphere, primarily in the form of carbon monoxide. Gasoline engines and diesel-powered vehicles differ in the quantity and quality of pollutants they generate. Engine type, type of fuel, mode of operation, traffic density, traffic patterns, local geography, and climate all affect the air pollution produced by mobile sources.

Most autos and trucks are powered by internal combustion engines that expel three major air pollutants: unburnt gasoline vapors, carbon monoxide, and nitrogen oxides, collectively referred to as tailpipe emissions. The unburnt or partially burnt gasoline vapors that evaporate from the gas tank and carburetor are hydrocarbons which are themselves thought to be innocuous at the concentrations found in the general atmosphere, but in combination with nitrogen oxides and sunlight, they create photochemical reactions that produce irritating compounds classed as oxidants. Oxidants cause smog in cities, Los Angeles being the most notorious example.

The auto's four major sources of pollution are the exhaust pipe, the carburetor, the crankcase, and the fuel tank. The exhaust emissions are composed of carbon monoxide (3.5 percent), hydrocarbons (900 ppm) and nitrogen oxides (1,500 ppm). An expert committee of the World Health Organization compared engine exhaust of cars idling, accelerating, cruising, and decelerating, and found that the amount of pollution emitted did not differ significantly. Major variations in emissions are due to engine efficiency and not to the way the vehicle is operated.

The fuel used in spark-ignition engines contributes significantly to total particulates and carbon monoxide emissions. Alkyl lead compounds used as antiknock fuel additives increase lead exposure for many city dwellers. As a result, some countries restrict the use of lead antiknock fuel additives.

Diesel-powered vehicles, increasingly popular, do not use a spark ignition, but heat the fuel-air mixture by compression. This high compression leads to less unburned fuel than gasoline engines. Comparisons between the two indicate that a properly maintained diesel engine emits smaller quantities of carbon monoxide and no lead. However, hydrocarbons are not reduced in diesels and nitrogen oxide emissions are greater. In addition, diesel fuels, which contain higher levels of sulfur, produce greater sulfur dioxide emissions. Diesel engines also emit visible, sootlike particles, and pungent odors due to irritants like acrolein and formaldehyde. Methods to trap these particulates are being investigated.

Autos and trucks also contribute particulate pollutants to the environment. The tires resuspend settled dust from the streets, and as tires, brakes, and mechanical parts age, they tend to abrade into particulate form. Keeping streets well washed is an effective means of minimizing the dust dispersion by automobiles.

WEATHER EFFECTS

Inversions

In an inversion, which occurs under certain topographic and weather conditions, a layer of cool air is trapped by the warmer air above it. The cool air stabilizes and is unable to rise or mix. During fall and winter nights, for example, valleys tend to collect cool air which is then trapped by warmer daytime air. In urban and industrialized areas where pollution is heavy, air stagnation prevents dispersion of pollution. The pollution episodes listed in table 11.1 were the direct outcome of such air inversions.

Fog

Fog is the condensation of natural water vapor in the air. The intensity of fog is determined by both air temperature and the amount of water vapor in it. Since warm air can contain more moisture than cooler air, fog occurs most frequently after dark when the daytime air is cooling. Fog may form if the temperature drops sufficiently during an inversion. This may be particularly hazardous because fog can convert harmful gases into even more harmful acids. For example, fog can convert sulfur dioxide, a by-product of coal or oil emissions, into sulfuric acid.

Smog

Smog is the word originally used to characterize the combination of smoke and fog in London. It has become a universal term to describe the condition of the air in places like Los Angeles. Its later connotation, however, generally refers to the atmospheric condition resulting from the photochemical action of sunlight on automobile emissions. The sun's radiant energy, absorbed by nitrogen dioxide in the presence of hydrocarbons from automobile exhausts, can produce a mixture of irritating chemical compounds.

Acid Rain

Rainfall is one way by which the sulfur and nitrogen from industry, automobiles, and home heating are returned to the earth. Since the 1950s, the acidity of rainfall in the U.S. has increased approximately 50-fold.

Acid rain is spread over the earth in air currents. Its fallout is currently confined to the northern hemisphere, with the largest concentrations in Canada, the northeastern U.S., and Scandinavia. But acid rain is expected to spread to the southern hemisphere eventually.

Acid rain is associated with (1) depletion and, in some instances, total elimination of fish in lakes and estuaries; (2) loss of crop productivity and forest yields; (3) damage to steel and stone structures and outdoor artworks; (4) harmful levels of trace metals in drinking water supplies from long-term leaching effects.

Greenhouse Effect

It is estimated that by the year 2000, manufactured emissions of carbon dioxide into the air will have increased 18-fold since 1890. Carbon dioxide absorbs heat energy from several sources (infrared radiation), and reflects that energy back to the earth. This trapping of the heat allows less of it to be released into outer space. At the same time the carbon dioxide permits ultraviolet energy from the sun to pass through, thus possibly creating a "greenhouse effect," raising air temperature on the earth. This process conceivably could have profound effects on the level of oceans and seas, the productivity of ocean fisheries, and agriculture. However, some scientists believe that increases in water vapor, dust particles, and other air pollutants block out or reflect away part of the sun's radiant energy, thus creating a cooling effect.

Health Effects

The effects of severe air pollution are generally limited to the respiratory tract, and the elderly and persons already troubled by heart and/or respiratory problems are the most adversely affected.

The hazards of air pollution should be viewed in relation to those of tobacco smoking. As table 11.3 shows, the concentration of general air pollution per cubic centimeter is much less than that of tobacco smoke. Thus tobacco smoking is far unhealthier than most air pollution (see chapter 4). Air sampled at one of New York City's busiest intersections shows a concentration of about 100,000 particles per cubic centimeter. However, a popular U.S. filter cigarette yielding about 15 mg. of condensate (tar) produces more than 1.5 billion particles per cubic centimeter, and a nonfilter cigarette produces twice as much again.

CHRONIC RESPIRATORY DISEASE

Chronic respiratory disease includes common lung diseases like chronic bronchitis, emphysema, and chronic obstructive lung disease. These highly prevalent pulmonary health problems involve 10 to 20 percent of the adult population. Unquestionably, the major contributing cause of chronic respiratory disease is cigarette smoking (see chapter 4, Tobacco), followed by occupational exposure to a wide variety of hazardous dusts, fumes, and gases. Not infrequently, populations at greater risk of chronic respiratory disease live in polluted areas, work in occupations involving hazardous dusts and fumes, more frequently are smokers, and have lower income levels. However, even when these factors are statistically allowed for, a relationship between high levels of local air pollution and chronic respiratory disease is repeatedly found.

Worldwide studies of air pollution also indicate a relationship between the sulfur oxide/particulate air pollution complex and the prevalence of chronic respiratory symptoms. The interrelationship between cigarette smoking, air pollution, and chronic bronchitis is well illustrated in the results of a British study shown in figure 11.1. The figure shows that the effect of cigarette smoking is considerably stronger than air pollution on the prevalence of chronic bronchitis, adjusted for age.

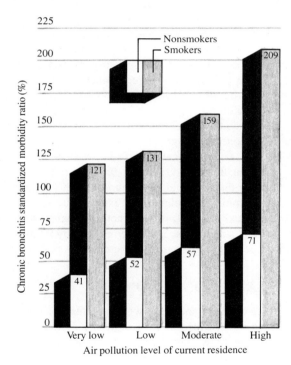

FIGURE 11.1

Prevalence of chronic bronchitis in relation to smoking and air pollution
SOURCE: *adapted from P.M. Lambert and D.D. Reid, "Smoking, Air Pollution, and Bronchitis in Britain,"* Lancet *1: 853–7, 1970*

BRONCHIAL ASTHMA

Asthma affects about 3 percent of the population with intermittent wheezing and shortness of breath, and air pollution is known to intensify its discomforts. Apparently, some pollutants, including photochemical oxidants and particulates, can provoke asthma attacks in susceptible people. Residents of the more polluted cities have more frequent asthma attacks, but the specific air pollutants responsible have not yet been identified. However, asthmatics are affected by other environmental stresses such as cold air, respiratory infections, psychological factors, and pollens, and it is therefore difficult to assess the added contribution of air pollutants.

CHRONIC BRONCHITIS AND EMPHYSEMA

Although it is difficult to separate the overwhelming effect of cigarette smoking from the effect of air pollution in causing chronic bronchitis, British studies have determined that air pollution is a distinct cause.

Among individuals already afflicted with chronic bronchitis or emphysema, there is considerable evidence that their underlying disease status can be worsened by high concentrations of sulfur dioxide, particulates, or photochemical oxidants. With decreasing concentrations of daily levels of the sulfur oxide/particulate complex, it is difficult to make a correlation between changes in affected individuals' symptoms and variations in air quality. For these specific diseases and for general mortality, it appears that the improved air quality of the 1970s has greatly diminished, if not completely removed, the readily demonstrable adverse health effects associated with uncontrolled combustion of fossil fuels that were so widely prevalent in the 1950s and early 1960s.

LUNG CANCER

There is no clear evidence that urban air pollutants actually contribute to an increased risk of lung cancer, although city air contains more carcinogens than does country air because of the higher levels of auto exhaust and industrial pollution. Even polluted city air does not contain the high concentration of carcinogens found in tobacco smoke; thus air pollution's independent effect on the development of lung cancer cannot be adequately evaluated without considering the effect of cigarette smoking. Cigarette smoking remains by far the strongest risk factor in the development of lung cancer in the general population (see chapter 4, Tobacco). Other well-documented risk factors include a number of occupational exposures to elements such as asbestos, uranium mining, arsenic, bis-chloromethyl ether, vinyl chloride, and coke oven emissions (see chapter 16, Occupational Health).

The carcinogen benzo(a)pyrene (BaP) is present in outdoor air, largely as a by-product of the incomplete combustion of fossil fuels, particularly coal. Since the major shift from coal to oil, natural gas, and electricity for heating homes took place, there has been, not surprisingly, a three- to tenfold decline in BaP levels of U.S. cities between 1950 and 1970. This decline, while not documented, has undoubtedly been continuing ever since 1940. Levels of BaP in urban air now are generally very low, several thousand-fold below BaP exposures of roofers, gas retort workers, and other occupational groups exposed to tars and incompletely burned coal or coal by-products.

Still, there is no reason for complacency about the presence of carcinogens in the air such as organic vapors from solvents and other industrial chemicals, additives in gasoline and other fuels, and many other organic compounds from consumer and industrial products that can be released.

RESPIRATORY DISEASES IN CHILDREN

During the first eight years of life, the lung continues to mature. If its development is compromised, the individual may well be affected for life.

During the five-day 1952 London smog episode, infants had a higher death rate than older children or young adults.

Children who live in more polluted communities suffer significantly more acute respiratory infections and diminished lung function when compared with children of the same age, sex, race, and socioeconomic level in less polluted communities. Very young children can average four to eight acute respiratory infections per year; air pollution exposure can increase this frequency by 10 to 50 percent.

Children living near busy roadways and lead smelters have higher than average blood lead concentrations. Although these lead levels are usually not high enough to cause outright poisoning, high levels in the outside air can increase total lead level in the body, and thereby add to the risk of harm from other sources like paint, pottery, and soil. Lead fallout from automotive exhaust onto soil and street surfaces can be ingested by infants and young children playing outdoors.

HEART CONDITIONS

Since the heart and lungs work together as a unit, anything that affects the respiratory system can also affect the heart. This includes air pollution. Impaired breathing makes the heart work harder to overcome the loss of oxygen. One effect can be an increase in the heart size. Persons suffering from heart disease or angina show a significant increase in sickness and death during periods of high air pollution.

OTHER EFFECTS

The nitrogen oxide and sulfur oxide components of smog and sulfur dioxide in the air are responsible for eye tearing and burning and nasal cavity irritations. Excess carbon monoxide in the air has been linked to bouts of dizziness, headaches, and blurred vision. Air pollution also reduces resistance to colds, flu, and pneumonia.

Prevention

INDIVIDUAL ACTION

The smoker chooses to inhale cigarette smoke, but the air we breathe is not a matter of choice. Therefore, it is important for each person to take all available measures to reduce air pollution's ill-effects.

The watchword is avoidance. For example, people should avoid jogging, running, and bicycling along busy roadways, especially when traffic is heavy.

Persons with heart or lung disease must be especially careful. They should avoid prolonged outdoor activity when pollution levels rise significantly above normal, as during summer stagnations or inversions, and be alert to worsening of their disease symptoms. They should avoid smoke from fireplace chimneys and exposure to burning leaves, a custom that is now illegal in some parts of the U.S.

In both home and indoor recreational areas, the worst form of pollution is sidestream tobacco smoke, which can lead to relatively high concentrations of carbon monoxide and particulate matter (see chapter 4, Tobacco). Proper ventilation can certainly help reduce indoor air pollution, particularly in the kitchen, and air conditioning helps to filter polluted air and control exposure to humidity and temperature.

In addition to the above actions, the government recommends these steps to help reduce air pollution and its detrimental health effects:

- Use mass transportation instead of cars, whenever possible.
- Join car pools to avoid contributing to already congested traffic.
- Keep cars tuned-up and eliminate unnecessary idling.
- Keep tires properly inflated to increase engine efficiency.
- Conserve electricity.
- Support Clean Air legislation.
- Learn, support, and obey an area's air pollution control laws and regulations.
- Install and maintain pollution control equipment in incinerators.

THE WORKPLACE

Air pollution in the workplace is apt to be thousands of times higher than that encountered out-of-doors. (See chapter 16, Occupational Health.) Most occupational diseases result from inhalation of toxic airborne dusts, vapors, or mists. The detrimental health effects of exposure to airborne toxic substances can be minimized by a variety of methods:

- Substitute less toxic or nontoxic materials where possible.
- Enclose and mechanize the process to avoid dispersion of potentially toxic substances into the atmosphere.
- Ventilate the workplace and industrial processes to avoid dispersion of the substances into the breathing zone of the operators.

Various kinds of respirators are available to protect the individual operator, but these should be used only in emergencies, or for unusual maintenance operations in which mechanical methods of control may not be feasible. Masks should be required for workers in areas where there are dusts, vapors, or mists.

AUTOMOBILES

Automobile manufacturers have reduced harmful emissions substantially in response to EPA regulations. Since 1960, emissions of hydrocarbons have been reduced by 89 percent, carbon monoxide (CO) by 82 percent, and oxides of nitrogen (NO) by 51 percent. With proper maintenance and care, such decreases can continue even though a car ages.

The major method used to achieve such reductions is the catalytic converter that changes the HC and CO in exhaust gases into harmless carbon dioxide (CO_2) and water (H_2O) through oxidation. In addition, the converter treats the exhaust gases after they leave the engine; thus, engine efficiency, vehicle drive-ability, and fuel economy are protected as long as the converter is maintained. Catalytic converters require the use of unleaded gas that helps to increase engine life. Maintenance requirements are lowered and lead emissions are reduced. As older cars are retired from the road, as more cars are equipped with catalytic converters and the use of unleaded gas is increased, lead pollution problems will abate.

Further progress in reducing harmful automobile emissions is expected from the development of improved converters and from devices that will reduce the sulfur content of unleaded gas at the refinery.

COMMUNITY AND LEGISLATIVE ACTION

In the mid-1930s, dust settled in New York City at a rate of 135 tons per square mile per month. By 1976, this was reduced to less than 25 tons. In the 1950s and 1960s, many cities had yearly average concentrations of sulfur dioxide and total particulate matter nearly ten times higher than yearly average levels in the late 1970s. Much of this improvement in air quality is due to the shift from use of coal to cleaner burning fuels such as oil and gas. Some areas now make substantial quantities of electricity in nuclear power plants. Nearly 50 percent of Chicago's electricity comes from nuclear sources. (The risks and benefits of nuclear energy are discussed in chapter 13, Radiation.) Much remains to be accomplished, however, and it is clear that air pollution must be controlled where it originates.

This can only be done through legislation. The Clean Air Act of 1970 established limitations for six major pollutants (table 11.4). It also directed the EPA to set acceptable air quality standards and establish emission levels for new pollutant sources. The method of attaining these standards was left up to the states. Each state was required to develop State Implementation Plans (SIPs), which detailed the ways in which the federal goals are to be met. The 1977 amendments to the Clean Air Act extended the deadlines for compliance with the original legislation and permitted the filing of new SIPs through July 1, 1979. While virtually no city in the U.S. exceeded allowable yearly average levels of particulate matter and sulfur dioxide by the late 1970s, automobile-related pollutants remained one of the most troublesome areas of control.

Control of automobile tailpipe emissions was first legislated in California in the early 1960s and subsequently applied nationally in the 1970 Federal Clean Air Act and its 1977 amendments. The controls were made increasingly stringent to reduce tailpipe emissions by 90 percent in 1975. In that year the regulations were expanded to include diesel-engine passenger cars, and beginning in motor year 1982, diesel engines will be further regulated so as not to exceed .6 particulate emissions per mile.

Pollution was further reduced when (1) the use of open fires for burning leaves, garbage, or construction wastes was prohibited or severely limited, (2) the use of incinerators in buildings was prohibited unless scrubbers or filters were provided to remove particulate matter, and (3) methods were adopted to assure proper combustion.

Desulfurization of flue gases is expected to become more widely used as more coal-burning power plants are built. In early 1980, sixty-five "sulfur scrubbers" were in use in the U.S., with forty-two under construction and another seventy-two planned. Most desulfurization processes depend on a reaction between flue gases and limestone. The finely powdered limestone is suspended in water and intimately mixed with exhaust gas; the sludge formed is dehydrated and removed from the system as solid waste. This process is expensive however and produces enormous volumes of sludge. The long-term environmental effects of sludge storage are not fully known. Thus, desulfurization can produce as many problems as it is intended to prevent.

New energy and chemical technologies are constantly evolving. They too will generate new kinds of pollutants, with as yet unknown health effects. The air quality standards for pollutants of the 1950s and 1960s may be irrelevant to the health aspects of today's pollution.

There is a danger that a combination of energy crises and inflation will weaken the national commitment to clean air. Nonetheless, the prospective shift to increasing quantities of coal need not necessarily be regarded with alarm. Particulates can be filtered from the stacks. It is possible that in the future coal will be desulfurized at the source. The best protection against air pollution is to support a national commitment to gain knowledge about its effects and to continue the program of air pollution control initiated with the Clean Air Act of 1970 and its 1977 amendments.

Table 11.4

NATIONAL AIR QUALITY STANDARDS
(Protective of Human Health)

Pollutant	Limitation
Sulfur dioxide	80 μg./m^3 (0.03 ppm) (a)
	365 μg./m^3 (0.14 ppm) (b)
Carbon monoxide	10 μg./m^3 (9 ppm) (d)
	40 μg./m^3 (35 ppm) (e)
Photochemical oxidants	160 μg./m^3 (0.08 ppm) (e)
Hydrocarbons	160 μg./m^3 (0.24 ppm) (f)
Nitrogen oxidants	100 μg./m^3 (0.05 ppm) (a)
Particulate matter	75 μg./m^3 (c)
	260 μg./m^3 (b)

(a)	=	Annual arithmetic mean
(b)	=	Maximum 24-hour concentration not to be exceeded more than once a year
(c)	=	Annual geometric mean
(d)	=	Maximum 8-hour concentration not to be exceeded more than once a year
(e)	=	Maximum 1-hour concentration not to be exceeded more than once a year. In 1979 this standard was revised to 0.12 ppm.
(f)	=	Maximum 3-hour concentration (6–9 AM) not to be exceeded more than once a year

SOURCE: Adapted from *Environmental Science and Technology*, vol. 5, page 503, 1971.

μg = microgram

CHAPTER
12

Water pollution

In spite of the fact that human beings cannot live without water, all too often they take the quality (and quantity) of their water supply for granted. Few of us have seen or been concerned about the distant reservoir that supplies water to our homes; few of us have wondered about possible contaminants in our wells or rivers.

As in many other areas of life, we need to compare the cost of the preventive measures to the benefits accruing to society. Appropriate legislative measures are being passed and need to be resolutely enforced to preserve and improve our water resources.

While the health benefit of such actions in the industrial countries may for the present be limited, it is clear that unless we act today, we run the risk of irreparably damaging our water supply and future quality of life.

Our rivers, lakes, and oceans must be kept safe for use by both sealife and humans.

Glossary

MINIMATA DISEASE   Mercury poisoning episode in the 1950s, affecting thousands of people exposed to mercury-containing wastes in Minimata Bay, Japan.

PCB   Polychlorinated biphenyl—a chemmical used for capacitators in the electric power industry. When released into the water supply, can interfere with the body's immunological system. Can cause cancer in laboratory rats.

POINT SOURCE   A specific, identifiable source of pollution.

NON-POINT SOURCE   Difficult-to-pinpoint source of pollution such as streams, eroded construction sites, or ground water contaminated by chemicals and/or sewage.

SLUDGE   Solid substance produced by water and sewage treatment processes.

History and Definitions

THE NEED FOR WATER

Water is an extraordinary substance. It is virtually everywhere, covering more than three-fourths of the earth's surface. Water is in the food we eat and the liquids we drink. We use it to bathe with as well as to wash our clothes and dishes. We cool ourselves with water and use it to grow crops and keep our lawns green.

Indeed, water is so pervasive that we often take it for granted. We shouldn't, for water is vital to our health. Depending on climate, we need about one or two quarts of water a day. We get water from our food, our beverages, and from our body's metabolic process, which produces water as a by-product. But the most important source is from drinking water. Most Americans get their water from municipal supplies that tap surfaces (rivers, lakes, or ponds) or ground water sources or from wells.

Unfortunately, in addition to the sample of uses listed above, water is also used to carry away our wastes. Since before the dawn of civilization, we have dumped refuse ranging from fecal matter to garbage to (more recently) industrial and chemical wastes into water. Even where dumping was not direct or intentional, wastes often are carried into lakes and streams by rainwater or by seeping into ground water. As a result, many of our waters have become polluted and a potential threat to our health. A 1970 survey of community water supplies in the U.S. found 360,000 people drank potentially dangerous water.

There is no such thing as "pure" water—all water contains some impurities. Even raindrops pick up dust and carbon dioxide as they fall to the ground. Water also collects organic matter that can cause disease, naturally occurring chemicals that in excess can be toxic, and industrial products, some of which are known or suspected causes of cancer, birth defects, and other illnesses.

Water can absorb most of these wastes, transform them into useful or innocuous substances, disperse them, and thus cleanse itself. Moving water stirs up waste matter, causing some to settle out or become diluted by fresh water. Dissolved oxygen in water metabolizes organic wastes much as our bodies burn food. The oxygen also sustains bacteria in water which feed on organic matter. The inoffensive residues are either dissolved and washed away or settle to the bottom.

Thus, given time and distance, water will stabilize its organic load. But our growing numbers and concentration in cities, plus the complexity of our manufacturing processes, have overburdened many lakes and streams beyond their self-cleansing capacity. Overloading water with organic wastes can exhaust its oxygen supply, prevent the elimination of wastes, and suffocate fish and other aquatic life.

HISTORICAL OUTBREAKS OF CHOLERA AND TYPHOID

Waterborne diseases and plagues are well known to history. But it was not until the 1850s that doctors and scientists began systematically to link diseases with contaminated water. In a now-famous case, an English doctor, John Snow, investigating a cholera outbreak in London in 1854, traced the epidemic to a well on Broad Street off Golden Square. He showed that people who got their water from the well became sick and died, while those who got their water elsewhere were largely unaffected. Once the Broad Street pump handle had been removed, thus cutting off the supply of contaminated water, the epidemic subsided. (See the Uses of Epidemiology, page 43.)

At about the same time, another English reformer, Edwin Chadwick, was campaigning for creation of local health boards to remove wastes and clean up the new industrial cities. Following

cholera outbreaks in 1832 and 1848, new sewers were laid in city after city in England. They were made of smooth ceramic pipe and built narrow enough so that a continuous flow of water could be maintained to flush sewage through the system.

Still, the sewage had to come out of the pipes somewhere. Usually it was into a lake or river, often with disastrous consequences. Only later, after scientists Louis Pasteur, Robert Koch, and others in the 1870s and 1880s had shown that many diseases were caused by minute microorganisms, did municipal authorities begin to build treatment plants to disinfect water and remove raw sewage. By the early twentieth century, most cities in the United States, Europe, and other advanced countries had or were building treatment facilities.

SOURCES OF POLLUTION

Pollutants enter water from a variety of sources (see table 12.1). Rainwater carries raw sewage along with human and animal feces from city streets, storm sewer overflows, or animal feedlots, as well as pesticides from farmer's fields. Industrial and chemical wastes buried in the ground leak out of their containers and collect in water. Phosphates from laundry detergents wash down the drain and eventually reach lakes and streams.

There are two types of water pollution. *Point sources* include wastes dumped into water by pipes, sewers, or other conduits from factories, sewage treatment plants, and waste and drainage disposal systems. Once identified, they are relatively easy to monitor and control. Because they are the most noticeable sources of water pollution, we have given point sources the greatest attention.

Nonpoint sources, on the other hand, are harder to pinpoint and have received less notice. They include the sewage, fecal matter, pesticides, fertilizers, and topsoil carried into streams and lakes by rainwater. Similarly, construction sites often leave bare ground, leading to erosion and pollution of nearby waterways. Septic tanks may deteriorate and leak contaminated water into the ground. Acids from abandoned mines may seep out and into water.

Quite recently, scientists have detected increasing acid levels in many lakes, particularly in the eastern part of the U.S. The acid comes from sulfur and nitrogen emissions of car and factory exhausts. The sulfur and nitrogen combine with oxygen, rise into the air, react with water vapor to become acids, and fall to earth with rain, known as "acid rain" (see chapter 11, Air Pollution). Acidic lakes may be incapable of supporting fish and other aquatic life.

Health Effects

Linking specific pollutants to human diseases is often difficult. Many sources of pollution are relatively recent, within the last twenty or thirty years. Many human cancers, like lung cancer, take that long to show symptoms. Therefore, if people were getting cancer from water pollution, they might not yet be showing the disease in measurable numbers. Additionally, water pollutants may not be great enough to cause a disease, but may combine with other sources of the same pollutant or different pollutants to bring about a cancer or other disease.

CHEMICAL POLLUTANTS

In some cases, however, specific illnesses have been traced to chemical water pollutants. In Japan in the late 1950s, for example, a fertilizer manufacturer dumped large quantities of mercury-containing wastes into Minimata Bay. The mercury settled, was picked up by bottom-dwelling organisms, and traveled up the food chain to fish, livestock, pets, and people. Hundreds and perhaps thousands of people were stricken with muscular paralysis, impaired vision, and/or mental retardation. Many died. All had eaten contaminated seafood. "Minimata disease" has since become a damning description of mercury poisoning.

In the 1960s and 1970s, Japanese living along the Jinzu River suffered excruciating bone disintegration caused by cadmium poisoning. Cadmium, a bluish metal used in electroplating, had seeped from mines and smelters upstream and settled in the soil and water along the river. Several hundred people got what is now called "Itai-Itai" disease. Cadmium occurs only in minute amounts in most U.S. waters. Its principal source is from discharges by the metallurgy, pesticide, electroplating, and photography industries. The most common source of cadmium in drinking water is from galvanized pipes and fixtures.

In the United States, doctors found serious trembling and other nervous system disorders among workers in a pesticide plant in Hopewell, Virginia in 1975. The plant made kepone, a deadly pesticide that causes neurological damage in humans and causes cancer in laboratory animals. Tests showed kepone had leaked from the plant and washed into the nearby James River, site of the famous Civil War battle between the ironclads Monitor and Merrimac. Because of its molecular structure, kepone resists breaking down into less lethal substances. In fact, it may persist in its toxic state for years or decades to come.

Table 12.1
PERCENTAGE OF WATER BASINS AFFECTED* BY TYPE OF POLLUTION PROBLEM

From point sources

Region (number of basins)	Thermal	Bacteria	Oxygen depletion	Nutrients	Suspended solids	Dissolved solids	pH	Oil and grease	Heavy metals	Nonmetal toxics
Northeast (40)	33	93	93	78	70	13	15	35	58	43
Southeast (47)	11	77	89	70	26	9	17	6	26	28
Great Lakes (41)	24	80	85	71	44	27	24	34	52	59
North Central (35)	11	89	80	74	23	20	14	0	57	23
South Central (30)	3	73	87	83	30	30	10	13	43	7
Southwest (22)	5	50	36	41	14	23	5	5	9	5
Northwest (22)	0	68	55	55	23	5	5	0	5	14
Islands (9)	33	89	78	56	33	11	0	44	22	11
Total (246)	15	78	79	69	35	17	14	16	38	28

From nonpoint sources

Region (number of basins)		Bacteria	Oxygen depletion	Nutrients	Suspended solids	Dissolved solids	pH	Oil and grease	Toxics	Pesticides
Northeast (40)	—	70	53	63	65	10	18	15	33	18
Southeast (47)	—	66	74	57	34	4	9	4	11	23
Great Lakes (41)	—	51	54	44	56	27	37	20	34	15
North Central (35)	—	69	66	83	80	51	20	0	51	37
South Central (30)	—	53	43	63	37	70	23	3	47	40
Southwest (22)	—	36	14	45	32	68	14	14	27	0
Northwest (22)	—	64	18	55	64	14	9	5	32	0
Islands (9)	—	89	44	44	100	0	0	0	22	44
Total (246)	—	61	51	56	54	30	18	9	32	22

* In whole or part.

SOURCE: Environmental Protection Agency, *National Water Quality Inventory.* EPA-440/4-78-001, October 1978.

Dredging the river may be difficult if not impossible because of the costs; dredging might also further disperse the kepone. The James River has been closed to fishing, disrupting the livelihoods of hundreds of people.

Another dangerous pollutant appearing in water across the country is polychlorinated biphenyl or PCB. Widely used for more than forty years in electrical capacitors, PCBs interfere with the body's immunological system and cause cancer in laboratory animals. Like kepone, PCBs resist breaking down. They have been found in human breast milk. Their discovery in the graceful Housatonic River, which flows through western Massachusetts and Connecticut, led the U.S. government to warn in 1976 that fish caught in the river were unfit to eat.

A recent study by the U.S. Environmental Protection Agency (EPA) linked high cancer rates in New Orleans with drinking water taken from the Mississippi River. Studies of other cities have found similar but less statistically significant results. While scientists cannot yet tie specific pollutants to particular cancers, EPA found in another survey that the water supplies of sixty-six U.S. cities contained small amounts of known or suspected cancer-causing agents.

MICROORGANISMS

If we cannot yet link chemical pollutants with specific cancers or other illnesses, we certainly can for waterborne microorganisms. In one of its undisputed triumphs, western civilization has eliminated devastating illnesses like cholera and typhoid as major causes of illness and death. These diseases, which still afflict people in less developed countries, are spread by water contaminated with organic pollutants, sewage, or fecal matter.

Today, 4,000 causes of waterborne illnesses strike Americans annually. They are caused by single-cell animals called protozoans, bacteria, viruses, or parasites that infest contaminated water. In particular, old or improperly maintained treatment facilities or sewer pipes can allow disease-causing microorganisms to invade the water we drink.

These diseases include *amoebic and shigella dysentery, schistosomiasis, giardiasis, hookworm, and salmonellosis* (see chapter 15, Infectious Diseases). All are common in warm regions with poor sanitation—open sewers, lack of running water, inadequate toilets, and lack of treatment facilities—and personal hygiene.

Almost unheard of in the United States and other countries with good sanitation, *amoebic dysentery* is prevalent in tropical countries, where more than half the inhabitants may have it at one time or another. Amoebic dysentery causes diarrhea, constipation, cramps, and, in more severe cases, soreness around the liver. Occasionally stools will contain mucus and blood. It is spread by touching hands with people who haven't washed their hands after using the bathroom or before handling food. When traveling abroad, one should heed public health instructions, boil drinking water if necessary, and avoid raw vegetables and meats.

Schistosomiasis is caused by a parasitic worm that infects the intestines and urinary tract of most mammals. You can get it by swimming in contaminated water. The worm enters the skin, travels through the blood first to the lungs and then to the liver, finally settling in the intestines. You may first notice a rash or itching around the site where the worm entered your body. Schistosomiasis can cause bleeding, chronic diarrhea, and tissue damage.

Schistosomiasis occurs only in the Caribbean, in Africa, in the Middle East, and in eastern Asia where certain snails are found to serve as intermediary hosts for the parasite. Avoid swimming in dirty waters when traveling in these areas.

While most common in countries with poor sanitation, *giardiasis* occurs in the United States where poorly disinfected water is used. It can be spread by touching the hands of an infected person. Although frequently causing no visible symptoms, giardiasis can produce severe diarrhea, stomach cramps and bloating, fatigue, and blood and weight loss. Your body may also fail to properly absorb fats and vitamins. Giardiasis can be prevented by adequate chlorination and filtering of our drinking water.

Several other diseases, including *hookworm, salmonellosis,* and *shigella dysentery,* are associated with poor sanitation and poor personal hygiene, although they are usually not transmitted directly by water. All three still occur in the United States, although they are more common in warmer regions. You can prevent them by washing your hands after using the bathroom and before and after handling food.

Preventive Measures
COMMUNITY

For years, we cleaned our municipal water by means of a maze of sewers leading to a primary treatment plant. In the treatment plant, water is filtered to remove the large, floating solids. In the next step, the smaller particles of sand, dirt, or other material settle to the bottom in large sedimentation tanks. Oxygen is then mixed into the water to kill bacteria and consume organic matter. Finally, chlorine is added to further kill the bacteria and make the water smell good.

This primary treatment, however, has been found to remove too little organic matter to restore the quality of our highly polluted waters. Many municipalities have now added secondary treatment to further purify the water. Following primary treatment, the water is passed through stone or other synthetic filters to remove additional solids. Next, bacteria-laden activated sludge is mixed with the water. The bacteria eat more organic matter, turning it into innocuous compounds that settle out of the water in sedimentation tanks. Finally, chlorine is once again added to the water to disinfect it.

Chlorine is the single most effective way to kill viruses in water. It has been used for more than sixty years in the United States. At very high doses, it can kill 99 percent of the viruses; the cost of such doses are high, however, and can kill aquatic life if the treated water is discharged directly into a lake or stream. Also, chlorine can mix with naturally occurring chemicals in water to produce chlorinated hydrocarbons which, in very large doses, cause cancer in laboratory animals. Thus, the chlorine content of treated waste water must be closely monitored, especially as it leaves the treatment plant.

Today, more advanced methods of treating water are being tested to handle the increasing amount and kinds of water pollution. Most methods rely on nonbiological processes. They can be adapted to primary or secondary treatment systems, and can be used in a series to achieve a desired level of waste treatment.

Coagulation, one such process, removes all suspended solids and more than 90 percent of the phosphates from water. Alum, lime, iron salts, and polyelectrolytes bunch particles together into larger masses that settle out of the water in basins. *Carbon absorption*, another advanced treatment method using activated charcoal, removes more then 98 percent of the dissolved organic matter and the taste- and odor-causing substances left by normal biological treatment. *Ozone*, a very active form of oxygen, is being tested as a replacement for chlorine.

Finally, *reverse osmosis, electrodialysis,* and *ion exchange* remove remaining dissolved solids from the water. In reverse osmosis, water is forced under pressure through a semipermeable membrane, leaving salts behind. Electrodialysis uses electric fields to get excess salts out of water. Ion exchange is absorption of undesirable electrically-charged atoms or molecules (ions) from the water onto plastic beads and replacement with harmless ions.

LEGISLATIVE CONTROL

Beginning in 1914, the U.S. government has set water quality standards to ensure that the water we drink is clean and free of disease-causing organisms. Acting out of concern over spreading cholera, typhoid, and dysentary, the government required cities to install filters in their water treatment plants to filter out bacteria. As a result typhoid and cholera have been almost eliminated in the United States. Whereas more than 35,000 people died of cholera in 1900, only 375 cases and no deaths were reported in 1975.

In 1962, the U.S. Public Health Service set standards for health-related chemical and biological pollutants and recommended standards for impurities causing color, taste, and odor changes in water. While these standards once applied only to drinking water on buses, trains, and airplanes, most states and large cities eventually adopted them.

Congress passed the first temporary water standards in 1948 and made them permanent in 1956. In 1965, a second act authorized water quality standards and a cleanup of all interstate and coastal waters. It also created the Federal Water Pollution Control Administration, EPA's predecessor.

In a major step, Congress created the Environmental Protection Agency (EPA) in 1970 and gave it authority to set and enforce drinking water standards. In the Federal Water Pollution Control Act of 1972, Congress declared water pollution to be undesirable and set 1983 as the target date by which all U.S. waterways should be clean enough for safe fishing and swimming. The act also provided funds for municipalities to build secondary treatment facilities and for industry to adopt the best practical technology to control discharges into waterways. By 1977, 40 percent of towns and cities and 80 percent of industrial dischargers had complied with the act.

To safeguard the water quality of the oceans, Congress passed the Marine Protection Research and Sanctuaries Act in 1972. It places strict limits on wastes that may be dumped into the oceans. This act responded to the call of an international conference in London in 1972 to control ocean pollution that posed a danger to human health or to our enjoyment of the oceans.

The Clean Water Act, first passed in 1972 and amended in 1977, made secondary waste treatment mandatory for all municipal waste water and placed controls on both point and nonpoint pollution. It gave the EPA power to protect wetlands (marshes, swamps, estuaries, tidal basins) from pollution.

Most important for our health, the Safe Drinking Water Act empowered the EPA to set national standards to protect the purity of our drinking water, including its underground sources. First passed in 1974 and amended in 1977, the act gave state governments primary responsibility for running drinking water programs. The EPA acts only if a state cannot or will not meet its responsibilities. As of July 1979, forty-one states had drinking water programs that met EPA minimum standards and another six were establishing such programs.

Under the act, EPA set interim national drinking water standards in 1977. The standards defined the maximum levels of pollutants that could be found in water used for drinking. While they deal with both organic and industrial pollutants, the latter are most important since this was the first time the government had set definite limits on them based on the health effects. For example, the EPA now allows no more than .05 milligrams of arsenic per liter of water. Arsenic, poisonous in large quantities, reaches water primarily from pesticides that run off agricultural land following a rainfall. Early symptoms of arsenic poisoning from polluted water include fatigue and loss of energy. The EPA standard for another mineral, cadmium, is .01 milligrams per liter of water.

One potential water pollutant is a chemical we add daily to water to protect our teeth from cavities—fluoride. In large amounts, it can cause brown spots to appear on the teeth of children under twelve. Adults can tolerate ten times more fluoride than young children. For fluoride, the standard is 2.4 milligrams per liter. The warmer the climate, however, the lower the standard since we drink more water in hot weather (see chapter 8, Dental Hygiene).

Selenium, a mineral that occurs naturally in soil and plants, causes some problems for the EPA's standards. It is found in some meats and other foods we eat, and it is believed to be es-

sential for proper diets (see chapter 1, Nutrition). Studies are underway to determine how much we need for good nutrition and the amount that might cause harm. In the meantime, the EPA has set a level of .01 milligrams per liter of water for selenium.

The EPA has also set limits on pesticide levels for drinking water. It would take a dose ten times greater than the maximum levels of each pesticide to cause harmful effects in people. The levels for some common pesticides are: endrin, .0002 milligrams per liter of water; lindane, .004 milligrams; methoxychlor, .1 milligrams; toxaphene, .005 milligrams; 2,4-D, .1 milligrams; 2,4,5-TP silvex, .01 milligrams.

Finally, under the Toxic Substances Control Act, the EPA regulates the disposal of toxic wastes created in manufacturing processes. The EPA is concerned that toxic substances could leak out of their containers and pollute water sources, as has happened in the Love Canal area of New York and elsewhere. Under the Resource Conservation and Recovery Act of 1976, the EPA controls hazardous wastes from where they are generated to where they are disposed of. The goal is elimination of all open dumps, upgraded waste disposal, and development of ways to manage solid wastes that are environmentally safe.

INDIVIDUAL MEASURES

Practice good personal hygiene. Wash your hands with soap and water every time you use the bathroom and before and after handling raw meats, vegetables, eggs, and other foods. Dispose of your garbage and sewage properly. Have your wells, cisterns, and septic tanks inspected regularly, including having water samples checked by health authorities.

As a concerned citizen, you can get involved in how your local, state, and federal governments maintain your water supplies. Learn who supplies your water, what sources it comes from, how it is treated, and how it is tested for safety. Let your officials know you are concerned about the health effects of polluted water and that you insist on clean water that is safe to use.

The quality of water depends on more than how it is treated—it is far easier and cheaper to prevent pollution than to clean it up later. Get involved in how your local and state governments set land use policies, regulate building codes, locate treatment facilities, decide where to dispose of wastes, and control sources of nonpoint pollution.

Resources

AGENCY/ORGANIZATION

PUBLICATION

U.S. Council on Environmental Quality
722 Jackson Place, N.W.
Washington, D.C. 20006

Report: "Environmental
Quality (1979)"

Environmental Protection Agency
401 M Street, S.W.
Washington, D.C. 20460

"Highlights of the Safe
Drinking Water Act of 1974";

"National Water Quality
Inventory: 1977 Report to Congress";

"What Everyone Should
Know about the Quality
of Drinking Water";

"Resources for the Future:
Carcinogenic Hazards
of Organic Chemicals
in Drinking Water"

AGENCY/ORGANIZATION	PUBLICATION
National Academy of Sciences/ National Research Council 2101 Constitution Avenue, N.W. Washington, D.C. 20418	"Drinking Water and Health" (both technical and summary reports available)
National Wildlife Federation 1412 Sixteenth St., N.W. Washington, D.C. 20036	"The Conservation Directory" (lists organizations, federal and state agencies, and officials concerned with natural resource use and management)

CHAPTER
13

Radiation

"It is the dose that makes a poison," Paracelsus stated some four centuries ago. The positive medical uses of ionizing radiation are well known but, in excess, radiation is detrimental to health.

Radiation can induce cancer and harm our reproductive systems. While nuclear energy as a source of electrical power is regarded by many as a necessary tool for survival, it is also a potential source of danger. And while most people perceive the tanned sunbather as the "picture of health," heavy exposure to the ultraviolet rays contributes to the aging process and to the risk of skin cancer.

With all the technological knowledge at hand, it should be possible for an informed society to harness radiation for the benefit of humankind without having to endure its harmful effects.

Glossary

ANGIOGRAPHY   X ray of the blood vessels for diagnostic purposes: A solution opaque to X rays is injected into arteries or veins revealing their ability to carry the blood where it is needed.

CHAIN REACTION   The splitting of uranium atoms whereby they emit neutrons that split other atoms in a continuing process. When the number of neutrons emitted is sufficient to keep this chain reaction going, a reactor is said to have reached criticality, thus releasing usable energy in the form of heat.

CURIE   The quantity of radiation produced by one gram of radium in one second. Used to denote the power of a source of radioactivity but not its effects, which depend on both duration and distance of exposure.

GONADS   The sex glands, ovaries in females, testes (testicles) in males.

ION   Chemically active atoms or groups of atoms with one or more normally present electrons absent or one or more in excess.

IONIZING RADIATION   A form of radiation powerful enough to knock electrons off atoms or molecules. Ions are thus formed which, in turn, may create harmful compounds in the body that can interfere with the normal working of cells.

ISOTOPE   Different forms of a single element having the same number of protons (positively charged particles) in the nucleus (and hence the same number of electrons, which are negatively charged particles) but differing in the number of neutrons in the nucleus. Unstable isotopes are said to decay when they emit radiation or particles. The half-life of an isotope, which may vary from seconds to centuries, is the time it takes for half of the remaining energy of decay to be emitted.

MAMMOGRAPHY   Diagnostic examination of the breast by X ray.

MELTDOWN   The worst disaster that can happen in a nuclear energy plant, second only in its effects to a nuclear weapon explosion. If the radioactive material in the core of a reactor is no longer jacketed by the cooling water that keeps its temperature under control, the core uranium rods melt into a radioactive mass that can sink deep into the ground, resulting in a massive release of radiation.

MICROWAVES   Short, nonionizing radio waves emitted by radar, TV transmitters, telephone relay systems, and microwave ovens, among other sources.

MELANIN   The pigment found in skin cells giving the epidermis a darker hue.

MUTATION   Any change, for better or for worse, in the DNA of the genes of cells that is passed along to their progeny, especially such changes in germ cells (reproductive cells such as sperm or ova) that will change the characteristics of succeeding generations.

NONIONIZING RADIATION   Radiation less powerful than ionizing radiation but which can harm cells by breaking chemical bonds. Example: microwaves, ultraviolet radiation.

PERMISSIBLE DOSE   The amount of radiation to which sensitive body tissues may be safely exposed over given periods of time. The National Council on Radiation Protection and Measurements recommends that cumulative exposure not exceed 5 rems multiplied by number of years over age eighteen for workers in jobs that expose them to ionizing radiation. The NCRPM recommends no more than 10 percent of such exposure for the general public.

(However, it must be remembered that no amount of radiation exposure can be considered totally innocuous. The developing fetus in the uterus is most sensitive, and there is still scientific debate as to just where the risk of cancer later in life begins to increase. Exposure to 100 rems over a short period produces changes in the blood and bone marrow in a small percentage of people; at 200 rems most will show such changes and a few will die. See definitions of Rad and Rem.)

RADIATION   Energy propagated through space or matter in the form of waves or particles.

RADIOACTIVITY   The emission of radiation due to the spontaneous rearrangement of the nucleus of an atom.

RADIOLOGY   The use of radiant energy in the diagnosis and treatment of disease.

RAD   The delivery of a given quantity of energy (100 ergs) to a given quantity of living tissue (one gram). This measure of radiation exposure, however, does not allow for the mass of the irradiating particles and the greater damage produced, for example, by protons. (A millirad is one thousandth of a rad.)

REM   This unit allows for the greater or lesser biological damage produced by various types of ionizing radiation. For purposes of this chapter and the exposures involved in nuclear power incidents, a rem is the dose equivalent of a rad. But for exposure to protons, neutrons, or alpha particles (two protons plus two neutrons, i.e., a nucleus of helium) one rad would produce dose equivalents of multiple rems. (A millirem is one thousandth of a rem.)

ROENTGEN   Amount of radiation producing a standard number of ions in a given volume of air. Named for Wilhelm Roentgen (1845–1923), discoverer of the X ray.

X RAY   High energy electromagnetic wave produced by bombarding a target in a vacuum tube with high velocity electrons. Used in diagnosis and in therapy because of its ability to penetrate solid matter and to act on photographic film.

History and Definitions

Radiation, the process whereby energy is propagated through space or matter in the form of waves, is not the creation of the twentieth century scientific curiosity. It has permeated the universe since the dawn of time. Natural radiation accounts for more than half the radiation exposure we receive. Radioactive particles and rays from the sun bombard the earth constantly. The earth itself subjects us to radiation from widely distributed materials—granite, natural gas, phosphates. Even our own bodies contain minute traces of radioactive elements (table 13.1).

There is little we can do about natural radiation. However, artificial, or man-made, radiation presents the human race with a fateful choice between great good and cataclysmic evil. Radiation has occupied a special role in the public consciousness in recent years due to the destructive potential of nuclear war and the potential risks in nuclear generation of power.

Table 13.1
SOURCES OF RADIATION
IN THE UNITED STATES

Sources	Average Dose Received (in millirem per year)
Environmental	
Natural	102
Global fallout	4
Nuclear power	0.003
Subtotal	106
Medical	
Diagnostic	72
Therapeutic	1
Subtotal	73
Occupational	0.8
Miscellaneous	2
Total	182

SOURCE: Jean St. Germain, M.S., Memorial Sloan-Kettering Cancer Center, New York, New York.

ELECTROMAGNETIC SPECTRUM

One system for organizing the various types of radiation is by their energy and wavelength. These properties are inversely related: the longer the wavelengths the less the energy; the shorter the wavelengths the greater the energy. All these radiations form the electromagnetic spectrum. They possess both electric and magnetic fields and are capable of transferring energy from one place to another (figure 13.1).

A wide variety of waves, each with differing characteristics, are found on the electromagnetic spectrum, including radio waves which oscillate at relatively low frequencies and travel over long distances. Faster oscillating waves appear as light visible to the human eye. Invisible, but powerful X and gamma rays occur at even higher frequencies.

All these forms of electromagnetic radiation are closely related and can often be converted from one form to another. Where conversion is practicable, a vital condition must be satisfied: the total amount of energy in the system must remain constant, a principle known as conservation of energy. The other basic principle, which was the foundation of nineteenth century physics, is the conservation of mass. These principles are still acceptable today with one important addition. Early in this century, Albert Einstein postulated his famous equation, $E = mc^2$ — energy equals mass multiplied by the speed of light squared. This equation says that it is possible to convert mass into energy and vice versa. Thirty years later, Lord Rutherford at Cambridge University verified the equation experimentally by performing an "atom-splitting" experiment.

Heat, one of the simplest forms of energy, is often produced as a by-product of energy conversions and is manifested as the random motion of the atoms or molecules of the heated object. The more rapid these motions, the higher the temperature. Since energy must always be conserved, the cooling of a heated material can only be achieved if the heat energy generated in a conversion process can be transferred to another place, or converted into another form. This transfer can be made by conduction, convection, or radiation. In the radiative process, rapid movement of atoms or molecules is converted into infrared radiation that travels out through space in all directions. The cooling rate obviously depends upon the differences in temperature between the hot object and its surroundings.

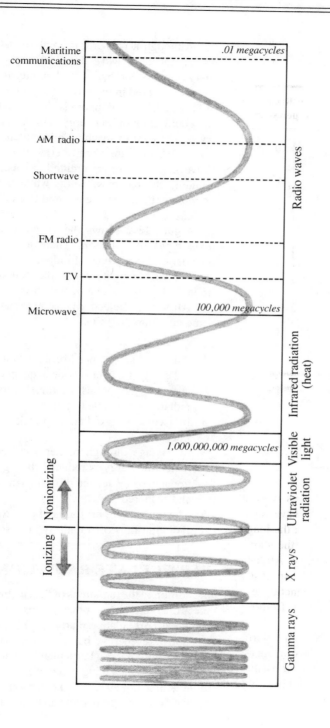

FIGURE 13.1

Variety of waves of the electromagnetic spectrum
SOURCE: Science 80

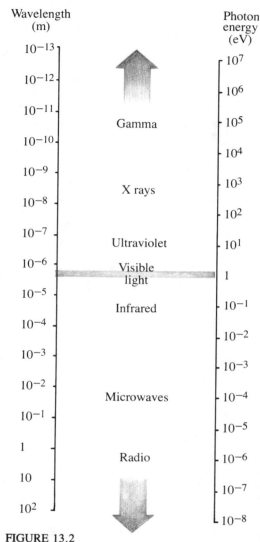

FIGURE 13.2

Wavelengths and photon energy of the electromagnetic spectrum
SOURCE: *American Health Foundation*

Although it is useful to think of radiation as waves, the term *wave* does not imply that the energy flow is continuous and uninterrupted. Energy is delivered in the form of separate packages of energy known as photons. To visualize this, one could think of an energy stream as the delivery of a stream of machine gun bullets. Gamma rays and X rays are often referred to as photons. However, the latter are emitted by electrons surrounding the nuclei of atoms while the former, more potent photons are emitted from the atomic nucleus itself.

Figure 13.2 shows the wavelengths of the main types of radiation. There are no precise boundaries for any type of radiation except in the case of visible light, where the boundaries are limited only by the eye of the observer.

All forms of electromagnetic radiation share some common properties:

1. All travel at the speed of light in a vacuum.
2. All energy transfer is done in quanta, or packages, of energy, which for electromagnetic radiations are called photons.
3. In free space, radiation travels in straight lines.
4. In passage through matter, the intensity of radiation energy is reduced through absorption and some deflected from its original path and scattered.
5. The intensity of all forms of electromagnetic radiation falls off rapidly with distance.

PARTICULATE RADIATION

In addition to the radiations of the electromagnetic spectrum, there are other forms of radiation known as particulate radiations. These radiations are not pure energy, but have some matter associated with them. Particulate radiations arise from interactions taking place within the nucleus of the atom. In 1897, J. J. Thompson discovered a negatively charged particle that was smaller than any atom and called it the electron. This discovery destroyed the view previously held that atoms were indivisible. Lord Rutherford and Niels Bohr postulated the existence of an atomic nucleus in 1911 and constructed the solar system model of the atom. In this model, the nucleus is the sun and most of the atom's mass is concentrated in the nucleus. The electrons, which are negatively charged, circle the central nucleus in orbits. Thus the large amount of empty space in the atom helps explain why radiation is able to pass unchanged through apparently solid matter.

Because the positive charge in the nucleus exactly balances the negative charge of its orbiting electrons, a normal atom is electrically neutral. Removal of an electron from an orbit upsets the balance, and the resulting particle will have an excess of positive charge. It has become a positive ion, carrying an electric charge.

If the displaced electron becomes attached to another atom, that particle now has an excess negative electric charge and is called a negative ion. Both positive and negative ions have a strong tendency to resume their electrically neutral status and, as a result, become chemically activated in living systems. Thus the production of ions by one of the effects of radiation can modify living cells, often injuriously.

In a process similar to the emission of X-radiation by the electrons around an atomic nucleus, an unstable nucleus itself can give off radiation as it decays to a more stable form. Instead of emitting X rays, a nucleus can give off either alpha particles, high-energy electrons called beta particles, or gamma rays, which are high energy electromagnetic radiation. (See Rem in glossary.)

The rate at which a radioactive material emits radiation diminishes with time as it decays to form a different isotope. Radioactive atoms decay at different rates, with half-lives varying from seconds to thousands of years. These rates of decay, or half-lives, are unique for each radioactive isotope of each element. (See Isotope in glossary.)

Sources and Health Effects of Radiation

NONIONIZING RADIATION

Nonionizing radiation, that part of the electromagnetic spectrum consisting of relatively low-frequency waves, includes radio waves, microwaves, infrared radiation, visible light, and ultraviolet radiation. All of these nonionizing radiations can heat by causing molecular vibrations within cells. Diathermy devices use radio waves to heat tissue and are now being employed experimentally in cancer treatment. At the other end of the nonionizing spectrum, painful sunburn is produced by the ultraviolet rays of the sun.

Ultraviolet radiation

Skin damage Almost all the energy of the invisible but biologically active ultraviolet radiation is absorbed in the skin. It is the most widespread form of radiation, and is hard to avoid.

All neutral ultraviolet radiation comes from the sun. As these rays enter the atmosphere, they are scattered and partially absorbed by air molecules, water droplets, and dust. Since the angle of the sun varies with time of day and the season, the distance that these rays have to pass through the atmosphere also varies. *Two-thirds of the biologically active ultraviolet light reaches us between 10 A.M. and 2 P.M.*; and, because there is less atmosphere between us and the sun, more ultraviolet light reaches us on high ground than at sea level. Furthermore, *about half of the ultraviolet radiation is so widely scattered that it comes from all directions, so that hats or umbrellas only reduce the radiation intensity by half at most.* Sand, snow, and ice are effective reflectors for this radiation. Water transmits most of it. Thus, it is possible to get a sunburn on a hazy or cloudy day in summer when infrared radiation is minimal, and the time spent swimming in a pool or in the ocean must be counted as nearly full exposure to ultraviolet in sunny weather.

Ultraviolet radiation causes relaxation (dilation) of the tiny blood vessels in the skin, which is what causes the redness of sunburn. Some skin cells are killed by the rays with the result that remaining skin cells start dividing rapidly to replace them. The repair process causes thickening of the outer, horny layer of skin, and blistering results when fluid from the dilated blood vessels leaks out under these layers.

With repeated injury, the inner layer of the skin, the connective tissue, is altered, resulting in thinning of the skin, formation of wrinkles, appearance of permanent freckles ("old age spots") and permanent dilation of superficial blood vessels—in other words, all the skin changes we call "aging." In some people with sensitive skin, precancerous lesions and skin cancers may appear after years of repeated ultraviolet insult.

Skin cancer Not everyone responds alike to the burning effect of ultraviolet radiation. The Celts (Irish, Scots, Welsh) and all others who freckle and burn easily are more likely to develop precancerous lesions and skin cancer after years of ultraviolet exposure than dark-skinned, deeply pigmented persons, because melanin, the skin pigment, protects the skin by absorbing ultraviolet light. In Australia, for example, the white-skinned European population is particularly susceptible to skin cancer, whereas the dark-skinned native population has virtually none.

The incidence of skin cancer, the most common malignant tumor of white-skinned people, has doubled in the U.S. since the 1960s. Each year there are about 300,000 new cases and 5,000 deaths due to nonmelanoma skin cancer, a relatively curable type of cancer. (There are 12,000 new cases of malignant melanoma, a much more lethal skin tumor, each year, with about 5,000 deaths.) In 1973, the National Academy of Sciences estimated that no less than 40 percent of the melanomas and 80 percent of the skin cancers in whites living at 40 degrees latitude (Philadelphia–Indianapolis–Denver–Red Bluff, Calif.) are caused by ultraviolet light. Nonmelanoma skin cancer is almost entirely caused by chronic exposure to solar ultraviolet radiation, and malignant melanoma is strongly related to it, as shown by the fact that melanoma mortality rates are about 75 percent higher in the southernmost states than in the northern ones. Where there is an increased rate, the cancer originates most frequently in areas of the body exposed to the sun.

Protecting the skin against ultraviolet radiation A tan, whether obtained painfully after a sunburn or gradually, is a response to injury to the skin and thus in the long run *is not good for the skin.*

The naive idea that sun-browned skin is a sign of health is based on the reversal of an old status symbol. In the courts of Europe in the seventeenth century and in the U.S. until early in this century, it was desirable to have pale skin. This signified that one was affluent enough to work indoors (or not to work at all). Now that most of us work indoors in artificially lighted offices and factories, a tan has become a symbol of leisure and affluence.

The beneficial effects—vitamin D production, pleasant "tense" feeling of the skin, and the satisfaction of a "beautiful tan"—are outweighed by the certain and cumulative damage, the excessive and premature wrinkling, thinning of the skin, and permanent cosmetic defects.

Here are some rules for protection against the acute damage of sunburn:

1. Take advantage of the sun's motion by minimizing exposure between 10 A.M. and 2 P.M. standard time. In bright sunlight it takes about fifteen minutes, on the average, for untanned skin to acquire a faint pink blush. Slight "touchiness" develops three to five hours later. One hour of exposure of untanned skin can result in a painful, flaming burn. Therefore, begin exposure gradually in early morning or late afternoon.

2. Increase exposure gradually—by fifteen minutes the first few days, and once the tan develops, by thirty minutes per day. *Count time in the water as exposure.*

3. Bear in mind that beach umbrellas and thin garments let ultraviolet radiation pass. A wet cotton T-shirt allows 20 to 30 percent of ultraviolet radiation to pass, and so do nylon stockings.

4. Use a good sunscreen. Apply it liberally; remember ears, back of neck, behind the knees, the instep. All sunscreens eventually wash or wear off. Put on the preparation as soon as you are out in the sun and repeat after every swim and frequently if perspiring actively. The best preparations contain either para-amino benzoic acid (PABA) or benzophenones or are white and opaque (zinc oxide paste). Most important: repeat applications of sunscreens often, particularly the first few days. Too much won't hurt, but too little will. Cocoa butter, baby oil, iodine, and similar preparations soften the skin and keep it from drying out, but they are not effective sunscreens.

5. The nose, top of ears, lower lip, and the top of the chest get the most radiation in the upright position (i.e., skiing, golfing, tennis playing, etc.). Protect them particularly well.

6. If you are redheaded or freckle easily or tan poorly, don't try to get a deep, even tan. The odds are your skin will never tan this way, for genetic reasons. All you will do is burn and burn. Use sunscreens liberally and frequently.

Follow these rules for avoiding long-term damage of chronic ultraviolet radiation exposure:

1. Don't let yourself get burned.
2. If you burn easily, are of Celtic background, or freckle easily, carry on your outdoor activities in the early morning or late afternoon.
3. If you wear makeup out-of-doors, use a good sunscreen as a makeup base, and apply it down to the neck below the ears and jaw and over the "V" of the neck, i.e., the area exposed by an open blouse or shirt. Do this any time of the year, but particularly in the summer or in the South. Wear gloves.
4. If you are past fifty, have your doctor check your skin once a year for sunlight-induced skin changes. Premalignant skin lesions can now be removed painlessly and without scarring, and much common skin cancer can be kept from developing.

By following these rules you can still be safe and attractive and enjoy the outdoors.

Eye damage The eye, particularly its cornea, is more vulnerable than the rest of the body to ultraviolet radiation, so special precautions are in order for anyone working under ultraviolet light or using the beam for tanning. After an eye exposure, complaints such as burning or itching should be treated by a physician. It is easy to protect the eye from ultraviolet radiation by means of glasses or goggles that selectively filter out the ultraviolet wavelengths.

Sunlamps Sunlamps for tanning emit ultraviolet radiation and must therefore be handled with utmost care. Hospitals treat thousands of sunlamp-related injuries annually, most of them skin burns and eye irritations. Many of these are the result of falling asleep while a sunlamp is on.

The U.S. Food and Drug Administration has drawn up a set of protective standards for all sunlamps manufactured after May 9, 1980. Every sunlamp must be equipped with a timer that automatically shuts it off within ten minutes or less. There must also be multiple timer settings adequate for the manufacturer's recommended exposure intervals for different distances specified on the label. A manual switch must also be provided.

Protective goggles must be provided for the maximum number of persons recommended by the manufacturer who can safely use the lamp at any one time. The label must also specify the recommended minimum distance and give directions for measuring this distance. Products covered by this regulation include sunlamps used in homes, tanning clinics, gyms, health clubs, and spas.

As with natural sunlight, overexposure can cause eye injury and sunburn; repeated exposure may cause premature aging of the skin and skin cancer. Medications and cosmetics applied to the skin may increase sensitivity to ultraviolet light. Consult your physician before using a sunlamp if you are taking any medication, or if you believe you are especially sensitive to sunlight.

Because of the germicidal properties of ultraviolet radiation, lamps have been used in specific areas in various industries to reduce germs in the environment. The safety systems of such installations must be inspected periodically to prevent accidental overexposure of industrial personnel working in the "germ-free" area. Those who work in such areas should be familiar with these systems and their fail-safe operation.

Laser beams

Ultraviolet radiation should not be confused with the much newer surgical and research tool, the laser, an acronym for Light Amplification by Stimulated Emission of Radiation. The energy concentrated in the narrow laser beam can burn through living tissue as if it were paper. Because the beam, unlike ultraviolet rays, is visible, prevention of injury is exceedingly simple. When in a laboratory or other area where a laser is in use, keep away from it and obey the warnings of those in charge of the device.

Microwave radiation

Microwaves are very short radio waves. (See figure 13.1.) They are emitted by radar, orbiting satellites, TV transmitters, telephone relay systems, burglar alarms, citizen's band radios, and diathermy units used to treat arthritis, bursitis, congested sinuses, and muscle and joint ailments.

Little is known about the subtle effects of microwaves on humans, but, as microwave ovens daily demonstrate, the concentrated energy of this form of radiation rapidly heats animal tissues. Studies show that exposure of the eye to intense microwave radiation results in opacities and, possibly, cataracts. However, a military survey of personnel operating a radar installation showed them not to have a higher rate of opacities than the general population.

Temporary or permanent sterility was reported as an effect of microwave radiation exposure in studies of radar personnel in the South Pacific in World War II. The effect was found to be due to heat damage to the testes of men who had worked around the intense microwave fields.

There is increasing concern that low-level exposure to microwaves may not be innocuous as was previously believed. There is a difference of opinion between U.S. experts and those of some Eastern European countries as to the permissible maximum level of microwave exposure. The Eastern European standard is stricter than that of the U.S. Survey programs have been conducted in the USSR and Poland of all workers in microwave installations. U.S. monitoring programs have not substantiated the European reports of ill effects.

Lawsuits have been instigated over radiation damage to workers in telecommunications installations. There has also been concern regarding exposure to the general public from television transmissions antennas on high buildings. Uniform exposure levels were found in the ten largest U.S. cities that were monitored by the Environmental Protection Agency. Exposure problems were found in buildings with a direct line of sight to these antennas.

Microwave ovens The safe operation of microwave ovens requires a number of precautions.

If the door interlock system, which turns off the current when the door is opened, is not properly adjusted, the nonionizing radiation can leak out. Ovens can be brought to dealers, service organizations, and some federal, state, and local programs to be tested for leakage while in operation. A leakage standard of 5 microwatts/cm² at 5 centimeters from the oven surface was established by the U.S. Food and Drug Administration for the lifetime of ovens manufactured after October 6, 1971.

The following safety precautions are recommended by the FDA:

- Follow manufacturer's directions.
- Make sure oven was not damaged in shipping.
- Have the oven serviced regularly by qualified technicians for signs of damage, wear, or tampering.

- Don't tamper with or inactivate the door interlock.
- Don't try to pry the door open with a screwdriver or other wedge around the seal.
- Don't operate the oven when it is empty.
- Clean the oven with water and a mild detergent. Don't use abrasives.
- If the oven was manufactured before the October, 1971 standard was in force, turn the oven off before opening the door and stay at least two feet away from the oven while it is on.

IONIZING RADIATION

The term *ionizing radiation* is used to describe high-energy packets and particles given off by the electrons or nuclei of atoms either spontaneously or with the stimulation of other particles or high-voltage electricity. Ionizing radiation encompasses X rays, gamma rays, and particulate radiations (see Curie, Isotope, Rad, Rem in Glossary).

Biological effects of ionizing radiation

As with chemical poisons, the effects of ionizing radiation on living things can be either acute, occurring in a matter of minutes or hours, or chronic, appearing only after days, weeks, and in some cases, years.

These effects can also be separated into those that affect the reproductive (or germ) cells and thus genetically affect the offspring of the injured animal or human, and those that affect the somatic cells such as the blood cells produced in the bone marrow, the skin, and the cells lining the digestive tract. When younger men and women are treated with high-energy radiation for cancer, radiotherapists take special precautions to shield their sex organs from the beam so that normal reproductive capacity can be preserved. This is because all ionizing radiation can cause aberrations in the molecules making up the chromosomes carrying our genes from one generation to the next. The deoxyribonucleic acid (DNA) making up the genes is considered a critical target for radiation, and the damage produced in DNA is believed to account for the emergence of cancer years later in persons exposed to critical doses of ionizing radiation.

Such high-energy radiation beams can also do harm to the cytoplasm of cells, the "jelly" surrounding the nucleus, where the chemical instructions of the DNA are carried out. When the sequence of chemical groups in the DNA is rearranged, either spontaneously or as a result of ionizing radiation, the resulting change is passed along to the progeny of the cells in question. When the cells involved are germ or reproductive cells, the change inherited by future generations of that organism is called a mutation. While the generally accepted explanation for the evolution of species depends upon such mutations, with those favorable to survival leading to new, enduring species and those unfavorable leading to extinction, it is also widely accepted that most mutations will turn out unfavorably. Since no one knows precisely how much radiation is needed to produce changes in somatic cells that can (in the case of bone marrow cells) lead to leukemia many years later, or in germ cells that can lead to mutations, (birth defects) in the ensuing generation, there are no absolute limits on tolerable doses of radiation. By and large, however, the less exposure the better.

Thus, since we are constantly exposed to some so-called background radiation from the sun and from terrestrial minerals without evident damage, the government has extrapolated evidence from such exposures (as well as from the atom bombed populations of the Japanese, ura-

nium miners, and other occupationally or inadvertently exposed populations such as physicians using X rays before the hazards of such exposure were fully understood) to place limits on "safe" exposure in terms of the rems of radiation we can safely tolerate over our lifetimes or shorter parts thereof.

Nuclear energy

Despite the fact that well over 99 percent of the general population have and will have received most of their ionizing radiation in the form of diagnostic or therapeutic X rays, concern over radiation today centers on the operation of nuclear power plants that produce steam from the heat of nuclear reactions and on the disposal of the wastes from such facilities. The March 28, 1979 incident involving the Three-Mile Island Nuclear Power Station in Pennsylvania has become a symbol for the fear and distrust of the public confronted with what was widely reported as the nearest miss to that date of an atomic core melt-down. Inept release of information by the operator of the facility, Metropolitan Edison, and confusion in the early reports of officials of the U.S. Nuclear Regulatory Commission (NRC) who went to the site, left many people convinced that serious exposure to radioactivity was suffered by many persons and animals within a fifty-mile radius of the Susquehanna River reactors in Dauphin County. Such was not the case, however, according to meticulous research conducted during and after the accident by the NRC and the Environmental Protection Agency (EPA).

The greatest danger to be anticipated in another such episode would be panic on the part of the public which could lead to accidents on clogged highways, fires in deserted structures, and looting and violence in suddenly deserted towns and cities. The Three-Mile Island episode alerted both the NRC and public officials to the need for better planning for evacuation of areas surrounding nuclear power stations and, for dissemination of information promptly in such a fashion as to merit public trust.

The release of information about radioactive emissions from nuclear power plants is complicated and rendered difficult precisely because of the public's fears of unknown, mysterious, and invisible radioactive particles in water courses and in the air they breathe. The NRC has reported that no excess radioactivity was released into the Susquehanna River during the 1979 episode or in the twenty months subsequent to the episode. The agency has also reported that for the year 1977 total release of radioactive materials into the Hudson River from the two nuclear reactors at Indian Point in Westchester County, N.Y., amounted to three curies in 112 million liters of waste water discharge. For purposes of comparison, the single reactor operating at Three-Mile Island in 1977 was responsible for the release of 0.19 curies of radioactivity into the Susquehanna in 3,410,000 liters of waste water.

As for the airborne plume from the Pennsylvania accident, it contained no surprising elements. The two major constituents, both fission products of uranium, were the radioactive isotope of iodine, I-131, and two radioactive isotopes of the chemically inert gas, xenon, Xe-135 and Xe-133. Fortunately, the isotopes of iodine and xenon have very brief half-lives, eight days in the case of I-131 and 5.3 days and nine hours in the cases of Xe-133 and Xe-135.

Measurements of exposure to radiation by persons living or working near Three-Mile Island were calculated by NRC and EPA from monitors, devices sensitive to both beta and gamma radiation required to be positioned by utilities operating nuclear plants at various distances from one-tenth of a mile to fifteen miles from the reactors. The monitoring devices can record exposures as low as one millirem and had been in place in Pennsylvania since December of the year preceding the March 28 accident. (In addition to the ground monitors, helicopters equipped with comparable devices flew through the plume soon after the radioactive releases from the plant.)

Wind direction obviously plays a role in exposing persons on the ground to the plume of radioactive particles and gases in a nuclear accident. In the Three-Mile Island accident, winds during the releases came predominantly from the southeast, the southwest, and the northwest, with the result that monitors northwest, northeast, and southeast of the site gave the highest readings.

Calculations by NRC and EPA scientists (aided by colleagues from the U.S. Food and Drug Administration and the Center for Disease Control) showed that the maximum cumulative exposure for a person remaining out-of-doors for the full period (March 29 to April 6) would have amounted to less than one-tenth of a rem, more precisely about 83 millirem. Since clothing protects against the beta component of the radiation as does shelter, most persons in the area received far less than this dosage. The investigators calculated that a man who spent ten hours on an island a little over a mile northwest of the plant during the period of maximum exposure received 37 millirem.

For comparative purposes, the most radiation-sensitive animal fetuses tested do not show developmental defects or stillbirths until exposed to about five rem (5,000 millirem) in the womb. And the normal "background" radiation exposure of residents of Dauphin County is estimated at 115 to 125 millirem per year.

In general, the inert (noble) gases such as xenon and krypton that might be released in a nuclear accident at the atomic power plant are the least worrisome since they are chemically inactive and are not taken up into body cells (though they do provide some lung radiation through inhalation). On the other hand, iodine-131 is taken up and concentrated by the thyroid gland and could be ingested by drinking milk from cows that have been grazing in pasture subjected to fallout. The most troublesome fission products are the isotopes of strontium and cesium since they are taken up into the bones. Air filters at nuclear power plants are specially designed to catch these particles, and the investigators at Three-Mile Island found no evidence that any had escaped into the air in the 1979 episode.

The best advice, then, during any real or potential nuclear accident would be:

1. Listen to the radio for news of the seriousness of the accident.
2. Remain indoors during periods of fallout and wear full clothing when you must go outdoors.
3. Don't eat plant or animal products derived from land under the fallout plume.
4. Don't panic, pack up, and leave. Wait for instructions.

Disposal of nuclear waste

In the U.S. there are at the moment only three burial sites for the disposal of radioactive waste. The states containing these sites have voiced their opposition to the receipt of wastes from all the other states. This opposition became particularly acute when the sites were closed for a short time in the fall of 1979. The problem of radioactive waste disposal is complicated by the fact that the sources of such wastes include military and industrial uses of radioactive materials as well as biological and medical uses of radioactive materials. The volume of waste generated from biomedical sources is approximately the same as that from industry. The radioactive materials contained in the biomedical wastes, however, are less toxic and shorter lived than wastes generated by nuclear facilities.

Nuclear weapon development

In the 1940s the Manhattan Project, under the direction of Dr. Robert Oppenheimer and Dr. Enrico Fermi, attempted to sustain the first chain reaction by splitting the uranium atom and releasing the tremendous energy of this process. This reaction required the construction of a nuclear reactor. The first one was built at the University of Chicago. The energy release of this first experiment was highly successful. The Manhattan Project produced the material that was used in the creation of the first atom bombs dropped on Hiroshima and Nagasaki, Japan in August 1945.

Subsequently, the U.S. and the Soviet Union engaged in atmospheric testing of nuclear weapons. These tests exposed native populations of the Pacific atolls as well as populations within the "worldwide" fallout belt in the Northern Hemisphere that corresponded with 45 degrees latitude and included a number of cities in the U.S. A series of sampling stations were established to monitor the fallout contamination of foodstuffs such as milk and drinking supplies. This network is still in existence. The test ban treaty between the U.S. and the USSR has eliminated atmospheric testing; although underground testing continues, and a number of other nations that are not signatories to this treaty have conducted atmospheric blasts. Over 1,000 nuclear devices are known to have been exploded since the Manhattan Project.

Following an aboveground blast, a certain amount of radioactive debris known as fallout is released into the stratosphere, the upper portion of the atmosphere. This debris is swept along the upper currents and is deposited at points along its path. Rain tends to bring down much of the material. Material that stays aloft for at least one or more transits of the earth will deposit less radioactivity since the shorter-lived isotopes will have decayed out by that time. Concern about fallout has focused on the radioactive materials, iodine-131 (I-131) and strontium-90 (Sr-90).

These two isotopes can be concentrated in milk and, because of this, they are likely to be absorbed by children who are more radiosensitive than adults.

The problems of disposal of radioactive nuclear waste generated by humans, from all sources—weapons testing, power plants, and biological and medical uses—have not been solved.

Armament policy—nuclear and otherwise—and energy policy—nuclear and otherwise—are issues of basic public policy beyond the province of medicine as medicine. However, the effects of radiation on health are the special concern of health professionals, and from this standpoint, the watchword must be the less radiation, the better.

Uranium mining

Uranium mines, located principally in the western states, supply the raw uranium for weapons production and for nuclear reactor fuel. They have employed large numbers of men over several decades. *The incidence of lung cancer among uranium miners is substantially higher than normal. For miners who smoke, this rate is more than four times as high.*

The cause of the increase is assumed to be the concentration of radon gas and related products in the mines, which represent a small but highly radioactive fraction found in uranium ore, particularly pitchblende. Standards for exposure in these mines are based on measured radon concentrations and have been gradually lowered. Minimum ventilation requirements have been established. Some critics maintain that these standards are inadequately enforced due to the shortage of federal inspectors.

Another potential hazard is presented by uranium mill tailings, the waste products of the mining operations. During the 1950s and early 1960s, large mounds of tailings accumulated near what may now be closed mines. These mounds have never been disposed of by the government. In fact, some of these tailings have been used by construction companies in the construction of homes and public buildings. Because of the restricted ventilation in such places, large quantities of radon gas can accumulate. In at least one instance, a public building had to be closed until more ventilation was supplied. The problem in private dwellings is still unsolved. The government has been severely criticized for the lax security around these dumps and for allowing such misuse to take place.

Cancer and ionizing radiation

Possibly no other effect of radiation on humans has received as much attention as radiation-induced cancer. Yet only a small part of cancer deaths in the U.S. can be blamed on radiation, 3 percent at most. Since at least half of all radiation is natural background radiation, we can do little about it.

Sufficient radiation delivered to any part of the body will increase the probability of cancer: skin cancers among radiologists and dermatologists, lung cancer among uranium miners, leukemia in those exposed to nuclear bomb blasts and fallout. Patients injected with a contrast medium called thorotrast, containing salts of the radioactive element thorium, used in diagnostic X rays between 1930 and 1950 had an increased risk for liver and bone cancer.

Leukemia is the most widely studied form of radiation-induced cancer. In the study of A-bomb survivors, an excess incidence of leukemia in the Japanese population appeared within two years after irradiation by bombing, and peaked between three and five years later. Persons within a mile of ground zero had significantly more leukemia. Surveys of this population have also suggested that there is an increased incidence of breast and thyroid cancer as well, indicating the particular sensitivity of these organs to ionizing radiation.

A second study covered a group of patients in the United Kingdom treated with X rays for an arthritic condition of the spine. Doses varied widely, but the areas treated were confined to limited parts of the body. These patients exhibited an increased incidence of leukemia at a risk of about 0.7 cases per million persons per rad per year. Persons exhibiting this risk received doses in the range of 300 to 2,000 rad.

In the 1940s it was reported that radiologists who regularly worked with X ray machines were ten times more likely to die of leukemia than were other physicians. A later study shows that the incidence of leukemia among radiologists has decreased. However, there appears to be an increase in incidence of melanoma (see Ultraviolet Radiation, page 527) among these radiation specialists.

Pregnancy and ionizing radiation

The greatest radiation exposure to pregnant women appears to be from medical X rays. Radiation has its greatest effects on rapidly multiplying cells. Since rapid cell replication is characteristic of the fetus, it is particularly radiosensitive. The radiosensitivity of the fetus is most acute during the first three months of pregnancy and decreases slightly thereafter, although some risks remain throughout pregnancy.

Sometimes a woman may not know she is pregnant at the time the X ray examination is conducted. It is the position of the American College of Radiology and the American College of Obstetrics and Gynecology that a therapeutic abortion is never justified solely on the basis of a radiologic diagnostic examination. If a woman is pregnant or thinks she may be, she should alert the technologist and the physician before the examination. It may be possible to modify the way in which the examination is done or it may be possible to postpone the examination until the question of pregnancy is clarified.

A heavy exposure of the conceptus to radiation during the period from conception to implantation (0–10 days) can result in the conceptus not implanting. This is unlikely to be noticed by the woman and will be followed by the conceptus being aborted during her next menstrual period. In any case, half of all conceptions result in spontaneous abortions without any known cause and these often occur before pregnancy is even suspected. Experimental results indicate that there may be a threshold of 10 rads for prenatal death.

During the implantation period, from 10–14 days after conception, the embryo is much more resistant to lethal effects of radiation. There is some risk of malformation, however. The level of risk during this period has been estimated as one case in 2,000 per rad.

During the period of major organ formation, abnormalities can be produced. This period extends from 14 to 50 days after conception, which would correspond to a period of 29–64 days since the onset of the last menses. There should be no problem in establishing pregnancy by the end of this time.

In studies on siblings it has been found that when the mother underwent X ray examination of the pelvic region to chart safe progress of her pregnancy, her child had a significantly greater risk of leukemia than babies who had not been irradiated in utero. As a result, the use of diagnostic ultrasound (nonionizing sound waves whose "echo" limns the fetus on a screen) for pelvimetry has replaced X rays for many pregnant women.

It is obvious that all radiation exposure during pregnancy should be avoided if at all possible (see chapter 6, Family Planning and Childbearing). If this is not feasible, then the upper limit of 0.5 rem recommended by the National Council on Radiation Protection and Measurements should be followed.

Medical and dental exposure

The U.S. Public Health Service has estimated that more than 200 million medical and dental X ray films were taken in the U.S. in 1970. These examinations and X ray therapy account for most non-natural radiation. In other words, the most promising way to reduce the total radiation exposure to the population is to reduce the X rays used in dentistry and medicine to the minimum, an effort that, according to the National Academy of Sciences, "must involve careful consideration of the balance between radiation benefits and risks."

Diagnostic radiology

X rays The discoverer of the X ray was a German physicist, Wilhelm Konrad Roentgen, who was working with unknown rays in his laboratory in 1895; he named them X rays. The first radiograph was a picture of the bones in his wife's hand taken that same year. Marie Curie, working in Paris in the same period, discovered the radioactive elements polonium and radium. The latter was found to emit a green light easily visible at night, and this property made it a novelty item.

Initially, radium was thought to be harmless, and radium salts were advocated for arthritis and other rheumatic ailments. However, many of the early radiation workers died of radiation injury. Because of the type of X ray film available in the early part of this century, radiologists held bare X ray tubes next to patients being radiographed for periods as long as fifteen minutes. Many of the radiologists developed radiation dermatitis or skin cancer from these exposures. It was also discovered that radium or its emanations could attack tumors, and one of the first uses of this new element was in cancer therapy.

X rays are indispensable as a medical diagnostic tool. Certain types of surgery cannot be considered without the use of one or more diagnostic X ray examinations. The benefit to mankind in the treatment of disease revealed by diagnostic X rays is immeasurable; however, this benefit does carry some risks. The doses from various types of X ray examinations differ and the repetitions of certain examinations is frequently unnecessary. The radiation doses to be expected from typical X ray examinations are summarized in tables 13.2 and 13.3.

In 1964 and 1970, the U.S. Public Health Service surveyed the population to determine the types of diagnostic examinations conducted, the number of films per examination, and the estimates of the dose delivered. Dose was expressed as the genetically significant dose (GSD), meaning the dose delivered to the gonads within the lifetime in both males and females. The data showed that the GSD decreased in the period between the two surveys. This was attributed at least in part to widespread programs of physician education aimed at dose reduction conducted in the intervening period by federal and professional agencies. The surveys demonstrated that simple adjustment of the diagnostic machine such as proper alignment or restricting the X ray beam to the size of the film were often not being performed properly. The educational programs sought to correct this problem, too.

In addition to educational programs, Congress gave the Food and Drug Administration the power to regulate the manufacturing of X ray equipment. As a result of these regulations, put into force in August 1974, all new equipment has to meet certain additional safety standards of operation.

However, by 1980, legislation had yet to be enacted that would require minimum federal standards for the education and training of radio-

Table 13.2
AVERAGE DOSES TO THE GONADS FROM
TYPICAL DIAGNOSTIC X RAY EXAMINATIONS

Type of Examination	Dose (mrad) male	Dose (mrad) female
Low gonad dose		
Head	less than 10	less than 10
Chest	" " 10	" " 10
Foot, hand	" " 10	" " 10
Arm (including forearm)	" " 10	" " 10
Moderate gonad dose		
Gallbladder series	5	150
Femur (thigh bone), lower two-thirds	400	5
Upper GI (gastrointestinal)	30	150
High gonad dose		
Lumbar spine	1,000	400
Pelvis	700	250
Urography (urinary tract)	1,200	700
Lower GI (gastrointestinal)	2,000	1,500
Pelvimetry (measuring pelvis to determine whether childbirth will be normal)	—	1,200 (1,000 fetal)

SOURCE: Jean St. Germain, M.S., Memorial Sloan-Kettering Cancer Center, New York, New York.

Table 13.3

AVERAGE* DOSES TO THE BODY FROM
TYPICAL DIAGNOSTIC X RAY EXAMINATIONS

Type of Examination	Dose (mrad) male	Dose (mrad) female
Low body dose:		
Chest	10	10
Hip	20	10
Shoulder	20	40
Moderate body dose:		
Pelvis	40	15
Skull	50	30
Cholecystogram	100	40
High body dose:		
Thoracic spine	180	315
Ribs	150	270
Lumbar spine	180	90
Upper gastrointestinal	230	150
Barium enema	250	135
Mammography	—	450

*average dose based on estimated average beam quality, organs exposed and the exposure level for each, frequency of examination, and sensitivity of exposed organs (by sex) to radiation carcinogenesis. Due to increasing concern about dosage exposure, these levels are being steadily reduced. For instance, in mammography, dosages as low as 200 mrad are possible with proper equipment.

SOURCE: data adapted from Seymour Jablon, and John C. Bailar, III. "The contribution of ionizing radiation to cancer mortality in the United States." *Preventive Medicine* 9, 219–226, 1980.

logical technologists. Several states now require them to undergo a formal two-year training program.

The American College of Radiology regularly conducts programs to educate physicians on the risks from diagnostic procedures and the methods by which they can be minimized.

Mammography Mammography is a relatively new and important way to detect early breast cancer, but it, too, has risks. Studies of A-bomb survivors demonstrate that the young female breast may be more prone to breast cancer due to irradiation than the older female breast. Therefore the dose delivered in mammography should be kept as low as possible. Table 13.4 gives the National Cancer Institute's current guidelines for screening. In making their recommendations, the NCI panel emphasized "the distinction between mammography used for diagnosis—the value of which was not in question—and mammographic screening to detect possible disease in women with no symptoms or other physical findings."

Special types of vacuum film packs are available that substantially reduce the dose to the skin from mammography films. Personnel can be specially trained to further reduce the dose.

Dental X rays Dental X rays also expose the patient to ionizing radiation. They should be employed only when special symptoms make X ray diagnosis necessary. It is no longer generally accepted that the annual taking of radiographs of the teeth is necessary without special reason.

Dental X rays are generally taken in the dentist's office, and therefore precautions against the effects of the radiation must be taken by the technician for himself as well as for the patient. The patient's body is covered with a lead apron to prevent the X rays from penetrating. The tech-

Table 13.4
CURRENT RECOMMENDATIONS
REGARDING MAMMOGRAPHY

1. Only in asymptomatic women, 50 years of age or older, should mammography examination be given as part of a routine screening process.
2. In asymptomatic women, 40–49 years of age, mammography should not be used for screening unless:

   There is a personal history of breast cancer *or* a history of breast cancer in the screenee's immediate family (mother/sisters).
3. Women 35–39 years of age should be given mammography only if they have a personal history of breast cancer.

SOURCE: National Cancer Institute, "Screening Guidelines for Breast Cancer Detection Demonstration Project" (BCDDP).

nician usually stands behind a lead door or shield while throwing a switch to take the picture. In order to expedite dental X rays with a minimum of hazard to all parties concerned, government recommendations include the use of the fastest film and shortest exposure time. For the patient, radiographs should be made of the entire set of teeth according to the patient's needs and age. A record of the patient's radiation history should be kept and special attention should be given to the patient who has radiographs at one office after another.(See table 13.5).

The operator should have a medical examination before employment and be checked annually by a physician experienced in radiation effects. The maximum permissible dose should not be exceeded. When a protective shield is not available, the operator should be positioned at least six feet from the patient at right angles to the beam or behind the machine. The operator should not hold the film during exposure or touch the tube or cone on the X ray machine during exposure. The X ray equipment and film should comply with government standards.

Table 13.5
RECORD CARD OF X RAY EXAMINATIONS

DATE	TYPE OF EXAM	REFERRING PHYSICIAN	ADDRESS WHERE X RAYS ARE KEPT

Radiation Therapy The number of patients treated by radiation therapy is fewer than 1 percent of the number of patients who will have some sort of diagnostic X ray examination during any given year.

The use of radioactive materials to treat tumors is nearly as old as the discovery of radiation itself. Early treatments involved inserting the radioactive material into a body cavity or into a space between tissues for set periods of time. Radium is still used in many institutions, though it is gradually being replaced by other radioactive materials such as cesium-137, iridium-192, and iodine-125. These substances emit radiations that are lower in energy than those emitted by radium and can be handled with less exposure by medical personnel.

The more familiar use of radiation therapy is teletherapy, in which the source of radiation is at some distance from the patient. The first widely available unit used cobalt-60 as the irradiating material. These machines are still in use, but others, known as accelerators, have been developed for this purpose. These devices use strong electric fields to produce high-energy rays. They have been installed in most major treatment centers in the U.S.

Radiation therapy does have some side effects, both transitory and long lasting. Patients should discuss any fears about radiation with their doctors. In many cases, these fears may be unjustified. As an example, some patients fear that as a result of this type of treatment, they will transmit some of the radiation that they receive to their family. This is not true, but unspoken fears can only contribute to the disease problem.

Nuclear medicine Nuclear medicine uses radioactive materials for both diagnosis and treatment. A nuclear medicine physician may be an internist, endocrinologist, or radiologist.

In nuclear medicine, radioisotopes are used to label nonradioactive compounds so that they are tracked as they move through the body by the radiation emitted at the spot where the radioisotope is concentrated.

One of the earliest compounds tagged with a radioactive label was sodium iodide (NaI), which was known to have a strong affinity for the thyroid gland. The nonradioactive iodine atom is replaced with a radioactive iodine atom, typically iodine-131 (I-131). The patient is given the labeled compound, and it is taken up by the thyroid. At some later time, typically twenty-four hours, a sensitive radiation detector is placed over the thyroid gland to detect how much of the administered activity has been absorbed by the thyroid and how the activity is distributed in the gland. The test tells if all or part of the thyroid is functioning normally. By using larger amounts of radioactive iodine, thyroid tumors can be selectively destroyed. Newer radioactive materials deliver a much smaller dose to the patient, among them a radioisotope known as technetium-99m (Tc-99m), which is used to detect cancer in the body. Iodine-131, however, is still used in treatment of thyroid cancer, hyperthyroidism, and Grave's disease (goiter accompanied by bulging eyeballs).

Because a nuclear medicine procedure may involve the injection of the compound containing the radioactive material, there is a possibility that the patient will retain some of it for some time afterward. Women who are breast-feeding and are to undergo such procedures should determine whether there are any specific precautions. Some, not all, radioisotopes may concentrate in breast milk, and this could be taken up by the child's thyroid, which is more radio-sensitive than the adult's. If there is any question, ask the nuclear medicine physician before the examination is conducted.

Precautions for medical and dental X rays

1. Ask your physician how the X ray will help with the diagnosis. You have a right to know why an X ray is suggested.
2. Tell your physician if you are, or might be, pregnant. Your doctor should know of even a possible pregnancy when considering an X ray for you.
3. Ask if a gonad shield can be used, if you or your children are to have X rays of the lower back or abdomen. A lead shield over the sex organs can keep X rays from reaching your reproductive cells. Remember, a shield cannot be used at all times, since it may cover an area that the doctor needs to see on the X ray.
4. Keep an X ray record card. A sample card is shown in table 13.5. Free cards are available from:
   Food and Drug Administration (HFX-28) Rockville, Maryland
   When an X ray is taken, have the date, type of exam, and where the X ray is kept filled in on the card. If other doctors suggest an X ray of the same part of the body, tell them about the previous X rays. Also, if a new X ray is needed, the previous one might help show any change in your medical problem.
5. Don't insist on an X ray. Sometimes doctors give in to people who ask for X rays even if they are not medically needed.

RESOURCES

Federal Agencies

Food and Drug Administration (FDA) Bureau of Radiological Health 5600 Fishers Lane Rockville, MD 20852	Regulation of consumer products, X ray equipment, lasers, microwave devices. Large variety of educational materials available free by mail.

Also at FDA:

Office of Consumer Inquiries

Occupational Safety and Health Administration (OSHA) (Dept. of Labor) (has ten regional offices in Atlanta, Boston, Chicago, Dallas, Denver, Kansas City, New York, Philadelphia, San Francisco, and Seattle)	Regulates occupational transport of radioactive materials across state lines.
Environmental Protection Agency (EPA) 401 M Street, S.W. Washington D.C., 20460 (has ten regional offices in same cities as OSHA)	Provides technical assistance to towns, states, and agencies having radiation protection programs; has a national surveillance and inspection program for measuring radiation levels in the environment.

Voluntary Organizations

National Council on Radiation Protection and Measurements 7910 Woodmont Avenue Bethesda, M.D. 20014	Develops standards; issues reports on specific topics.
Public Citizen, Inc. Health Research Group 2000 P Street, N.W. Washington, D.C. 20036	Citizen's interest group. Publishes consumer guide.
Nat'l. Academy of Sciences/ Nat'l. Research Council 2101 Constitution Avenue, N.W. Washington, D.C. 20036	Issues reports on research priorities, recommendations on standards for exposure of public in reports.

CHAPTER
14

Noise

While we all appreciate the silence and tranquility of a quiet countryside, science has only now begun to measure the unhealthful effects of a noisy environment upon the human mind and body. The advent of rock music played through powerful amplifiers has confirmed what industrial health workers had long suspected: chronic exposure to loud noise damages hearing acuity and may pose other health dangers as well.

Thanks to our industrial progress and to our increasingly urban population, and thanks to jet aircraft, subways, larger trucks, and the din of construction, noise has indeed become part of modern life.

While we can accurately measure hearing loss, we have not yet been able to assess the damage to health done by the stress of sudden, earsplitting noises. Nor can we easily measure the effects of chronic inability to concentrate or to sleep soundly, caused by the insistent racket of today's environment.

Noise is as much a pollutant of our homes and working places as are any of the chemicals we read about in the daily newspaper. Far greater efforts than are now being made will be required to control it.

Glossary

DECIBELS Fourteen Bels (named after Alexander Graham Bell) represent the human intensity range of hearing. Each Bel is divided by ten into decibels that are calculated logarithmically. An increase of ten decibels (dB) represents a tenfold increase in acoustic energy but is perceived by the human ear as a doubling of loudness.

DIFFRACTION Bending of sound.

FREQUENCY The rate of occurrence of an air particle's displacement back and forth about its resting position—expressed in Hertz (Hz).

HERTZ One Hertz (Hz) is one complete cycle of movement back and forth about an air particle's resting position.

INTENSITY The extent or amplitude of a particle's displacement away from its resting position—expressed in decibels (dB).

PITCH The perception of sound on a scale of high to low musical tonality.

REVERBERATION Multiple reflection of sound.

History and Definitions

FROM SOUND TO NOISE

Throughout history noise has exerted powerful influences on people, both good and bad. It has been used to frighten, to inspire, and to entertain. One belief held that the devil was allergic to noise; hence church bells, bells on ships, the clinking together of glasses, and the general hullabaloo associated with weddings were intended to drive away evil forces. Noise was always strongly associated with praising the deity too. There are many references to loud sounds of praise in the Psalms. Psalm 33, verse 3 says, "Sing unto him a new song; play skillfully with a loud noise."

Little is known about how noise was regarded in the Middle Ages, or what its health effects might have been, beyond the superstitions about its effects on evil forces. Noise played a role among soldiers as rallying and battle cries to hearten themselves and frighten the enemy, but it was not until the invention of gunpowder and powerful explosives that hearing problems became associated with military action.

With the industrial revolution and advanced forms of mechanization, noise became increasingly recognized as an occupational health hazard. Ironworkers have repeatedly been cited as particularly vulnerable, and boilermaking probably ranks as the favorite high-risk skill among twentieth century observers dealing with occupational hearing loss. The term *boilermaker's ear* came to apply to such loss of hearing and, as early as 1713, Remazzini noted in *DeMorbis Artificum* that men engaged in the hammering of copper "Have their ears so injured by the perpetual dinn... that workers of this class become hard of hearing and, if they grow old at this work, completely deaf." Perhaps the earliest recorded public constraint on making noise is one attributed to Julius Caesar, who tried to ban daytime chariot racing because of the clatter of hooves and wheels on the uneven paving stones of the streets of Rome.

Noise pollution has now become so widespread that its adverse effects on health and the quality of life have become a major public concern. Environmentalists and various scientific professions have become vitally interested in reversing its unhealthy effects. The professions of audiology and otology are providing new approaches to noise abatement. They see noise as a threat not only to hearing but also to the maintenance of the other basic communicative functions—voice, language, and speech—and to the quality of life.

THE NATURE OF SOUND

Sound is a minute disturbance of the particles of air or any other substance that surrounds or touches a vibrating object. These tiny changes in normal atmospheric pressure occur at very rapid rates and quickly progress through the air in all directions from the source. They move outward in alternating waves of compression and expansion until they strike against something where they can be absorbed or reflected, depending on the resistance of what is struck. If what is struck is a living creature's healthy ear, this organ will pick up the vibrations and convert them into patterns of nerve impulses that are transmitted to the brain, where they will be perceived as sounds that are unique to the specific patterns of the original vibrations.

The three most important physical elements of a sound wave are (1) frequency, the rate of occurrence of an air particle's displacement back and forth about its resting position; (2) intensity, the extent or amplitude of a particle's displacement away from its resting position; and (3) time, the length and variation of sound patterns over time.

Frequency and Pitch

One complete cycle of movement back and forth about an air particle's resting position is called one Hertz (abbreviated Hz). The number of Hertz or cycles per second is called the frequency of sound, and it is the physical quality that gives rise to the psychological sensation of pitch. Pitch is the word for the way we perceive a sound on a scale of high to low musical tonality. If the frequency of a sound is exactly doubled, say from 220 to 440 cycles per second, the pitch will be perceived as going up exactly one octave on the musical scale (from A below middle C on the piano to A above middle C).

The total frequency range to which the normal young healthy human ear is responsive extends from a low of 16 Hz. to a maximum high frequency of about 20,000 Hz. The important frequencies of speech lie within a reduced range from about 300 to 3,000 Hz., and their most critical range for comprehension extends from 500 to 2,000 Hz.

Intensity and Loudness

The amount of force exerted on the vibrating particles of air by a sound source determines the extent of their displacement from positions of rest. Measurements of this factor, in terms of sound pressure changes above existing atmospheric pressure, provides a convenient way of describing sound intensity. This physical stimulus gives rise to the sensation of loudness which is the psychological manifestation of intensity. The louder the sensation, the greater the amount of sound pressure required to achieve it.

Within the 16 Hz.–20,000 Hz. range lie all of the sounds that are audible to humans, including all those known to be hazardous to health. Sounds must be capable of being heard in order

Sound levels in decibels (dB) are calculated on a logarithmic basis. An increase of 10 decibels represents a 10-fold increase in acoustic energy while an increase of 20 decibels corresponds to a 100-fold increase in acoustic energy.

However, the human ear also works logarithmically. Hence, our perception of the noise increase (loudness) works in such a way that each 10 dB increase in sound level is perceived as approximately a doubling of loudness. The noise produced by a heavy truck (90 decibels), for example, seems twice as loud as an alarm clock (80 decibels), but four times as loud as freeway traffic (70 decibels).

The weighted A scale approximates the frequency response of the human ear by placing most emphasis on the frequency range of 1000 to 6000 Hertz. Sound levels measured using A-weighting are often expressed as dBA. The chart below shows how sound interferes with speech.

Noise level

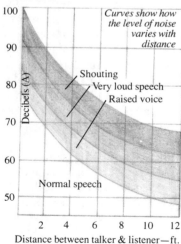

Distance between talker & listener—ft.

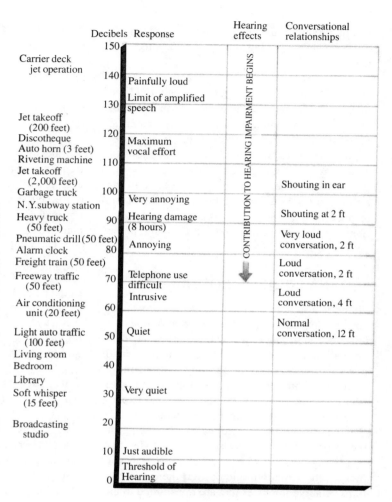

FIGURE 14.1

Sound levels and human response
SOURCE: *Environmental Protection Agency*

to be damaging. The range of sound pressure from the loudest sound that can be tolerated by the normal human ear down to the weakest that can be detected is a scale of more than ten million to one.

The growth of intensity is described by a notation system that compresses the enormous range of audible sound intensities into a much more convenient scale. Each successive unit represents a point that has ten times more energy than the preceding point. Each unit is called a Bel in honor of Alexander Graham Bell, the inventor of the telephone and great teacher of the deaf. The human range of hearing encompasses an intensity scale of 14 Bels, with each Bel divided by ten into decibels, abbreviated dB (see figure 14.1).

Time and Duration

Time is the physical aspect of a sound that gives rise to the sensation of duration. Sounds can be steady over time, unvarying in frequency and intensity, or they can be continuous, while fluctuating rapidly or slowly in frequency and/or intensity. Sounds that are discontinuous may also be fluctuating or nonfluctuating when they are present, and they may be intermittent regularly or irregularly.

Sound is classified as impulse or impact noise when it lasts for less than one second and is characterized by a sudden rise in power, often to an unmeasurably high peak followed by a rapid decay. Time is an important ingredient along with frequency and intensity when considering the effects of noise on hearing because it is the length of exposure to intense sounds that ultimately determines the extent and severity of permanent noise-induced hearing impairment.

THE SENSE OF HEARING

Hearing lets us acquire and maintain language and enables us to express it in speech. Persons who are born deaf or become so at an early age cannot acquire language skills without extraordinary educational measures. Even hearing impairment sustained after language and speech are learned can result in imprecise production of speech due to the altered ways in which the deafened persons hear their own spech.

The complete hearing mechanism consists of the interaction of many different parts. The process begins with the two separate ears. Each acts as a microphone or filter of extraordinary sensitivity to variations in sound pressure in the surrounding air. When functioning properly, each is capable of sensing sounds ranging from the gentlest footsteps of a gnat to the gigantic thrust of a rocket engine. Together they provide us with our natural stereophonic acoustic image of the world of sound that surrounds us.

The hearing mechanism's nerve cells are highly specialized cells responsive to touch. Their very sensitive endings are located in the inner ear section or cochlea, so-called because it is coiled in the manner of a cockle or snail shell. (See figure 14.2).

The two-and-a-half tiny turns of this bone-encapsulated space contain up to sixteen thousand individual hearing receptor cells. They are called hair cells because of the microscopic hairlike projections extending from the ends of each one into the endolymph—the fluid that bathes them all.

When a sound wave in the air strikes the eardrum, the membrane vibrates causing the three small bones (ossicles) of the middle ear to move. The movements of the innermost bone actuate the inner ear fluids (perilymph and endolymph) which, in turn, cause movements of the basilar membrane in the cochlea on which the hair cells are located. This makes the hairs bend, causing

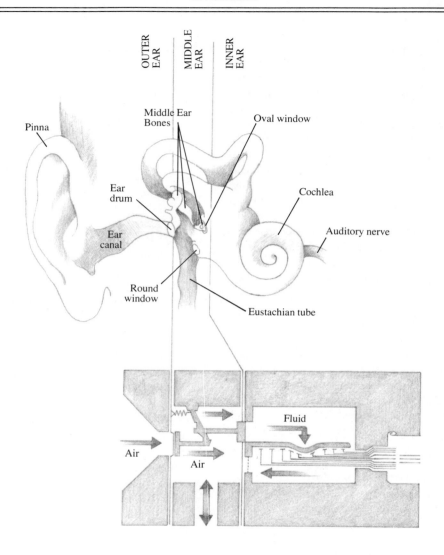

FIGURE 14.2

Functional diagram of the ear.
Sound waves impinge on outer ear and cause ear drum to vibrate. Vibrations are conducted via lever action of middle-ear bones (ossicles) to oval window, which actuates fluid-filled inner ear. Inner ear portion shows cross section of unrolled cochlea with nerve endings distributed along basilar membrane of cochlea. Frequency-selective excitation initiates nerve impulses which are carried via discrete fibers of the auditory nerve to the brain.
SOURCE: *Adapted from Cyril Harris,* Handbook of Noise Control, *2d ed., (New York: McGraw-Hill, 1979)*

the individual cells to become activated according to the patterns of movement.

Each hair cell is especially sensitive to a particular sound frequency. Altogether, their range of sensitivity is from 16 Hz. through 20,000 Hz. As a back-up system, a few adjacent hair cells are sensitive to the same frequency. Also, each cell interconnects with a number of adjacent ones. This assures that a signal will get through if possible even though some cells may be too fatigued to respond at a given moment or may have been destroyed.

This precautionary interconnection makes it possible for us to tolerate a certain amount of exposure to damaging noise levels. Depending on the severity of each exposure, most of the cells recover, but a few are probably lost forever. The more intense the sound and the longer the exposure time, the greater the number of hair cells destroyed during each exposure.

The two ears are connected to the brain by a complex system of interrelated nerve tracts. Beginning in the cochlea of each ear, the thousands of tiny nerve endings are precisely organized according to frequency sensitivity. Each hair cell extends from its location in the cochlea via its elongated cell body directly to the brain stem. As they leave the cochlea, these cell bodies, or nerve fibers, twist together into bundles that form the auditory branch which, together with the vestibular branch from the balance receptors, comprise the eighth cranial nerve. These two nerve trunks enter directly into the brainstem, one from each ear. Most of the fibers of each nerve trunk cross over to the opposite side of the brain stem and rise through its several sections up through the midbrain to the auditory cortex in the temporal lobe of the cerebrum, where the signal patterns they transmit are perceived as sound.

Language and Speech Development

Speech is made up of patterns of sound. It is the most important signal we hear. We acquire the ability to speak by hearing the speech of those around us from the time of birth. Slowly and laboriously we learn that these utterances have meaning, and we finally organize them into systematic patterns that ultimately become our native language.

Speech is our primary form of language usage and appears only after our language acquisition process has progressed considerably, normally by the age of two. Language acquisition seems to reach its peak and begins to taper off at about four-and-a-half years of age. Thus, the longer it is put off, the more difficult acquiring a second language becomes. Reading and writing usually come long after speech development is well under way. It is a simple and profoundly important fact that the hearing is the foundation for normal acquisition and development of language and speech. Hearing health should be of primary concern from birth onward.

Health Effects

PRENATAL

A baby's ear is well developed at birth, having been so for some time in the womb. Since the speed of sound is greater in water than in air, there is no natural barrier to the transmission of the mother's bodily noises and vibrations to the fetus. Her voice, breathing, digestive functions, heartbeat, and pulse sounds are very familiar to the baby.

The fluidborne sounds reaching the fetus in utero probably arise for the most part from within

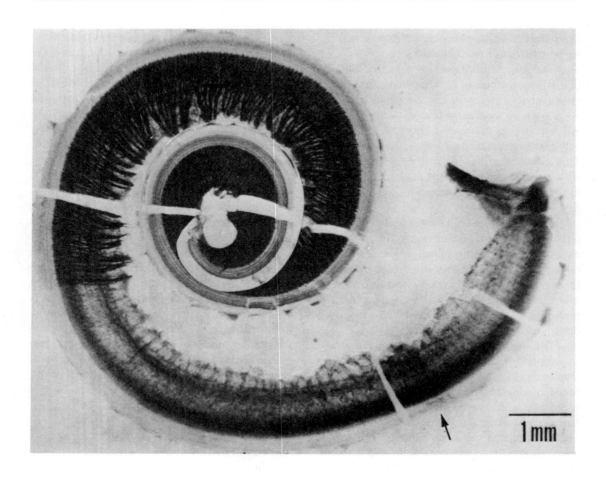

FIGURE 14.3

Organ of Corti.
Surface preparation of the organ of Corti from a human cochlea that has been
exposed to damaging noise. The darkly stained radials (hair-like projections)
are nerve fibers leading from the hair cells. The fibers in the lower turn have
been destroyed by the noise.
SOURCE: *David M. Lipscomb, ed.,* Noise and Audiology. *(Baltimore: University Park Press,*
1978)

the mother's body. But very intense external airborne sounds can set the mother's body into sympathetic vibration and would, of course, be transmitted to the fetus in the same manner as maternally generated sounds. Fetal heart rate changes occur in response to loud noises in the mother's environment, and late in pregnancy the fetus will respond with bodily movements like kicking.

Studies of babies born of women living near large airports show a remarkable and predominant effect of the noise levels present there: low birth weight. This is probably due to the constricting effect of the noise on the mother's circulatory system and the consequent reduction of oxygen and nutrients to the fetus.

There is some evidence that birth abnormalities like cleft lip, cleft palate, and spinal defects have also been linked to the noise around airports. The most critical period for fetal damage from such causes is very early during pregnancy—from about fourteen to sixty days following conception. During this time, important developments are taking place in vital organs, anatomical structures, and the central nervous system. Often, women are not aware of their pregnancy until well into this period and will not have taken any extra precautions.

It is difficult to say at what level noise becomes dangerous to pregnant women, but any level that creates extreme stress in the mother should definitely be avoided.

EARLY CHILDHOOD

Young children have often been observed sleeping blissfully through most noise levels. Except under conditions of profound exhaustion and sickness, deep sleep appears to be related to serenity. Whereas young adults will be awakened from deep sleep by a steady noise of from 50 to 55 decibels, young children and infants will require an average of 65 decibels.

During waking hours, however, noise in the home can have adverse effects on language and speech acquisition. Noise can interfere with attention and distort speech models so that imitation of speech sounds becomes imprecise. The louder the noise levels are in a child's surroundings, the louder, but shorter, are the child's speech responses.

Such noise also promotes unvocal behavior in general. Consistent relationships have been shown between the psychological development of infants aged seven to twenty-two months and a noisy household that interferes with the opportunity to hear vocal signs or words for specific objects, actions, and relationships. The excessively loud noise levels and variations in input are generally negatively related, whereas the opportunity to hear words being spoken in conjunction with what they mean has a positive effect. Thus, a noisy, overcrowded slum would overwhelm casual conversation, and speech models would be degraded. It has been suggested that the adverse effects of slum rearing on psychological development may lie in stimulus bombardment of the child rather than in stimulus deprivation. In any case, excessive noise may be a factor in the almost universally observed language deficiencies of disadvantaged children.

In young school children, negative effects on speech sound discrimination and reading abilities are produced by traffic noises. Poorer reading scores correlate with longer residence in such noisy environments. A study comparing reading scores of children in classrooms next to a noisy and busy elevated rapid transit line with the scores of those in classrooms on the quieter, opposite side of the building showed significantly poorer scores among the former. The study was repeated after the installation of quieting materials on the elevated lines and in the classrooms, and the reading score differences disappeared.

Children who live in noisy homes and play in noisy areas may never have the chance to develop the ability to listen well enough to become good pupils once they get to school. If the school is also noisy, the effects are still worse. Children with even mild hearing impairments can be at such a disadvantage in even moderately noisy situations that they will always be behind in language and speech skills without special help.

School hearing screening tests may not identify all such children for a variety of reasons: the fluctuation of hearing sensitivity in and out of the normal range; poor testing facilities; well-intentioned but inadequately trained testers; poorly calibrated equipment; or simply too many children to test by the available staff.

Parents should have their children's hearing tested by a qualified audiologist. They should know that a hearing test alone will not establish the presence or absence of ear abnormality and, by the same token, a physician's ear examination alone will not establish the presence or absence of hearing impairment. The two conditions are not the same, and each requires its own examination by its own specialist. However, it is preferable to have them done in conjunction so that findings may be shared by both specialists.

If hearing impairment is present at birth or during childhood, it should be identified at the earliest possible time so audiological and educational management can be provided throughout the language and speech acquisition period. Since this begins at birth, there is *no* time to waste on well-intentioned but distinctly ill-informed advice that is often given, such as "wait for the child to become old enough to test." Competent audiologists can test the child from birth onward. Governmental agencies, usually at state level, are prepared to assist parents of hearing-impaired children who require aid in the form of proper medical and audiological care, including providing and maintaining a hearing aid. Parents owe their children an environment that helps rather than hinders the acquisition of language and speech skills and that provides surroundings quiet enough to further the development of attentive awareness and listening.

NOISE-INDUCED HEARING IMPAIRMENT

The most obvious consequence of continuous or frequent exposure to hazardous noise is impairment of hearing. Damage to the inner ear structures can also result from sudden, violently powerful sounds. This is called "acoustic trauma" and may involve pain. It is different from slowly encroaching painless damage due to less violent stimuli: "noise-induced hearing impairment."

Long-term exposure to very loud stimuli probably destroys specific areas in the cochlea due to excessive local stimulation. Exposure to less loud levels induces vasoconstriction and a consequent temporary reduction in the amount of oxygen and nutrients available to the hair cells. Most of the hair cells survive this deprivation and are revived by the reappearance of oxygen and nutrients after the noise exposure stops and the vasoconstriction ceases. Damage to the ear resulting from long exposure to noise usually first afflicts the hair cells responsive to the frequency of about 4,000 Hz. Damage then gradually spreads both upward and downward through the frequency range until it invades the speech frequencies, and interferes with hearing for speech.

Most of this damage can be prevented if caught early enough. Hearing impairment due to noise exposure is definitely the most preventable of all forms of hearing disability. It need not happen.

Although it usually takes years of exposure for the permanent effect of noise-induced hearing loss to appear, there are early warning signs and they should be heeded. These warning clues are the same whether the exposure takes place at work, at home, or at play. Genuinely hazardous noise levels are by no means restricted to the workplace. Household and recreational noises can also induce hearing impairment. These are the most important clues to be on the alert for:

1. Having to talk louder in order to converse face to face in noise. This is the best rule-of-thumb indicator that the noise is hazardously loud.

2. Hearing any ringing, buzzing, or roaring in your ears after exposure to noise. This phenomenon, known as *tinnitus*, may be a symptom of damage to specific hair cells.

3. Experiencing diminished hearing sensitivity following noise exposure. With rest, it goes away, although never completely. If exposure continues on a regular basis, it can develop into a serious hearing impairment. The fact that it can take as long as twenty years to develop makes it difficult for victims to perceive that anything is happening to them.

Regardless of the exposure location, some people seem to be invulnerable to this problem. Various theories have been advanced to explain why different people exposed to the same levels of noise for the same length of time show markedly different susceptibility to hearing loss. "Tough and tender ear" theories have not been easy to prove and structural differences are difficult to demonstrate.

One fascinating recent theory attempts to explain why, in some instances, people exposed to loud music at rock concerts may have different physiological reactions on the basis of different attitudes toward the noise stimulus. The musicians themselves take frequent breaks and have a chance to recover before the next exposure, but most of the audience happily and eagerly remains throughout a series of performances by one band after another. The theory proposes that those who are favorably disposed to the sound experience strongly positive stress, or eustress, which is thought to be enhancing rather than destructive. Those who are negatively disposed to the sound

experience distress, which is thought to be destructive. This theory does not mean that some of the rock fans do *not* experience hearing damage.

SLEEP DISRUPTION

Sleep is a crucial part of our life maintenance. People differ in the amount of sleep needed to recover from fatigue, but it must be deep sleep not fitful or superficial sleep, for at least part of the time. Noise lifts a sleeper from the deeper levels, where recovery from fatigue takes place, to lighter levels that are much less restorative. Naturally, noise can also waken sleepers, or even prevent the tired from falling asleep.

The effects of noise on health and the ability to work can be serious if sleep interference occurs too frequently. For example, people who live next to noisy elevated trains may spend little time in restful sleep. Sometimes people get so accustomed to recurring noise that it does not waken them or they do not remember awakening. But the uncontrollable shift from deep to light levels that nevertheless occurs is enough to interfere with their recovery from fatigue, and they will habitually begin the next day unrested.

Attitudes toward noise, probably shaped by upbringing, are powerful governors of response to noise when asleep as well as when awake. Some people are never awakened by noise, while others can never actually get to sleep. Mild feelings of anger that might dissipate in restful surroundings can make even moderate noises substantially annoying while rage can keep a person wide awake even in a quiet place. Either situation can ruin any chance of recovery from fatigue.

Older people, along with the sick, are much more easily awakened and have more trouble getting back to sleep. They therefore require special protection from noises. Other age groups do not appear to be as affected by noise while asleep. However, this may be due to failure to recall being awakened. People tend to underestimate the number of times they awaken.

Noise forces sleepers to adapt, whether it actually wakes them or just changes the depth of their sleep. The body responds to noise by moving into a state of preparedness for action of some kind. The release of hormones and the shift in blood pressure and heart rate to higher levels put the body under stress.

STRESS

Stress produced by noise is the same as that resulting from any other stressor. Yet, the way noise may affect cardiovascular diseases or other stress-related illnesses (see chapter 7, Stress) has had little study. Practically no research has been carried out on humans in the United States. Studies in Europe, however, suggest that working in high noise conditions is associated with permanently elevated blood pressure and cardiovascular episodes. These suggestions are supported by some animal data. In one research study, a chimpanzee was exposed to twenty-four hours of ordinary traffic noises recorded outside the hospital of the University of Miami medical school. The animal's blood pressure rose and has remained elevated ever since. Continuing experiments indicated that heart rate and blood pressure remained elevated for months after the twenty-four-hour exposure, and suggested that the condition might be permanent.

Obviously, the same stress-related illness can have multiple causes. But noise is, without doubt, a potent stressor.

Noise does not affect the heart directly. Increasing evidence shows, rather, that stress following noise causes an increase in adrenalin re-

lease, an elevation in heart rate, constriction of blood vessels, and a resultant increase in blood pressure. All of these changes may aggravate an existing heart condition.

Animal studies have also shown a significant increase in blood cholesterol levels of rabbits exposed for ten weeks to noise levels commonly found in noisy workplaces. Unexposed rabbits on the same diets remained normal.

To determine the effects of noise on children, a study was conducted on grade school pupils exposed to aircraft noise both at school and at home. Preliminary results showed that they had higher blood pressures than similar children in quieter areas.

The effects of noise on cardiovascular disease and hypertension are hard to evaluate. Noise exposure is difficult to measure in the average person's life. Persons exposed to high levels of noise may have other risk factors for cardiovascular disease such as smoking cigarettes and eating high-fat diets. Doctors frequently try to guard their heart disease patients from noise's stressful effects; hence it is only good sense for all people to protect themselves from these effects as a preventive measure.

Prevention and Reduction of Noise

Preventing and reducing noise are essential in our highly mechanized societies. Our homes should be havens from noise, a place where one can find daily relief. Manufacturers are capable of producing acceptably quiet household equipment of all kinds. In order to get quiet equipment, all we need to do is insist upon it in the competitive marketplace. Noise in the home as well as in the workplace can and should be controlled.

Three elements are involved in reducing or preventing noise—the sound source, the sound path, and the sound receiver. Each element can be dealt with separately or together.

IDENTIFY THE SOURCE

In most cases, the source is all too obvious: mechanical, hydraulic, aerodynamic, magnetic, electric, or electronic devices that create acoustic or vibratory energy by setting other potential sound sources in motion. These may be machines, appliances, air and water handling devices, sound producing and reproducing devices such as musical instruments and amplifiers, radios, tape recorders, and television sets. The source may also, of course, be living creatures.

Consider the following guidelines for controlling noise at the source. First of all, an attempt should be made to select quiet equipment. Look for low-noise certification and advertising claims such as "sound treated," "sound conditioned," or "quiet operating." While these terms can be less than accurate, they do suggest that the manufacturers are aware of the consumer's interest.

Before buying a product, compare the actual sound output of several, side-by-side if possible, keeping in mind that where and how the device is actually installed will also affect the sound. Look for devices that emphasize "lower" and "slower" operating characteristics. Try to visit other installations of the equipment to make your own evaluation.

Quiet operation of equipment. If noisy equipment has already been installed, a careful analysis of the moving parts, the radiating surfaces, the direct contacts, and the mounting surfaces should be made. Corrective measures can be taken, such as,

1. cushioning the impact or impulsive forces;
2. reducing the speed in machines, and the flow velocities and pressures in air, gas, or fluid systems;
3. balancing rotating parts;
4. reducing frictional resistance by lubricating, aligning, and polishing contacting parts and surfaces;

5. isolating vibrating elements within the machine by using resilient or flexible connectors and mountings;
6. reducing the sound radiating surface, e.g., replace a large vibrating sheet metal safety guard on a machine with one of wire mesh or webbing;
7. applying vibration damping materials such as liquid mastics, pads of absorptive material, and viscoelastic laminates to vibrating surfaces;
8. reducing noise leakage from the interior of the appliance by sealing or covering all openings and applying acoustical materials to inner surfaces; and
9. treating moving air and fluid "kindly" by reducing the pressure, streamlining the flow, and smoothing boundary surfaces to reduce turbulence.

Quieter replacements. Choose quieter machinery when replacing appliances or parts. Use:

1. heavy glass rather than plastic blender containers;
2. rubber or plastic rather than metal trash cans;
3. wood or fiberboard rather than metal cabinets;
4. wood or laminate rather than metal sliding or folding closet doors;
5. smooth rather than corrugated vacuum cleaner hose to reduce whistling noise;
6. large low-speed, rather than small high-speed fans;
7. squirrel cage or centrifugal rather than propeller or vane axial fans;
8. a belt-driven furnace blower operated by a resiliently mounted motor rather than a motor-coupled blower.

If the noise source is beyond direct control because of unresponsive or unsympathetic ownership, inaccessibility, jurisdictional considerations, or inadequate or ineffectual laws governing noise emission limits, control measures will have to take the form of civil actions, political pressures, or efforts of citizen action groups.

IDENTIFY THE SOUND PATH

Tracking the pathway of noise is one important way of locating an unknown sound source. When the source is known, it is possible to determine if its transmission has changed the quality of the sound reaching the receiver, and thus to tell whether it is entering by air or through a structure.

Airborne sounds usually arrive with their high-frequency components intact, and may reach the receiver over many paths. The most direct path is a line-of-sight airpath from the source to the receiver, such as from an airplane overhead to a person on the ground. But a person practicing on an amplified guitar in the apartment next door can cause the sound to travel through large or small openings. Looking for light leaks around a closed door in a darkened room is one way of detecting openings.

Structure-borne sounds are more likely to seem muffled since they are transmitted directly, along with their vibrations, through massive, rigid building supports. Such sounds cause room surfaces to vibrate and radiate noise into other areas, but the mass absorbs the high frequencies, giving rise to the muffled effect. Thus, listening to the type of intruding sound can help to locate both sources and pathways of the noise.

In many locations, a stethoscope or a large mailing tube will help detect surface vibrations or noise leaks. One simple technique is to turn on a noisy appliance such as a vacuum cleaner or blender, close the door, go into the next room, and listen with the tube along the cracks and surfaces of the other side of the wall. The noise increases as you approach a leak or radiating surface. Caulking or gasketing minor leaks as you discover them makes finding the dominant leaks or vibrating surfaces easier, and they must be found before any appreciable overall noise reduction can be obtained.

When control of noise at its source is neither possible nor effective, the pathway should be controlled by setting up barriers or deflectors to absorb, block, divert, or otherwise reduce the flow of sound energy before it reaches the receiver. The most effective technique will depend on the size and type of the source, the frequency and intensity range of the noise, and the nature of the environment.

There are several factors which affect sound transmission. One of these is, *absorption: soaking up sound*. In the outdoors, air absorbs high-frequency sounds quite well; over great distances low frequencies are effectively absorbed, as in the case of a roaring high-flying jet aircraft that can be seen from its contrails but cannot be heard at all from the ground.

Inside ordinary buildings, air absorbs little or no sound. Properly selected and installed material will absorb most airborne sound energy striking it. Soft, porous materials such as heavy, pleated draperies and thick, padded carpeting help soak up sound generated within. Upholstered furniture, paintings on the walls, acoustical tiles on the ceilings, and even people are excellent sound absorbers for high frequencies, but great mass and bulk are required to absorb the lows. Such mass and bulk is not always practical in the average house. For this reason, heavy masonry, brick, or stone are quieter than houses built of those constructed of more flimsy materials.

Sound reflection: bouncing of sound. Sound waves striking a flat solid surface that is larger than the wavelength of the sound will be reflected at an angle equal to the one at which it struck the surface. Some of its energy will be absorbed by the reflecting surface, but if the surface is hard, most of it will be reflected, like a light beam striking a mirror. Using a hard reflective surface can effectively channel, or direct sound toward or away from a particular location.

Reverberation: multiple reflection of sound. In a fairly small room with hard reflective surfaces, direct and reflected sound waves tend to merge and amplify the sound beyond its original energy level. Properly used in an auditorium, reverberation can enhance music, and in a band shell it helps to amplify and direct the music to the outdoor audience. Placing a loudspeaker in a corner does the same thing. Too much reverberation, however, can create so many echoes that sound is badly distorted. Singing in such acoustically "live" rooms as tiled bathrooms can fool us into pondering a musical career. It is all

a matter of reverberation and absorption. A simple way to test a room for excessive reverberation is to time the length of a handclap. If it takes longer than a second or two to die away, the room requires absorptive acoustic treatment.

Diffraction: bending of sound. Sound can bend around or over an obstacle such as a wall, or squeeze through an opening, provided the wavelength of the sound is comparable to the size of the obstacle or opening. Diffraction occurs when sound waves strike the solid edge of a barrier. The edge generates a new train of waves of the same frequency but reduced sound pressure. The new wave fronts progress spherically away from their new points of origin along the edge, which means that the original sound is now being

---

Steps in quieting the path of sound:

1. Separate the noise source and the receiver by as great a distance as possible.
2. Use sound-absorbing materials installed as close as possible to the noise source.
3. Use sound barriers and deflectors that are large enough in size and appropriate for the frequency range of the noise.
4. When the sound source is external, increase the sound insulation of the exterior shell of the house. Windows and doors are common leaks for both noise and heat. The intrusion of outdoor sounds can be reduced along with heat transfer by installing properly sealed and fitted solid core doors and double-glazed storm windows.
5. Use acoustical lining on the inside surfaces of air ducts, pipe channels, or electrical channels to control high-frequency sounds.

6. Install mufflers or silencers on all gasoline or diesel engines regardless of size, and wherever large amounts of high-pressure, high-velocity gasses, liquids, steam, or air are discharged into the open air.
7. Structure-borne noise transmission paths may be interrupted by the use of vibration isolators such as resilient mountings and flexible couplers. Expansion joints along the outer edges of mechanical equipment room floors can reduce the transmission of vibration to building walls and structural frames.
8. Massive enclosures that are airtight and insulated on the inside can be used to isolate noisy existing machinery that would be difficult to quiet by alteration. Structural contact between the noise source and the enclosure must be carefully avoided.

propagated in all directions on the *other* side of the wall. This explains how sound striking the top edge of a wall will bend downward on the other side.

Much the same thing happens when sound encounters a small hole or crack in the wall. That part of the sound that gets through is regenerated as a new spherical wave by encountering the inside edge of the opening, from which it then progresses to all parts of the room on the other side, now weaker, but definitely there. It is because of diffraction that small holes and cracks, especially around loose windows and doors, should be sealed if sound treating is to succeed.

Care should be taken to consider the effects of diffraction if exterior walls are to be erected to control noise. Because of diffraction, the wall could actually bend the noise in the direction of the location intended to be quieted. A qualified sound engineer should be consulted before committing such an expensive error.

IDENTIFY THE RECEIVER

Resentful receivers of unwanted noise are unlikely to be alone in their resentment. To make a case for controlling a problem, as many receivers as possible should be identified in families, tenant groups, classrooms, office forces, community and civic organizations, neighborhoods, or even entire communities.

When source, pathway, and receivers have been located and appraised, the nature of the solution should begin to become apparent. In most cases, solutions will involve some combination of (1) modifying the source to reduce or remove its noise output; (2) altering or controlling the transmission path and the environment to reduce the noise level reaching the receiver; and (3) providing the listener with personal protective equipment. In a few cases, attention to only one of these elements will suffice.

Protecting the receiver

Ear plugs, ear muffs, or both together, are essential when exposed to the operation of excessively noisy equipment such as power tools, firearms, or inadequately mufflered engines on trucks, stock cars, boats, snowmobiles, motorcycles, mopeds, model airplanes, and the like. Such protection should also be worn consistently when riding on noisy public transportation.

Properly fitted devices can prevent noise-induced hearing impairment, and guard against stress-related disorders associated with noise exposure. Comfortable compressible ear plugs can help ward off sleep disruption due to noise.

People who wear ear plugs frequently, however, should have their ears examined by an otologist or otolaryngologist—physicians who specialize in the care of the ear—to determine whether there are any medical reasons for not using them. This should be followed by frequent checkups to be on guard against a buildup of ear wax in the ear canal. Ear wax is natural and protective, but since an ear plug pushes the daily accumulations down toward the eardrum membrane, an impaction of this material could cause a temporary hearing loss, and possibly a more serious condition if neglected. Impacted earwax should only be removed under the direction of a physician. Simple hygiene and preventive checkups can make the consistent use of ear plugs an effective personal weapon in the battle against noise.

The soft, compressible, polymer foam ear plugs that expand in the ear canal to achieve an excellent fit are the most effective type, especially while sleeping. They tend to stay in place, give with external pressure, and do not feel as uncomfortable after a period of wear as more rigid varieties. Wax-impregnated cotton plugs are unhygienic and should not be used. Whether or not ear plugs enable sleepers to remain in deep level sleep states is not known, but some persons say they feel more rested after their use.

In the case of persons with normal or near normal hearing, any emergency warning that could be heard without hearing protection devices will be heard as well or better with such devices in place. The only sounds totally eliminated are the very quiet sounds that could not be heard easily because of the noise. Most of the disruptive and damaging noise will be reduced to safe levels.

Persons with moderate to severe hearing impairments should seek professional advice before wearing such devices in places where danger signals must be heard.

Another means of protecting the receiver is to alter the work schedule. When all possible sound control has been achieved on a noise source around which people live, and the source still makes noise, its use should be scheduled to cause the least disturbance to all affected. For instance, you should operate a noisy power mower only when the neighbors agree to tolerate the distraction. If you have conferred with them, chances are they will understand. If the noise causes them disruption, work in blocks of time with frequent rest intervals, at reasonable hours of the day, avoiding the early and late hours, especially on Saturday and Sunday. And don't forget to wear ear plugs.

Masking noise is useful in altering the way we perceive noise in specific locations. While it does not protect the receiver from the noise, it may make it possible to forget about it.

It works because certain sounds may be masked by other sounds that are similar in frequency and intensity. Since people's attitudes toward sound varies widely, the notion of a universally appealing background sound makes little sense. Masking noises are most effective when personal choice is exercised. For example, a broad-spectrum noise generator in the bedroom may be used to obscure distant but distracting sound at sleep time. Such devices are available in steady or gently pulsating modes reminiscent of rainfall or surf. Often a fan or air conditioner can provide adequate masking noise.

On the other hand, masking can compound the problem by merely adding more noise. If the intruding noise approaches the level of conversational speech, an effective masking noise will surely make communication difficult or impossible. In short, it is not possible to create a peaceful environment in an already noisy place by obscuring the sounds with an equally loud stimuli. The idea of "acoustical perfume" has been vastly overworked; many consider background music as another intrusion or as outright noise pollution.

Legislative Measures

Congress enacted noise legislation for the first time in the Walsh-Healey Public Contract Acts of 1936. They remained in force until 1969 when a revised standard was set, establishing a maximum permissible eight-hour exposure to a level of 90 decibels. This regulation was incorporated without change into the Occupational Safety and Health Act (OSHA) of 1970 that became effective in 1971. Efforts to reduce the permissible level to 85 decibels have met with strong opposition from industry, chiefly on economic grounds.

In 1976, 40 percent of the over 14 million workers then exposed to noise in production industries were exposed to levels between 85 and 90 decibels. Thirty percent were exposed to levels less than 85 decibels. Reduction to 85 decibels would thus bring at least 70 percent of the exposed workers under mandatory protection. The percentage of exposed workers who show increases in permanent hearing impairment actually doubles as the noise exposure increases from 80 to 85 decibels and from 85 to 90 decibels.

According to a 1974 "Levels Document" of the Environmental Protection Agency (EPA), when an average exposure level reaches 70 decibels at the ear over a twenty-four-hour period, it is necessary to protect the public from significant adverse effects on their hearing, with an adequate margin of safety. Of course, many people are exposed to levels of noise significantly above 70 decibels in their places of employment, in public transportation, in their recreational activities, and some even in their own homes, especially those near airports, traffic arteries, and rapid transit conduits. Those who are exposed to higher levels for 40 or more years risk losing some hearing. The EPA cautions that this is not a regulatory goal, but rather a recommended level defined by scientific consensus.

CHAPTER
15

Infectious diseases

The greatest and best known triumphs of twentieth century science and medicine have been the eradication or effective control of many of the infectious diseases that were the major causes of death and disability less than a century ago.

Because of our ability to immunize people against many diseases, and through the development of a whole spectrum of antibiotics that destroy or control the growth of disease-causing organisms, we have achieved a historic advance against the scourge of infections, particularly those affecting infant mortality.

Yet, there remain a number of infections against which neither immunizations nor drug therapy are totally effective. Thus, avoiding contact with the germs that cause these diseases still remains our first line of defense. But people with a lower standard of living still suffer a higher incidence of various infectious diseases than the rest of us. Better, less crowded housing, improved nutrition, and greater health knowledge will help to reduce the risk in these groups. To accomplish this goal, the assistance of all of society is required.

Glossary

ANTIBODY A protein substance either produced by the body in response to a foreign substance (antigen) such as a bacterium or toxin, or a substance normally present in the circulation that exerts a specific restrictive effect against an antigen. Antibodies may be transferred from the mother to the fetus or may develop over time by undetected contact with disease-causing agents.

ANTIGEN A substance that stimulates the formation of antibodies. Examples are bacteria, foreign blood cells, etc.

ANTISEPSIS Prevention of infection by inhibition of the growth and multiplication of microorganisms.

ASYMPTOMATIC Without symptoms.

CARRIER An infected person who is capable of transmitting a disease but lacks any signs or symptoms of the illness.

EPIDEMIC Increase in the occurrence of an event such as an infectious disease beyond the expected number of cases at the same time within the same population or geographic area.

IMMUNOSUPPRESSIVE AGENT A chemical compound used to control immunological disorders such as rheumatoid arthritis. However, such an agent also reduces the body's ability to fight infection.

INCUBATION PERIOD The period of time elapsing between the introduction of a disease-causing organism into the body and the onset of symptoms.

MICROBE Microorganism.

MUTATE To alter genetic characteristics.

VECTOR An animal carrier transmitting infectious agents from host to host.

History and Definitions

Perhaps the most impressive medical achievement of modern times is the conquest of most infectious diseases in the developed nations of the world. Until recently, infections were the major causes of death, and epidemics were common. Today, a combination of social, scientific, and medical advances has dramatically reduced the toll of these diseases in the United States and other developed countries.

Until these advances were achieved, epidemics were a depressingly predictable factor in human history. The Athenian plague that altered the course of the war with Sparta, the Black Death that killed more than a third of the population of medieval Europe, and the seven cholera pandemics that have swept the world since 1800 are only a few examples of such epidemics.

A first major medical victory against infectious disease was the discovery by William Jenner in the late eighteenth century that cowpox virus could immunize individuals against smallpox—an achievement that culminated in 1980 with the worldwide elimination of smallpox. The tide began to turn against many other infectious diseases during the nineteenth century. One important factor was a general improvement in living standards and in sanitation. Another was the development of the germ theory of infection, which enabled scientists and physicians to mount effective attacks against many diseases.

While Louis Pasteur played the most important part in establishing the principle that specific infectious agents are responsible for specific diseases, many others made important contributions. Ignaz Semmelweiss helped to make childbirth safer for women by advising physicians to disinfect their hands and clothing. Joseph Lister made surgery safer by applying the principle of antisepsis in the operating room. Robert Koch showed how to identify the causes of diseases by growing colonies of bacteria in the laboratory and by establishing the basic rules that still are used to prove that an infectious agent is responsible for a specific illness.

Such biomedical advances led to the development of vaccines against diphtheria, rabies, and other infectious illnesses. The incidence of other diseases, such as tuberculosis and typhoid fever, declined at the same time, more because of improvements in living conditions and in sanitation than because of specific medical measures.

Progress has accelerated in the twentieth century. Perhaps the most important single effort has been the development of drugs that are effective against a wide range of infectious bacteria. No such drugs were available until the 1930s, when German scientists showed that a class of synthetic compounds, the sulfonamides, were active against streptococcal infections. In the 1940s, British researchers developed penicillin, the first antibiotic derived from a living organism. Many other antibiotics since then have been isolated from microbes and are in common medical use.

Recent decades have seen the development of vaccines against many viral diseases. The Salk and Sabin vaccines have virtually eliminated polio, and vaccines against measles, mumps, rubella, and other childhood diseases.

Nonetheless, the fight against infectious diseases is not over. Such diseases as measles, which are well on the way to extinction in the developed nations, remain major killers in areas where living conditions and nutrition are primitive. Venereal diseases such as syphilis and gonorrhea still are widespread in the developed countries. Parents must continually be reminded of the need to have their children immunized against infectious diseases. And several of the diseases listed in this chapter remain beyond the reach of modern medicine, although there is hope of progress through basic and applied research.

Types of Infectious Agents

Infectious agents can be divided roughly into two classes. One class consists of single-cell organisms that are relatively complex. This class includes the bacteria, protozoa, fungi, and rickettsia. The second class contains the viruses, much simpler organisms that are on the borderline between the animate and the inanimate.

Bacteria. These are single-cell microbes which, like the cells of the human body, have cell walls, and carry on relatively complex metabolic functions. Disease-causing bacteria can reproduce within the body, destroying healthy tissues, most often by releasing toxic compounds. Antibiotics combat bacterial infections by interfering with the essential life processes of the organisms. Penicillin, for example, prevents the production of bacterial cell membranes, the protective cell wall without which bacteria cannot exist. Bacterial diseases include cholera, diphtheria, gonorrhea, and typhoid fever.

Protozoa. These are parasitic organisms, usually one-celled, which take up residence in the body's organs and tissues and compete with the body's cells for nutrients. Protozoal diseases include amebiasis (see page 575).

Rickettsiae. These are microbes which have cell walls and require oxygen like bacteria, but which like viruses depend on living cells for growth. The rickettsiae are carried by insects. Once they enter the body, they multiply in the cells of small blood vessels. Rickettsial diseases include Rocky Mountain spotted fever and typhus.

Fungi. These organisms include molds, mildews, yeasts, and other one-celled microbes. Fungal infections include candidiasis, ringworm, and athlete's foot.

Viruses. These organisms are much smaller than bacteria. A virus consists of a core of genetic material surrounded by a protein coat. To reproduce, the virus must enter a living cell and transform the cell's activity so that more viruses are produced. Antibiotics generally are not effective against viral diseases, although they may be prescribed to prevent bacterial infections that sometimes accompany these diseases. A few antiviral drugs now are available, but the most effective weapon against viral diseases is prevention, generally by the use of vaccines. Viral diseases include polio, influenza, measles, mumps, and the common cold.

Modes of Transmission

Inhalation of airborne microbes. Infectious organisms can be exhaled by an infected individual and travel to another person in droplets of moisture, which may cling to dust or other particles. Diseases spread in this way include measles, chickenpox, smallpox, scarlet fever, diphtheria, mumps, whooping cough, influenza, tuberculosis, the common cold, and meningococcal and streptococcal infections.

Contamination of food or water. Diseases that are spread from person to person by food or water include amebiasis, cholera, hepatitis, polio, salmonellosis, and typhoid.

Personal contact. Contaminated fingers can carry microbes to the face and mouth, or to open wounds that allow them to enter the body. Diseases spread by direct contact include hepatitis, boils, and rabies, which is spread by animal bites.

Sexual contact. Sexually transmitted diseases include gonorrhea, herpes progenitalis, nongonococcal urethritis, and syphilis. All forms of intimate body contact, including kissing and oral-genital practices, can spread these diseases.

Insects. Diseases spread by biting insects include malaria, dengue, and yellow fever.

Prevention

The prevalence of infectious disease is related to the standard of living. Both the prevention and the control of infectious disease are easier when individuals have good diets, clean water, effective sanitation, and decent housing. The severity of an illness, once it is contracted, depends on the patient's overall state of health. Persons who are fatigued, undernourished, or chronically ill are especially likely to contract infectious diseases. Thus, prevention requires action both by individuals and by society.

Sanitation. Sanitary improvements in the nineteenth century helped cause a sharp decline in deaths from infectious diseases before vaccines and antibiotics were available. Cholera and typhoid fever were virtually eradicated by programs to prevent contamination of food and water. Yellow fever and malaria have been combatted by mosquito control. Diphtheria and tuberculosis death rates went down as housing conditions improved and overcrowding was reduced. However, occasional outbreaks of disease still can occur when sanitary precautions are neglected.

Today sanitation is partly a governmental function and partly an individual responsibility. Governmental agencies work to prevent contamination of the food and water supplies. Individuals can prevent infectious diseases by such measures as washing hands before eating or preparing foods; covering the mouth when coughing or sneezing; and properly disposing of human wastes. Infected individuals can protect others by seeking prompt medical attention and completing the prescribed course of treatment.

Vaccination. There are two basic types of vaccine in use against viral diseases. A killed-virus vaccine contains viruses that have been killed by chemical treatment. There is no danger of acquiring infection from the vaccine, but booster shots of vaccine are required periodically. The Salk polio vaccine is a killed-virus vaccine.

A live-virus vaccine uses a strain of virus which has been weakened by careful breeding in the laboratory but which is still alive. Live-virus vaccines confer longer immunity than killed-viruses vaccines, but there is a slight danger that the vaccine can cause the illness if the treated virus reverts to the virulent type. The Sabin polio vaccine is a live-virus vaccine.

Vaccination is valuable for the community as well as for the individual. When a large proportion of a community is immunized against a disease, the rest of the people in the community benefit from what is called "herd immunity": the disease does not spread because carriers are lacking. Thus, there is a constant need for vigilance to prevent the loss of herd immunity by neglecting to have children immunized against preventable diseases.

Travel Vaccinations

No vaccinations are required of persons traveling from the U.S. to Europe, Canada, Mexico, and the Caribbean.

In all other parts of the world, countries have individual requirements. Consult the nearest Department of Health for specific requirements.

No vaccinations are required of residents reentering the U.S.

Childhood Diseases

Chickenpox is an acute viral illness that causes mild fever and a distinctive skin rash. It is transmitted by direct contact or by airborne spread of viruses from the respiratory tract of the patients. Symptoms appear two to three weeks after infection occurs. One attack usually gives permanent immunity.

Prevention: An infected child should be isolated for at least one week after the onset of symptoms. Soiled articles should be disinfected.

Diphtheria is a viral disease that attacks the mucous membranes of the tonsils, nose, and throat. It usually occurs in winter. The disease is spread from the oral, nasal, and skin discharges from an untreated patient in the two- to four-week incubation period. Symptoms appear two to five days after infection and include low fever, swollen glands, and sore throat with whitish membranes. A throat culture should be taken as diphtheria can resemble other infections such as scarlet fever and tonsillitis.

Prevention: An effective vaccine is available. Children should be immunized in the first year of life and should receive a booster dose before entering school.

Measles is a highly communicable viral disease that causes fever, conjunctivitis, a runny nose, and a characteristic rash. It can cause pneumonia and, in some cases, serious complications that can be fatal. It is most frequently transmitted by direct contact with secretions from the nose or throat of an infected person. Symptoms appear about ten days after infection. One attack usually gives permanent immunity.

Prevention: A live-virus vaccine is available. Vaccination is recommended at fifteen months of age.

Mumps is a viral disease whose characteristic signs are inflammation of the salivary glands, headache, fever, and vomiting. It can be spread by direct contact with the saliva of an infected person. Symptoms appear twelve to twenty-six days after infection. Although the disease usually does no permanent harm to children, it has been known to cause sterility when contracted by adult males.

Prevention: A live-virus vaccine is available. Immunization is recommended at any time after twelve months of age.

Poliomyelitis is a viral disease that can cause paralysis that may lead to respiratory failure and death. It can be spread by direct contact with an infected individual. Symptoms appear seven to twelve days after infection occurs. There is no specific treatment for the disease.

Prevention: The use of polio vaccine has virtually eliminated poliomyelitis from the United States. The disease is so rare that some parents neglect to have their children immunized. All infants should have their first polio shot at two months of age (see table 15.1).

Table 15.1
RECOMMENDED SCHEDULE FOR ACTIVE IMMUNIZATION
OF NORMAL INFANTS AND CHILDREN

Repeat at these intervals

2 months	DTP (diphtheria, tetanus, and pertussis vaccine)
	TOPV (trivalent oral poliovirus vaccine)
4 months	DTP, TOPV
6 months	DTP
1 year	Mumps, rubella*
15 months	Measles
1½ years	DTP, TOPV
4–6 years	DTP, TOPV
12 years	TD (tetanus, diphtheria vaccine)—repeat every 5–10 years thereafter

*Mumps and rubella may be given in combination with measles at 15 months.
SOURCE: *The Merck Manual*, Merck & Co., 1977.

Rubella (German measles) is a mild viral disease characterized by a spotty rash that first appears on the face and then spreads to the torso and limbs. Symptoms appear two to three weeks after infection. Rubella generally is harmless to children, but it can cause severe birth defects if it is contracted by a woman during the first three months of pregnancy. Damage to the newborn may include cataracts, deafness, heart disease, and abnormalities of the nervous system, bones, liver, spleen, and blood.

Prevention: A live-virus vaccine is available. Immunization of all children after the first year of life is recommended. Women of childbearing age who have never contracted the disease should also receive the vaccine. However, the vaccine should not be given to any woman who is pregnant or who is trying to become pregnant.

Whooping cough (pertussis) is a viral disease that often occurs before the age of seven. It starts with loss of appetite, lethargy, and a hacking cough, which is followed in one or two weeks by violent coughing episodes accompanied by the characteristic "whoop." Pertussis may be transmitted by direct contact with an infected individual or by contact with articles contaminated by discharges from a patient. Symptoms appear about ten days after infection occurs.

Prevention: An effective vaccine is available. Children should be given the vaccine at two, four, and six months after birth, with booster shots a year later and before entering school.

Waterborne and Foodborne Diseases

Amebiasis is a protozoal disease that causes abdominal dicomfort and diarrhea, sometimes accompanied by fever and chills. It is prevalent in areas of poor sanitation and is transmitted by the ingestion of contaminated water or of food contaminated by the feces of infected persons. Symptoms appear three to four weeks after infection occurs.

Prevention: Amebiasis can be prevented by careful attention to the basic rules of sanitation, such as washing the hands before handling food.

Botulism is a severe, often fatal food poisoning caused by a toxin released by a bacterium that grows only in the absence of oxygen. Signs of illness—fatigue, dizziness, digestive complaints, progressing to paralysis of the central nervous system, cardiac and respiratory systems—appear within twenty-four hours of eating contaminated food. Prompt use of an antitoxin can prevent the respiratory failure that often causes death.

Prevention: Most cases of botulism are caused by failure to observe safety rules when canning fruits and vegetables at home. The toxin is destroyed by heating, so that all foods canned or bottled at home should be boiled for at least three minutes. Any food that shows signs of contamination should be discarded. Do not eat food from cans that show visible bulges.

Cholera is a bacterial disease most commonly contracted by drinking water that is contaminated by infected feces. It causes vomiting, diarrhea, and dehydration that can be fatal unless large amounts of replacement fluid are given to the patient. Symptoms appear as soon as a few hours or as long as five days after infection occurs.

Prevention: Improved sanitation has virtually eliminated cholera from the United States. Outbreaks still occur in western Asia, the western Pacific, and in areas where sanitary measures are neglected. A cholera vaccine is available, but it is relatively ineffective and its use is not recommended. The most effective preventive measures for an individual are thorough washing of the hands before eating and drinking only treated or boiled water. Also, avoid raw fruits or vegetables washed in untreated water.

Salmonellosis is a form of bacterial food poisoning that causes acute diarrhea, abdominal pain, vomiting, and fever. It occurs most often in the summer and frequently is due to the presence of the bacteria in undercooked meat, egg products, and unpasteurized dairy foods. The bacteria do not affect the appearance, taste, or smell of the food. Symptoms appear a few hours after eating contaminated food.

Prevention: Proper handling and treatment of food is essential. All persons who handle food should wash their hands thoroughly. Hot foods should be kept hot and cold foods should be kept refrigerated for as long as possible before eating, since the bacteria grow most rapidly at medium temperatures.

Shigellosis is a highly contagious bacterial disease that is transmitted either by contaminated water or milk or by direct person-to-person contact. The symptoms appear one to seven days after infection, and include headache, fever, loss of appetite, abdominal discomfort, and, occasionally, vomiting and diarrhea. Two-thirds of all cases and most of the deaths occur in children under ten years of age.

Prevention: Observance of good sanitary measures with water, milk, and food is essential. Hands should be washed before eating or pre-

paring food. The disease is most common in less developed areas of the world. In such areas, the traveler should eat only food that is cooked and served hot. Salads should be avoided, and all raw fruits and vegetables should be washed thoroughly and peeled before eating.

Staphylococcal food poisoning is the most common kind of food poisoning. It is caused by a bacterial toxin. Symptoms begin one to six hours after eating contaminated food and include vomiting and abdominal cramps. Recovery usually occurs quickly.

Prevention: The rules described for prevention of salmonellosis apply to staphylococcal food poisoning.

Typhoid fever is a severe form of salmonellosis characterized by fever, headache, weakness, loss of appetite, skin rash, and either constipation or diarrhea. It is transmitted via food and water contaminated by patients and carriers. Symptoms appear one to three weeks after infection occurs. Prompt antibiotic therapy is recommended.

Prevention: Milk pasteurization and purification of drinking water have sharply reduced the incidence of typhoid fever in the United States. A vaccine that gives partial protection is available and is recommended for individuals traveling to areas where typhoid fever is endemic.

Sexually Transmitted Diseases

Gonorrhea is a bacterial disease that has become a major public health problem. There is a gonorrhea epidemic in the United States (figure 15.1), but the true incidence is almost certainly higher than the statistics show, since many cases are unreported. One reason for this is that about 85 percent of infected women have no apparent symptoms, and so do not seek treatment. In women, gonorrhea can spread into the cervix and pelvic cavity, scarring the fallopian tubes and impairing fertility. If a pregnant woman has gonorrhea, the child's eyes may be infected during delivery. Untreated, the infection can cause corneal ulcers and blindness in the child. The major symptom of gonorrhea in men is a discharge of pus from the penis, accompanied by a burning sensation during urination. The symptoms appear three to nine days after infection occurs.

Prevention: Barrier methods of contraception, such as the condom, reduce the likelihood of contracting gonorrhea (see chapter 6, Pregnancy and Childbirth). Washing the genitals with soap and water before and after sexual contact is also recommended. But it is more urgent that any person who suspects infection should seek treatment immediately, and should also warn all sexual partners of the possibility of infection. Gonorrhea can be cured by treatment with penicillin and other antibiotics; treatment is the best prevention, since it stops the spread of the disease.

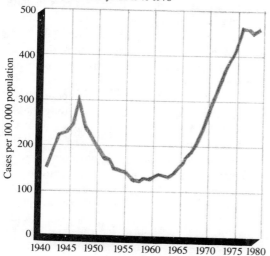

GONORRHEA—reported civilian case rates by year, United States, calendar years 1941-1978

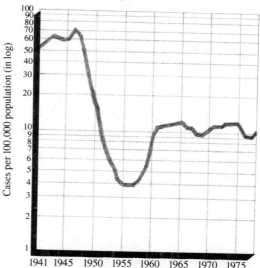

SYPHILIS (primary and secondary)—reported civilian case rates by year, United States, 1941-1978*

*1941-1946 fiscal years: twelve month period ending June 30 of year specified; 1947-1978 calendar years.

FIGURE 15.1

*Reported civilian case rates
of gonorrhea and syphilis*
SOURCE: *U.S. Department of Health and Human Services, Center for Disease Control*, Reported Morbidity and Mortality in the United States, *Annual Summary, 1978*

Pregnant women should be tested for gonorrhea during the first visit to the obstetrician and again just before delivery; a gonorrhea test should be part of the gynecological examination of any sexually active woman. A vaccine against gonorrhea is in the experimental stage.

Herpes simplex II or *herpes progenitalis*, is caused by a virus that is related to the one responsible for cold sores. Genital herpes has become a major problem in recent years, in large part because there is no effective treatment for the disease. Many individuals who contract genital herpes have outbreaks of fluid-filled blisters on the genitals periodically for many years. The disease is transmitted by sexual contact during such an outbreak. If a pregnant woman delivers during an outbreak of herpes progenitalis, the newborn infant may contract the disease. In newborns, genital herpes can cause severe problems and can be fatal. Caesarian delivery is recommended for any woman with active lesions. In addition, women with genital herpes should have a Pap smear every six months, since the Herpes simplex II virus is associated with an increased incidence of cervical cancer.

Prevention: The best way to prevent spread of the disease is to abstain from sexual activity during an outbreak. The use of condoms also helps prevent spread of genital herpes.

Syphilis is a bacterial disease whose incidence has increased in recent years. The course of the disease can be deceptive. About three weeks after sexual contact with an infected person, a small, painless, open sore appears at the site of contact. Syphilis can be cured if it is treated promptly with antibiotics when the sore, called a *chancre*, appears. If the disease is not treated, the chancre will disappear in about six weeks, but the disease remains in the body. The next symp-

tom in an untreated case is a body rash, which also goes away spontaneously. Skin lesions may appear later. Left untreated, syphilis can cause severe damage to the brain and other organs over a period of years. The disease can be transmitted from mother to child during pregnancy, and can cause major damage or death (figure 15.1).

Prevention: The most effective preventive measure is to have the disease cured by antibiotic treatment, stopping the chain of infection. It is urgent for an infected person to notify all recent sexual partners, so that they can seek treatment. The use of condoms during sexual intercourse reduces the risk of infection.

Other Common Diseases

The *common cold* is a blanket term for any upper respiratory infection caused by more than one hundred different viruses. The symptoms include coughing, sneezing, and a runny nose. Antibiotics often are prescribed for the common cold, although there is no evidence to support their use. Bed rest, hot liquids, and aspirin can ease the symptoms.

Prevention: Overcrowding and poor ventilation appear to help spread colds, so they should be avoided. Handkerchiefs and tissues used by anyone with a cold should be disposed of quickly. Infected individuals should avoid contact with vulnerable persons, such as infants and people with chronic bronchitis. Some studies indicate that relatively large doses of vitamin C can reduce the duration of the symptoms, although the results remain controversial. (See chapter 1, Nutrition.)

Hepatitis is a viral disease that can be contracted by person-to-person contact, by ingesting contaminated food or water, and by blood transfusion. Several types of hepatitis are known to exist. Type A, once known as infectious hepatitis, usually has a sudden onset and causes fever, fatigue, loss of appetite, abdominal discomfort, and jaundice. Type B, once known as serum hepatitis, causes similar symptoms but has a slower onset. A third type, detected in human blood, is known as "non-A, non-B hepatitis" and is believed to be caused by several different viruses. The incubation period for Type A hepatitis is about one month; for Type B it is two to three months.

Prevention: Tests are available to detect the hepatitis virus in transfused blood, but they are not totally effective. Hepatitis A patients should be isolated during the infectious period, which begins a few days after the onset of jaundice. A dose of immune serum globulin is recommended for anyone who had close contact with a patient.

Careful attention to hygiene can help prevent spread of hepatitis B. A vaccine to prevent hepatitis B in high-risk groups is being tested.

Influenza is a viral disease that most often occurs in the winter months and causes fever, chills, headache, muscle aches, a runny nose, a sore throat, and coughing. It can be dangerous to individuals who are weakened by old age or the presence of chronic illness. Influenza is transmitted by person-to-person contact and by contact with contaminated clothing. Symptoms appear twenty-four to seventy-two hours after infection occurs.

Prevention: Influenza vaccine is available and is recommended for the elderly, for persons with chronic diseases, and for other vulnerable individuals. The influenza vaccine must be changed constantly, because the flu virus mutates—that is, changes its genetic characteristics—so that the vaccine may not provide protection against the currently active strain. Use of amantadine, an antiviral drug, has been found to help prevent infection with Type A influenza virus, which has been responsible for most epidemics.

Malaria is caused by a parasite that lives in the blood. It is transmitted by mosquitoes or, less commonly, by a transfusion of infected blood. The symptoms include fever, chills, sweating, headache, and jaundice. They begin twelve to fourteen days after infection occurs. Effective drug therapy is available for most forms of malaria, although some cases of drug-resistant malaria have been contracted by Americans in Vietnam or other areas where the disease is endemic.

Prevention: Persons traveling to malaria-ridden areas should take medication that prevents the disease and should use malaria nets and repellents. No vaccine is available. A worldwide malaria eradication program, aimed at eliminating disease-carrying mosquitoes, has been set back by the growth of insecticide-resistant mosquitoes.

Meningitis is an inflammation of the meninges, or membranes of the spinal cord and brain, that can be caused either by bacteria or by viruses. Viral meningitis is a common, usually nonfatal, disease, which causes a stiff neck and headache. It occurs most commonly in the late summer and early fall. Bacterial meningitis is a much more serious disease that occurs most commonly in children and young adults, generally during the spring and winter. It starts abruptly with fever, headache, nausea, a stiff neck and, in some cases, a rash all over the body. The disease can cause delirium, coma, collapse, and death. It is transmitted by direct contact with discharges of infected persons. Symptoms appear three to four days after infection occurs.

Prevention: Good personal hygiene and avoidance of contact with infected individuals can help prevent bacterial meningitis. A vaccine is available for the form called meningococcal meningitis, and it is recommended for individuals who are considered to be at high risk.

Mononucleosis is a viral disease that often occurs in college populations. The disease is believed to be spread from person to person by an oral-respiratory route. The symptoms include high fever, fatigue, swollen glands, and a sore throat; they appear two to six weeks after infection occurs. Mononucleosis is believed to be caused by an agent called the Epstein-Barr virus, although details of the relationship are not entirely clear.

Prevention: No preventive method is available other than avoidance of contact with infected individuals.

Pneumonia is an inflammation of the lung that can be bacterial or viral. Symptoms include chills, fever, chest pains, and a cough. The onset of bacterial pneumonia is more sudden than that of viral pneumonia. Legionnaire's disease, so-called because it was detected through an outbreak at a 1976 American Legion convention, is a newly discovered form of bacterial pneumonia.

The incidence of pneumonia usually increases during outbreaks of influenza, because resistance is lowered in many individuals. Bacterial pneumonia often can be treated effectively with antibiotics, which have reduced the mortality rate significantly.

Prevention: Crowded and poorly ventilated quarters should be avoided, because the infection is spread by droplets from or in close contact with an infected person. A vaccine against bacterial pneumonia is available and should be given to vulnerable individuals, including the elderly and those suffering from chronic diseases.

Rabies is an acute viral infection of the brain that is almost always fatal unless it is treated in time. The incubation can be as short as two weeks and as long as six months. The disease usually is transmitted by animal bites, and the incubation period depends on the site and severity of the bite. Among the animals known to have transmitted the disease are dogs, foxes, skunks, racoons, bats, and rats.

In case of an animal bite, the wound should be washed thoroughly and a physician should be seen immediately. If the animal is known or suspected to have rabies, it is imperative that the patient receive a series of antirabies injections. A new rabies vaccine that requires fewer injections and causes fewer side effects than the conventional vaccine is becoming available.

Prevention: Animals suspected of having rabies should be avoided. Domestic pets should be immunized against rabies.

Rocky Mountain spotted fever is a rickettsial disease that is spread by the bites of infected ticks. Despite its name, the disease now is widespread and often occurs in the eastern United States. Symptoms appear about one week after infection occurs, starting with fever, headache, and chills. A rash develops on the limbs, hands, and feet three days later and soon spreads to the rest of the body. Antibiotics are used to treat the disease.

Prevention: Persons in tick-infested areas should examine the body for ticks after possible exposure. Pets should also be examined for ticks after being outdoors. A tick repellent can be useful. A vaccine is available.

Strep throat is a severe form of sore throat caused by streptococcal bacteria. It is transmitted by direct contact, and the sore throat usually develops within three days. One form of the disease is *scarlet fever*, which usually affects children aged three to thirteen. The symptoms include tonsillitis, fever, vomiting, and headache, followed by a rash that appears one to five days later. The tongue also takes on a "strawberry" appearance in color and texture. Both strep throat and scarlet fever respond well to antibiotic treatment. Recovery usually occurs within two weeks.

The real danger of streptococcal infection is rheumatic fever, which can cause permanent heart damage. A course of antibiotic therapy can prevent rheumatic fever. Persons who have been in close contact with patients should be tested to determine whether preventive antibiotic therapy is needed.

Prevention: Contact with infected persons should be kept to a minimum, and materials used by patients should be disposed of properly. Patients should cover their mouths when coughing or sneezing.

Tetanus is a dangerous disease caused by a bacterium that is anaerobic—that is, it lives where oxygen is not present. The bacteria usually enter the body through wounds that are contaminated by soil or animal feces. The first symptom is painful tightening of the jaw muscles (lockjaw), which appears within fourteen days after infection occurs and is followed within twenty-four hours by painful contractions in the rest of the body. Medical attention is essential when a wound occurs.

Prevention: A tetanus vaccine is available and is a recommended part of routine childhood immunization (table 15.1). Booster shots are recommended for persons in agriculture-related jobs or who work where the risk of injury or wounds is large.

Tuberculosis is a bacterial disease that can affect many parts of the body but is best known as a lung infection. It is usually transmitted through the air by the sputum of infected individuals, but can also be contracted by ingestion of unpasteurized dairy products from an infected cow. Tuberculosis was the second leading cause of death in the United States in 1900, but it declined to the twentieth leading cause of death in 1970. Nonetheless, tuberculosis still occurs, primarily in crowded slum areas of cities. Effective antibiotic therapy is available.

Prevention: The first line of defense against tuberculosis is good nutrition and good housing. Persons who have been in contact with an infected individual should be tested and, if necessary, should be treated with a drug such as isoniazid.

Typhus is a rickettsial disease that is transmitted to humans by the bite of head lice. Symptoms, which appear one to two weeks after infection occurs, include fever, headache, and a rash on the body. Typhus can be treated effectively with antibiotics.

Prevention: Typhus vaccines are available, but the disease is best prevented by keeping the body free of lice.

Athlete's foot is a common fungal infection that causes scaling and blisters between the toes. It is transmitted by contact with an infected person or with contaminated objects.

Prevention: Carefully clean and dry feet after swimming or bathing and wear sandals and absorbent socks. Antifungal compounds are available without prescription.

Candidiasis also called *thrush*, is caused by a fungus called *Candida albicans*. The fungus often can live in the body without doing harm, but it can proliferate abnormally, invading the mouth or other organs such as the vagina, which becomes inflamed, producing a white discharge. Candidiasis is more common in women than in men; use of oral contraceptives or of antibiotics increases the risk. It is spread by contact with feces or saliva of an infected person, or by vaginal contact. It can be transmitted from mother to newborn during childbirth, so early detection during pregnancy is essential.

Prevention: Some physicians recommend that female patients taking antibiotics eat a small amount of yogurt with active cultures daily. Bacteria in the cultures can offset the effect of the antibiotics which kill the protective strains of vaginal bacteria that normally resist the fungus. Once contracted, candidiasis is treated with the antifungal drug nystatin.

Ringworm is a fungal skin disease characterized by ring-shaped lesions on all parts of the body but the scalp, the feet, or the beard area. It occurs more often in males than in females, and it is transmitted by contact with an infected person or with contaminated articles.

Prevention: Ringworm can be prevented by careful laundering of clothing and towels, good personal hygiene, and proper maintenance of showers, baths, and gymnasiums.

CHAPTER
16

Occupational health

More than 2,000 years ago, Hippocrates first noted the effects of the environment on individual health. Even the founder of the practice of medicine could not have foreseen an environment—especially a work environment—as complex and potentially threatening to the individual as that which the modern technological-industrial society has created. Today, a separate branch of medicine designed to treat and prevent occupational-induced illness has developed. As there are comparatively few mysteries about how workplace injuries and illnesses take place, prevention can be the most effective way of "treating" them.

Society—management, labor, and the individual worker—can and must collaborate to make technology work for us without causing injury and disease. It is within our grasp, with the help of appropriate and cost-effective measures, to reach such a goal.

Glossary

ALVEOLI Air cells in the lung.

BYSSINOSIS (BROWN LUNG DISEASE) An allergylike lung disease caused by inhaling dusts of cotton, hemp, and flax.

CARCINOGENS Cancer-causing substances.

DERMATITIS Inflammation of the skin.

ERGONOMICS The study of human factors in the design and operations of machines and the physical environment.

FARMER'S LUNG Acute lung disease caused by dust from moldy hay and other vegetable products.

MESOTHELIOMA A rare form of cancer affecting the membrane lining of the chest or abdomen, linked with exposure to asbestos.

PPM Concentration of a chemical in *parts per million*.

THRESHOLD LIMITING VALUE (TLV) Legal limit of exposure to toxic chemicals.

History

In 1700, Bernardino Ramazzini, generally known as the father of occupational medicine, published a book summarizing all the existing knowledge about occupational disease. Ramazzini's book was an important landmark in medicine because for the first time it was recognized that the patient's occupational and social condition had to be known before diagnosis and treatment could begin.

Ramazzini was blessed with prescience. Some 400,000 new cases of occupationally related diseases are now reported annually, and it is estimated that 100,000 Americans die of them each year, according to the National Institute for Occupational Safety and Health. Although it is difficult to pinpoint specific occupations as causative factors in many instances, the extent of occupational disease is thought to be underestimated because the connection between job and disease often goes unrecognized or unreported. In addi-

tion, more than 13,000 workers are killed and nine million injured each year in work-related accidents. It is also probable that an additional 25 million work-related accidents occur each year but are not reported.

The U.S. Department of Labor has estimated that 20 million workers face exposure to potentially toxic substances. At the present time more than 60,000 different kinds of chemicals are in general use in industry. Some 47,000 commercial substances are listed in the Environmental Protection Agency's Toxic Substance Inventory. So far, standards of exposure have not yet been set for most of these chemicals. U.S. production of synthetic (carbon-based) organic chemicals has been doubling every seven to eight years, and now approaches 200 billion pounds a year. At a given concentration, some of these chemicals are poisonous and cause cancer. Therefore, they should be tested for toxicity and carcinogenicity, and standards of exposure should be set for workers. We also need better information to determine the ways in which workers are exposed to hazardous substances and the duration and severity of the exposure. Monitoring of specific occupational environments and the maintenance of health records for all workers are also essential steps in combating occupation-related disease.

Since 1970, these and other activities essential to an effective program of prevention and control have been centralized under the Occupational Safety and Health Administration (OSHA), created by Congress to deal with the problem on a national basis (see Worker Protection, page 611).

Health Effects of the Workplace

CHEMICALS AND THEIR POTENTIAL TOXICITY

Since World War I, American and worldwide industry has rapidly increased its use of chemicals both in quantity and in variety.

Every chemical, even table salt, can be detrimental to health under certain circumstances. The detrimental or untoward effects of chemicals are termed "toxic reactions." For a chemical to produce a toxic reaction it must reach a site in the body where that reaction can be produced, and it must reach that site in adequate quantities. *The dose/response relationship is fundamental to the understanding of diseases caused by chemical substances. That is, as the dose or quantity of a chemical absorbed by the body increases, the toxic effects of that chemical will also increase.* A companion concept important to the protection of all people working with chemicals is that it is possible to find a level of exposure that is small enough not to produce a toxic response. The search for the safe or "no effect" level of exposure is the province of the occupational health spe-

cialists. The knowledge that the toxicologist provides serves as the foundation for the protection of workers who must use chemicals.

Chemicals produce either acute or chronic effects or combinations of both. Acute effects have rapid onset; the affected people either recover or die. Chronic effects usually appear a long time after initial exposure, and their consequences are likely to be irreversible.

Of the approximately 60,000 chemicals in general use in industry today, toxicity data adequate for the establishment of standards for protection exist for only some 600 chemicals. These chemicals, however, are the ones most widely encountered by workers, and the standards serve an important role in the prevention of chemically induced occupational disease. Initially, the standards for protection of workers exposed to chemicals were based upon prevention of the acute effects of chemical exposure; in recent years, especially since the passage of the Occupational Safety and Health Act of 1970, emphasis in the development of worker protection standards has also been placed on the elimination of chronic effects.

Chronic toxicity may occur at exposure levels considerably below those necessary to produce acute effects. As a consequence of the greater attention being paid today to chronic effects, the standards for worker protection have become increasingly more stringent. The search for chronic detrimental effects is increasing both at the level of animal studies, where lifetime exposure research is going on, and at the level of workers, where increasing efforts are being made to maintain close medical surveillance of worker populations.

Standards for the protection of industrial workers exposed to chemicals principally provide information about the concentrations of chemicals in the air and focus concern on the lungs as the primary route for entry into the body. (See Worker Protection, page 611.) Other routes of exposures are also of concern, however. For instance, many chemicals enter the body through the mouth and digestive tract as a result of the contamination of hands, of food, and of smoking materials.

Not only is it important for people handling chemicals to understand the ways in which chemicals enter the body, but it is also important for them to understand the effects that chemicals will have on their bodies. Further, it is important that they understand that the transport of chemicals on contaminated clothing and shoes to the home can poison the family. Information about the effects of chemicals should be available to all persons handling chemicals in the course of their work. Such information can be obtained from the manufacturer of chemicals in the form of material safety data sheets. In the following section on health effects of chemicals, we list potential toxic chemicals by name. While these lists will seem of no interest to the average reader, they will be of help to those with known exposures.

OCCUPATIONAL DISEASES

The diseases of occupations are generally classified according to the organs or organ systems involved. Thus, the major occupational diseases are those of the skin, lungs, nervous system, liver, and kidneys. Occupational cancers are usually considered as a separate group.

Cancer

Certain occupational exposures have long been known to increase the risk for certain cancers. In the nineteenth century, the reported high rate of lung cancer recorded among certain miners in Eastern Europe was probably due to inhalation of radioactive ores. In 1895, an increased risk of

bladder cancer among dye workers was observed, and it was suggested that carcinogenic aromatic compounds were the cause. The cancers in radium dial painters and the leukemias of early radiologists were due to excessive radiation exposure. An excess of skin cancers reported among farmers in 1894 was considered to be due to prolonged exposure to sunlight (see chapter 13, Radiation).

More recently, heavy asbestos exposure has been shown to increase the risk of lung cancer, particularly in cigarette smokers. The risk of lung cancer is estimated to be more than ninety times greater in asbestos workers who smoke than in workers not exposed to asbestos who never smoked. Asbestos alone is an established cause of another form of lung cancer called *mesothelioma*.

Processing of vinyl chloride in polymerization plants induced the normally rare *angiosarcoma* of the liver. Bis(chloromethyl) ether (BCME) used in research in industry is a powerful carcinogen for nasal passages and the lungs.

Of the many chemicals in the workplace, some have been tested in experimental animals and found to be carcinogenic.

Table 16.1 is OSHA's list of those chemicals reported or suspected of being carcinogenic to humans. Evaluation of carcinogenicity is made more easily if the effect is large and the work force easily identifiable as, for example, lung cancer among asbestos workers and uranium miners, or if the cancer is normally rare, such as liver cancer in vinyl chloride workers. It is difficult to evaluate the risk if a cancer is common and the effect is small.

Estimates for the effect of occupation on cancer risk vary. Although some have estimated the percentage of work-related cancers to be as high as 20 percent, *our estimate is that at present about 5 percent of current cancers in men and less than 1 percent of cancers in women are due to occupational exposures.* Some of the variation in risk estimates is explained by the fact that not all

Table 16.1

COMMONLY USED INDUSTRIAL SUBSTANCES
REGULATED BY OSHA
AS CARCINOGENIC TO HUMANS

Asbestos
4-Nitrobiphenyl
alpha-Naphthylamine
Methyl chloromethyl ether
3,3' - Dichlorobenzidine (and its salts)
bis-Chloromethyl ether (BCME)
beta-Naphthylamine
Benzidine
4-Aminodiphenyl
Ethyleneimine
beta-Propiolactone
2-Acetylaminofluorene
4-Dimethylaminoazobenzene
N-Nitrosodimethylamine
Vinyl chloride
Coke oven emissions
Inorganic arsenic
Benzene

SOURCE: OSHA (Occupational Safety and Health Administration), U.S. Department of Labor

workers in a given high-risk occupation are exposed to the same extent or for the same length of time.

Exposure to toxic substances, of course, may extend beyond the workplace into the community in many ways (see chapters 11 and 12). A worker's clothes can transport toxic substances and dusts to his home. In one study, more than a third of the people living with asbestos workers had lung abnormalities characteristic of asbestos exposure.

Another complication is the relationship of occupational exposure to other risk factors, especially smoking. Some workers are known to be particularly heavy smokers, and because their work requires the use of both hands, the lit cigarette is kept in the mouth and deeply inhaled.

Unless smoking is taken into account, the independent effect of work exposure is often difficult to evaluate, particularly in lung and bladder cancers.

Table 16.2 lists occupations that are thought to carry an increased risk for cancer. The occupations are listed for exposure to asbestos, arsenic, radiation, and known chemical carcinogens, and also for exposure to known specific substances, such as wood dust and paint, where specific chemical agents have not as yet been identified. Not all of the occupations listed in table 16.2 have been well established as increasing the risk of cancer in humans. In those workers where the evidence of a causal relationship is strong, the risk is related to the intensity and length of exposure. Primary sites most commonly affected are the lung and bladder—the sites where environmental agents enter and their metabolites exit. Exposure to radiation and certain chemicals causes leukemias because of the sensitivity of the bone marrow to these agents.

To properly investigate occupational risk factors for cancer, we need to keep careful records for the worker's entire life, including details of occupational exposure and variations in lifestyle. With proper care by management and workers in respect to limiting or avoiding exposure to carcinogens and suspected carcinogens as preventive measures, we can do much to reduce occupational cancers. Current laboratory tests permit the rapid assessment of possible carcinogenic risks. It should be possible through proper engineering to design production lines to limit exposure to suspected carcinogens or otherwise toxic chemicals. Carcinogenic chemicals with limited benefits or advantages might be considered for phasing out. For occupational carcinogens as well as environmental hazards and toxicants in general, costs and benefits of each commercial action also have to be determined.

Table 16.2
CARCINOGENS AND PARTIAL LISTING OF WORK GROUPS AT RISK

Carcinogens	Work groups at risk	Primary site
Acrylonitrile	Synthetic fur and wig makers; acrylic fiber, plastic product resin makers; textile workers	colon, lung
4-Aminobiphenyl (no longer made for industrial use in U.S.)	Chemical research workers; formerly dyestuff manufacturers	bladder
Arsenic and certain arsenic compounds	Arsenic, Babbit metal, printing ink, typemetal workers; aniline color, brass, bronze, ceramic, fireworks, herbicide, insecticide, lead shot, paint, pigment, rodenticide, semiconductor compound makers; copper smelters; gold refiners; lead smelters; painters; silver refiners; taxidermists; textile printers; tree sprayers, water weed controllers; weed sprayers	lung, skin
Asbestos	Rubber tire industry workers; asbestos miners; textile makers; auto brake repairers; construction workers; cutters, layers of water pipes; insulation cord makers; insulators; shipyard workers	lung,* mesothelioma, gastrointestinal tract
Benzene	Shoe manufacturing, styrene makers—adhesive, glue, linoleum, maleic acid, nitrobenzene, putty, rubber, rubber tire; asbestos product impregnators; petrochemical workers—benzene hexachloride, chlorinated benzene, dry battery; burnishers; chemists; furniture finishers; shoemakers; distillers	acute leukemia, erythroleukemia
Benzidine	Clinical chemists; dye workers; plastic and rubber workers; wood chemists	bladder
N,N-Bis (2-chloroethyl)-2-napthylamine (chlornaphazine)	Research workers	bladder

Table 16.2
CARCINOGENS AND PARTIAL LISTING OF WORK GROUPS AT RISK

Carcinogens	Work groups at risk	Primary site
BCME and technical grade chloromethyl methyl ether (CMME)	Anion exchange resin production; lab. workers; organic chem. synthesizers; polymer manufacturers	lung
Chromium and certain chromium compounds	Anodizers. copper etchers; electroplaters; glass, pottery, metal, stainless steel and textile workers; lithographers; oil purifiers; photo engravers; process engravers; welders	lung, nasal sinuses
Coke oven emissions	Coke oven workers	lung, kidney
Mustard gas	Mustard gas workers	respiratory tract
2-Naphthylamine	Researchers, dyestuff manufacturers, producers of antioxidants	bladder
Nickel dusts and nickel carbonyl	Battery, ceramic, ink, magnet, paint, spark plug varnish makers; chemists; dyers; enamelers; foundry, Mond process, petroleum refinery workers; gas platers; oil hydrogenators; organic chemical synthesizers; textile dyers	lung, nasal passages
Soots, tars, and mineral oils	Cable layers; coal, gas, coke, petroleum industry, coal tar, and pitch, electrical equipment workers; fabric proofers; net fixers; optical lens grinders; waterproofers; wharfmen; wood preservers	skin, scrotum, lung, bladder
Vinyl chloride	Organic chemical synthesizers; polyvinyl resinmakers; rubber workers	liver, lung, brain, blood systems
Wood dusts	Furniture makers; wood and sawmill workers	nose, lung, colon, brain
Radon daughters (products of radioactive decay of radon)	Uranium workers	lung

*Mainly cigarette smoking *and* asbestos exposure

SOURCE: Adapted from Schottenfeld, D. and Haas, J.F. "The Workplace as a Cause of Cancer" Parts 1 and 2, *Clinical Bulletin* 8, pp. 54–60 and 107–119, 1978, and from "Improving the Quality of the Work Environment," *in* Phyllis E. Lehmann and Vicki Kalmar, M.P.H., *"Healthy People: The Surgeon General's Report on Health Promotion and Disease Prevention, Background Papers"* U.S. Dept. of Health, Education and Welfare, U.S. Gov't Printing Office, Wash., D.C.

Table 16.3
SEVERE LUNG IRRITANTS

Acrolein	Ketene
Ammonia	Maleic anhydride
Antimony	Methyl bromide
ANTU	Methylene bisphenyl isocyanate
Beryllium and beryllium compounds	Methyl iodide
Boron trifluoride	Methyl isocyanate
Bromine	Methyl mercaptan
Butyl mercaptan	Nickel carbonyl
Cadmium dust/fume	Nitric acid
Chlorine	Nitroethane
Chlorine dioxide	Nitrogen dioxide
Chlorine trifluoride	2-Nitropropane
1-Chloro–1–nitropropane	Oxygen difluoride
Chloropicrin	Ozone
Chromium acid and chromates	Paraquat
Chromium, metal and insoluble salts	Perchloromethyl mercaptan
Cotton dust, raw	Perchloryl fluoride
Diazomethane	Phosgene
Diborane	Phosphine
1,1-Dichloro–1–nitroethane	Phosphorus trichloride
Dichloroethyl ether	Phthalic anhydride
Diisopropylamine	Selenium hexafluoride
Dimethylamine	Silicone tetrafluoride
Dimethyl sulfate	Sulfur dioxide
Ethanolamine	Sulfuric acid
Ethylene chlorohydrin	Sulfur pentafluoride
Ethyleneimine	Tellurium hexafluoride
Ethylene oxide	Toluene 2,4–diisocyanate
Ethyl mercaptan	Tributyl phosphate
Fluorine	Uranium (natural), soluble and
Hydrogen chloride	insoluble compounds
Hydrogen fluoride	Vanadium pentoxide
Hydrogen sulfide	Zinc chloride fume
Iodine	

SOURCE: adapted from *Chemical Hazards of the Workplace* by Nick H. Proctor. J.B. Lippincott Co., 1978.

Lung disease

Chemicals and dust to which people are exposed in the workplace produce disease in the airways that conduct air to the parts of the lung where oxygen is absorbed and carbon dioxide is given off, and in the respiratory bronchioles, the alveoli, and the lung tissue separating the alveoli. Damage to the airways makes it difficult for air to enter and leave the lungs. Damage to the alveoli and interalveolar tissue impairs the ability of the lungs to take up oxygen from the air and release carbon dioxide. Diseases of the lungs affecting the airways are termed *obstructive lung diseases*. The diseases involving the alveoli and interalveolar lung tissue are termed restrictive lung diseases. Severe lung irritants are shown in table 16.3.

The term *restrictive* derives from the fact that the tissue of the lungs becomes stiff or has reduced compliance, usually as a result of increased fluid or collagen fibers in the interalveolar tissue. The effect on the airways can produce either constriction of those airways or chronic bronchitis in which cells in the lining of the airways produce increased amounts of mucus. Inflammatory responses may lead to increased susceptibility to infection.

The best-known of the occupational lung diseases are those produced by certain dusts. These diseases are called *pneumoconioses*; silicosis and asbestosis are classic examples. Particles of silica or asbestos deposited in the lungs have the ability to stimulate the production of fibrous tissue in the lungs. Other dusts capable of producing restrictive lung disease through fibroses are listed in table 16.4.

A variety of dusts produce benign pneumoconioses that affect the respiratory tract but do not impair the functioning of the lung. It is important therefore to distinguish between the benign pneumoconioses and those produced by fibrogenic dust. Agents causing benign pneumoconiosis are listed in table 16.5.

Table 16.4
DUSTS CAUSING LUNG FIBROSES

Aluminum powder (stamped)
Asbestos
Coal dust
Cobalt, metal fume and dust
Hematite
Kaolin (when contaminated with crystalline silica)
Silica, amorphous including diatomaceous earth (when contaminated with crystalline silica)
Silica, crystalline
Yttrium

SOURCE: adapted from *Chemical Hazards of the Workplace* by Nick H. Proctor. J.B. Lippincott Co., 1978.

Table 16.5
AGENTS CAUSING
BENIGN PNEUMOCONIOSIS

Aluminum powder
Barium and compounds
Cobalt, metal fume, and dust
Graphite, natural
Hematite
Iron oxide fume
Kaolin
Mica
Silica, amorphous, including natural diatomaceous earth
Soapstone
Stannic oxide
Talc, nonasbestos form

SOURCE: adapted from *Chemical Hazards of the Workplace* by Nick H. Proctor. J.B. Lippincott Co., 1978.

Table 16.6
LUNG SENSITIZERS

Castor bean pomace	Phthalic anhydride
Cobalt, metal fume, and dust	Platinum salts
Enzymatic detergents	Polyvinyl chloride (fume from heated film:
Grain dusts	meat wrapper's asthma)
Maleic anhydride	Toluene 2,4–diisocyanate
Methylene bisphenyl isocyanate	Tungsten carbide
Methyl isocyanate	Western red cedar dust
Nickel, metal	Wood pulp dust
p- Phenylenediamine	

SOURCE: adapted from *Chemical Hazards of the Workplace* by Nick H. Proctor. J.B. Lippincott Co., 1978.

Organic dust can produce two types of pulmonary response. The first is *allergic*, leading to the constriction of airways and producing symptoms and signs typical of asthma. The second involves the lower airways and the alveoli associated with oxygen absorption, producing a condition known as *hypersensitivity pneumonitis* or *extrinsic allergic alveolitis. Farmer's lung*, produced by bacterial spores found in moldy hay, is a well-known example. Occupational asthma is also produced by a number of chemicals capable of producing pulmonary sensitization (table 16.6). The best known of these is toluene 2,4-diisocyanate, the compound used in the manufacture of polyurethane.

Another lung disease having signs and symptoms similar to asthma but probably not having an allergic mechanism as its cause is *byssinosis*, (or brown lung disease) seen in workers exposed to the dust of cotton, hemp, and flax. As to be expected, these occupationally induced lung conditions are worsened if the workers also smoke. Since occupational lung disease can be very severely disabling and since methods for treatment are for the most part inadequate, the major focus should be on prevention.

Disease of the nervous system

Many chemicals produce damage or dysfunction in both the brain and the peripheral nerves. The site of action of chemicals depends principally upon the distribution of the chemical within the body and the biological processes affected by the chemical. In general, lipid or fat-soluble chemicals such as anesthetic gases and organic compounds like tetraethyl lead, can enter the substance of the brain with little difficulty. Materials such as calcium arsenate and inorganic lead are less easily transported from the blood to the brain and mainly affect the peripheral nervous system.

Other compounds such as methyl butyl ketone and normal hexane (n-hexane) affect both the brain and the peripheral nervous system. These chemicals have been used widely in industry for many years and, only recently, studies of exposed workers have demonstrated the damage that they are capable of doing to the peripheral nervous system. The brain and peripheral nervous system are remarkably complex biological structures; consequently, it is not surprising to note that these systems respond to industrial chemicals in a wide variety of ways. Many industrial solvents act as anesthetic agents, depressing the function of the brain (table 16.7).

Table 16.7
CENTRAL NERVOUS SYSTEM DEPRESSANTS

Acetaldehyde	Ethyl bromide
Acetone	Ethyl butyl ketone
Acetylene dichloride	Ethyl chloride
Allyl glycidyl ether	Ethylene dibromide
n- Amyl acetate	Ethylene dichloride
sec- Amyl acetate	Ethylene oxide
Benzene	Ethyl ether
Bromoform	Ethyl formate
1,3- Butadiene	Ethyl mercaptan
n- Butyl acetate	Ethylidene chloride
sec- Butyl acetate	Furfuryl alcohol
tert- Butyl acetate	Glycidol
n- Butyl alcohol	*n-* Heptane
sec- Butyl alcohol	Hexachloroethane
tert- Butyl alcohol	*n-* Hexane
n- Butyl glycidyl ether	*sec-* Hexyl acetate
Butyl mercaptan	Isoamyl acetate
Carbon disulfide	Isoamyl alcohol
Carbon tetrachloride	Isobutyl acetate
Chlorobenzene	Isobutyl alcohol
Chlorobromomethane	Isopropyl acetate
Chloroform	Isopropyl alcohol
Cresol, all isomers	Isopropyl ether
Cumene	Mesityl oxide
Cyclohexane	Methyl acetate
Cyclohexanol	Methyl acetylene
Cyclohexanone	Methyl acetylene, propadiene mixture
Cyclohexene	Methylal
Decaborane	Methyl amyl ketone
Diacetone alcohol	Methyl butyl ketone
Dichlorodifluoromethane	Methyl cellosolve acetate
Dichloroethyl ether	Methylcyclohexane
Difluorodibromomethane	Methylcyclohexanol
Diglycidyl ether	*o-* Methylcyclohexanone
Diisobutyl ketone	Methylene chloride
Dipropylene glycol methyl ether	Methyl ethyl ketone
2- Ethoxyethyl acetate	Methyl formate
Ethyl acetate	Methyl iodide
Ethyl alcohol	Methyl isobutyl carbinol
Ethyl amyl ketone	Methyl isobutyl ketone
Ethylbenzene	Methyl mercaptan

Table 16.7
CENTRAL NERVOUS SYSTEM DEPRESSANTS *(continued)*

	Methyl propyl ketone		Sulfuryl fluoride
alpha-	Methyl styrene	1,1,1,2-	Tetrachloro–2, 2–difluoroethane
	Naphtha, coal tar	1,1,2,2-	Tetrachloro–1, 2–difluoroethane
	Naphtha, petroleum distillates		Tetrachloroethane
	Nitroethane		Tetrachloroethylene
	Octane		Tetrahydrofuran
	Pentaborane		Toluene
	Pentane	1,1,1-	Trichloroethane
	Phenyl glycidyl ether	1,1,2-	Trichloroethane
	Propyl acetate		Trichloroethylene
n-	Propyl alcohol		Trichlorofluoromethane
	Propylene dichloride	1,2,3-	Trichloropropane
	Propylene oxide	1,1,2-	Trichloro–1,2,2–trifluoroethane
	Pyridine		Turpentine
	Stoddard solvent		Vinyltoluene
	Styrene		Xylene

SOURCE: adapted from *Chemical Hazards of the Workplace* by Nick H. Proctor. J.B. Lippincott Co., 1978.

Table 16.8
CONVULSANTS

	Aldrin	Methyl iodide
2-	Aminopyridine	Methyl mercaptan
	Camphor	Monomethylhydrazine
	Chlordane	Nicotine
	Crag herbicide	Nitromethane
	DDT	Oxalic acid
	Decaborane	Pentaborane
2,4-	Dichlorophenoxyacetic acid	Phenol
	Dieldrin	Rotenone
1,1-	Dimethylhydrazine	Sodium fluoroacetate
	Endrin	Strychnine
	Heptachlor	Tetraethyllead
	Hydrazine	Tetramethyllead
	Lindane	Tetramethylsuccinonitrile
	Methoxychlor	Thallium, soluble compounds
	Methyl bromide	Toxaphene
	Methyl chloride	

SOURCE: adapted from *Chemical Hazards of the Workplace* by Nick H. Proctor. J.B. Lippincott Co., 1978.

Table 16.9
TOXINS PRODUCING PERIPHERAL NEUROPATHY

Acrylamide	Mercury
Arsenic and compounds	Methyl bromide
Calcium arsenate	Methyl butyl ketone
Carbon disulfide	Thallium, soluble compounds
n- Hexane	2,4,6- Trinitrotoluene
Lead and inorganic lead compounds	Tricresyl phosphate
Lead arsenate	

SOURCE: adapted from *Chemical Hazards of the Workplace* by Nick H. Proctor. J.B. Lippincott Co., 1978.

Convulsions and other manifestations of brain stimulation are produced by a large number of chlorine-and bromine-containing organic chemicals as well as certain chemicals that have specific effects on enzyme systems (table 16.8). Both the anesthetic and convulsant effects of chemicals are largely acute, and the affected person usually will recover completely from such episodes.

Severe carbon monoxide poisoning or childhood lead poisoning produce effects that are less reversible. Signs and symptoms may include severe difficulty in walking, persistent vomiting, intermittent lethargy and stupor, followed by convulsions, hyperactivity, and coma. Approximately 25 percent of the survivors may have severe brain damage. Tetraethyllead and carbon disulfide can produce mental aberration and psychosis. These are usually reversible in the case of tetraethyllead poisoning, but may not be reversible in the case of carbon disulfide poisoning.

Chronic manganese poisoning may produce a condition similar to Parkinson's disease with a masklike face, muscle rigidity, tremor of the upper extremities and head, and impaired gait. The effects of chemicals on the peripheral nervous system may be seen in either the sensory nerves or the motor nerves or in a combination of sensory and motor nerves. Either the fatty myelin sur-

rounding the nerve or the body or the fibers of the nerve cells themselves may be damaged. The peripheral nerve effects caused by occupational exposure to chemicals are generally bilaterally distributed and more frequently seen in the lower extremities than in the upper extremities.

The effects of lead are principally on the motor nerves, usually in the arms more than in the legs, with the arm most frequently used being more affected. Other chemicals used in industry tend to affect both motor and sensory nerves. A list of chemicals found to affect the peripheral nerves is provided in table 16.9.

Since many of the neurotoxins are absorbable through the skin, special precautions beyond those of control of air concentrations must be taken to protect workers. Some of these chemicals are capable of penetrating rubber gloves and, consequently, the proper selection of skin protection materials must be made. Since the brain and peripheral nervous system are susceptible to many diseases and to the effects of many pharmaceutical agents, the diagnosis of occupationally caused nervous system disease must be made with great care.

Liver disease

In past years the major cause of occupational liver disease was carbon tetrachloride, widely used in industry as a degreaser and as a dry cleaning agent in dry cleaning establishments. Because it produced liver disease in some people, but not in others, it took a number of years to convince industry that it was indeed a dangerous substance. This variability in response is related to an important characteristic of the liver itself.

The liver has the capability to metabolically convert a wide number of substances. Liver metabolism causes compounds such as carbon tetrachloride to change to a more toxic substance. This metabolic change is caused by enzymes in the liver, whose activity can be greatly enhanced by other substances, e.g., barbiturates and DDT. Alcohol also markedly enhances the toxicity of carbon tetrachloride and other chlorinated hydrocarbons such as chloroform, trichloroethylene, and 1,1,2-trichlorethane. Chemicals used in industry produce two principal changes. One is the accumulation of fatty materials, principally triglycerides, within liver cells. This process appears to be reversible. The other is the death of liver cells. Because of the regenerative capability of liver cells, recovery from all but massive cellular destruction also occurs. Table 16.10 provides a list of chemicals used in industry capable of producing liver disease. The liver disease produced by industrial chemicals is clearly related to dose, and the dose-response relationship of industrial chemicals makes it possible for the prevention of liver disease by the control of exposure.

Table 16.10
LIVER TOXINS

Acetylene tetrabromide	Hexachloronaphthalene
Carbon disulfide	Kepone
Carbon tetrachloride	Nitroethane
Chlorodiphenyl, 42% chlorine	Octachloronapthalene
Chlorodiphenyl, 54% chlorine	Pentachloronaphthalene
Chloroform	
p- Dichlorobenzene	Picric acid
Dimethylacetamide	Tetrachloroethane
Dimethylformamide	Tetrachloroethylene
Dioxane	Tetrachloronaphthalene
Ethylene chlorohydrin	Tetryl
Ethylene dibromide	Trichloronaphthalene
Ethylene dichloride	2,4,6- Trinitrotoluene

SOURCE: adapted from *Chemical Hazards of the Workplace* by Nick H. Proctor. J.B. Lippincott Co., 1978.

Kidney disease

Occupational kidney disease can occur either acutely or chronically, with the kidney tubule as the site where toxic materials are most likely to be concentrated. Before carbon tetrachloride was recognized as a serious industrial hazard, it caused a significant amount of acute hidden damage. Excessive exposure to heavy metals can cause *chronic kidney damage*. Of these, cadmium and lead constitute the most serious sources. Complications of lead-induced kidney disease include *gout* and *hypertension*. Fortunately, modern control methods for protecting lead and cadmium workers have significantly reduced the instance of kidney disease. Table 16.11 lists a number of industrial chemicals capable of producing kidney disease.

Skin disease

Occupational skin diseases are seldom life threatening; however, they lead to discomfort and loss of time on the job, and are by far the most frequently occurring of all the occupational diseases. Often, affected workers must be transferred from one job to another and, occasionally, they are no longer able to continue work in a given industry (table 16.12). The most frequent are those caused by direct contact with primary irritant chemicals—those that react directly on the site of contact. These can be strong acids or strong alkalies, solvents, oxidizing and reducing agents, and the salts of certain metals (see table 16.13). How these materials produce *primary irritant contact dermatitis* is not well understood.

Another form of contact dermatitis results from direct exposure to chemicals capable of producing an *allergic response* within the skin. Approximately 20 percent of occupational contact dermatitis is the result of this sort of allergic re-

Table 16.11
KIDNEY TOXINS

4- Aminodiphenyl
Carbon disulfide
Carbon tetrachloride
Chloroform
Dioxane
Ethylene chlorohydrin
Ethylene dibromide
Mercury
Oxalic acid
Picric acid
Tetrachloroethane
2,4,6- Trinitrotoluene
Turpentine
Uranium (natural), soluble and insoluble compounds

SOURCE: adapted from *Chemical Hazards of the Workplace* by Nick H. Proctor. J.B. Lippincott Co., 1978.

sponse. Chemicals such as the amine hardeners for epoxy resins, nickel, and formaldehyde have a marked capability for producing allergic responses, and a very large number of other chemicals used in industry are also allergenic (see table 16.14).

It is frequently difficult to determine whether or not a patient's contact dermatitis is due to primary irritation or to sensitization leading to an allergic response. Clinically, they may be quite similar, and yet the distinction between these two forms of occupational skin disease is important. Once the dermatitis has been treated and the skin has cleared, the worker with primary irritant dermatitis can in most cases be returned to the former job with precautions to reduce the amount of exposure through the use of gloves or to change the methods of handling the primary irritant chemical. These precautions may not be helpful for the worker who has become sensitized, however. It is frequently very difficult to return such a person to the former job situation. Once sensitized, the

Table 16.12
WORK GROUPS EXPOSED TO PRIMARY
SKIN IRRITANTS AND ALLERGIC SENSITIZERS

Primary skin irritants	Work groups
Acids	
Nitric (fuming nitric acid)	Rocket fuel handlers, nitroglycerine makers, aircraft workers
Phosphoric	Fertilizer and animal feed manufacturers; rust inhibitors, wax and rubber latex makers
Acetic	Drycleaners, tannery workers
Alkalies	
Soaps	Cloth preparers, laundry workers, ink makers, athletes, bartenders, household workers, restaurant workers
Cement	Cement workers, brick masons, tunnel builders
Butylamines	Chemists, insecticide workers, dye and rubber makers
Metal salts	
Chromium and alkaline chromates	Textile dye and steel workers
Zinc chloride	Battery makers, cotton sizers, disinfectant makers, dyers, electroplaters, embalmers, galvanizers, mordanters, nickel platers, print makers, plumbers, rubber workers, solderers, taxidermists, wood preservers
Solvents	
Alcohol methyl	Bronzers, furniture polishers
Chlorinated trichloroethylene	Dry cleaners, degreasers
Coal tar benzol	Bronzers, coal tar workers, histology technicians, rubber workers, shoemakers
Ketones acetone	Bronzers, painters
Petroleum benzene	Furniture polishers

Primary skin irritants	Work groups
Gasoline	Automobile assembly workers, auto mechanics, construction workers, garage workers, petro refinery workers, rocket fuel handlers
Turpentine	Bronzers, dry cleaners, furniture polishers, ink makers, print makers, optical workers, printers, photographers, rubber workers
Allergic sensitizers	
Metals	
Mercury	Battery makers—alloy, pigment, mercury vapor lamp, fungicide, herbicide, antiseptics, latex paint, electrical industry; nuclear industry (waste purification); chemical industry workers, dentists, and dental technicians
Plants	
Anacardiaceae *toxicodendron radicans* (poison ivy)	Forest rangers, farmers, gardeners
Resin systems	
Epoxy	Aircraft workers, automobile mechanics, brick masons, cable splicers, cement workers, electric apparatus workers, electricians, garage workers, histology technicians, road workers
Rubber chemicals	
Hexamethylene-tetramine	Drug, explosives, fuel tablet, resin, rubber, phenol and urea-formaldehyde resin workers; textile makers

SOURCE: Adapted from *Patty's Industrial Hygiene and Toxicology,* 3d ed. Vols. I, II, III (Clayton, G.D. and Clayton, F.E., eds) John Wiley and Sons, N.Y. 1978 and *Occupational Diseases: A Guide to Their Recognition.* Rev. ed. June 1977. U.S. Dept. Health, Education and Welfare (NIOSH) Pub. No. 77–181. Public Health Service Center for Disease Control.

Table 16.13
PRIMARY IRRITANTS OF THE SKIN

Acetaldehyde	Chlorobromomethane
Acetic acid	Chlorodiphenyl, 42% chlorine
Acetic anhydride	Chlorodiphenyl, 54% chlorine
Acetone	Chloroform
Acrolein	Chloropicrin
Acrylamide	Chloroprene
Acrylonitrile	Chromic acid and chromates
Allyl alcohol	Chromium, soluble chromic and
Allyl chloride	chromous salts
Allyl glycidyl ether	Coal tar pitch volatiles
Ammonia	Copper dust and mists
n- Amyl acetate	Crag herbicide
sec- Amyl acetate	Cresol, all isomers
Antimony	Crotonaldehyde
Arsenic and compounds	Cumene
Barium and compounds	Cyanides (alkali)
Benzene	Cyclohexane
Benzoyl peroxide	Cyclohexanol
Benzyl chloride	Cyclohexanone
Beryllium and beryllium compounds	Cyclohexene
Boron oxide	DDT
Boron trifluoride	Diacetone alcohol
Bromine	Dibutyl phosphate
n- Butyl acetate	*o-* Dichlorobenzene
sec- Butyl acetate	*p-* Dichlorobenzene
n- Butyl alcohol	1,1- Dichloro-1-nitroethane
sec- Butyl alcohol	Diethylamine
tert- Butyl alcohol	Diethylaminoethanol
n- Butylamine	Diglycidyl ether
n- Butyl glycidyl ether	Diisobutyl ketone
Calcium arsenate	Dimethylamine
Calcium oxide	Dimethylformamide
Carbaryl	1,1- Dimethylhydrazine
Carbon disulfide	Dimethyl sulfate
Carbon tetrachloride	Dioxane
Chlorinated diphenyl oxide	Epichlorhydrin
Chlorine	Epoxy resins
Chlorine trifluoride	Ethanolamine
Chloroacetaldehyde	2- Ethoxyethanol
alpha- Chloroacetophenone	2- Ethoxyethyl acetate
Chlorobenzene	Ethyl acetate
o- Chlorobenzylidene malononitrile	Ethyl acrylate

Ethylamine
Ethyl amyl ketone
Ethylbenzene
Ethyl bromide
Ethyl butyl ketone
Ethylenediamine
Ethylene dibromide
Ethylene dichloride
Ethyleneimine
Ethylene oxide
Ethyl ether
Ethyl formate
Ethylidene chloride
Ethyl silicate
Fluoride
Fluorine
Formaldehyde
Formic acid
Furfural
Glycidol
n- Heptane
Hexachloronaphthalene
n- Hexane
Hydrazine
Hydrogen bromide
Hydrogen chloride
Hydrogen fluoride
Hydrogen peroxide, 90%
Iodine
Isoamyl acetate
Isobutyl alcohol
Isophorone
Isopropylamine
Isopropyl ether
Isopropyl glycidyl ether
Ketene
Lead arsenate
Lithium hydride
Maleic anhydride
Mercury
Mercury, alkyl compounds
Mesityl oxide

Methyl acetate
Methyl acrylate
Methylal
Methyl alcohol
Methylamine
Methyl bromide
Methyl butyl ketone
Methyl chloride
Methylcyclohexane
Methylcyclohexanol
o- Methylcyclohexanone
Methylene bisphenyl isocyanate
Methylene chloride
Methyl ethyl ketone
Methyl iodide
Methyl isobutyl ketone
Methyl isocyanate
Methyl methacrylate
Methyl propyl ketone
$alpha$- Methyl styrene
Monomethylhydrazine
Morpholine
Naled
Naphtha, coal tar
Naphtha, petroleum distillates
Nickel, metal
Nitric acid
Nitrobenzene
Nitroethane
Nitromethane
Octachloronaphthalene
Octane
Osmium tetroxide
Oxalic acid
Pentaborane
Pentachloronaphthalene
Pentachlorophenol
Pentane
Perchloromethyl mercaptan
Phenol
p- Phenylenediamine
Phenyl ether

Table 16.13
PRIMARY IRRITANTS OF THE SKIN *(continued)*

Phenyl ether-biphenyl mixture	Tellurium
Phenyl glycidyl ether	Terphenyls
Phenylhydrazine	Tetrachloroethane
Phosgene	Tetrachloroethylene
Phosphoric acid	Tetrachloronaphthalene
Phosphorus (yellow)	Tetranitromethane
Phosphorus pentachloride	Tetryl
Phosphorus pentasulfide	Thiram
Phosphorus trichloride	Tin, organic and inorganic
Phthalic anhydride	compounds
Picric acid	Toluene
Platinum, soluble salts	Toluene 2,4-diisocyanate
Portland cement	*o-* Toluidine
Propyl acetate	Toxaphene
n- Propyl alcohol	Tributyl phosphate
Propylene dichloride	1,1,1- Trichloroethane
Propylene imine	Trichloroethylene
Propylene oxide	Trichloronaphthalene
Pyrethrum	2,4,5- Trichlorophenoxyacetic acid
Pyridine	1,2,3- Trichloropropane
Quinone	1,1,2- Trichloro-1,2,2-trifluoroethane
Rotenone	Triethylamine
Selenium compounds	2,4,6- Trinitrotoluene
Silver, metal and soluble compounds	Turpentine
Sodium hydroxide	Uranium (natural), soluble and
Stoddard solvent	insoluble compounds
Styrene	Vanadium pentoxide
Sulfur dioxide	Vinyltoluene
Sulfur monochloride	Xylene
Sulfuric acid	Zinc chloride fume

SOURCE: adapted from *Chemical Hazards of the Workplace* by Nick H. Proctor. J.B. Lippincott Co., 1978.

Table 16.14
SKIN SENSITIZERS

Acetaldehyde	Iodine
Acetic acid (rare)	Isopropyl glycidyl ether
Acetic anhydride	Maleic anhydride
Allyl glycidyl ether	Mercury
Arsenic and compounds	Naphthalene
Benzoyl peroxide	Nickel, metal
Beryllium and beryllium compounds	Nitrobenzene
n-Butyl glycidyl ether	p-Phenylenediamine
Chromic acid and chromates	Phenyl glycidyl ether
Cobalt, metal fume and dust	Phenylhydrazine
Copper dusts and mists	Phthalic anhydride
Cresol, all isomers	Picric acid
o-Dichlorobenzene	Platinum, soluble salts
Epoxy resins	Pyrethrum
Ethyl acrylate	Selenium compounds
Ethylenediamine	Tetryl
Ferbam	Thiram
Formaldehyde	Toluene 2,4–diisocyanate
Formic acid	2,4,6- Trinitrotoluene
	Vanadium pentoxide

SOURCE: adapted from *Chemical Hazards of the Workplace* by Nick H. Proctor. J.B. Lippincott Co., 1978.

worker may develop a repeated episode of allergic dermatitis with remarkably small levels of exposure. Information about the exposure, the relationship of exposure to onset of signs and symptoms, and the distribution over the body of the dermatitis will frequently help the dermatologist with special knowledge about occupational skin disease to differentiate between the forms of contact dermatitis. Occasionally, diagnostic patch testing by a dermatologist will be required.

Prevention of occupational dermatitis depends upon control of exposure and provisions for good personal hygiene. Frequent cleansing of the skin with solvents may destroy the normal protective mechanisms of the skin and paves the way for both forms of contact dermatitis. Certain chemicals known as photosensitizers are capable of producing dermatitis only after exposure to light.

ACCIDENTS

For every one hundred workers in private industry, there were 9.4 occupational injuries and illnesses in 1978, according to the Labor Department's Bureau of Labor Statistics. Their data was obtained from a selected sample of businesses regulated by the Occupational Safety and Health Administration.

However, the Bureau of Labor Statistics does not receive data from businesses employing fewer than eleven workers—those companies that do not have to report to OSHA—nor does it cover public sector jobs.

The causes of work-related accidents are shown in table 16.15. Certain types of industry are more accident-prone. The incidence of deaths by industry is listed in table 16.16.

Table 16.15
CAUSES OF WORK-RELATED DEATHS*

Causes	Percentage
Over-the-road motor vehicles	29
Falls	13
Industrial vehicles and equipment	9
Heart attacks	9
Electrocutions	7
Aircraft crashes	7
Struck by objects other than vehicles or equipment	5
Caught in, under, or between objects other than vehicles or equipment	4
Explosions	4
Plant machinery operations	3
Fires	3
Gas inhalations	3
Gun shots	3
All other	2
Total	100

*in private sector companies with 11 or more employees
SOURCE: U.S. Department of Labor, Bureau of Labor Statistics, 1978.

Injuries to the back and trunk represent 26 percent of all worker compensation cases in the U.S. and account for the largest amount of compensation insurance payments, according to the National Safety Council. Many back and trunk injuries are caused by inappropriate lifting, sitting, or carrying. Swelling and inflammation of joints often result from extended improper use of the body. Many of these injuries can be prevented through proper design of the worker's equipment and work setting (see Ergonomics, page 615). Cramped work settings are exacerbated by obesity, which also reduces agility and increases fatigue.

Alcohol is thought to be a factor in about 10 percent of all fatal work-related accidents. In addition, a problem drinker is likely to have many more accidents on the job than a non- or moderate drinker. Drugs and industrial chemicals like toluene, as well as alcohol, can impair the worker's judgment and reflexes, causing accidents. (See chapters 2 and 3.)

The fact that serious injury afflicts nearly 10 percent of the work force and threatens many more indicates the low priority given to safety standards in the workplace.

PHYSICAL AGENTS

As with the chemicals found in industry, the physical agents occupy a wide spectrum. They range from the mechanical forces of vibration and atmospheric pressures including those rapid changes in atmospheric pressure that are perceived by the ear as noise, to segments of the electromagnetic spectrum, which range from radio waves, at one end to radiant heat and visible and ultraviolet light, X rays, and gamma radiation at the other end. The relationship between health and the important segments of the electromagnetic spectrum are discussed in chapter 13, Radiation. The occupational health aspects of temperature extremes, noise, and vibration are discussed below.

Temperature extremes

The human body functions comfortably within a very narrow range of external temperatures: an average temperature of 73°F and 45 percent humidity. Depending on the nature of the work done, the further the temperature moves away from the comfort average, the harder the body has to work to maintain its internal temperature.

In seeking to control internal temperature, the body uses certain mechanisms in response to varying temperatures and humidities. Environmental heat is offset by sweating through the body's two-and-a-half million sweat glands. Excess body heat is evaporated from the skin sur-

Table 16.16
INCIDENCE OF DEATHS BY INDUSTRY

Type of industry	Private sector annual average employment Percentage of work force	Fatalities Percentage of fatalities
Manufacturing	33	26
Construction	5	20
Transportation and public utilities	8	18
Wholesale and retail trade	24	14
Service	21	8
Mining	1	8
Finance, insurance, and real estate	6	4
Agriculture, forestry, and fishing	1	2
Total	100	100

SOURCE: U.S. Department of Labor, Bureau of Labor Statistics, 1978.

face. In addition, the small blood vessels of the skin dilate, thus bringing body heat to the surface where it can be dissipated.

Cold air is dealt with in two ways: (1) the blood vessels leading to the skin, hands, and feet constrict in order to minimize blood flow and body heat loss through such surfaces; (2) shivering helps to generate compensatory heat. In responding to conditions of the heat and cold, the body is stressed: heart and pulse rates increase, and body chemistry changes.

Where physical exertion is required in high outside temperatures (farming, steel mills), the body is increasingly inefficient at maintaining its internal temperature balance. The body, however, is more efficient at dissipating excess heat than in coping with extreme cold. There are three increasingly severe reactions to heat stress. The mildest, resulting from excessive loss of salt, are heat cramps—spasms of voluntary muscles and

severe abdominal pain. *Heat exhaustion* or fainting is another reaction to unaccustomed high temperatures. Signs of heat exhaustion include dizziness, profuse sweating, fainting, and clammy skin. Dehydration and loss of salts are the cause of this condition. *Heat stroke,* the most serious form of heat stress, requires hospitalization; it is precipitated by extreme physical exertion or heat exposure and is seen most often in the elderly or those with chronic illnesses. Symptoms include very high body temperature, hot and dry skin without sweat, and confused, disoriented behavior leading to delirium, collapse, and coma.

It is extremely important to have an adequate supply of drinking water in a hot work environment. Thirst is an inadequate stimulus to fluid intake under heat stress conditions, and workers must be encouraged to drink increased amounts of fluids. Salt intake should be increased through the salting of food, not through the use of salt tablets. Unacclimatized workers should be allowed five to seven days of increasing activity in hot environments to allow for acclimatization to occur.

Temperatures too low for comfort (in outdoor construction work, fishing, telephone line repairing, etc.) can produce effects ranging from muscular numbness and stiffness and acute emotional distress to frostbite. Chilled and desensitized hands and fingers increase the probability of malfunctioning and accident. Workers continually exposed to cold without freezing combined with damp, even submersion into water, may get trench foot, or immersion foot. Below normal body temperatures may also result from prolonged cold exposure and the risk is increased by drugs or alcohol. Cold can aggravate existing vascular problems. Those working outdoors in extreme winter temperatures without adequate protection run the risk of frostbite.

Noise

The main threat of industrial noise is prolonged exposure gradually resulting in permanent reduction of hearing ability. This generally occurs at sound levels higher than 80 decibels as shown in table 16.17 (see chapter 14, Noise). The higher the sound level, the greater the danger of hearing impairment, whether the noise pollution is steady or intermittent.

In 1976, of the more than 14 million industrial workers exposed to noise in U.S. production industries, forty percent were exposed to noise of 85–90 decibels; 30 percent to levels higher than 90 decibels; and 30 percent to levels lower than 85 decibels. The percentage of workers whose hearing is permanently impaired doubles as their exposure to noise increases from 80–85 decibels, and doubles again from 85–90 decibels.

Table 16.17
SELECTED WORK PROCESSES AND LOCATIONS WITH WORK LEVELS OF 80 DECIBELS AND ABOVE

Decibels*	Work processes
over 130	jet engines
	pneumatic hammer riveting on steel tank
up to 129	propeller airplane engines
	riveting guns
	horns
	pneumatic chippers
up to 119	pneumatic air hoist
	corrugating machines
	internal combustion engine testing
	sandblasting
	subways
up to 109	gas, oil, and electric furnaces
	lathes (automatic wood, turret ram type)
	pneumatic equipment
	riveting, chipping operations
	forging, hammering
	sawing (circular, cutting metal, and wood, friction, cutting steel)
up to 99	steel making, foundries
	mill processing, grinding
	welding (butt electric, gas on steel, and tube-welding machines)
	wood sanding and sawing
	lathes (engine, turret, other than ram type)
	shot blast room
	operating medium to heavy trucks, snowmobiles, and diesel locomotives
	furniture making
	directing traffic
up to 89	machine and woodworking
	grinding
	automatic lathes
	arc welding
	laundries
	spraying and varnishing

*Each 10 decibel increase represents an increase of 10 *times* the intensity; thus, 99 decibels is 10 times louder than 89 decibels.
SOURCE: data adapted from Jeanne M. Stellman and Susan M. Daum, *Work is Dangerous to Your Health*, Vintage Books, New York, 1973.

The Occupational Safety and Health Administration permits an upper limit of 90 decibels, and has proposed a reduction to 85, which would bring at least 70 percent of the exposed workers under mandatory protection. The change has been strongly opposed by industry on economic grounds.

Noise also produces effects beyond reduction of hearing ability. As in any environment, noise at work fosters stress. It heightens tensions, adds to fatigue, interferes with concentration, makes communication difficult, and in general detracts from the quality of life.

In an office, noise distractions can produce stress without inducing hearing loss. Masking systems have been instituted in some work environments. Called "white" or "pink" noise, the masking sound resembles a sustained hiss. These systems were designed to eliminate distracting noises by covering them up. However, the long-term effects of the masking sounds are not yet known.

Noise also intensifies any existing dangers to safety and health. For example, warnings or instructions may not be heard or fully understood. Workers may not hear abnormal sounds that indicate possible danger in operating machinery or equipment. In addition, noise can adversely affect other sensory systems and result in reduced ability to perform tasks, not only competently, but also safely.

Vibration

About 8 million U.S. workers are exposed to some form of vibration. It can affect the whole body, as in the case of drivers and operators of heavy equipment, or vibration can be segmental, affecting the hands and arms, as do vibrating hand tools such as chain saws and pneumatic drills.

Whole-body vibration Not much is known about the chronic health effects of whole-body vibration, although it may be considered to induce stress. At some frequencies, the human body may be in resonance with the vibration, thus amplifying it. When the body is in resonance it is thought to be most susceptible to the vibration effects. Whole-body vibration can cause an *increase in oxygen consumption, increased breathing, and short bursts of rapid heart rate*. People exposed to intense low-frequency vibration occasionally feel unstable. The long-term health effects of whole-body vibration have been alleged to include *injury to the bone structure, gastrointestinal tract problems, varicose veins, enlargement of scrotal veins, and piles*. Workers also report weakness, loss of appetite, nausea, and irritability. However, these effects have not been documented in long-term scientific studies. Occupations where workers may be at risk to whole-body vibration include:

- Truck drivers and terminal workers
- Farm vehicle and tractor operators
- Intercity and local bus drivers
- Heavy equipment operators
- Foundry workers
- Metal stamping operators
- Steel mill and blast furnace workers
- Printing and publishing press operators
- Fork lift operators
- Lumber mill and wood product manufacturing operators
- Underground miners
- Railway workers
- Autobody stamping workers
- Textile machine operators

Segmental vibration The most pronounced effect of hand-arm vibration is Raynaud's phenomenon, or vibration white finger (VWF), an *episodic disturbance of blood flow in the fingers*. The first symptom of VWF is bouts of blanching of the fingers. These become more frequent, longer, and more severe as the disease progresses. Other effects are numbness and some loss of muscle control, and reduction of sensitivity to heat, cold, and pain. Eventually, the person with VWF loses the ability to use the fingers in fine tasks, such as picking up coins or buttoning clothing. VWF is often not recognized as compensable as an occupational disease, although it may severely restrict the victim's employment opportunities. The latent period between beginning work with vibrating tools and onset of symptoms can be as short as several months. The extent of the problem in most industries using vibrating tools is not known.

Other effects of segmental vibration include bone changes, muscular weaknesses, and degenerative alterations, inflammation of the tendons, bone cysts, and vascular changes.

REPRODUCTIVE HEALTH

Incomplete information and lack of research surround the issue of reproductive health and the effects of the workplace. Until very recently, efforts by employers to preserve and protect the reproductive health of workers have primarily been directed to women of childbearing age, specifically within industries where heavy metals such as lead were used. The method used to protect these women was to transfer them to different jobs and to prohibit them from working with the known toxic substances. This practice not only discriminated against the women, but it also did not protect the men who worked with the same substances. In some cases, women wanting to retain their jobs were voluntarily sterilized.

To compound the problem of limited research to date there is very little data associating reproductive problems with employment histories. The need is acute for employers to keep good records on workplace substances and employee's contact with them. This requires development and maintenance of a comprehensive monitoring system.

The pregnant worker

It is generally accepted by scientists that the greatest period of risk in pregnancy occurs in the first three months when the fetus undergoes organ development. It is estimated that at least half of American women with two children are employed up to the seventh month of pregnancy. Nearly 60 percent of all women bearing a first child are employed.

Under healthful conditions there is no reason for the pregnant woman not to work. However, the large number of working women coupled with much wider use of toxic substances in the workplace means that the need for identification and assessment of risks to reproductive health becomes pressing.

At present, little information is available on the association between reproductive history and workers in the field of medicine, which employs a large number of women. Many workers in this field are exposed to radiation from X-ray machines and radioactive chemicals. Exposure to radiation is known to be extremely hazardous in pregnancy, and at high-dosage levels it causes *sterility* and *infertility* in males and females. However, the effects of long-term exposure to low levels of radiation typical of the exposure of workers in the medical field are not yet known. The long latency period involved in low-level exposure to radiation is particularly significant in reproduction. Subtle damage to genetic material may result in *birth defects* not directly traceable to the employment experience (see chapter 13, Radiation; see also chapters 6, 4, 1, and 2 on Family Planning and Childbearing, Tobacco, Nutrition, and Alcohol where the interrelationships of smoking, caffeine, alcohol, and pregnancy are discussed.)

STRESS

The work environment—including noise, restricted space, lack of ventilation, time constraints—may all be stressful at some time to some people, particularly in extreme situations. Other factors such as working hours, boredom, the commuter trip, employee-employer relationship, job security, upward mobility, are all common stressful experiences.

Their effect on health, however, is difficult to measure in part because stress is difficult to standardize (see chapter 7, Stress), and in part because stress has an impact on personal habits such as smoking, eating, drinking, alcohol, and drugs. If individuals become overstressed by their work environment, possibly because they feel entrapped by it, they may seek relief from their frustrations by overeating or excessive smoking or drinking, thus putting themselves at increased risk for certain diseases.

Whether a reduction of a stressful environment can lead to an improvement of personal habits is discussed in chapters 1, 2, 3, and 4 on Nutrition, Alcohol, Drugs and Tobacco. There is much the employer and the employee can do to reduce stress at the workplace, especially by the establishment of good communication.

Preventive Strategies for Worker Protection

Preventive medicine recognizes no distinction between the work and home environments. The good or bad health habits acquired by an individual in one setting are inevitably carried over to the other. But the prevention of occupationally-related illness, disease, and disability requires much more than the individual worker's vigilance. The potential hazards of the workplace cannot always be controlled by the men and women who work there. Thus, an effective program of prevention requires a comprehensive ap-

proach involving government, management, and labor. To some extent, the interests of these three forces are in conflict. Management is necessarily committed to maximum profit, whereas labor is inevitably committed to maximum safety. This divergence of objectives creates honest differences over questions of the cost of preventive measures versus the benefits derived from them. Government, committed to the welfare of the nation as a whole, must take the role of regulator and mediator.

The role of preventive medicine, as always, is to provide the hard data from which decisions can be made. Table 16.18 lists the measures that can be taken to protect workers' health.

The basic principles for preventing occupational illness, disease, and disability include:

- Monitor toxic substance exposure in work environment
- Monitor individual worker's health with timely notification of findings to worker
- Keep ongoing occupational health record for each worker
- Provide basic information routinely to worker about pertinent toxic substances and effects in understandable language using generic names of hazardous agents
- Restructure existing workplace and jobs to eliminate and reduce hazardous health conditions according to standards set by governing agencies
- Initiate engineering design for equipment, machinery, and work structure that is conducive to good health and minimizes hazardous environments
- Practice healthful lifestyles to promote general well-being—smoking cessation, weight reduction, a physical fitness program, moderate or no drinking, 7–8 hours of sleep, and controlled blood pressure. Follow the American Health Foundation Food plan on page 158.

Table 16.18
MEASURES TO PROTECT WORKERS' HEALTH

Condition	Means for Control
Cancer	• Contain or eliminate exposure to carcinogens • Substitute less toxic substances when possible • Reduce levels of exposure • Require protective equipment until problem controlled
Reproductive health	• Avoid and/or eliminate hazardous substances • Substitute safe substances • Assure full benefits, seniority, and work rights if pregnancy necessitates temporary transfer
Respiratory conditions	• Use proper ventilation • Eliminate or reduce exposure to harmful substances • Use correct respirator type, well fitted to each worker
Skin	• Avoid irritants, sensitizers • Use barrier creams • Use appropriate personal protective equipment • Follow correct cleaning procedures using soaps or solvents
Stress	• Maintain clean facilities, proper lighting • Limit noise level to less than 80 decibels • Rotate jobs • Promote job enlargement, job enrichment, autonomous work groups • Develop and encourage body tension/stress reduction mechanisms and techniques • Redesign workplace if necessary • Analyze human factors of jobs to ease stress of physical tasks
Infection	• Avoid infectious agents • Vaccinate, innoculate • Give immediate attention to bites, cuts, scratches

Table 16.18
MEASURES TO PROTECT WORKERS' HEALTH *(continued)*

Condition	Means for Control
	• Use gloves
	• Wash affected areas with soap and water
	• Use disinfectants
	• Handle specimen properly
	• Sterilize equipment
	• Ventilate adequately
	• Correct maintenance and waste disposal
	• Isolate infected person or animal
Accidents and injuries	• Maintain equipment properly
	• Use equipment and machinery designed for human factor
	• Assure appropriate job design
	• Handle equipment properly
	• Follow correct housekeeping procedures
	• Make sure lighting is adequate
	• Establish engineering controls oriented to good health
Noise	• Use hearing protectors (muffs or plugs)
	• Screen workers
	• Use noise absorbent materials in environment
	• Use noise reduction shield
	• Use equipment designed to reduce noise levels
	• Conform work environment to meet maximum noise exposure levels of 90 decibels for 8 hours to 105 decibels for one hour
Vibration	• Use equipment designed to absorb vibrations
	• Use suspension seats in transport vehicle
	• Use absorbent rubber padding
	• Rotate tasks requiring hand-arm vibration tasks
	• Limit workday exposure to vibration
Temperature extremes	• Rotate jobs to reduce time exposure
	• Assure adequate climate control
	• Wear proper clothing without safety interference

SOURCE: Division of Occupational Health and Toxicology, American Health Foundation, New York, New York.

LABOR'S ROLE

Labor unions, which represent about one-quarter of the American work force, are firmly committed to obtaining the maximum amount of protection for workers on the job. The unions support OSHA, seek to strengthen its powers and its purse, and monitor its work. Unions negotiate health and safety provisions in their collective bargaining agreements with management, and participate in worker-management health and safety committees. The unions provide training for their members in industrial hygiene and proper work procedures. In case of disputes, the unions represent workers who have complaints.

Naturally, these activities can be undertaken by any group of workers, whether organized as a labor union or not.

THE WORKER'S ROLE

You as an individual worker have the highest stake in occupational health and safety.

Take an intelligent interest in your work surroundings. Join the plant's health and safety committee. Be on the lookout for hazards and call them to the attention of the appropriate authorities; follow up until they are properly dealt with. Make suggestions.

If, for whatever reason, your job is causing you stress, try to eliminate the reasons. If you can't, try to get shifted to another function or even to get another job.

Conduct yourself sensibly in your work. If personal protection equipment is called for in your job, use it—and use it properly and consistently no matter what it is—respirators, safety shoes, safety goggles and glasses, hard hats, gloves, ear muffs and plugs, or protective clothing. Don't cut corners. If the equipment is cumbersome, uncomfortable, or doesn't fit, try to get it improved, but in the meantime use it.

Maintain a sensible lifestyle outside your workplace. If you are in good health generally, you are less likely to be harmed by workplace hazards. If you are an asbestos worker and smoke cigarettes, your chance of getting lung cancer is far greater than that of a nonsmoker. If you are a problem drinker, your chance of having an on-the-job accident is three and one-half times greater than that of a nondrinker.

Know your right to complain. You have the right to complain to OSHA about work hazards without fear of reprisal. OSHA protects the identity of complainants who request it and will seek redress for workers who have been discriminated against by their employers for complaining to OSHA. You can file your complaint through your union or some other group of workers.

Know your right to information. You—or your union or your designated representative with your written permission—have the right to examine and copy your employer's records of exposures to toxic substances, your personal medical records and analyses based on these records. Exposure records include environmental and biological monitoring information, including your past and present exposure to harmful substances. Medical records include your medical history, examinations and test results, medical opinions and diagnoses, descriptions of treatments and prescriptions, and your medical complaints. You are entitled to all this information within fifteen days, at no cost to you.

MANAGEMENT'S ROLE

On large-scale work sites, the most important step management can take to reduce occupational hazards is to employ a well-trained industrial hygienist in the plant and provide him or her with all possible support.

An industrial hygienist surveys the plant's operations, identifies any problems, isolates the causes, and develops corrective measures.

One of the often neglected, but significant, contributions to worker health is the provision of a work setting that enhances health and productivity by making furnishings and equipment idealized for human use. This field of study is called *ergonomics*. A well-designed workshop makes positive use of the human form and human movement as well as of psychological motivation. The result is improved work output. In poor design human physiology, anatomy, and psychology are in fact ignored. The consequences are stress, illness, injury, inefficiency, and reduced output.

Any equipment that requires awkward, unnatural use of the human body invites injury to the operator and inefficient performance. This would include not only the design of the equipment itself—its size, shape, and accessibility—but also the location and operation of its controls. The idea is to make the equipment work with rather than against the operator.

The body needs to be considered in construction of working surfaces, seating, and the most suitable relationship between them. A table or desk too high or low or too distant from seating can produce strain, tension, and fatigue, and hence, error or reduced output. A seat designed with no regard for the human shape can lead to similar negative results.

Intelligent design of the workplace will also take into consideration the effects of light, color, sound, and internal climate in relation to the kind of tasks performed. When human comfort is rationally planned as a variable of production, the result will be improved efficiency and output, as well as better worker health.

All of these rules apply to the office as well as to the plant or factory. A typing table at the wrong height, a chair without rollers for the worker who must move around, a chair that does not swivel for the worker who must turn around, a crowded but partitionless office without sound-proofing, a frequently used but remotely located piece of equipment—all these illustrate poor design that will inevitably have negative effects on efficiency and output.

GOVERNMENT'S ROLE

The federal government recognized its overall responsibility in 1980 when Congress passed the Occupational Safety and Health Act creating the Occupational Safety and Health Administration (OSHA) "to assure as far as possible every working man and woman in the nation safe and healthful working conditions and to preserve our human resources."

OSHA, which operates within the Department of Labor, was given two main functions: the setting of safety and health standards and the enforcement of those standards.

Setting standards

To serve OSHA's research arm, OSHA established the National Institute for Occupational Safety and Health (NIOSH) in the Department of Health and Human Services. NIOSH identifies job hazards and recommends steps to abate them. By 1980, NIOSH had issued more than one hundred "criteria documents" dealing with occupational exposure to hazardous substances as well as with the psychological, motivational, and behavioral factors involved in efforts to improve job safety and health.

Initially, OSHA adopted as its health standards a number of threshold limiting values (TLV) set by the American Conference of Governmental Industrial Hygienists—values generally accepted as appropriate limits for workplace exposure to toxic substances. Since then OSHA has established, through the federal rule-making process, twenty-four comprehensive health standards dealing with carcinogens, cotton dust, and lead. In addition to determining permissible exposure limits, the comprehensive health standards include requirements for engineering controls limiting worker exposure, monitoring levels of exposure for each worker, and keeping accurate records. They require work practice controls, setting aside of regulated areas, the use of protective clothing and equipment, and routine medical examination for workers. The agency has also promulgated a standard covering future standards for occupational carcinogens.

OSHA requires all employers with eleven or more workers to record all occupational injuries and illnesses and post a summary of them annually for their employees.

National statistics in these job hazards are compiled by the Department of Labor's Bureau of Labor Statistics based on an annual survey of employers. OSHA's standard-setting role is also assisted by the Toxic Substances Control Act of 1976, which authorizes the Environmental Protection Agency to obtain information from manufacturers on the production, use, and health effects of chemicals, and to regulate their manufacture, processing, commercial distribution, and disposal.

Enforcing standards

Once OSHA sets a health and safety standard, all affected employers are required by law to comply with it. Effective compliance requires adequate inspection of workplaces. OSHA's authority covers 71 million private workers in nearly 5 million workplaces. Federal government workers are covered by their own agencies; state and local officials are covered in the twenty-four states that operate their own programs under OSHA guidelines. The special needs of one of the most hazardous occupations are dealt with by the Mine and Safety Act of 1977.

Since routine inspections of all workplaces are impossible, OSHA has established inspection priorities. Top priority is given to imminent danger situations. Next come catastrophes and fatal accidents, which must be reported to OSHA within twenty-four hours. Then come legitimate employee complaints, then special emphasis programs, and finally random inspections designed to focus on high-risk industries. OSHA may conduct follow-up inspections of serious violations.

Citations, including proposed penalties, are issued to employers found in violation of OSHA standards. Employers can appeal OSHA's findings to an Occupational Health and Safety Review Commission for adjudication.

As enforcement becomes stricter, especially in highly hazardous workplaces, more and more citations are contested. In 1979 there was an increase of 400 percent over 1973 contested enforcement cases. Labor claims that many settlements leave workers unprotected. Management says that they often admit "guilt" regardless of the circumstances to avoid the costs of contesting citations.

OSHA offers a free on-site consultation program, primarily for smaller firms, to aid employers in reviewing potential hazards and correcting any problems. The program involves no citations or penalties, but employers must agree in advance to correct any serious hazards the consultants find in their workplaces. Long-term Small Business Administration Loans may be used to meet the costs of complying with OSHA standards.

OSHA issues a wide variety of publications and training materials, and provides grants to labor, business, academic and non-profit groups to develop worker and employer programs designed to reduce workplace hazards.

All of OSHA's various activities, however, cannot by themselves insure a safe and healthful workplace. The regulatory process, by its nature, is lengthy, and the agency's resources and powers are limited. Months or years may pass from the identification of a health hazard until appropriate standards are promulgated and effective controls actually instituted in the workplace. In the meantime, workers remain at risk, but, as we have seen, there is much management and labor can do about safety on the job without government. The goal of a safe work environment is the responsibility of both management and labor.

SELECTED SOURCES OF INFORMATION

U.S. GOVERNMENT

Department of Labor

Occupational Health and Safety Administration (OSHA)
3rd St. and Constitution Ave., N.W.
Washington, D.C. 20210

Bureau of Labor Statistics
441 G Street, N.W.
Washington, D.C. 20212

Consumer Product and Safety Commission
Washington, D.C. 20207 (mailing address)

Dept. of Health and Human Services
(formerly Health, Education and Welfare)

National Institute for Occupational Safety and Health (NIOSH)
5600 Fishers Lane
Rockville, MD 20852

Food and Drug Administration (FDA)
Rockville, MD 20857

National Institute of Environmental Health Sciences
Research Triangle Park, NC 27709

National Cancer Institute
Bethesda, MD 20014

Health Resources Administration
National Center for Health Statistics
3700 East-West Highway
Hyattsville, MD 20708

Environmental Protection Agency (EPA)

Office of Toxic Substances (TSCA)
Washington, D.C. 20460

Federal Mine Safety and Health Review Commission

1730 K Street, N.W.
Washington, D.C. 20006

ORGANIZATIONS

AFL-CIO Standing Committee on Occupational Safety and Health
815 16th Street, N.W.
Washington, D.C. 20006

United Automobile, Aerospace, and Agricultural
    Implement Workers of America (UAW)*
8000 East Jefferson Avenue
Detroit, MI 48214

International Brotherhood of Teamsters, Chauffeurs,
    Warehousemen and Helpers of America*
25 Louisiana Avenue, N.W.
Washington, D.C. 20001

United Mine Workers of America*
900 15th Street, N.W.
Washington, D.C. 20005

*not in the AFL-CIO

SRI International
Center for Occupational and Environmental Safety and Health
1611 N. Kent Street
Arlington, VA

Public Citizen, Inc.
Health Research Group
2000 P Street, N.W.
Washington, D.C. 20036

National Safety Council
425 Michigan Avenue
Chicago, IL 60611

American Industrial Hygienist Association
475 Wolf Ledges Parkway
Akron, OH 44311

Women's Occupational Health Resource Center
School of Public Health, Columbia University
60 Haven Avenue, #B-1
New York, NY 10032

CHAPTER
17

Legislative medicine

To the extent that some of us knowingly injure our own well-being and that of others, society must consider the need for appropriate legislative action. "No man is an island, entire of itself," wrote the poet John Donne. If our action, premeditated or not, serves to harm our fellow human beings or unnecessarily adds to the cost of health care, society has a right to intervene.

The laws of various countries view the subject matter with varying degrees of severity. Different societies possess markedly different attitudes toward alcohol abuse (especially related to driving), drug abuse, regulation of food and food additives, occupational health and safety, and environmental pollution.

It is apparent that we need to give more consideration in our laws to the economic and physical health of society as a whole, foregoing our individual rights to damage ourselves, when others are called upon to pay the bill. There are, indeed, thorny questions of civil rights involved in these areas where individual rights come in conflict with the rights of society at large. Ultimately, the well-being of the majority should prevail over the pleasure of the minority.

Role of the Government

In the past several years, an important political and legislative phenomenon has emerged in the United States and in the industrialized nations in general, involving the ever-increasing role of government in protecting the health of its constituents. Thus, while no inalienable right to health is guaranteed by the American Constitution or the Declaration of Independence, an unwritten "law" has recently evolved about government's responsibility for society's health. Implicit in the superstructure of modern society is the duty of government to intervene in our lives to protect us from the harmful aspects of life in our society.

The trend toward government regulation began in earnest after World War II. With the prevailing mood of unlimited economic and social progress, we developed a heightened awareness of the importance of the quality of life. We were no longer content just to have a job; we demanded a clean and safe workplace. We were no longer content to accept our susceptibility to disease. As the death rate declined with the development of wonder drugs, we came to believe that science could keep us well and alive.

In response to this mood, Congress vastly enlarged budgetary allocations to existing regulatory agencies such as the *Food and Drug Administration*, created completely new agencies such as the *Environmental Protection Agency* and the *Occupational Safety and Health Administration*, and enacted broadly defined legislation providing the agencies with sweeping powers. These agencies tended strongly toward conservatism (i.e., protection of human health) even in the face of inadequate scientific information. This tendency can be seen in the tighter environmental standards enacted, in the stricter interpretation of laws, and in acceptance of standards mandated by Congress rather than by scientists.

The decision of when and what to regulate is more often a political and sociological one rather than a strictly medical or scientific one. In brief, there are two elements to the question: (1) What is the impact of environmental influences on human mortality and morbidity, the avoidance of which would enhance the well-being of society at large? and (2) What should the response of government be when environmental influences on health are identified? For example, regulation of known or implied hazards to which we are *involuntarily* exposed have generally been politically acceptable up to now. Thus, clean air, clean water, and pure food and drug laws, as well as noise control laws, have been relatively successful.

By contrast, government intervention in areas of exposure to which we *willingly* and knowingly submit ourselves have generally been unsuccessful politically. For example, efforts to legislate speed limits, seat belt usage, alcohol consumption, and even the use of helmets by motorcyclists have been seen by many as an unwarranted intrusion by government into their private lives.

These apparent contradictions have become even more complex as the economic costs of actual or proposed regulations are projected onto the economy. When unemployment rises, and when inflation shrinks the spending power of workers, government regulation increasingly is perceived as impinging upon economic growth. The resultant prevailing mood builds pressure for less regulation, or at least regulation that is demonstrably cost-beneficial. In response to this mood, Congress has begun to limit the scope of power of the regulatory agencies and to enact legislation that defers enforcement of strict environmental standards.

Clearly, we are still struggling to strike a delicate balance between the goal of creating a safe and healthy society with the goal of maintaining a stable economy. Thus, the laws that are catalogued in the following pages should not be seen as immutable, but as part of a continuing process of growth. It is hoped that a society will emerge in which prevention is not seen as a luxury to be indulged in only during periods of robust economic activity. On the other hand, we must accept the fact that zero risk is not an attainable goal and that our health, to a large extent, is directly related to our willingness to accept a greater degree of responsibility for our individual well-being and to make those lifestyle choices that will reduce the risk of developing avoidable illness. In addition, if we are all parties to a social contract, then we must all be responsible for our own actions and must be aware of the social and economic ramifications of our actions vis-à-vis our ultimate societal goals.

Summary of Laws Affecting Prevention

Below are excerpts taken from the main body of this book, added here to provide a ready reference guide of the extent to which regulation by federal, state, and local laws affects various areas of prevention.

NUTRITION

In 1906, the Pure Food and Drug Act marked the beginning of the general enactment of complementary laws by local governments. The original statute was limited to the manufacture, sale, or transportation of adulterated food and drugs. In 1938 and several times thereafter, the law was amended to expand its scope.

Of singular importance was the passage of the so-called Delaney Clause in 1958. Named after its chief congressional sponsor, this amendment to the Food, Drug, and Cosmetic Act has had a significant impact on food safety and has been highly controversial. Surprisingly, it contains only five lines:

No additive shall be deemed to be safe if it is found to induce cancer when ingested by man or animal, or if it is found, after tests which are appropriate for the evaluation of food additives, to induce cancer in man or animals.

The Delaney Clause has been invoked, largely on the basis of animal tests, several times: in hearings on allegedly dangerous food additives in 1960; with regard to the cyclamate ban in 1969; in the partial banning of DES in 1969; and in the debate over saccharine's alleged role in causing cancer of the bladder in 1978–1979.

Delaney, it should be remembered, deals only with food additives and does not apply to toxins that are natural ingredients in foods, such as aflatoxin mold sometimes present in peanuts, which is a carcinogen.

The future interpretation and enforcement of the Delaney Clause will provide valuable insights into the future direction our society is moving vis-à-vis our willingness to accept risks as an inherent part of life in our times. (See chapter 1, Nutrition.)

ALCOHOL

The production of alcohol is governed by federal law, specifically the Treasury Department's Bureau of Alcohol, Tobacco, and Firearms. In general, these regulations are confined to the taxes to be paid as a result of the production of liquor. The consumption of alcohol comes under the jurisdiction of local and state governments. Thus minimum drinking age, licensure of liquor stores, minimum price regulations, and intoxicated driving laws, vary from state to state, even from municipality to municipality. Such an absence of uniformity may be a significant contributing factor to the lax enforcement of alcohol-related laws, especially those pertaining to drunk drivers. In those states (and foreign countries) where there is strict enforcement of these laws, a dramatic decrease in the incidence of alcohol-related death and disability has been noted. (See chapter 2, Alcohol.)

DRUGS AND DRUG ABUSE

As early as 1909 the federal government sought to control the use of narcotics for other than medicinal purposes. In 1914 the Harrison Narcotics Act was passed. It strengthened and extended existing legislation regarding the importation, manufacture, and use of narcotics. Subsequently, the Controlled Substances Act was enacted and established a comprehensive set of standards for drugs of different categories.

In addition, each state government has enacted legislation to deal with the use of illicit drugs and each has a single office responsible for drug abuse, intervention, and treatment.

Legal drugs that may be used for illicit purposes are controlled by the Food and Drug Administration. The FDA oversees the approval of all new drugs and subjects them to rigorous tests before permitting them to be publicly marketed. First passed in 1906, the Food and Drug Act established the role of the government in protecting the general population from dangerous, untested drugs.

The Federal Trade Commission has authority over claims for "patent medicine" and other nostrums and closely regulates the pronouncements made by manufacturers about their products. (See chapter 3, Drugs.)

SMOKING

The production, use, and distribution of cigarettes (and all tobacco products) are specifically excluded from the Food and Drug Act. Rather, tobacco use comes under the jurisdiction of the Treasury Department's Bureau of Alcohol, Tobacco, and Firearms, which is mainly concerned with the taxation of such use.

In 1964 the Surgeon General of the United States issued a report on the harmful effects of cigarette smoking. Subsequently, in 1969, the Federal Trade Commission issued regulations requiring manufacturers of cigarettes to place a warning label on every package of cigarettes, as well as on all advertisements appearing in magazines, billboards, flyers, and so forth. In 1972 Congress banned the advertising of cigarettes on television and radio.

In addition, as of 1980, some thirty states have enacted restrictions on smoking in public places. These so-called clean indoor air acts have been met with vigorous opposition from the tobacco industry, as well as from restaurateurs and other merchants. Various agencies of the federal government have also implemented regulations limiting smoking in such places as federal buildings and on airplanes.

There are substantial federal excise taxes imposed on cigarettes, as well as state and local taxes. These provide revenue and are believed to impede the purchase of cigarettes. In this regard, many local governments seek to prevent the onset of smoking among children by prohibiting the sale of cigarettes to children below a certain age.

In contrast to the United States, there has been a great deal of recent legislation and regulations enacted abroad which prohibit smoking in public places, impose high taxes on tobacco products and restrict the sale of cigarettes to young people. (See chapter 4, Tobacco.)

TRAFFIC ACCIDENTS

Although the United States Department of Transportation has issued regulations for the installation of automobile restraint systems, highway safety is generally the responsibility of local and state government agencies. As a result, there exists a myriad of state and local regulations regarding minimum driving age, license requirements, seat belt usage, and intoxicated driver laws. Until a national consensus develops on the standardization and enforcement of these laws, we will continue to see a high rate of accidents and fatalities on our roads. As noted with regard to alcohol, in counties and localities where strict enforcement of rules about drunk driving, seat belt use, and the use of helmets pertains, the rate of injury and death is noticeably lowered. (See chapter 10, Traffic Accidents.)

AIR POLLUTION

In 1970 the Federal Clean Air Act was enacted by Congress, authorizing the Environmental Protection Agency to set acceptable air quality standards and establish emission limitations for pollutants. The most dramatic effect of the Clean Air Act has been in the reduction of air pollution in our major cities. This has been achieved by limiting (and in some cases banning) the use of certain fuels and upgrading the efficiency (from a pollution perspective) of automobiles.

Many local and state governments have enacted stringent air pollution legislation of their own. Perhaps most notable among these has been the large number of "clean *indoor* air acts," which relate to the banning of cigarette, pipe, and cigar smoking in public places. (See chapter 11, Air Pollution.)

WATER POLLUTION

Since 1914 the federal government has been cognizant of the importance of ensuring the continued existence of safe drinking water, water free of disease-carrying mechanisms. In 1962 the U.S. Public Health Service established new and more stringent standards as it became apparent that our lakes and streams were endangered.

A major step toward further ensuring the safety of our water supply occurred in 1970 with the establishment of the Environmental Protection Agency. It is empowered to set and enforce drinking water standards. Subsequently, in 1974, the Safe Drinking Water Act set national standards for water purity, leaving state governments with the responsibility to enforce these standards.

As for the nation's waterways, Congress enacted the Federal Water Pollution Control Act of 1972. The specific goal of this legislation was to clean up the lakes, rivers, and streams by 1983. Paralleling this, the Marine Protection Research and Sanctuaries Act sought to control the pollution of our oceans, especially the dumping of waste matter.

Finally, the Toxic Substances Control Act grants the Environmental Protection Agency the authority to control the disposal of industrial toxic wastes into inland waterways. Under the Resource Conservation and Recovery Act of 1976, EPA has the power to control hazardous wastes from generation site to disposal site, and to enforce the law when necessary through fines and other measures. (See chapter 12, Water Pollution.)

RADIATION

The manufacture of X-ray equipment has been regulated, since 1974, by the Food and Drug Administration. It establishes and enforces regulations for all new equipment, including microwave devices. As of 1980, however, federal standards for the education and training of radiological technologists have not been enacted.

The Environmental Protection Agency provides technical assistance to states and local agencies having radiation pollution programs and maintains a national surveillance and inspection program for measuring radiation levels in the environment. (See chapter 13, Radiation.)

NOISE

In 1936 Congress enacted the Walsh-Healy Public Contacts Act. This was the first effort to control noise through federal legislation and is noteworthy because it reflects the fact that noise has been recognized as an environmental hazard for almost half a century. In 1976 a greatly expanded standard for noise pollution was enacted by the Congress and was incorporated into the provisions of the Occupational Safety and Health Act. Though the federal government has been active in noise control for some time, local and state governments have adopted a broad array of parallel legislation. (See chapter 14, Noise.)

OCCUPATIONAL HEALTH

Perhaps nowhere has the role of the federal government been more pronounced in the past decade than in the identification and elimination of health hazards in the workplace. In 1970 Congress enacted the Occupational Safety and Health Act, which gave rise to the Occupational Safety and Health Administration. The sole function of OSHA is to protect the safety and health of workers in the workplace. To achieve this, OSHA has established a complex and often controversial set of standards. Empowered with substantial enforcement powers by the government, OSHA has been one of the most aggressive government agencies vis-à-vis health and safety promotion.

In 1976 the Toxic Substances Control Act was passed by Congress, authorizing the Environmental Protection Agency to collect information on the harmful effects of chemicals and to regulate their manufacture, use, and even disposal.

In 1977 Congress passed into law the Mine and Safety Act, designed to deal specifically with the health and safety problems associated with the most hazardous of occupations in the country. (See chapter 16, Occupational Health.)

PART

III

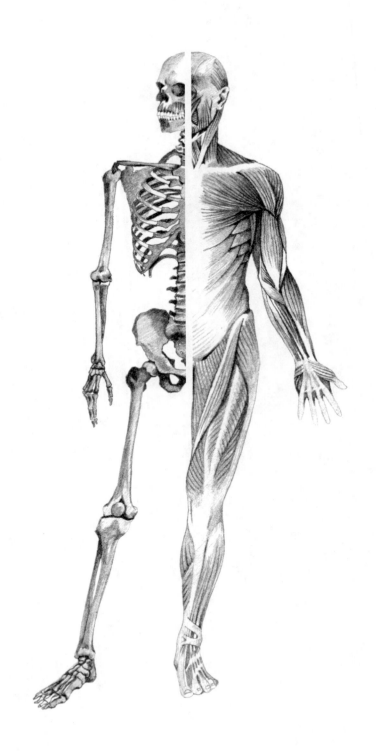

KNOWING YOUR BODY

Anatomy of the body and its systems

The Book of Health explains how certain lifestyles or exposures can lead to disability or death and, conversely, how reducing risk factors for disease can lead to a longer, healthier, more useful life.

In order to *act* on the advice in the preceding chapters, each of us should know how risk factors operate, how they affect specific parts of the body, how the various organs interact, and how the organ systems are structured.

To accomplish this last task, schematically detailed illustrations of the major organ systems of the human body are presented in this chapter. Smokers can see the various parts of the upper alimentary and respiratory tracts that are affected by smoke. Those concerned about heart attacks can visualize from the illustration of the cardiovascular system how the buildup of fatty deposits

(plaques) in the arteries can lead to a loss of blood supply to sections of the heart and cause a heart attack.

Most of us are not very knowledgeable about the relative positions of our internal organs—the liver, spleen, pancreas, stomach, and colon. The following illustrations will help the reader to picture where these organs are. While knowing the body's anatomy will not necessarily help us to change bad health habits, such insight can help us to understand what areas of the body can be harmed by certain risk factors or hazards. If we understand and appreciate the intricacies of our own bodies, we might be more inclined to preserve them.

The skeletal system (front view)

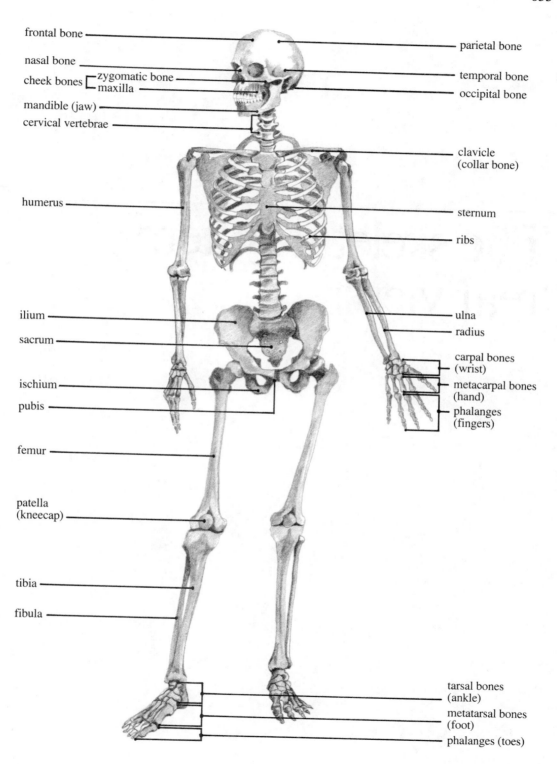

frontal bone — parietal bone

nasal bone — temporal bone

cheek bones ⌈ zygomatic bone — occipital bone
⌊ maxilla

mandible (jaw)

cervical vertebrae — clavicle (collar bone)

humerus — sternum

ribs

ilium — ulna

sacrum — radius

carpal bones (wrist)

ischium — metacarpal bones (hand)

pubis — phalanges (fingers)

femur

patella (kneecap)

tibia

fibula

tarsal bones (ankle)

metatarsal bones (foot)

phalanges (toes)

The skeletal system (rear view)

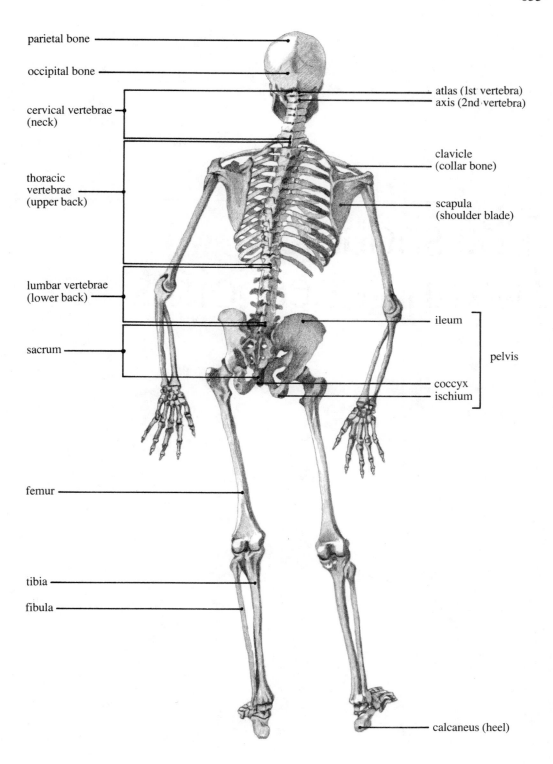

parietal bone

occipital bone

atlas (1st vertebra)
axis (2nd vertebra)

cervical vertebrae
(neck)

clavicle
(collar bone)

thoracic
vertebrae
(upper back)

scapula
(shoulder blade)

lumbar vertebrae
(lower back)

ileum

sacrum

pelvis

coccyx
ischium

femur

tibia

fibula

calcaneus (heel)

The shoulder, hip and knee joints

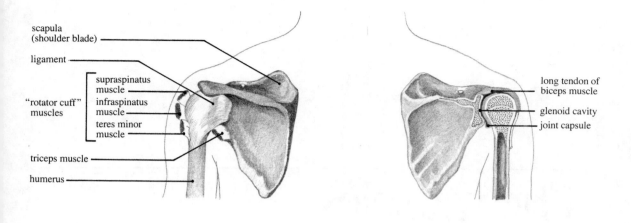

scapula (shoulder blade)

ligament

"rotator cuff" muscles
- supraspinatus muscle
- infraspinatus muscle
- teres minor muscle

triceps muscle

humerus

long tendon of biceps muscle

glenoid cavity

joint capsule

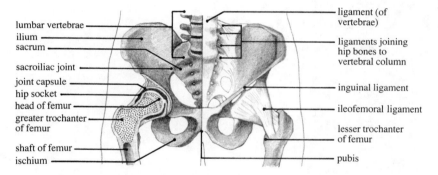

lumbar vertebrae

ilium

sacrum

sacroiliac joint

joint capsule

hip socket

head of femur

greater trochanter of femur

shaft of femur

ischium

ligament (of vertebrae)

ligaments joining hip bones to vertebral column

inguinal ligament

ileofemoral ligament

lesser trochanter of femur

pubis

(LIGAMENTS REMOVED) (SHOWING LIGAMENTS)

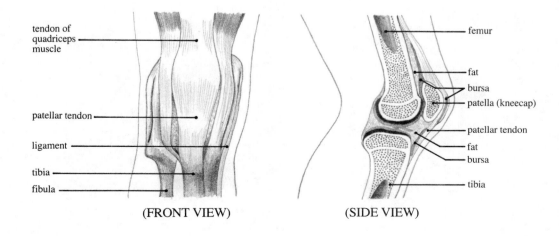

tendon of quadriceps muscle

patellar tendon

ligament

tibia

fibula

femur

fat

bursa

patella (kneecap)

patellar tendon

fat

bursa

tibia

(FRONT VIEW) (SIDE VIEW)

The muscles (front view)

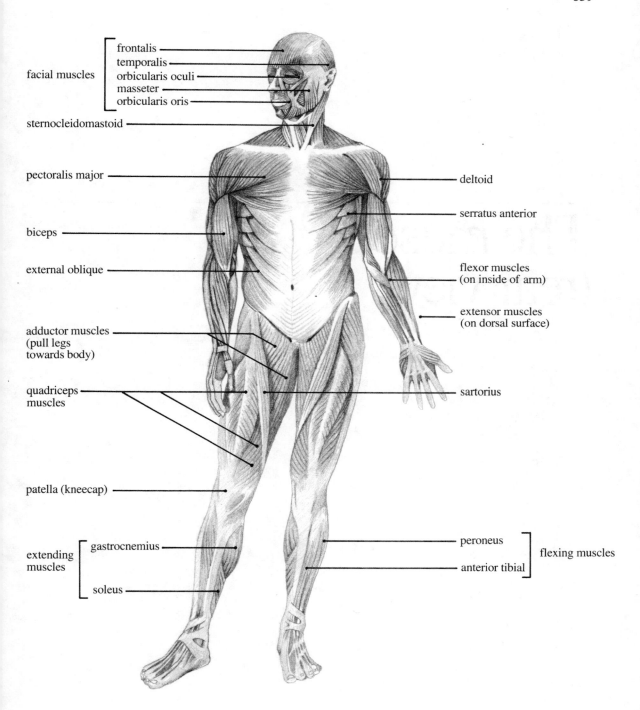

facial muscles
- frontalis
- temporalis
- orbicularis oculi
- masseter
- orbicularis oris

sternocleidomastoid

pectoralis major

biceps

external oblique

adductor muscles
(pull legs
towards body)

quadriceps
muscles

patella (kneecap)

extending
muscles
- gastrocnemius
- soleus

deltoid

serratus anterior

flexor muscles
(on inside of arm)

extensor muscles
(on dorsal surface)

sartorius

peroneus
anterior tibial
} flexing muscles

The muscles (rear view)

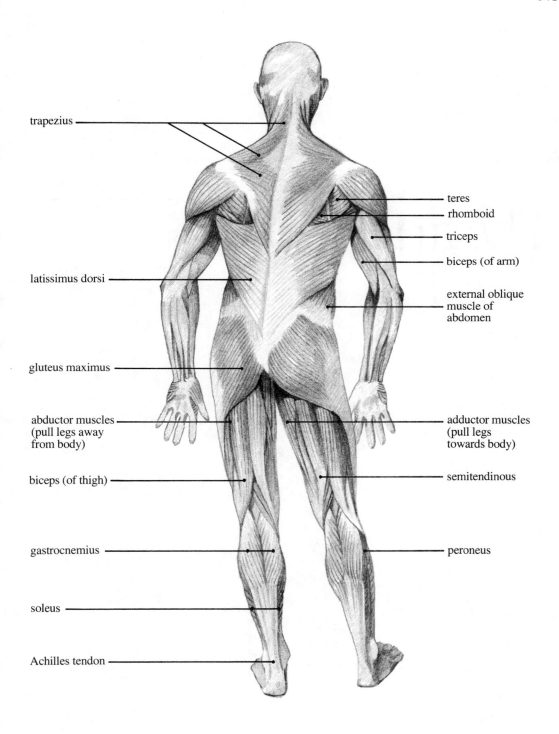

trapezius

teres

rhomboid

triceps

biceps (of arm)

latissimus dorsi

external oblique muscle of abdomen

gluteus maximus

abductor muscles (pull legs away from body)

adductor muscles (pull legs towards body)

biceps (of thigh)

semitendinous

gastrocnemius

peroneus

soleus

Achilles tendon

The arteries

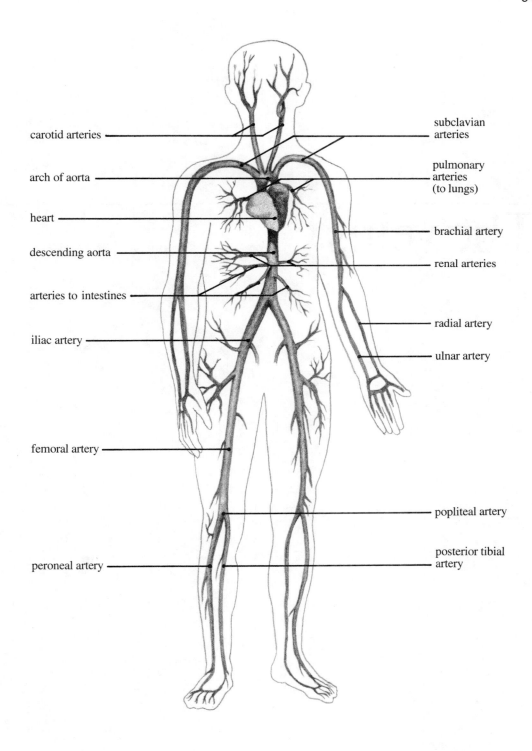

carotid arteries

subclavian arteries

arch of aorta

pulmonary arteries (to lungs)

heart

brachial artery

descending aorta

renal arteries

arteries to intestines

radial artery

iliac artery

ulnar artery

femoral artery

popliteal artery

posterior tibial artery

peroneal artery

The veins

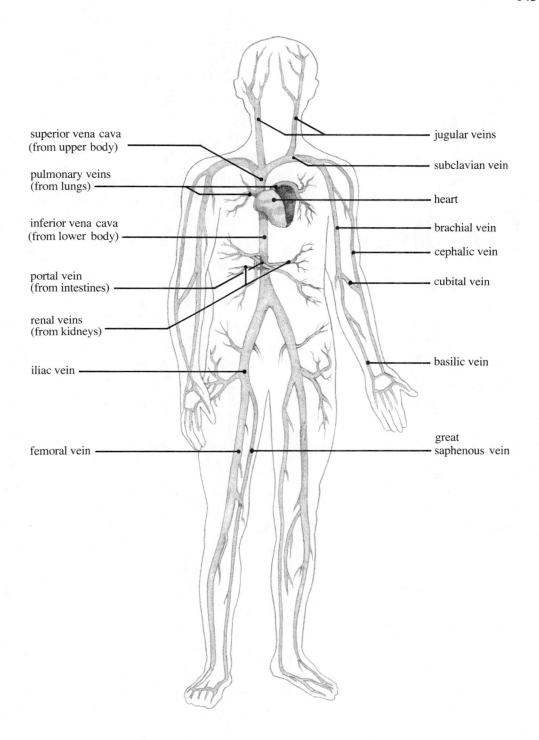

superior vena cava (from upper body)

pulmonary veins (from lungs)

inferior vena cava (from lower body)

portal vein (from intestines)

renal veins (from kidneys)

iliac vein

femoral vein

jugular veins

subclavian vein

heart

brachial vein

cephalic vein

cubital vein

basilic vein

great saphenous vein

The heart

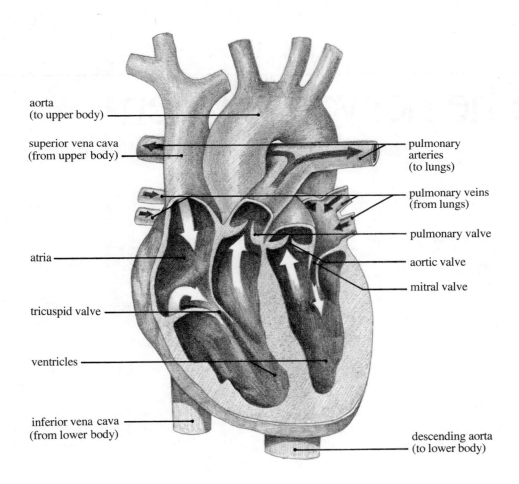

aorta
(to upper body)

superior vena cava
(from upper body)

pulmonary
arteries
(to lungs)

pulmonary veins
(from lungs)

pulmonary valve

aortic valve

mitral valve

atria

tricuspid valve

ventricles

inferior vena cava
(from lower body)

descending aorta
(to lower body)

The nervous system

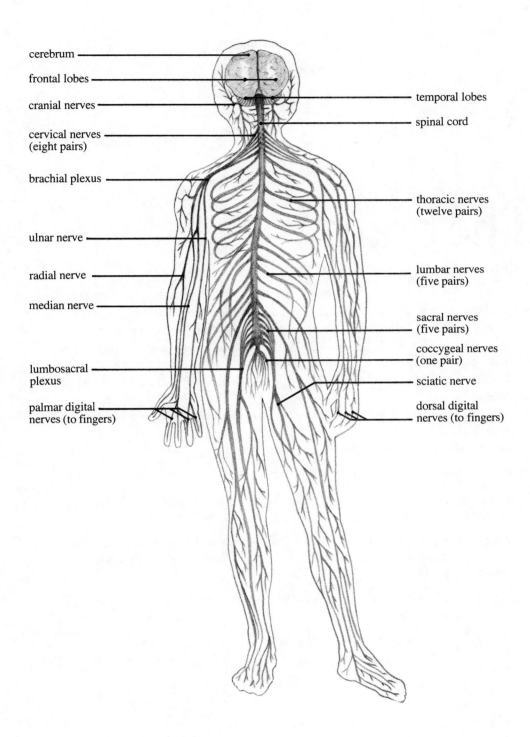

cerebrum

frontal lobes

cranial nerves

cervical nerves
(eight pairs)

brachial plexus

ulnar nerve

radial nerve

median nerve

lumbosacral
plexus

palmar digital
nerves (to fingers)

temporal lobes

spinal cord

thoracic nerves
(twelve pairs)

lumbar nerves
(five pairs)

sacral nerves
(five pairs)

coccygeal nerves
(one pair)

sciatic nerve

dorsal digital
nerves (to fingers)

The brain

The CEREBRAL CORTEX, the "thinking" part of the brain, incorporates:

frontal lobe: associational area, where various thoughts and feelings are linked.

parietal lobe: sensory and motor areas (shared with part of frontal lobe; controls feelings on body surface and movement of skeletal muscles).

temporal lobe: speech area (shared with parietal lobe) hearing area, and areas related to emotion and smell.

occipital lobe: visual cortex, where light impulses received by eye are decoded into meaningful image.

corpus callosum: connects right and left halves of cerebral cortex.

CEREBELLUM—muscular coordination.

MEDULLA OBLONGATA—pathway for nerve fibers between brain and rest of body; continuous with spinal cord.

HYPOTHALAMUS—controls release of hormones by pituitary; involved in regulation of some basic functions such as appetite, sleep patterns, body temperature, sexual activity, and rage responses.

PITUITARY—releases hormones that regulate function of other organs of endocrine system throughout body.

PINEAL—function not well understood. Responds to light; possibly involved in biological rhythms.

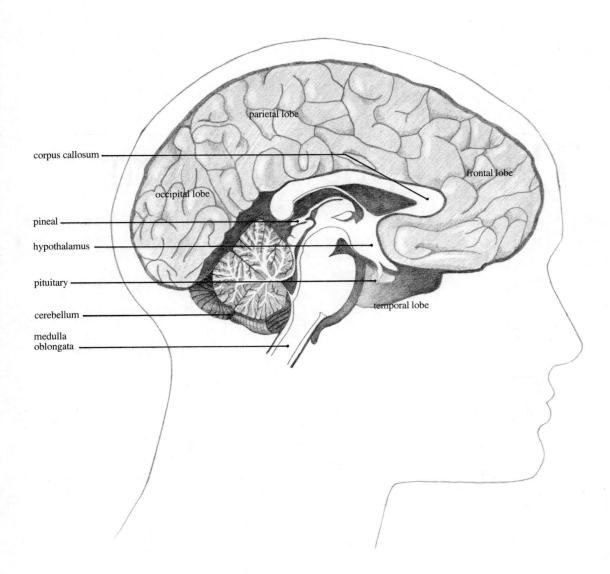

parietal lobe

corpus callosum

frontal lobe

occipital lobe

pineal

hypothalamus

pituitary

cerebellum

medulla oblongata

temporal lobe

The lymphatic system

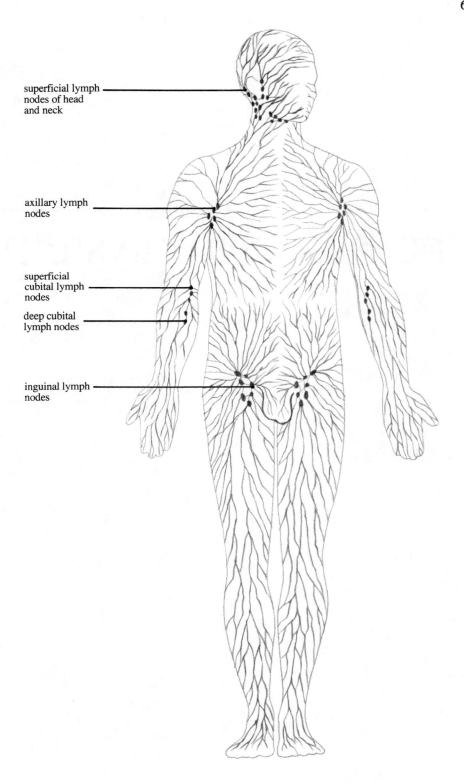

superficial lymph nodes of head and neck

axillary lymph nodes

superficial cubital lymph nodes

deep cubital lymph nodes

inguinal lymph nodes

The endocrine system

Thyroid gland

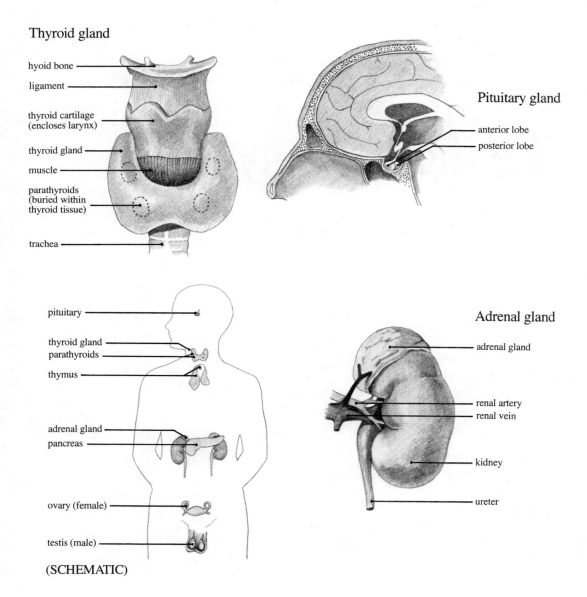

hyoid bone

ligament

thyroid cartilage
(encloses larynx)

thyroid gland

muscle

parathyroids
(buried within
thyroid tissue)

trachea

Pituitary gland

anterior lobe

posterior lobe

pituitary

thyroid gland

parathyroids

thymus

adrenal gland

pancreas

ovary (female)

testis (male)

(SCHEMATIC)

Adrenal gland

adrenal gland

renal artery

renal vein

kidney

ureter

The digestive system

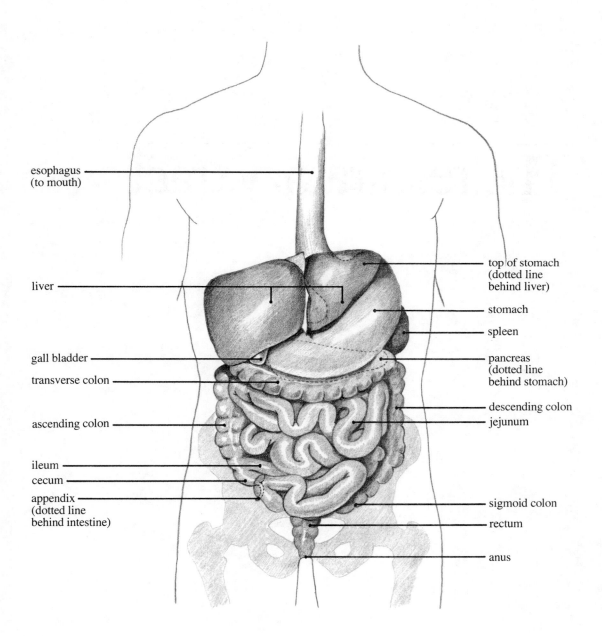

esophagus (to mouth)

top of stomach (dotted line behind liver)

liver

stomach

spleen

gall bladder

pancreas (dotted line behind stomach)

transverse colon

descending colon

ascending colon

jejunum

ileum

cecum

appendix (dotted line behind intestine)

sigmoid colon

rectum

anus

The respiratory tract

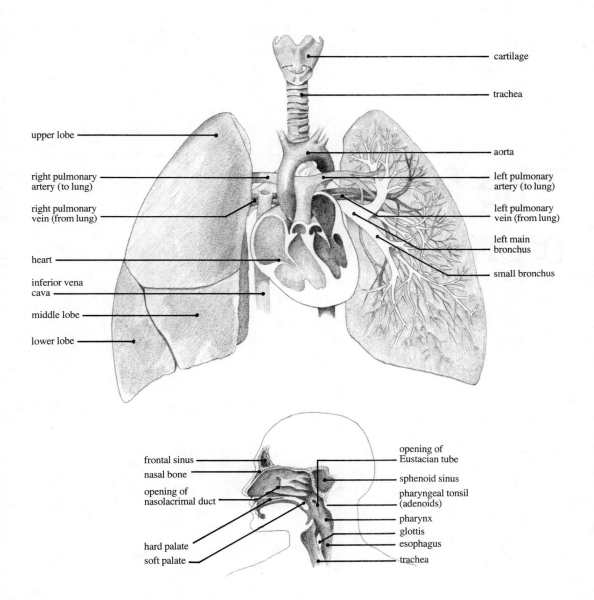

cartilage

trachea

upper lobe

aorta

right pulmonary artery (to lung)

left pulmonary artery (to lung)

right pulmonary vein (from lung)

left pulmonary vein (from lung)

left main bronchus

heart

small bronchus

inferior vena cava

middle lobe

lower lobe

frontal sinus

opening of Eustacian tube

nasal bone

sphenoid sinus

opening of nasolacrimal duct

pharyngeal tonsil (adenoids)

pharynx

hard palate

glottis

soft palate

esophagus

trachea

The female reproductive organs

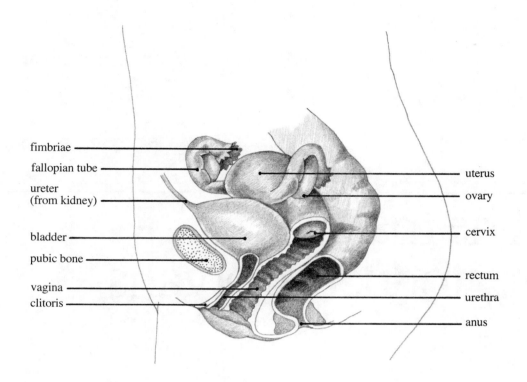

fimbriae — fallopian tube — ureter (from kidney) — bladder — pubic bone — vagina — clitoris — uterus — ovary — cervix — rectum — urethra — anus

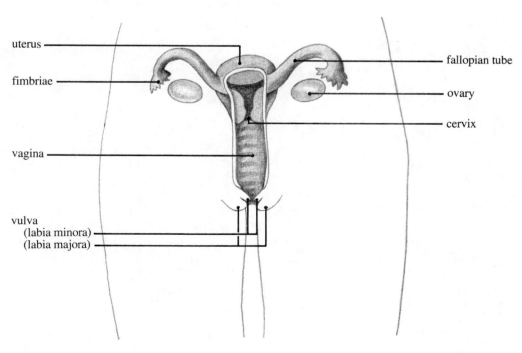

uterus — fimbriae — vagina — vulva (labia minora) (labia majora) — fallopian tube — ovary — cervix

The male reproductive organs

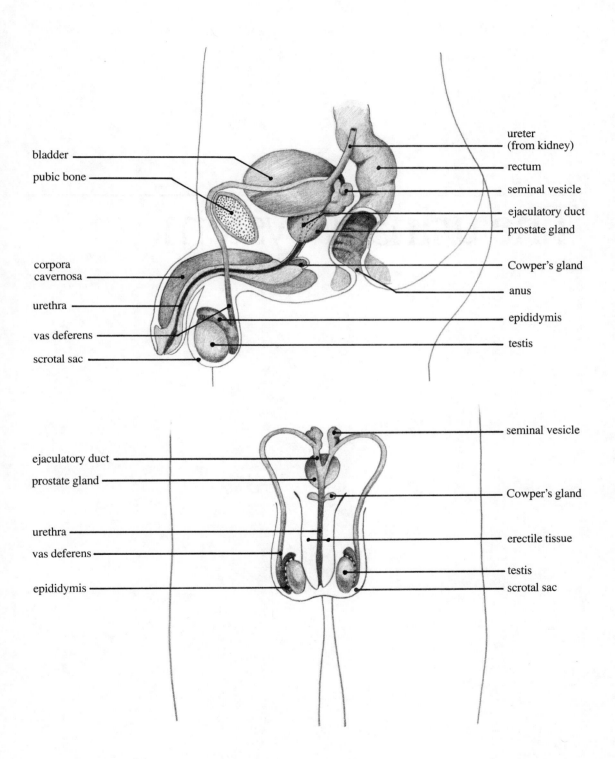

bladder

pubic bone

corpora
cavernosa

urethra

vas deferens

scrotal sac

ureter
(from kidney)

rectum

seminal vesicle

ejaculatory duct

prostate gland

Cowper's gland

anus

epididymis

testis

ejaculatory duct

prostate gland

urethra

vas deferens

epididymis

seminal vesicle

Cowper's gland

erectile tissue

testis

scrotal sac

The urinary system

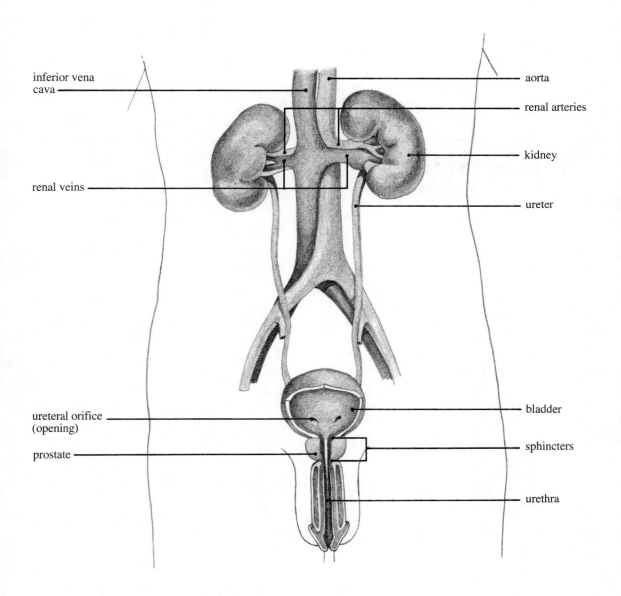

inferior vena cava

aorta

renal arteries

kidney

renal veins

ureter

ureteral orifice (opening)

bladder

prostate

sphincters

urethra

The eye

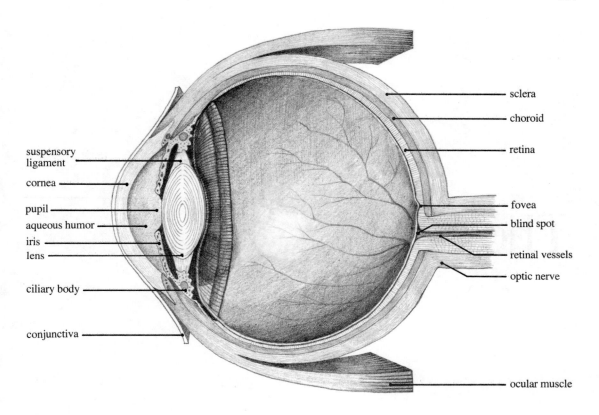

sclera

choroid

retina

suspensory ligament

cornea

pupil

aqueous humor

iris

lens

fovea

blind spot

retinal vessels

optic nerve

ciliary body

conjunctiva

ocular muscle

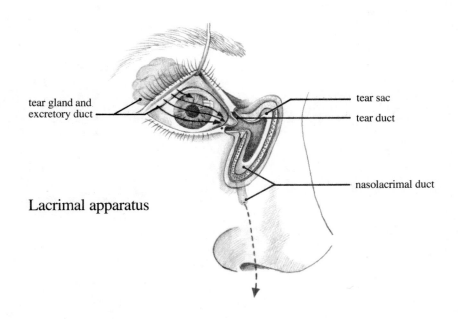

tear gland and excretory duct

tear sac

tear duct

nasolacrimal duct

Lacrimal apparatus

The ear

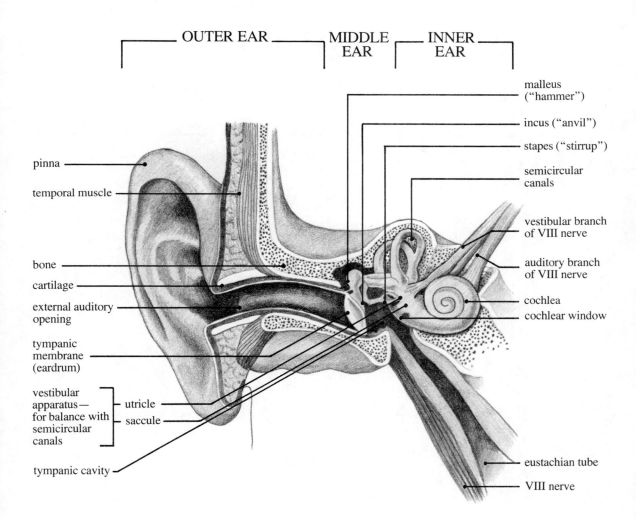

OUTER EAR — MIDDLE EAR — INNER EAR

malleus ("hammer")

incus ("anvil")

stapes ("stirrup")

semicircular canals

vestibular branch of VIII nerve

auditory branch of VIII nerve

cochlea

cochlear window

pinna

temporal muscle

bone

cartilage

external auditory opening

tympanic membrane (eardrum)

vestibular apparatus— for balance with semicircular canals

utricle

saccule

tympanic cavity

eustachian tube

VIII nerve

The skin

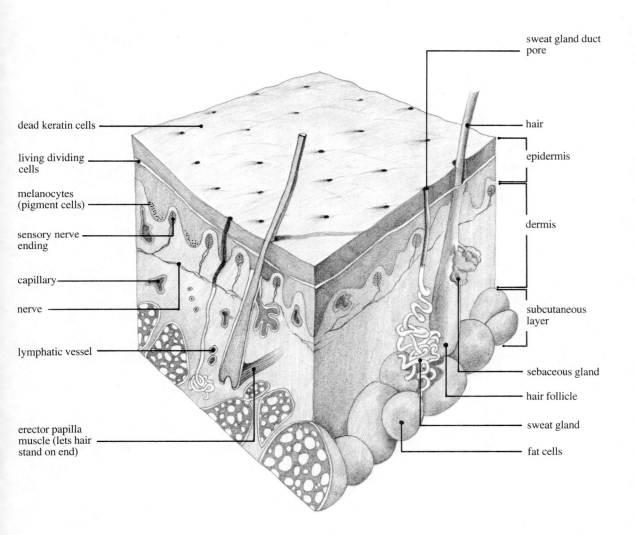

dead keratin cells

living dividing cells

melanocytes (pigment cells)

sensory nerve ending

capillary

nerve

lymphatic vessel

erector papilla muscle (lets hair stand on end)

sweat gland duct pore

hair

epidermis

dermis

subcutaneous layer

sebaceous gland

hair follicle

sweat gland

fat cells

Passports to health

Most adults are remarkably uninformed as to their blood cholesterol level or, for that matter, what an *optimal* blood cholesterol level is (see Figure 1.2, chapter 1, Nutrition). Many do not know their blood pressure or the *optimal* weight for their height (see Table 1.12, chapter 1). How can we expect to safeguard our health if we do not know the risk factors that affect it?

> Health knowledge is an important pre-requisite for changing health behavior.

For this reason, starting in the first grade of school, children should know the basic risk factors for disease—particularly those that are largely under their own control. Such risk factors can be determined and recorded for lifelong reference in a *Health Passport*. The message on the cover is: "Nobody takes better care of you than you."

Students in grades one through three should each have their own Health Passport that teaches them the significance of risk factors and also records their immunizations and allergies. When the students enter the fourth grade, specific values for certain risk factors are recorded in a new Health Passport. Based on these entries, the risks can be monitored continuously throughout the child's school life.

Both documents are part of the American Health Foundation's *Know Your Body* child health education program. Because risk factors for chronic diseases such as heart disease, cancer, and stroke can be detected as early as childhood, the American Health Foundation has developed the *Know Your Body (KYB)* screening designed to be administered in schools by registered nurses and medical technicians. Children are given a short examination that measures their blood pressure, blood cholesterol, height, weight, and skin-fold thickness (to measure percentage of body fat), and are questioned about their health behavior. The results are recorded in the student's Health Passport. The KYB health education curriculum, taught by the children's classroom teachers, provides them with current health information and encourages them to take responsibility for their own health. Family involvement and participation is integrated throughout the program. The KYB curriculum includes instruction on:

- self-care and self-responsibility
- health decision-making
- accident prevention
- lifestyle decisions
- substances such as alcohol and drugs
- heart disease and cancer prevention
- nutrition
- exercise and physical fitness
- dental health

Through questionnaires and discussions in class about health knowledge, behavior, and attitudes, the program promotes decision-making and positive action by making health education personalized and individually relevant to the students. The KYB program increases children's knowledge about early risk factors that can contribute to major diseases in adulthood, enables early detection of these factors, and promotes self-responsibility for maintaining their own health.

The school KYB program has an adult counterpart. Upon undergoing a mini-screening at the doctor's office, at work, or in the military, for example, adults can have a medical history including blood pressure, height, weight, and blood cholesterol recorded in an adult Health Passport.

On the basis of the various risk factors as recorded in the Health Passport, we can proceed to correct any abnormal findings and change health behavior. Again, knowledge is the key. All adults should know and—based on the contents of this book—understand at least the risk factors listed in the adult Health Passport and, if necessary, act accordingly to make recommended changes.

Often, after having a test for blood cholesterol and blood pressure, an individual may not understand what the results mean. "My doctor says not to worry; my cholesterol is normal." However, the doctor's acceptance of "normal" may not agree with the idea of "optimal" as described in Figure 1.2 in chapter 1, Nutrition. "Nobody takes better care of you than you," the adult Health Passport says, but it is difficult to accomplish this when the appropriate health knowledge is not available.

With the help of a Health Passport kept in a secure place and updated regularly, all of us have an excellent opportunity to safeguard and improve our health.

A.

Health Passport

Wise Bird says:
Nobody takes better
care of you
than you!

KYB

© AMERICAN HEALTH FOUNDATION

Date _____

Identification No. ☐☐☐☐☐☐

This passport belongs to:

_____

School

_____

212 953 1900

HEALTH PASSPORT

B.

HEALTH PASSPORT

C.

A. Health Passport for 1st, 2nd and 3rd grades;
B. Health Passport for 4th-12th grades;
C. Health Passport for adults.

Figure 1. Health Passport for 1st, 2nd and 3rd Grades

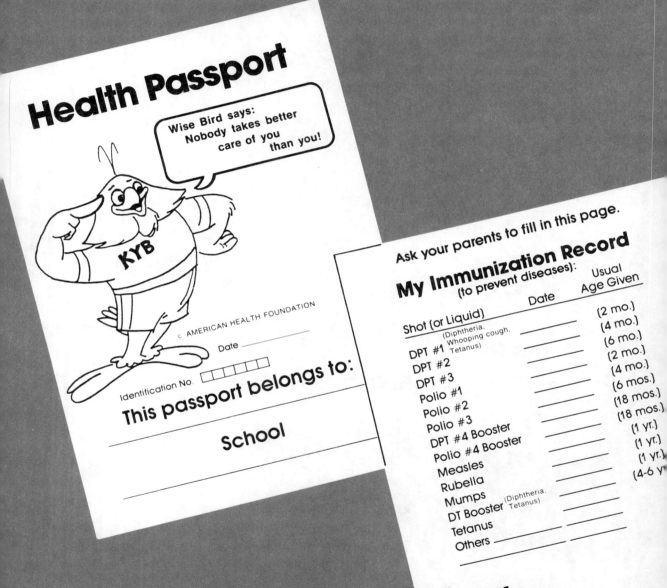

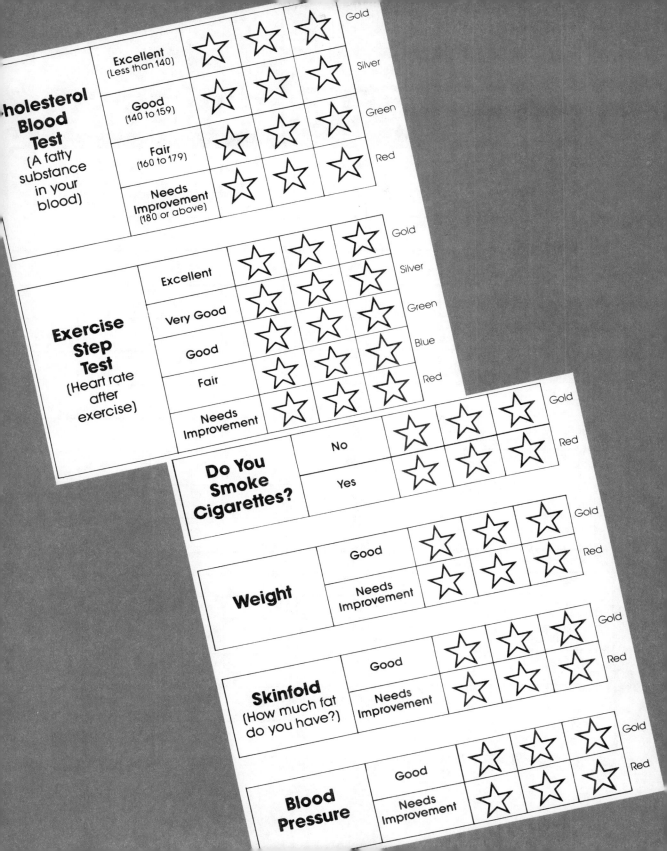

Cholesterol Blood Test (A fatty substance in your blood)

Excellent (Less than 140)	☆	☆	☆	Gold
Good (140 to 159)	☆	☆	☆	Silver
Fair (160 to 179)	☆	☆	☆	Green
Needs Improvement (180 or above)	☆	☆	☆	Red

Exercise Step Test (Heart rate after exercise)

Excellent	☆	☆	☆	Gold
Very Good	☆	☆	☆	Silver
Good	☆	☆	☆	Green
Fair	☆	☆	☆	Blue
Needs Improvement	☆	☆	☆	Red

Do You Smoke Cigarettes?

No	☆	☆	☆	Gold
Yes	☆	☆	☆	Red

Weight

Good	☆	☆	☆	Gold
Needs Improvement	☆	☆	☆	Red

Skinfold (How much fat do you have?)

Good	☆	☆	☆	Gold
Needs Improvement	☆	☆	☆	Red

Blood Pressure

Good	☆	☆	☆	Gold
Needs Improvement	☆	☆	☆	Red

Figure 2. Health Passport for 4th-12th Grades

KNOW YOUR BODY

Date						
Grade						
Age						
HEALTH PROFILE						
Height						
Weight						
Skinfold*						
Blood Pressure						
Recovery Index**						
Cholesterol***						
HEALTH HABITS						
Cigarette Smoking						
Smoke Now						
Smoked but quit						
Never Smoked						
Snack I eat most often						
Exercise I do most often						
HEALTH KNOWLEDGE						
Health Knowledge Score (percent of right answers)						

PERSONAL IMMUNIZATION RECORD

Shot (or Liquid)	Dates Given
DPT (Diphtheria, Whooping Cough, Tetanus)	
DT (Diphtheria, Tetanus)	
Polio (Oral Vaccine)	
Measles	
Mumps	
Rubella (German Measles)	
Influenza	
Tetanus	

Name _____

Address _____

_____

Telephone No. _____

Birth Date _____

A profile result I would like to change or maintain

_____

_____

_____

ALLERGIES

DRUGS _____

FOODS _____

(PHOTO)

Figure 3. Health Passport for adults

Height/weight table (Women)

height (no shoes)   'ideal' weight range

4'10".	95-104 lbs.
4'11".	98-107
5'.	101-110
5'1".	104-113
5'2".	107-117
5'3".	110-120
5'4".	114-124
5'5".	117-128
5'6".	120-131
5'7".	123-134
5'8".	126-137
5'9".	129-141
5'10".	132-144
5'11".	135-147

This range takes into account variations in body build. These figures are based on Metropolitan Life Height-Weight tables.

Operations & immunizations

date	operation or immunization

Annual check-up record *(Women)

date	exam	results	remarks
	breast exam		
	pap smear		
	breast exam		
	pap smear		
	breast exam		
	pap smear		
	breast exam		
	pap smear		
	breast exam		
	pap smear		

* Don't forget a monthly breast self-exam; also be lookout for irregularities, lumps, or unusual discha

Annual health record

	date	current year	year 2	year 3	year 4	year 5
height	weight					
lbs. over/under ideal weight *						
blood pressure						
serum cholesterol **						
blood glucose						
other						

* for optimal body weight, see Table 1.12 chapter 1, Nutrition.
** for optimal cholesterol level, see Fig. 1.2, chapter 1, Nutrition.

Annual tobacco & alcohol consumption

	date	current year	year 2	year 3	year 4	year 5
cigarettes daily						
cigars/pipes daily						
shots of liquor daily						
glasses of wine daily						
beer daily (ozs.)						

Health record

Each of us should complete and keep a Health Record that can be updated periodically like a diary. Often, when trying to diagnose or treat an illness, a physician is hampered by the patient's faulty memory. For the purpose of furthering this book's basic aim, which is the prevention of disease and disability, it is useful, for example, to know the cause of death of one's parents and grandparents. Family history may affect one's risks, particularly for various diseases like heart attacks, breast cancer, or genetic diseases (see chapter 6, Family Planning and Childbearing). Our consumption of drugs, exposure to radiation, sunlight, or occupational hazards, usage of alcohol, usage of seat-belts, and surgical and medical history are among the many factors that can have an effect on health, as we have described in the preceding chapters.

Following is a Health Record form containing Health History and Health Habits sections, for each member of the family (fathers, mothers, and children) to be updated as medical conditions or health habits change. Keeping a Health Record will prove useful for the family physician in diagnosing and treating a disease, and will help to remind us about the existence of risk factors that affect our health.

Such a complete record, even more than the briefer Health Passport, will help us to be more aware of the status of our health and how we can improve it. Family members should fill out these forms together, update them as the need arises, and be conscious of the fact that to a large extent we can control our well-being and our health.

The Health Record, the Health Passport, and knowledge about the structure of our own bodies should help us in our resolve "to make health last a lifetime."

Health Record

HEALTH HISTORY

Name_____ Date of birth_____

Family History

Names of: Grandmothers	Age (if alive)	Any major illness	Age at death	Cause of death

Grandfathers

Mother

Father

Sisters/brothers

Personal History

Blood type _____   Rh factor _____

	date	date	date	date	date
Height					
Weight					
Blood cholesterol level					
Blood pressure *systolic*					
diastolic					

Illnesses (check appropriate boxes)   present   past   at what age/date

☐ ☐

☐ ☐

☐ ☐

☐ ☐

☐ ☐

☐ ☐

☐ ☐

☐ ☐

☐ ☐

☐ ☐

☐ ☐

☐ ☐

☐ ☐

☐ ☐

☐ ☐

Surgical history

type of operation	date or age at surgery	Physician	Hospital (if hospitalized)
_____	_____	_____	_____
_____	_____	_____	_____
_____	_____	_____	_____
_____	_____	_____	_____
_____	_____	_____	_____
_____	_____	_____	_____
_____	_____	_____	_____
_____	_____	_____	_____

Procedures

type of procedure	date or age	Physician	Hospital (if hospitalized)
blood transfusions	_____	_____	_____
	_____	_____	_____
	_____	_____	_____

diagnostic x-rays (see Chapter 13, Radiation)

_____	_____	_____	_____
_____	_____	_____	_____
_____	_____	_____	_____
_____	_____	_____	_____

x-ray therapy

_____	_____	_____	_____
_____	_____	_____	_____
_____	_____	_____	_____

Medical check-ups (check appropriate boxes)

frequency of general physical ☐yearly ☐every 3–5 yrs. ☐rarely/never

date of last checkup _____,_____,_____,_____,_____

FOR WOMEN

*frequency of breast exam** ☐self-exam monthly ☐examination by physician yearly ☐rarely/never

date of last physician examination_____,_____,_____,_____,_____

frequency of Pap test ☐more than once/year ☐yearly ☐rarely/never

date of last Pap test _____,_____,_____,_____,_____

*see Chapter 13, Radiation, for guidelines for mammography

HEALTH HABITS

LIFESTYLE—Section 1 (check appropriate boxes)

Nutrition (see Chapter 1)

snack habits ☐ daily ☐ frequently ☐ infrequently ☐ rarely/never

Alcohol (see Chapter 2)

present
amount   *hard liquor* (1½ oz. shot)   *wine* (4 oz. glass)   *beer* (12 oz. can or bottle)
                  _____per day   _____per day   _____per day
                  _____per week   _____per week   _____per week
age when quit   _____   _____   _____
amount before   _____per day   _____per day   _____per day
quitting   _____per week   _____per week   _____per week

Drugs (see Chapter 3)

type of drug

painkillers

_____ ☐daily ☐1–2 times per week ☐less than once/week ☐rarely/never

_____ ☐ ☐ ☐ ☐

tranquilizers

_____. ☐ daily ☐ 1–2 times per week ☐ less than once/week ☐ rarely/never

_____ ☐ ☐ ☐ ☐

sleeping pills

_____ ☐ ☐ ☐ ☐

_____ ☐ ☐ ☐ ☐

other medications

_____ ☐ ☐ ☐ ☐

_____ ☐ ☐ ☐ ☐

_____ ☐ ☐ ☐ ☐

_____ ☐ ☐ ☐ ☐

oral contraceptives (see below, Family Planning)

Tobacco (see Chapter 4)

	cigarettes	*cigars*	*pipes*	*snuff*	*chewing tobacco*
present amount	_____per day	_____per day	_____per day	_____per day	_____per day
age when quit	_____	_____	_____	_____	_____
amount before quitting	_____per day	_____per day	_____per day	_____per day	_____per day

Physical exercise that raises pulse rate (see Chapter 5, Physical Fitness)

☐ regularly (3+ times/week)   ☐ frequently (1+ times/week)   ☐ infrequently (less than once/week)   ☐ rarely/never

Family Planning (see Family Planning/Childbearing, Chapter 6)

use of oral contraceptives   ☐ present ☐ past ☐ never

*Type*_____*no. of years*_____ *Type*_____*no. of years*_____

Stress levels (See Chapter 7, Stress)

see Table 7.1, The Social Readjustment Rating Scale to rate life events

Dental Hygiene (see Chapter 8, Dental Hygiene)

brushing ☐ after every meal ☐ daily ☐ more than once/week ☐ rarely/never

flossing ☐ ☐ ☐ ☐

checkups ☐ every 6 months ☐ yearly ☐ every 3–5 years ☐

Home accidents (see Chapter 9, Home Accidents)

complete check for electrical and other hazards

☐ living room ☐ bedroom _____ ☐ yard
☐ dining room ☐ bedroom _____ ☐ pool
☐ kitchen ☐ bedroom _____ ☐ barn
☐ playroom/den ☐ bedroom _____ ☐ garage
☐ attic ☐ bathroom _____ ☐ fireplaces
☐ basement ☐ bathroom _____ ☐ other _____
☐ workshop ☐ hallways ☐ _____

learned fire escape route ☐ yes ☐ no

practiced fire escape route ☐ yes ☐ no

Traffic accidents (see Chapter 10, Traffic Accidents)

wear seat belts ☐ always ☐ usually ☐ infrequently ☐ never

drive after drinking ☐ ☐ ☐ ☐

ENVIRONMENT—Section 2

Radiation (see Chapter 13, Radiation)

exposure to sun

☐ daily at peak hours ☐ several times/week at peak hours ☐ less than once/week at peak hours ☐ rarely

☐ fair skinned ☐ medium skinned ☐ dark skinned

Noise (see Chapter 14, Noise)

regular exposure to_____decibels at work (see Figure 14.1, Noise chapter)
(on average)
_____decibels at home (use highest level shown)

Infections (see Chapter 15, Infectious Diseases)

Immunizations   age or date

childhood   _____   _____

              _____   _____

              _____   _____

              _____   _____

              _____   _____

adult   _____   _____

              _____   _____

              _____   _____

Occupation (see Chapter 16, Occupational Health)

exposure to chemicals, pollutants, radiation   years exposed

_____   _____

_____   _____

_____   _____

_____   _____

_____   _____

_____   _____

use of safety equipment and safety procedures

☐ always   ☐ usually   ☐ infrequently   ☐ never

knowledge of chemicals, pollutants, and other hazards at work

☐ completely informed ☐ partially informed ☐ don't know

Health Record

HEALTH HISTORY

Name _____ Date of birth _____

Family History

Names of: Grandmothers	Age (if alive)	Any major illness	Age at death	Cause of death

Grandfathers

Mother

Father

Sisters/brothers

Personal History

Blood type_____   Rh factor_____

	date	date	date	date	date
Height	_____	_____	_____	_____	_____
Weight	_____	_____	_____	_____	_____
Blood cholesterol level	_____	_____	_____	_____	_____
Blood pressure *systolic*	_____	_____	_____	_____	_____
diastolic	_____	_____	_____	_____	_____

Illnesses (check appropriate boxes)   present   past   at what age/date

	present	past	at what age/date
_____	☐	☐	_____
_____	☐	☐	_____
_____	☐	☐	_____
_____	☐	☐	_____
_____	☐	☐	_____
_____	☐	☐	_____
_____	☐	☐	_____
_____	☐	☐	_____
_____	☐	☐	_____
_____	☐	☐	_____
_____	☐	☐	_____
_____	☐	☐	_____
_____	☐	☐	_____
_____	☐	☐	_____
_____	☐	☐	_____

Surgical history

type of operation	date or age at surgery	Physician	Hospital (if hospitalized)

Procedures

type of procedure	date or age	Physician	Hospital (if hospitalized)

blood transfusions

diagnostic x-rays (see Chapter 13, Radiation)

x-ray therapy

Medical check-ups (check appropriate boxes)

frequency of general physical   ☐yearly ☐every 3–5 yrs. ☐rarely/never

date of last checkup _____,_____,_____,_____,_____,_____

FOR WOMEN

frequency of breast exam*   ☐self-exam monthly ☐examination by physician yearly ☐rarely/never

date of last physician examination_____,_____,_____,_____,_____

frequency of Pap test   ☐more than once/year ☐yearly ☐rarely/never

date of last Pap test _____,_____,_____,_____,_____,_____

*see Chapter 13, Radiation, for guidelines for mammography

HEALTH HABITS

LIFESTYLE—Section 1 (check appropriate boxes)

Nutrition (see Chapter 1)

snack habits   ☐ daily   ☐ frequently   ☐ infrequently   ☐ rarely/never

Alcohol (see Chapter 2)

	hard liquor (1½ oz. shot)	*wine* (4 oz. glass)	*beer* (12 oz. can or bottle)
present amount	_____per day	_____per day	_____per day
	_____per week	_____per week	_____per week
age when quit	_____	_____	_____
amount before	_____per day	_____per day	_____per day
quitting	_____per week	_____per week	_____per week

Drugs (see Chapter 3)

type of drug

painkillers

_____ ☐daily ☐1–2 times per week ☐less than once/week ☐rarely/never

_____ ☐ ☐ ☐ ☐

tranquilizers

_____ ☐daily ☐1–2 times per week ☐less than once/week ☐rarely/never

_____ ☐ ☐ ☐ ☐

sleeping pills

_____ ☐ ☐ ☐ ☐

_____ ☐ ☐ ☐ ☐

other medications

_____ ☐ ☐ ☐ ☐

_____ ☐ ☐ ☐ ☐

_____ ☐ ☐ ☐ ☐

_____ ☐ ☐ ☐ ☐

oral contraceptives (see below, Family Planning)

Tobacco (see Chapter 4)

	cigarettes	*cigars*	*pipes*	*snuff*	*chewing tobacco*
present amount	_____per day	_____per day	_____per day	_____per day	_____per day
age when quit	_____	_____	_____	_____	_____
amount before quitting	_____per day	_____per day	_____per day	_____per day	_____per day

Physical exercise that raises pulse rate (see Chapter 5, Physical Fitness)

☐ regularly (3+ times/week)   ☐ frequently (1+ times/week)   ☐ infrequently (less than once/week)   ☐ rarely/never

Family Planning (see Family Planning/Childbearing, Chapter 6)

use of oral contraceptives   ☐ present   ☐ past   ☐ never

Type_____no. of years_____   Type_____no. of years_____

Stress levels (See Chapter 7, Stress)

see Table 7.1, The Social Readjustment Rating Scale to rate life events

Dental Hygiene (see Chapter 8, Dental Hygiene)

brushing	☐ after every meal	☐ daily	☐ more than once/week	☐ rarely/never
flossing	☐	☐	☐	☐
checkups	☐ every 6 months	☐ yearly	☐ every 3–5 years	☐

Home accidents (see Chapter 9, Home Accidents)

complete check for electrical and other hazards

☐ living room	☐ bedroom _____	☐ yard
☐ dining room	☐ bedroom _____	☐ pool
☐ kitchen	☐ bedroom _____	☐ barn
☐ playroom/den	☐ bedroom _____	☐ garage
☐ attic	☐ bathroom _____	☐ fireplaces
☐ basement	☐ bathroom _____	☐ other _____
☐ workshop	☐ hallways	☐ _____

learned fire escape route	☐ yes	☐ no
practiced fire escape route	☐ yes	☐ no

Traffic accidents (see Chapter 10, Traffic Accidents)

wear seat belts	☐ always	☐ usually	☐ infrequently	☐ never
drive after drinking	☐	☐	☐	☐

ENVIRONMENT—Section 2

Radiation (see Chapter 13, Radiation)

exposure to sun

☐ daily at peak hours	☐ several times/week at peak hours	☐ less than once/week at peak hours	☐ rarely
☐ fair skinned	☐ medium skinned	☐ dark skinned	

Noise (see Chapter 14, Noise)

regular exposure to _____ decibels at work (see Figure 14.1, Noise chapter)
(on average)
_____ decibels at home (use highest level shown)

Infections (see Chapter 15, Infectious Diseases)

Immunizations   age or date

childhood _____   _____

_____   _____

_____   _____

_____   _____

_____   _____

adult _____   _____

_____   _____

_____   _____

Occupation (see Chapter 16, Occupational Health)

exposure to chemicals, pollutants, radiation   years exposed

_____   _____

_____   _____

_____   _____

_____   _____

_____   _____

_____   _____

use of safety equipment and safety procedures

☐ always   ☐ usually   ☐ infrequently   ☐ never

knowledge of chemicals, pollutants, and other hazards at work

☐ completely informed ☐ partially informed   ☐ don't know

Health Record

HEALTH HISTORY

Name_____ Date of birth_____

Family History

Names of: Grandmothers	Age (if alive)	Any major illness	Age at death	Cause of death
_____	_____	_____	_____	_____
		_____		_____
_____	_____	_____	_____	_____
		_____		_____
Grandfathers				
_____	_____	_____	_____	_____
		_____		_____
_____	_____	_____	_____	_____
		_____		_____
Mother	_____	_____	_____	_____
		_____		_____
Father	_____	_____	_____	_____
		_____		_____
Sisters/brothers	_____	_____		
_____	_____	_____	_____	_____
		_____		_____
_____	_____	_____	_____	_____
		_____		_____
_____	_____	_____	_____	_____
		_____		_____

Personal History

Blood type_____ Rh factor_____

	date	date	date	date	date
Height	____ ____	____ ____	____ ____	____ ____	____ ____
Weight	____ ____	____ ____	____ ____	____ ____	____ ____
Blood cholesterol level	____ ____	____ ____	____ ____	____ ____	____ ____
Blood pressure *systolic*	____ ____	____ ____	____ ____	____ ____	____ ____
diastolic	____ ____	____ ____	____ ____	____ ____	____ ____

Illnesses (check appropriate boxes)   present   past   at what age/date

Surgical history

type of operation	date or age at surgery	Physician	Hospital (if hospitalized)
_____	_____	_____	_____
_____	_____	_____	_____
_____	_____	_____	_____
_____	_____	_____	_____
_____	_____	_____	_____
_____	_____	_____	_____
_____	_____	_____	_____

Procedures

type of procedure	date or age	Physician	Hospital (if hospitalized)
blood transfusions	_____	_____	_____
	_____	_____	_____
	_____	_____	_____

diagnostic x-rays (see Chapter 13, Radiation)

_____	_____	_____	_____
_____	_____	_____	_____

x-ray therapy

_____	_____	_____	_____
_____	_____	_____	_____
_____	_____	_____	_____

Medical check-ups (check appropriate boxes)

frequency of general physical   ☐yearly ☐every 3–5 yrs. ☐rarely/never

date of last checkup_____,_____,_____,_____,_____,_____

FOR WOMEN

*frequency of breast exam**   ☐self-exam monthly ☐examination by physician yearly ☐rarely/never

date of last physician examination_____,_____,_____,_____,_____

frequency of Pap test   ☐more than once/year ☐yearly ☐rarely/never

date of last Pap test _____,_____,_____,_____,_____,_____

*see Chapter 13, Radiation, for guidelines for mammography

HEALTH HABITS

LIFESTYLE—Section 1 (check appropriate boxes)

Nutrition (see Chapter 1)

snack habits   ☐ daily   ☐ frequently   ☐ infrequently   ☐ rarely/never

Alcohol (see Chapter 2)

present amount	*hard liquor* (1½ oz. shot) _____per day _____per week	*wine* (4 oz. glass) _____per day _____per week	*beer* (12 oz. can or bottle) _____per day _____per week
age when quit	_____	_____	_____
amount before quitting	_____per day _____per week	_____per day _____per week	_____per day _____per week

Drugs (see Chapter 3)

type of drug

painkillers

_____ ☐daily   ☐1–2 times per week   ☐less than once/week   ☐rarely/never

_____ ☐   ☐   ☐   ☐

tranquilizers

_____ ☐daily ☐1–2 times per week ☐less than once/week ☐rarely/never

_____ ☐ ☐ ☐ ☐

sleeping pills

_____ ☐ ☐ ☐ ☐

_____ ☐ ☐ ☐ ☐

other medications

_____ ☐ ☐ ☐ ☐

_____ ☐ ☐ ☐ ☐

_____ ☐ ☐ ☐ ☐

_____ ☐ ☐ ☐ ☐

oral contraceptives (see below, Family Planning)

Tobacco (see Chapter 4)

present	*cigarettes*	*cigars*	*pipes*	*snuff*	*chewing tobacco*
amount	_____per day	_____per day	_____per day	_____per day	_____per day
age when quit	_____	_____	_____	_____	_____
amount before quitting	_____per day	_____per day	_____per day	_____per day	_____per day

Physical exercise that raises pulse rate (see Chapter 5, Physical Fitness)

☐ regularly (3+ times/week)   ☐ frequently (1+ times/week)   ☐ infrequently (less than once/week)   ☐ rarely/never

Family Planning (see Family Planning/Childbearing, Chapter 6)

use of oral contraceptives   ☐ present   ☐ past   ☐ never

Type_____no. of years_____   Type_____no. of years_____

Stress levels (See Chapter 7, Stress)

see Table 7.1, The Social Readjustment Rating Scale to rate life events

Dental Hygiene (see Chapter 8, Dental Hygiene)

brushing ☐ after every meal ☐ daily ☐ more than once/week ☐ rarely/never

flossing ☐ ☐ ☐ ☐

checkups ☐ every 6 months ☐ yearly ☐ every 3–5 years ☐

Home accidents (see Chapter 9, Home Accidents)

complete check for electrical and other hazards

☐ living room ☐ bedroom _____ ☐ yard

☐ dining room ☐ bedroom _____ ☐ pool

☐ kitchen ☐ bedroom _____ ☐ barn

☐ playroom/den ☐ bedroom _____ ☐ garage

☐ attic ☐ bathroom _____ ☐ fireplaces

☐ basement ☐ bathroom _____ ☐ other _____

☐ workshop ☐ hallways ☐ _____

learned fire escape route ☐ yes ☐ no

practiced fire escape route ☐ yes ☐ no

Traffic accidents (see Chapter 10, Traffic Accidents)

wear seat belts ☐ always ☐ usually ☐ infrequently ☐ never

drive after drinking ☐ ☐ ☐ ☐

ENVIRONMENT—Section 2

Radiation (see Chapter 13, Radiation)

exposure to sun

☐ daily at peak hours ☐ several times/week at peak hours ☐ less than once/week at peak hours ☐ rarely

☐ fair skinned ☐ medium skinned ☐ dark skinned

Noise (see Chapter 14, Noise)

regular exposure to____decibels at work (see Figure 14.1, Noise chapter)
(on average)
____decibels at home (use highest level shown)

Infections (see Chapter 15, Infectious Diseases)

Immunizations   age or date

childhood   _____   _____

_____   _____

_____   _____

_____   _____

_____   _____

adult   _____   _____

_____   _____

_____   _____

Occupation (see Chapter 16, Occupational Health)

exposure to chemicals, pollutants, radiation   years exposed

_____   _____

_____   _____

_____   _____

_____   _____

_____   _____

_____   _____

use of safety equipment and safety procedures

☐ always   ☐ usually   ☐ infrequently   ☐ never

knowledge of chemicals, pollutants, and other hazards at work

☐ completely informed ☐ partially informed ☐ don't know

Health Record

HEALTH HISTORY

Name _____ Date of birth _____

Family History

Names of: Grandmothers	Age (if alive)	Any major illness	Age at death	Cause of death

Grandfathers

Mother

Father

Sisters/brothers

Personal History

Blood type _____   Rh factor _____

	date	date	date	date	date
Height	____ ____	____ ____	____ ____	____ ____	____ ____
Weight	____ ____	____ ____	____ ____	____ ____	____ ____
Blood cholesterol level	____ ____	____ ____	____ ____	____ ____	____ ____
Blood pressure systolic	____ ____	____ ____	____ ____	____ ____	____ ____
diastolic	____ ____	____ ____	____ ____	____ ____	____ ____

Illnesses (check appropriate boxes)   present   past   at what age/date

_____ ☐ ☐ _____

_____ ☐ ☐ _____

_____ ☐ ☐ _____

_____ ☐ ☐ _____

_____ ☐ ☐ _____

_____ ☐ ☐ _____

_____ ☐ ☐ _____

_____ ☐ ☐ _____

_____ ☐ ☐ _____

_____ ☐ ☐ _____

_____ ☐ ☐ _____

_____ ☐ ☐ _____

_____ ☐ ☐ _____

_____ ☐ ☐ _____

_____ ☐ ☐ _____

Surgical history

type of operation	date or age at surgery	Physician	Hospital (if hospitalized)
_____	_____	_____	_____
_____	_____	_____	_____
_____	_____	_____	_____
_____	_____	_____	_____
_____	_____	_____	_____
_____	_____	_____	_____
_____	_____	_____	_____

Procedures

type of procedure	date or age	Physician	Hospital (if hospitalized)
blood transfusions	_____	_____	_____
	_____	_____	_____
	_____	_____	_____

diagnostic x-rays (see Chapter 13, Radiation)

_____	_____	_____	_____
_____	_____	_____	_____
_____	_____	_____	_____

x-ray therapy

_____	_____	_____	_____
_____	_____	_____	_____
_____	_____	_____	_____

Medical check-ups (check appropriate boxes)

frequency of general physical   ☐yearly ☐every 3–5 yrs. ☐rarely/never

date of last checkup _____,_____,_____,_____,_____

FOR WOMEN

*frequency of breast exam**   ☐self-exam monthly ☐examination by physician yearly ☐rarely/never

date of last physician examination_____,_____,_____,_____,_____

frequency of Pap test   ☐more than once/year ☐yearly ☐rarely/never

date of last Pap test _____,_____,_____,_____,_____

*see Chapter 13, Radiation, for guidelines for mammography

HEALTH HABITS

LIFESTYLE—Section 1 (check appropriate boxes)

Nutrition (see Chapter 1)

snack habits   ☐ daily   ☐ frequently   ☐ infrequently   ☐ rarely/never

Alcohol (see Chapter 2)

present amount	*hard liquor* (1½ oz. shot)	*wine* (4 oz. glass)	*beer* (12 oz. can or bottle)
	_____per day	_____per day	_____per day
	_____per week	_____per week	_____per week
age when quit	_____	_____	_____
amount before	_____per day	_____per day	_____per day
quitting	_____per week	_____per week	_____per week

Drugs (see Chapter 3)

type of drug

painkillers

_____ ☐daily   ☐1–2 times per week   ☐less than once/week   ☐rarely/never

_____ ☐   ☐   ☐   ☐

tranquilizers

_____ ☐daily ☐1–2 times per week ☐less than once/week ☐rarely/never

_____ ☐ ☐ ☐ ☐

sleeping pills

_____ ☐ ☐ ☐ ☐

_____ ☐ ☐ ☐ ☐

other medications

_____ ☐ ☐ ☐ ☐

_____ ☐ ☐ ☐ ☐

_____ ☐ ☐ ☐ ☐

_____ ☐ ☐ ☐ ☐

oral contraceptives (see below, Family Planning)

Tobacco (see Chapter 4)

	cigarettes	*cigars*	*pipes*	*snuff*	*chewing tobacco*
present amount	_____per day	_____per day	_____per day	_____per day	_____per day
age when quit	_____	_____	_____	_____	_____
amount before quitting	_____per day	_____per day	_____per day	_____per day	_____per day

Physical exercise that raises pulse rate (see Chapter 5, Physical Fitness)

☐ regularly (3+ times/week)   ☐ frequently (1+ times/week)   ☐ infrequently (less than once/week)   ☐ rarely/never

Family Planning (see Family Planning/Childbearing, Chapter 6)

use of oral contraceptives   ☐ present   ☐ past   ☐ never

Type_____ no. of years_____   Type_____ no. of years_____

Stress levels (See Chapter 7, Stress)

see Table 7.1, The Social Readjustment Rating Scale to rate life events

Dental Hygiene (see Chapter 8, Dental Hygiene)

brushing	☐ after every meal	☐ daily	☐ more than once/week	☐ rarely/never
flossing	☐	☐	☐	☐
checkups	☐ every 6 months	☐ yearly	☐ every 3–5 years	☐

Home accidents (see Chapter 9, Home Accidents)

complete check for electrical and other hazards

☐ living room	☐ bedroom _____	☐ yard
☐ dining room	☐ bedroom _____	☐ pool
☐ kitchen	☐ bedroom _____	☐ barn
☐ playroom/den	☐ bedroom _____	☐ garage
☐ attic	☐ bathroom _____	☐ fireplaces
☐ basement	☐ bathroom _____	☐ other _____
☐ workshop	☐ hallways	☐ _____

learned fire escape route	☐ yes	☐ no
practiced fire escape route	☐ yes	☐ no

Traffic accidents (see Chapter 10, Traffic Accidents)

wear seat belts	☐ always	☐ usually	☐ infrequently	☐ never
drive after drinking	☐	☐	☐	☐

ENVIRONMENT—Section 2

Radiation (see Chapter 13, Radiation)

exposure to sun

☐ daily at peak hours	☐ several times/week at peak hours	☐ less than once/week at peak hours	☐ rarely
☐ fair skinned	☐ medium skinned	☐ dark skinned	

Noise (see Chapter 14, Noise)

regular exposure to____decibels at work (see Figure 14.1, Noise chapter)
(on average)
____decibels at home (use highest level shown)

Infections (see Chapter 15, Infectious Diseases)

Immunizations	age or date
childhood	
adult	

Occupation (see Chapter 16, Occupational Health)

exposure to chemicals, pollutants, radiation	years exposed

use of safety equipment and safety procedures

☐ always ☐ usually ☐ infrequently ☐ never

knowledge of chemicals, pollutants, and other hazards at work

☐ completely informed ☐ partially informed ☐ don't know

Index

production of, 54, 107; in saturated fat, 107, 131, 173, 253; sources of, 107, *table* 110; stress-related effects, 393, 394. *See also* Blood cholesterol

Chromium, 58, 116, 496, *table* 591, *tables* 600–601

Chromosomes, disorders of, 346, 362, 363

Chronic obstructive pulmonary disease, 256–257, 277, 498

Chronic respiratory disease, air pollution and, 498–499, 500

Cigar smoking, 246, 247, 435; cancer and, 249, 251–253

Cigarettes and cigarette smoking, 37, 38, 43; adolescent, 260–261; air pollution and, 249, 257, *table* 496, 498–501; alcohol and, 251, 252; cancer and, 44–45, 118, 135–136, 199, 247, *table* 248, 249, *fig.* 250, 251–253, 277, *fig.* 278, 279, 393, 500, 588, 589; cholesterol level and, 132, 133, 253; circulatory disease linked to, *table* 248, 256; coughing, 249, 256, 257, 275; death and, 247, *table* 248, 249, 252–253, 255–256; filter, 45, 271, 276–277, *fig.* 278, 279, *table* 279, 280; heart disease and, 247, *table* 248, 253, *fig.* 254, 255–257, 277; legislative measures, 626–627; nicotine in, *see* Nicotine; pregnancy and, 144, 258–259, 360, *table* 361, 370; preventing use, 260–276; pulmonary disease and, 247, *table* 248, 256–257, 277, 498, *fig.* 499; quitting methods, 262–276; smoke, *see* Smoke, tobacco; social use, 260–262; stress and, 393, 394, 401; tar, *see* Tar; ulcers and, *table* 248, 257; withdrawal, 247, *table* 262, 263, 272, 274, 275–276

Circulatory disease, *table* 248, 252, 253, 255, 256

Circulatory system, 268, 431; exercise and, 287, 288, 335

Cirrhosis of the liver, 37, 139, 184, 196, *fig.* 197, *table* 248

Coal, and air pollution, 492, 493, 495, 496, 500, 503

Cobalt, 58, 116, 542

Cocaine, 212, 213, 216, 218–219

Cochlea, 553, *fig.* 554, 555, 558

Coconut oil, 171, *table* 173

Codeine, 212, 215–217, 230

Coffee, 118, 119, 215

Coitus interruptus, 346, *table* 349, 354

Colon, 140, 392

Colon cancer, 56, 110, 138–139, 156, *table* 248

Common cold, *table* 372, 572, 579; vitamin C and, 111, 578

Condom, 346–349, 354, 577, 578

Constipation, 217, 275, 369, 370, 392–393; fiber intake helpful to, 103, 140, 157

Consumer Reports, 449, 452, 465

Contaminants, food, 119–121, 124, 445, 464

Contaminants, particulate, 495–496

Convulsants, chemical, 594, *table* 596, 597

Cooking: equipment, 174, *table* 175; fats and oils, compared, *tables* 172–173, 174; methods, low-fat, 160, *tables* 172–173, 174, *table* 175; mineral loss in, 145; oil, 171–173, 437

Copper, 58, *table* 113, 116, 117, 142, 351

Corn oil, 54, 58, 106, 107, *table* 172, 174, 176

Coronary heart disease, 57; angina pectoris, 132, 255; atherosclerosis causing, 131–132, 253, 255; cigarettes and, *table* 248, 253; exercise and, 285, *table* 288, 289–290, 303, 333, 336; high blood cholesterol risks, 110, 131, 132; stress-related, 393–394. *See also* Cardiovascular disease

Cottonseed oil, *table* 173, 174, 176

Cyclamates, 120–121, 625

Cyst, ovarian, 355, 359

Cystic fibrosis, *table* 364, 364

Dairy products, 55, 174; child needs, *table* 154, 155; cholesterol in, 107, *table* 110; cooking methods of, *table* 175; fat in, 58, *table* 108, 131, 138; minerals in, *table* 113, 114, 116, 117, 143, 145; nutritional value of, *table* 60–62; pregnancy needs, 145, 146, *tables* 148–149; saturated fatty acids in, 58, 107, *table* 108, 131; substitutes for, *tables* 176–177. *See also* Butter; Cheese; Eggs; Milk

DDT, 119, 445, *table* 596, *table* 602

Dental: disease, 198, 420–422, 425; hygiene, 420–425; X rays, 537, 540, 542, 543. *See also* Teeth; Tooth decay

Depressant drugs, 188, 208, 212, 272; central nervous system, 220–222,

table 596, 597. *See also* Alcohol; Barbiturates; Hypnotics; Sedatives; Tranquilizers

Depression, 290; causes of, 187, 188, 192–193, 276, 351, 394–395, 397, 398, 399; drug relief for, 213, 219

Dermatitis, 537, 586, 599, 605

DES, 124, 625

Deterrent drugs, 207

Diabetes, 37, 53, 121, 135, 157, 197; carbohydrates and, 103, 135, 289, 396; and cardiovascular illness, 132, 135; cigarettes and, *table* 248; and failure of blood glucose regulation, 103, 135, 289; hypoglycemia, 103, 396; insulin deficiency causing, 103, 135, 289, 396: mellitus, 103, 286, *table* 286, 396; obesity and, 125, 128, 135, 396; pregnancy and, 358, *table* 361, 367, 374, 376, 377

Diagnostic radiology, 360, 371–374, 523, *table* 524, 532, 537–542. *See also* X rays

Diagnostic ultrasound, 346, 365, 374, 536

Diaphragm, 346, 347, *table* 348–349, 353

Diarrhea, 112, 114, 116, 147, 151, 392

Diet: adolescent, 156; American Health Foundation Food Plan, 128, 139, 158, *tables* 159–170; cancer linked to, 135, 137, 138–139, 158; childhood, 153, *table* 154, 155; elderly, 157–158; excesses in, *see* Obesity; food labeling in, 54, 171, *tables* 171–173; food substitutes in, *tables* 176–177; habits in, 56–57, 126–129, 135, 137, 138–139, 153, 155, 158; high-fat, 127, 139; infant, 59, 126, 147, 150, *table* 150, 151–152, *table* 152; low-fat, 107, 137–139, 171, *tables* 172–173, 174, *table* 175; pregnancy, 144, 145, *table* 145, *tables* 148–149, 367–368. *See also* Food; Nutrients; Nutrition

Digestive enzymes, 54, 114, 197

Digestive system: alcohol affecting, 195–198; carbohydrate digestion, 103; fats in, 106; protein in, 100, 147, 150. *See also* Esophagus; Intestines; Stomach

Digestive system, disorders of, 112, 142, 392–393. *See also* Abdominal pain; Intestinal disease; Ulcers

Diphtheria, 571, 572, 573–574